D1502956

Attention-Deficit Disorders and Comorbidities in Children, Adolescents, and Adults

Provided as an educational service by Shire Richwood.

Attention-Deficit Disorders and Comorbidities in Children, Adolescents, and Adults

Edited by

Thomas E. Brown, Ph.D.
Associate Director, Yale Clinic for Attention and Related Disorders; Assistant Clinical Professor of Psychiatry, Yale University School of Medicine, New Haven, Connecticut

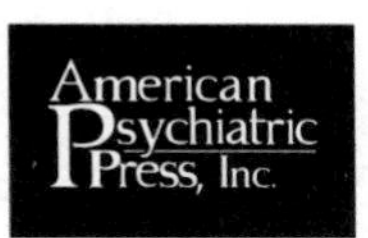

Washington, DC
London, England

Note: The authors have worked to ensure that all information in this book concerning drug dosages, schedules, and routes of administration is accurate as of the time of publication and consistent with standards set by the U.S. Food and Drug Administration and the general medical community. As medical research and practice advance, however, therapeutic standards may change. For this reason and because human and mechanical errors sometimes occur, we recommend that readers follow the advice of a physician who is directly involved in their care or in the care of a member of their family.

Manufactured in the United States of America on acid-free paper
First Edition
03 02 01 00 4 3 2

American Psychiatric Press, Inc.
1400 K Street, N.W.
Washington, DC 20005
www.appi.org

Library of Congress Cataloging-in-Publication Data
Attention-deficit disorders and comorbidities in children, adolescents, and adults / edited by Thomas E. Brown.—1st ed.
p. ; cm.
Includes bibliographical references and index.
ISBN 0-88048-711-9 (alk. paper)
1. Attention-deficit hyperactivity disorder. 2. Comorbidity. I. Brown, Thomas E., Ph.D.
[DNLM: 1. Attention Deficit Disorder with Hyperactivity.
2. Comorbidity. WS 350.8.A8 A883 2000]
RC394.A85 A88 2000
616.85′ 89—dc21

99-047756

British Library Cataloguing in Publication Data
A CIP record is available from the British Library.

To my wife, Bobbie,
With love and gratitude for all you are,
all you give, and all we share together.
TEB

Perhaps the most indispensable thing we can do as human beings, every day of our lives, is remind ourselves and others of our complexity, fragility, finiteness and uniqueness.

Antonio R. Damasio (1994)
Descartes' Error: Emotion, Reason and the Human Brain

Contents

Assessment and Interventions for Attention-Deficit Disorders

Contributors

Howard Abikoff, Ph.D.
Director of Research, Child and Adolescent Psychiatry, New York University Medical Center; Professor of Clinical Psychiatry, New York University School of Medicine, New York, New York

Joseph Biederman, M.D.
Director, Pediatric Psychopharmacology Unit, Massachusetts General Hospital, Boston; Professor of Psychiatry, Harvard Medical School, Boston, Massachusetts

Thomas E. Brown, Ph.D.
Associate Director, Yale Clinic for Attention and Related Disorders; Assistant Clinical Professor of Psychiatry, Yale University School of Medicine, New Haven, Connecticut

Alice S. Carter, Ph.D.
Associate Professor, Department of Psychology, University of Massachusetts, Boston, Massachusetts

Jennifer E. Cohen, M.A.
Doctoral Student in Clinical Psychology, City University of New York, New York, New York

David E. Comings, M.D.
Director, Department of Medical Genetics, City of Hope Medical Center, Duarte, California

Martha Bridge Denckla, M.D.
Director of Developmental Cognitive Neurology, Kennedy-Krieger Institute; Professor of Neurology, Pediatrics, and Psychiatry, Johns Hopkins University School of Medicine, Baltimore, Maryland

George J. DuPaul, Ph.D.
Professor of School Psychology, College of Education, Lehigh University, Bethlehem, Pennsylvania

Christopher Gillberg, M.D., Ph.D.
Professor of Child Neuropsychiatry, Sahlgren University Hospital, Göteborg University, Göteborg, Sweden

Jeffrey M. Halperin, Ph.D.
Professor of Psychology, Queens College of the City University of New York; Professorial Lecturer, Mount Sinai School of Medicine, New York, New York

Margaret Harding-Crawford, B.A.
Research Assistant, Pediatric Psychopharmacology Unit, Massachusetts General Hospital, Boston, Massachusetts

Lily Hechtman, M.D., F.R.C.P.
Professor of Psychiatry and Pediatrics and Director of Research, Division of Child Psychiatry, McGill University; Director of Adolescent Psychiatry, Montreal Children's Hospital, Montreal, Quebec, Canada

James J. Hudziak, M.D.
Associate Professor of Psychiatry and Medicine (Division of Human Medical Genetics), Department of Psychiatry, College of Medicine, University of Vermont, Burlington

Peter S. Jensen, M.D.
Director, Center for the Advancement of Children's Mental Health, Department of Psychiatry, Columbia University; Professor of Psychiatry, Columbia University College of Physicians and Surgeons, New York, New York

Björn Kadesjö, M.D.
Head, Neuropsychiatric Unit for Children and Adolescents, Central Hospital, Karlstad, Sweden

Stephen P. McDermott, M.D.
Director, Cognitive Therapy and Research Program, Department of Psychiatry, Massachusetts General Hospital; Clinical Instructor in Psychiatry, Harvard Medical School, Boston, Massachusetts

Edward J. Modestino, A.L.B., M.L.A.
M.Phil. Candidate in Psychobiology, University of Pennsylvania; Research Assistant, Department of Neurology, University of Pennsylvania School of Medicine, Philadelphia

Jeffrey H. Newcorn, M.D.
Director, Child and Adolescent Psychiatry, Mount Sinai Medical Center; Associate Professor of Psychiatry and Pediatrics, Mount Sinai School of Medicine, New York, New York

Thomas J. Power, Ph.D.

Assistant Professor of School Psychology in Pediatrics, University of Pennsylvania School of Medicine, Philadelphia, Pennsylvania; Co-Director, Center for Attention and Learning Problems, Children's Hospital of Philadelphia

Donald M. Quinlan, Ph.D.

Professor of Psychiatry and Psychology and Director, Clinic for Attention and Related Disorders, Department of Psychiatry, Yale University School of Medicine, New Haven, Connecticut

Beth A. Shepard, Ph.D.

Assistant Professor of Psychology, St. Mary's University, San Antonio, Texas

Thomas J. Spencer, M.D.

Assistant Director, Pediatric Psychopharmacology Unit, Massachusetts General Hospital, Boston; Associate Professor, Harvard Medical School

Rosemary Tannock, Ph.D.

Senior Scientist, Brain and Behaviour Research Program, Research Institute of The Hospital for Sick Children; Associate Professor of Psychiatry, University of Toronto, Toronto, Ontario, Canada

Timothy Wilens, M.D.

Staff Psychiatrist, Pediatric Psychopharmacology Unit, Massachusetts General Hospital, Boston; Associate Professor, Harvard Medical School, Boston, Massachusetts

Janet Wozniak, M.D.

Staff Psychiatrist, Pediatric Psychopharmacology Unit, Massachusetts General Hospital, Boston; Assistant Professor, Harvard Medical School, Boston, Massachusetts

Acknowledgments

The idea for this book emerged in casual conversation over lunch with colleagues. Several were complaining of their difficulty in locating persons with uncomplicated attention-deficit/hyperactivity disorder (ADHD) to participate in a research project. Heads nodded agreement when someone commented on the irony that most research studies focused on "pure" ADHD cases, while the ADHD of most children, adolescents, and adults seen in our clinical practices is complicated by multiple comorbidities. That was 7 years ago.

In the intervening years, we have learned much more about the complexities of ADHD and its comorbidities across the life span. Some of our understanding has come from research, some from conversations with colleagues, and much of it from talking with thousands of boys and girls, men and women who have come seeking assessment and treatment for their frustrating struggles with ADHD and related disorders. I am deeply grateful to my patients, whose sharing of their unfolding life experiences continues to teach me about the amazingly complex interaction of human impairments and strengths.

Many colleagues have enriched and helped to refine my understanding of ADHD and its comorbidities. I appreciate the contributions of Dr. G. Davis Gammon to my earlier work and am grateful for ongoing collaboration and support from Dr. Don Quinlan, Director of the Clinic for Attention and Related Disorders at Yale. I am also grateful to Dr. Tom Spencer, Dr. Rosemary Tannock, and Dr. Tim Wilens, from whom I have learned much as we have worked together in teaching many courses and symposia.

Many thanks are due to all of the colleagues who contributed chapters to this book. Every one of these outstanding researcher–clinicians is overworked in an extremely demanding schedule of research, teaching, and clinical practice. Their generosity in giving precious time, effort, and care to prepare and revise their chapters is deeply appreciated.

A special word of thanks is due to the very competent staff at American Psychiatric Press, Inc., for their support and hard work in moving this book from a germinating idea to a finished volume. Special thanks to Dr. Carol Nadelson, Editor-in-Chief and CEO, and Claire Reinburg, Editorial Director, for their kind support and their patience with multiple delays; to Pam Harley, Managing Editor, Books, who has skillfully coordinated the production process; to Greg Kuny and Beth Rosenfeld, who have done a masterful job of editing the manuscript; to Pam Maher and Abdul Kargbo for their careful preparation of the manuscript for press; and to Bob Pursell, for his insight and expertise in marketing.

Most of all, I am grateful to my wife, Bobbie, for her boundless love, delightful wit, and generous support in the lengthy vicissitudes of this project and throughout our many years together. In countless ways, our daughter and son, Liza and Dave, as well as my mother and mother-in-law, Dorothy and Rose, have also provided love and support that nurtures my work and sustains and enriches my life. For all my family, I am continuingly grateful.

Thomas E. Brown, Ph.D.
Hamden, Connecticut
October 15, 1999

Introduction

For many years assessment and treatment of the disorder currently known as attention-deficit/hyperactivity disorder (ADHD) seemed relatively simple. Typically, the diagnosis was made by a pediatrician when parents or teachers reported a child, usually a young boy, to be disruptive, with extraordinarily hyperactive and impulsive behavior. Such children were usually placed on a regimen of stimulant medication, to be continued until puberty, at which time it was expected that the disorder would naturally remit.

Over the past decade extensive research and clinical experience have dramatically altered our understanding of this disorder. We now know that ADHD afflicts not only young boys who are hyperactive but also a much wider segment of the population. It results in impairment in a substantial percentage of children, adolescents, and adults of both genders, probably at least 5% of the population, many of whom are not hyperactive (Barkley 1990; Gaub and Carlson 1997). For over 50% of those who have ADHD in childhood, these impairments persist into adulthood, although often they do so with a changing profile of complex symptoms (Biederman et al. 1993; Spencer et al. 1994; Weiss and Hechtman 1993; Wender 1995).

No longer can ADHD be viewed as a simple or insignificant behavioral disorder. Recent studies demonstrate that for many of those affected, the ADHD diagnosis encompasses chronic impairments in cognitive functions that are essential to consistent, effective adaptation in school, work, and family and social relationships. Severity of these impairments can range from chronic frustration and underachievement to devastating inability to complete one's education, to hold a job, or to maintain a relationship.

"Inattention" impairments of ADHD encompass not just chronic difficulties in listening to a speaker but also significant problems in a wide variety of cognitive functions, including ability to activate and organize for work, ability to sustain alertness and effort for work, and ability to utilize short-term "working memory" effectively (Barkley 1996, 1997; Brown 1995, 1996; Douglas 1988, 1999; Pennington et al. 1996; Pennington and Ozonoff 1996).

Some of these attention impairments are included or adumbrated in current diagnostic criteria for ADHD, but emerging findings suggest that persons with ADHD, particularly affected adolescents and adults, have a wider range of chronic cognitive impairments than those incorporated in DSM-IV.

Increasingly, researchers in this field are recognizing that ADHD inattention symptoms overlap with "executive functions," which play critical and complicated roles in integrating, regulating, and managing ongoing mental activity (Barkley 1997; Castellanos 1999; Tannock and Schachar 1996).

Since this complicated set of ADHD-related cognitive impairments is linked to attention but is not essentially linked to hyperactive-impulsive behavior, the persistence of the term "hyperactivity" in the name of this disorder may be misleading. The title of this book uses the term *attention-deficit disorders* to emphasize the centrality of attention impairments, with or without hyperactivity, in the disorder. The plural form is utilized in the title to emphasize the diversity of ways in which attention-deficit disorders are manifest in children, adolescents, and adults. Within the book the terms *attention-deficit disorder* and *attention-deficit/hyperactivity* are used interchangeably.

Attention-deficit disorders are complex not only because of the variegated cognitive functions impaired in inattention. Very often these disorders are further complicated by comorbidities. The term *comorbidities* refers to other psychiatric disorders that impair an individual concurrent with his or her primary diagnosis. Many studies have found that over 50% of persons diagnosed with an attention-deficit disorder also meet the diagnostic criteria for one or more additional psychiatric disorders—for example, mood disorder, anxiety disorder, substance use disorder, learning disorder, or behavior disorder. The problem is not only that persons with an attention-deficit disorder can have other concurrent psychiatric disorders; there is evidence that individuals with an attention-deficit disorder have a markedly increased probability of having one or more additional psychiatric disorders (Biederman et al. 1991; Jensen et al. 1997).

Researchers and clinicians are now recognizing that appropriate assessment and treatment of persons with attention-deficit disorders requires careful attention to a wide range of cognitive impairments and also to the extensive variety of other psychiatric disorders that may be comorbid. Comorbid disorders may mask or be masked by symptoms of an attention-deficit disorder and thereby confuse the diagnostic process. Comorbidities, recognized or unrecognized, may also seriously complicate the process of treatment for attention-deficit disorders.

Those who assess, treat, educate, and care for children, adolescents, or adults with attention-deficit disorders need to appreciate and understand the complexity of these disorders and their comorbidities. It is not sufficient for evaluation of a person with an attention-deficit disorder to include only an assessment of possible attention-deficit disorder symptoms. Nor is it sufficient in the treatment of persons with attention-deficit disorders to focus only on symptoms of the attention-deficit disorder without regard for possible psychiatric comorbidities. Clinicians who provide assessment and treatment for attention-deficit disorders need to be well informed about the complexities of attention-deficit disorders and their comorbidities as well as about the implications of these complexities for effective therapeutic and educational interventions.

This book is an effort to consolidate what is currently known about attention-deficit disorders and their common comorbidities as they occur in children, adolescents, and adults. The chapters are written by outstanding clinical researchers, many of whom work on the cutting edge of current research in this field. Each chapter summarizes what its author or authors see as important in what is currently known about its particular topic, but all of the chapters should be regarded as reports of current understandings that await elaboration and correction by findings from additional research.

Each chapter incorporates many references to the relevant scientific literature so that readers can examine directly the details of the studies being summarized. The authors have attempted to focus their discussion of research toward practical implications for clinicians, educators, and others concerned with direct service to individuals with attention-deficit disorders. Although there are similarities among the views of many of these authors, there is also considerable diversity within the group in the way that they currently conceptualize attention-deficit disorders and comorbidities and their assessment and treatment.

OVERVIEW OF THE BOOK

The first section of this book begins with two chapters in which the authors describe the emerging understandings of the nature of attention-deficit disorders and of genetic factors implicated in their transmission. These are followed by 10 chapters, in each of which is described a specific cluster of psychiatric disorders often found to be comorbid with attention-deficit disorders, including mood disorders; anxiety disorders; learning disorders; oppositional defiant, conduct, and aggressive disorders; obsessive-compulsive disorder; sleep disorders; substance abuse and substance use disorders; tic disorders; and developmental coordination disorders. Each of these chapters describes what is currently known about a particular cluster of comorbidities and how such comorbidities may have an impact on the patient and modify the process of assessment and treatment. The section concludes with one chapter describing problems in assessing and treating attention-deficit disorders in preschoolers and another summarizing various types of outcomes of individuals with attention-deficit disorders as these have been reported in existing longitudinal studies.

The second section of the book focuses on assessment and treatment interventions for attention-deficit disorders and comorbidities in children, adolescents, and adults. Beginning with a chapter on clinical assessment, the section also includes chapters on pharmacotherapy, psychosocial interventions, cognitive therapy, and educational interventions for individuals with attention-deficit disorders and comorbid disorders. The volume concludes with a chapter on tailoring of interventions for individuals with attention-deficit disorders, in which is emphasized the need for individualizing treatment to take into account comorbidities and combinations of comorbidities as well as other specifics of the individual, his or her family, and their social setting.

Thomas E. Brown, Ph.D.

REFERENCES

Barkley RA (ed): Attention-Deficit Hyperactivity Disorder: A Handbook for Diagnosis and Treatment. New York, Guilford, 1990

Barkley RA: Linkages between attention and executive functions, in Attention, Memory, and Executive Function. Edited by Lyon GR, Krasnegor NA. Baltimore, MD, Paul H Brookes, 1996, pp 307–325

Barkley RA: ADHD and the Nature of Self-Control. New York, Guilford, 1997

Biederman J, Faraone SV, Lapey K: Comorbidity of diagnosis in attention-deficit disorder, in Attention-Deficit Hyperactivity Disorder. Edited by Weiss G. Philadelphia, PA, WB Saunders, 1991, pp 335–360

Biederman J, Faraone SV, Spencer T, et al: Patterns of psychiatric comorbidity, cognition, and psychosocial functioning in adults with attention deficit disorder. Am J Psychiatry 150:1792–1798, 1993

Brown TE: Differential diagnosis of ADD vs. ADHD in adults, in A Comprehensive Guide to Attention Deficit Disorder in Adults. Edited by Nadeau KG. New York, Brunner/Mazel, 1995, pp 93–108

Brown TE: Brown Attention Deficit Disorder Scales. San Antonio, TX, Psychological Corporation, 1996

Castellanos FX: Psychobiology of attention-deficit/hyperactivity disorder, in Handbook of Disruptive Behavior Disorders. Edited by Quay HC, Hogan AE. New York, Kluwer Academic/Plenum, 1999, pp 179–198

Douglas VI: Cognitive deficits in children with attention deficit disorder with hyperactivity, in Attention Deficit Disorder: Criteria, Cognition, Intervention. Edited by Bloomingdale LM, Sergeant J. New York, Pergamon, 1988, pp 65–81

Douglas VI: Cognitive control processes in attention-deficit hyperactivity disorder, in Handbook of Disruptive Behavior Disorders. Edited by Quay HC, Hogan AE. New York, Kluwer Academic/Plenum, 1999, pp 105–138

Gaub M, Carlson CL: Gender differences in ADHD: a meta-analysis and critical review. J Am Acad Child Adolesc Psychiatry 36:1036–1045, 1997

Jensen PS, Martin D, Cantwell DP: Comorbidity in ADHD: implications for research, practice, and DSM-V. J Am Acad Child Adolesc Psychiatry 36:1065–1079, 1997

Pennington BF, Ozonoff S: Executive functions and developmental psychopathology. J Child Psychol Psychiatry 37:51–87, 1996

Pennington BF, Bennetto L, McAleer O, et al: Executive functions and working memory, in Attention, Memory, and Executive Function. Edited by Lyon GR, Krasnegor NA. Baltimore, MD, Paul H Brookes, 1996, pp 327–348

Spencer T, Biederman J, Wilens T, et al: Is attention deficit hyperactivity disorder in adults a valid disorder? Harv Rev Psychiatry 1:326–335, 1994

Tannock R, Schachar R: Executive dysfunction as an underlying mechanism of behavior and language problems in attention deficit hyperactivity disorder, in Language, Learning, and Behavior Disorders. Edited by Beitchman JH, Cohen NJ, Konstantareas MM, et al. New York, Cambridge University Press, 1996, pp 128–155

Weiss G, Hechtman LT: Hyperactive Children Grown Up: ADHD in Children, Adolescents, and Adults, 2nd Edition. New York, Guilford, 1993

Wender PH: Attention-Deficit Hyperactivity Disorder in Adults. New York, Oxford University Press, 1995

Attention-Deficit Disorders With Comorbidities

1 Emerging Understandings of Attention-Deficit Disorders and Comorbidities

Thomas E. Brown, Ph.D.

Over the past 10 years, interest in attention-deficit disorders (ADDs) has burgeoned throughout North America. Once seen simply as behavioral disorders in young boys, ADDs are now being more widely recognized in females (Arnold 1996; Biederman 1999; Gaub and Carlson 1997; McGee and Feehan 1991), in adolescents (Barkley 1990; Biederman et al. 1996b, 1998; Schaughency et al. 1994; Weiss and Hechtman 1986, 1993; Wilson and Marcotte 1996), and in adults (Biederman et al. 1993; Millstein et al. 1997; Spencer 1994; Wender 1995).

Increasing numbers of boys and girls, and men and women, are being diagnosed with and treated for chronic attention problems and related difficulties that have seriously disrupted their functioning in school, at work, and in their family and social relationships. Many patients report that treatment has produced dramatic and continuous improvement in their long-standing ADD symptoms. Anecdotal reports on the usefulness of medications for alleviating ADD symptoms are supported by research evidence of the efficacy of medication treatment for preschoolers (Musten et al. 1997), children (Spencer et al. 1996), adolescents (Smith et al. 1998), and adults (Spencer et al. 1995).

Some question the reasons for the increased number of people who are reporting ADD symptoms, suggesting that this may simply be a passing fad in psychiatric diagnosis. Yet clinical experience in assessing those who seek treatment for and are diagnosed with ADDs makes clear the substantial impairments and genuine suffering experienced by persons with these disorders, and clinical experience in the treatment of them makes clear the substantial and continuous improvements in multiple life functions that result from effective treatment of ADD symptoms.

Moreover, clinical impressions on the validity of the diagnosis of attention-deficit/hyperactivity disorder (ADHD) and the efficacy of ADHD treatment are substantially supported by empirical research. Clearly, more people are being recognized as having ADHD and are being successfully treated for it. This has led to increasing concern among some professionals and laypeople, who wonder why the number of persons with ADHD has been increasing so rapidly.

It seems likely that what has been increasing is not the number of persons who have inattention problems, but the number of such persons who recognize these impairments as symptoms of a treatable disorder that occurs in females as well as males and in adolescents and adults as well as young children. Individuals, male and female, both young and old, with chronic attention impairments have probably existed in every generation; however, they may have been seen simply as underachieving, lazy, immature, or unmotivated. Among those who erratically demonstrated the ability to perform well in school or at work or to have successful social relationships but seemingly lacked the ability or motivation to sustain success may have been many who had the disorder currently recognized as ADHD.

Such individuals now may seek treatment for ADHD because they have heard that this disorder can be treated effectively with medication. As increasing numbers of children, adolescents, and adults have achieved significant improvement from ADHD treatment, reports of their diagnosis and successful treatment have spread, reaching family members, friends, and acquaintances who have struggled with similar difficulties.

As teachers, psychologists, and physicians witness improvements obtained by treatment of ADHD symptoms, many are becoming more alert to these symptoms and are suggesting appropriate assessment and treatment for those who might benefit. Educational and advocacy efforts by support groups such as CHADD (Children and Adults with Attention Deficit Disorder) and the National Attention Deficit Disorder Association, as well as books and widespread media coverage, have further expanded public and professional awareness of ADHD as a treatable disorder. Yet increasing popular interest in ADHD appears to be sustained not so much by the media but by expanding awareness of the successful treatment of ADHD symptoms in adults as well as in children.

Recognition of the validity of ADHD and the effectiveness of its treatment was supported by a recent report from the American Medical Association (AMA). In response to public and professional concern regarding possible overdiagnosis of ADHD and possible overprescription of stimulant medications used to treat the disorder, the AMA commissioned a study to review relevant evidence. The study concluded, "ADHD is one of the best-researched disorders in medicine, and the overall data on its validity are far more compelling than for most mental disorders and even for many medical conditions" (Goldman et al. 1998, p. 1105). In addition, the report noted the potentially deleterious impact of this disorder: "ADHD is associated with significant potential comorbidity and functional impairment, and emotional problems at subsequent stages of life" (p. 1106). The AMA report also noted the effectiveness of medications used to treat ADHD, concluding: "Medications have been unequivocally shown (i.e., by double blind, placebo-controlled studies) to reduce core symptoms of hyperactivity, impulsivity, and inattentiveness. They improve classroom behavior and academic performance; diminish oppositional and aggressive behaviors; promote increased interaction with teachers, family and others; and increase participation in leisure time activities" (Goldman et al. 1998, p. 1103). The report further noted, "Adverse effects from stimulants (used to treat ADHD symptoms) are generally mild, short-lived, and responsive to dosing or timing adjustments" (p. 1104).

Although researchers and clinicians in the United States and Canada have pioneered the assessment and treatment of ADDs, recognition of these disorders as a significant public health problem has been gradually expanding worldwide. Differences in cultural expectations, diagnostic criteria, and ascertainment methods cause variability in reported incidence rates from one country to another (Mann et al. 1992), but significant rates of ADDs have been recognized in countries as diverse as New Zealand (Anderson et al. 1987; Fergusson et al. 1993), Germany (Baumgaertel et al. 1995), Italy (Gallucci et al. 1993), China (Leung et al. 1996; Tao 1992), Japan (Kanbayashi et al. 1994), India (Bhatia et al. 1991), as well as in Puerto Rico (Bird et al. 19885).

As increasing numbers of medical and educational professionals in other countries have become aware of ADDs among their patients and students, and laypeople recognize these disorders in their offspring, interest has been growing steadily in learning about the disorders and their treatment. Well-attended national conferences on ADDs have been held recently for medical and educational professionals, as well as laypeople, in England, Norway, Sweden, Venezuela, India, and many other countries. With increasing recognition of these disorders internationally, there has been increasing interest worldwide in improving assessment and treatment services for children, adolescents, and adults with ADDs.

One important result of the burgeoning numbers of people being assessed and treated for ADDs is an increase in efforts to identify and understand ADD impairments and why they often respond to existing treatments. As more information about ADDs has accumulated, particularly in adolescents and adults, understanding of these disorders has begun to shift from an emphasis on disruptive behavior, which has long characterized them.

FORMER UNDERSTANDING OF ADDS AS DISRUPTIVE BEHAVIOR DISORDERS

Currently, the diagnosis for chronic symptoms of inattention remains closely linked to problems with hyperactive/impulsive behavior, even though research has demonstrated that many individuals with ADDs are not hyperactive. This linkage has persisted from early studies of young children who were hyperactive and disruptive in school. Researchers studying these children noticed that many had chronic problems with sustaining attention. As a result, attentional problems were incorporated into diagnostic criteria for hyperactive/impulsive behavior disorders and have remained closely linked to disruptive behavioral diagnoses ever since.

The first major recognition of inattention symptoms as central to ADDs came with the publication of DSM-III (American Psychiatric Association 1980), which shifted emphasis to inattention as the primary symptom of the disorder known until then as "hyperactivity." In DSM-III the name of the diagnosis changed from "hyperkinetic reaction of childhood" to "attention deficit disorder" and diagnostic criteria for ADD with and without hyperactivity were established. For 7 years, criteria for diagnosing ADD without hyperactivity were included in DSM.

Recognition of attentional impairments as central to ADDs was lost in DSM-III-R (American Psychiatric Association 1987). The revision committee challenged the notion of ADDs without hyperactivity because of a lack of supporting research. In DSM-III-R, diagnostic criteria for ADDs without hyperactivity were dropped and inattention symptoms were combined into a single list, along with symptoms of hyperactivity and impulsivity. This hybrid diagnosis was then named "attention-deficit hyperactivity disorder" and remained classified as a disruptive behavior disorder.

Although numerous research studies in the late 1980s clearly demonstrated the validity of the diagnosis of ADD without hyperactivity, there were no officially accepted diagnostic criteria for this type of ADD from 1987 until

DSM-IV was published (American Psychiatric Association 1994). DSM-IV recognized a "predominantly inattentive type" of ADD, which required no symptoms of hyperactivity or impulsivity, but the name of the diagnosis remained "attention-deficit/hyperactivity disorder". The slash between the defining terms was introduced to allude to the separability of symptoms of the hybrid disorder ADHD.

Despite these changes in the official definition of this diagnosis, much of the professional and lay literature about ADHD continues to describe the disorder as characterized by three cardinal symptoms: inattention, hyperactivity, and impulsivity. Few publications focus on attention impairments of ADHD without linking these to hyperactive and impulsive behavior. As a result, the disruptive behavioral focus continues and individuals whose significant attention impairments are not accompanied by hyperactive-impulsive symptoms are less likely to be recognized as having ADHD.

INATTENTION

Inattention Without Hyperactivity

Lahey and Carlson (1991) reviewed the substantial research supporting the validity of the diagnosis ADD without hyperactivity. Among studies reviewed were several that demonstrated, by factor analysis, that ADD symptoms yielded two separate factors: one comprising chronic inattention and the other including combined hyperactivity and impulsivity. These studies showed that children whose ADDs were with hyperactivity-impulsivity (ADD/H) differed from children whose ADDs were without hyperactivity (ADD/WO) in their emotional and behavioral patterns, peer relationships, and cognitive functioning.

Using this base of research, the DSM-IV committee on ADHD conducted a field study to test new diagnostic criteria for ADDs with and without hyperactivity-impulsivity. Results of this study led the committee to recognize that an individual may have an ADD without symptoms of hyperactivity or impulsivity. The name given to this diagnosis was "attention-deficit/hyperactivity disorder, predominantly inattentive type" (Lahey et al. 1994).

In addition to the inattentive type of ADHD, another new diagnosis, "predominantly hyperactive-impulsive type," was introduced in DSM-IV. This category was added primarily to identify preschool children who were extremely hyperactive, though their young age precluded identification of significant problems of inattention. This category may turn out to identify a prodromal form of combined type ADHD.

"Attention-deficit/hyperactivity disorder, combined type" is offered in DSM-IV to diagnose individuals with significant problems with both inattention and hyperactivity-impulsivity. Although DSM-IV introduced the predominantly inattentive type of ADHD, this name perpetuated the continuing linkage of inattention to hyperactivity.

Subsequent research on the incidence of the various types of ADHD identified in DSM-IV has indicated significant differences in frequency of each type, depending on the setting. In clinical psychiatric settings, the combined type is found with the greatest frequency: 45%–62% of clinical samples of patients with ADHD (Eiraldi et al. 1997; Faraone et al. 1998; Paternite et al. 1995). Probably for this reason, the combined type has claimed the largest share of attention in most research done on ADHD. Yet, in the wider community, the predominantly inattentive type is most common. According to epidemiological studies, prevalence of the predominantly inattentive type ranges from 4.5% to 9.0% of the general population of children, whereas the combined type occurs at frequencies ranging from 1.9% to 4.8%. The predominantly hyperactive-impulsive type is even less common, ranging from 1.7% to 3.9% (Baumgaertel et al. 1995; Gaub and Carlson 1997; Wolraich et al. 1996).

Shortly after DSM-IV was published, additional research documented significant differences in the life course of the two primary types of ADHD. A 4-year longitudinal study by Hart et al. (1995) demonstrated, in a sample of boys diagnosed with DSM-III-R ADHD, that inattention symptoms tended to persist, whereas hyperactivity-impulsivity symptoms tended to diminish. In Australia, Levy et al. (1997) found a similar pattern in a 3-year study of a large sample of male and female children with ADHD. Together, these studies highlight the developmental separability of inattention symptoms from hyperactivity-impulsivity, even when both symptom sets initially coexist (e.g., a child with combined-type ADHD).

Persistence of Inattention Into Adolescence and Adulthood

The phenomenon of hyperactivity symptoms diminishing with age may account for the long-held assumption that children with ADDs tend to outgrow these disorders in their teens. When only behavioral symptoms are considered, many individuals with ADDs in childhood may be seen as outgrowing their symptoms in adolescence. Yet when attention impairments are present in childhood, with or without hyperactivity, they tend to persist into adolescence and adulthood, often in ways that create problems for individuals at school, at work, and in social relationships (Biederman et al. 1998; Millstein et al. 1997).

Achenbach et al. (1995) published results of a large 6-year national study of male and female adolescents making the transition into adulthood. Results indicated that childhood attention deficits tend to persist into early adulthood, usually without persistence of significant problems with hyperactivity-impulsivity. Attention problems were found to be not only more persistent into adulthood than hyperactivity-impulsivity symptoms but also more impairing. In young adulthood, attention problems were found to be associated with significant impairments in employment and social relationships.

Increasingly, research is establishing the validity and importance of inattention not only as separate from hyperactivity-impulsivity but also as the most persistent and impairing of the two symptom sets in the current understanding of ADHD. Yet identification of which cognitive impairments should be included within "inattention" continues.

A Broad Concept of Inattention

The concept of inattention referred to in DSM-IV is a broad one; it involves much more than simply not paying attention while someone is speaking. DSM-IV criteria refer also to excessive problems with distractibility and chronic difficulties in organizing tasks and activities, attending to details, following instructions and completing tasks, and undertaking tasks that require sustained mental effort, as well as to problems with losing things and excessive forgetfulness. This broad range of impairments encompassed within the DSM-IV criteria for inattention delineates impairment of not a single unitary function but a composite of diverse, but related, cognitive functions subsumed under the concept of "attention" (see Parasuraman 1998).

Consistent with the broad DSM-IV list of inattention symptoms, patients diagnosed with ADDs tend to report chronic impairments across a wide range of cognitive functions. From interviews with adolescents and adults diagnosed with ADDs, Brown (1995, 1996) derived 40 self-report items regarding aspects of inattention. These items clustered into five independent, but related, factors: 1) organizing and activating for work, 2) sustaining attention and concentration, 3) sustaining energy and effort for work, 4) managing affective interference, and 5) utilizing working memory and accessing recall. Persons diagnosed with ADDs who reported chronic difficulties in one of these factors tended to report similar levels of impairment in the other four.

Symptoms in Brown's patient-derived factors extend beyond DSM-IV inattention criteria by incorporating several functions adumbrated, but not explicitly included, in DSM. For example, items related to activation for work tasks extend the DSM-IV item "often avoids tasks that require sustained mental effort" and are closer to the item "often seems unmotivated" used in the DSM-IV field studies (Lahey et al. 1994).

Some items on the Brown ADD scales are not directly linked to DSM-IV criteria but do reflect aspects of inattention identified by other studies of ADDs. For example, items related to managing affective interference are similar to reports by Wender (1995) that adults with ADDs but with no diagnosable mood disorders often have marked impairment in their ability to manage affective responses to stress or frustration to avoid excessive disruption in their work and relationships.

Executive Function

Inattention as Impairment of Executive Function

The broader view that inattention is an impairment of executive function is consistent with current neurological and neuropsychological understandings of attention. Unlike the psychiatric model, in which inattention has been linked primarily to disruptive behavior, neurological models tend to emphasize linkage of attention to memory and to a cluster of other cognitive functions often labeled "executive function" (Lyon and Krasnegor 1996).

Denckla (1996a, 1996b; see also Chapter 8 in this volume) has described how ADHD often overlaps with the neurological diagnosis of impairments in executive function. Executive function refers to a wide range of central control processes in the brain that connect, prioritize, and integrate operation of subordinate brain functions. Taylor (1995) highlighted the need to distinguish between modular and executive processes of attention wherein modular processing is integrated by executive functioning into strategically appropriate programs to complete necessary tasks. Denckla emphasizes that this central management system, often attributed to operations in the prefrontal cortex, is crucial to organizing and integrating cognitive processes over time and plays an increasingly important role as the young child matures and takes on more complex tasks and more independent activities.

Although the concept of executive function has not yet been rigorously defined, it provides a framework for recognizing that some brain functions manage other functions. These management, or executive, functions might be compared to the functions of the conductor of a symphony orchestra, the chief of a large city fire department, or the management team of a corporation.

One metaphor for executive function might be the conductor of a symphony orchestra, who does not play a musical instrument in the orchestra but does play a critical role by enabling the orchestra to produce complex music. The conductor organizes, activates, focuses, integrates, and directs the musicians as they play. With his or her instructions and motions, the conductor weaves together the sounds of the various instruments, controlling the musicians' pace and signaling them to bring in and fade out their particular sounds to bring each musical score to life. The brain's executive functions, like the functions of the conductor, organize, activate, focus, integrate, and direct, allowing the brain to perform both routine and creative work.

Executive function might be compared to the chief of a large city fire department, who carries no hoses or ladders but does play an essential role in planning how firefighters should respond to a wide range of emergencies and in providing moment-to-moment directions to those who lay the hoses, climb the ladders, and enter burning structures to save life and property. The chief's role involves rapidly assessing unexpected dangers as they arise, deploying needed equipment and personnel, and carefully monitoring the situation, being alert to collapsing structures, sudden wind changes, and hazardous materials. Like the fire chief, the brain's executive functions respond to unexpected situations as they arise, by selecting from a variety of problem-solving tactics stored in long-term memory, implementing them, monitoring their execution, and changing them as needed to meet challenges.

Executive function might also be compared to the management team in a corporation. The corporation might have many divisions: procurement, human resources, manufacturing, marketing, and distribution. These separate divisions, however competent, could not function as a corporation without effective management to organize, integrate, monitor, and modify their functions to meet constantly changing needs. Likewise, the managers could not produce and profit from the corporation's products without support from these divisions. Such is the relationship between executive function and other components of the working brain.

These metaphors cannot do justice to the complexity of the brain's executive functions, but they may help illustrate the important multiple roles involved in managing complex human activities. Executive function refers to the wide variety of functions within the brain that activate, organize, integrate, and manage other functions to allow the individual to function effectively. Many of the symptoms classified as ADD symptoms of inattention are actually symptoms of executive function impairments.

Developmental Demands on Executive Function

Impairments in executive function may not become apparent until the individual is required to use this particular function. Preschool children, for example, are not expected to manage much for themselves; there is little demand on them for self-management beyond complying with parental directions. Usually, parents or other caretakers are responsible for starting, directing, and stopping most of the young child's activities. These adults often adapt their demands to the wishes and moods of the particular child, but they typically provide most of the child's "executive management."

Entry into nursery school or other group care situations gradually introduces the child to more demands for self-regulation and accommodation to the needs of caretakers and other children. Kindergarten and first grade increase demands for the child to regulate behavior (e.g., to sit still, refrain from talking, complete tasks within given time frames). The school environment also increases demands for the child to regulate cognition (e.g., to maintain focus on specific tasks, organize and prioritize activities, remember particular concepts and skills). Children whose executive function impairments include severe difficulties with inhibiting impulsive behavior are likely to be identified very early in their school careers. Children who can manage basic behavioral self-control adequately, but who have significant impairments in the inattention spectrum of ADDs, may not be identified until they advance to the upper grades.

Demands on executive function usually escalate rapidly in junior high school, high school, and the first 2 years of college. This is when most individuals are faced with the widest range of demands to organize and direct themselves in the broadest range of cognitive and social activities, with the least opportunity to escape from activities for which they are not well suited. Moreover, early and middle adolescence is when parents and teachers are expected to decrease their management efforts and gradually require the teenager to take primary responsibility for self-management (i.e., for the exercise of executive function).

Another important fact about executive function is that it becomes progressively more necessary and complex as an individual gets older. Denckla (1996b) suggested that growing up is essentially the development of competence in executive function. Complex tasks such as dealing with multiple courses and different teachers in high school, driving a car, managing finances, and providing day-to-day parenting for children are a few of the many tasks that place strong demands on executive function. The increasing challenges to executive function as an individual matures may explain why inattention symptoms of some individuals with ADDs, particularly those who are bright and not hyperactive, are noticed not in early childhood but in middle to late adolescence or early adulthood, as demands on executive function increase.

Viewing ADDs as developmental impairments in executive function, which may not be recognizable until an individual confronts the demands of the upper grades, has important implications for determining the age at onset of ADD symptoms. DSM-IV diagnostic criteria for ADHD stipulate that at least some of the symptoms must have been present before age 7 years. Recently, the validity of this age requirement has been challenged by further analysis of the empirical field study data on which it presumably was based (Applegate et al. 1997). Barkley and Biederman (1997), following this same reasoning, argued that the age-at-onset criterion for ADHD should be either abandoned or "generously broadened" because it has no sound scientific basis and may impede recognition of ADD cases in which the onset of symptoms was not apparent as early as age 7.

Among the most important aspects of executive function as an individual matures is "working memory" (see below). Neuropsychologists (e.g., Pennington and Ozonoff 1996; Pennington et al. 1996) have highlighted working memory as a central aspect of executive function.

ATTENTION

Short-Term Memory as a Critical Element of Attention

The linkage of attention to memory has long been recognized (see R. A. Cohen 1993; Cowan 1995). Recent developments on this linkage, however, focus on the role of working memory, a construct introduced into the psychological literature by Miller et al. (1960, p. 65) in their groundbreaking book on the organization of human behavior.

The concept of working memory has been developed by Baddeley (1986) and elaborated by Goldman-Rakic (1987, 1991, 1994, 1995) and others (see Richardson et al. 1996) to refer to a subset of short-term memory functions that hold and manipulate information currently being processed. Working memory holds the focus and immediate context of current attention and refers to the brain's capacity to keep "online" and actively use bits of information crucial for current functioning, while carrying on other functions.

What separates current understandings of working memory from earlier notions of short-term memory is the recognition that working memory is not just a temporary storage system but an active processing system that helps the mind deal with immediate situations, whether novel or routine, in light of relevant information remembered from the immediate and/or distant past. Kosslyn and Koenig (1995, p. 388) described working memory as comprising "activated information in the long-term memories, the information in short-term memories, and the decision processes that manage which information is activated in long-term memories and retained in short-term memories."

Kosslyn and Koenig's point of view follows that of Anderson and Bower (1973), cited in Richardson (1996, p. 121), who emphasized that working memory is not structurally separate from long-term memory but rather is a currently active partition of long-term memory. Much remains to be learned about the nature and functioning of working memory, but two characteristics are generally agreed on: 1) working memory has a limited capacity and there are functional constraints on how much information can be activated simultaneously in it, and 2) individuals differ in the effective capacity of their working memory (Richardson 1996, p. 124). In many ways, working memory is similar to the random access memory (RAM) in a computer.

Neuropsychologists and neuroscientists are still at an early stage in conceptualizing, operationalizing, and testing models of working memory. It is clear that many of the attention impairments associated with ADD are closely tied to chronic ineffectiveness of working memory. Yet several other cognitive functions, which extend beyond working memory, apparently are impaired in persons with ADD. These include problems with insufficient arousal, energy, and effort for work tasks, which tie directly to the role of activation and emotion/affect in cognition.

Activation/Arousal Aspects of Attention

Although neuropsychological concepts of working memory and executive function are as complex as the wide-spectrum concept of attention, existing models seem overly intellectualized and detached from the varying intensities of arousal and energy, which are crucial elements of attention. Sergeant (1996, 1999) noted that an adequate model of attention must incorporate elements of arousal, activation, and effort. Attention involves not only the flow of information within the cortex but also varying intensities of arousal and activation, engaged with and disengaged from a constant flow of internal and external stimuli. Arousal and activation may vary considerably from one individual to another and within persons from one situation to another (cf. Revelle 1993).

Two DSM-IV inattention symptoms address problems related to insufficient arousal, activation, and sustained effort for work tasks. The later-revised item "often seems unmotivated to do schoolwork or homework" from the DSM-IV field study picks up the problem of chronic procrastination regarding work tasks. "Often does not follow through . . . and fails to finish schoolwork, chores or duties in the workplace" alludes to chronic problems in sustaining effort for timely completion of work tasks. Several other inattention symptoms (e.g., "difficulty sustaining attention" and "easily distracted") can also be understood as reflecting problems with insufficient arousal/engagement or possibly excessive arousal.

Affective/Emotional Aspects of Attention

Although the DSM-IV diagnostic criteria for ADHD include no affective symptoms, Wender's pioneering work (1987, 1995) and more recent formulations of ADD symptoms (e.g., Barkley 1997; Brown 1996; Conners 1997) recognize modulation of affect as a significant aspect of executive function that is often impaired as a result of ADDs. Moreover, as Rothbart et al. (1995) noted, processing of emotional information is an important aspect of attentional neural networks.

Energetic and arousal aspects of attention involve emotion as well as cognition. In *The Emotional Brain,* LeDoux (1996) argues that there is no unified emotional system in the brain. He argues that, instead, there are a variety of ways cognitive and emotional arousal may be activated, sustained, or modulated by a rapid flow of unconscious linkages in working memory between current stimuli and activated memories unconsciously assumed to be relevant. Regardless of whether LeDoux's specific formulations become widely accepted, his argument highlights the critical influence of unconscious emotional associations, often virtually inseparable from perceptions, as activators and modulators of attention. What remains to be clarified is the variety of mechanisms by which emotional influences (e.g., terror, longing, affection, jealousy, rage) both facilitate and impair the exercise of attention.

It is important to note that emotion affects attention not only as an internal influence that may disrupt attention and need to be managed but also as a vital element in generating and sustaining attention. This was highlighted by Taylor et al. (1997), who discussed emotions as "readiness for action" and "motivators and organizers of behavior." The researchers noted that "interest," probably the most frequently experienced positive emotion, "is an extremely important motivation in the development of skills, competencies and intelligence" (p. 11). The motivating power of such "interest" may be most apparent when it is absent, as described in the chronic complaints of many adults with ADDs who report that although they can "hyperfocus" on activities in which they have special interest, they chronically find themselves unable to mobilize effort for tasks in which they do not feel any special immediate interest, even when they are fully aware that their failure to do that uninteresting task may cause significant problems later.

Negative impact of emotion/affect on attention is also apparent in many emotional disorders. Wells and Matthews (1994, p. 320) argued that emotional disorders of anxiety, depression, and obsessionality are all associated with a general core dysfunctional attentional syndrome upon which features of the specific disorder and the individual personality and cognitive style are superimposed. The authors described this dysfunctional attentional syndrome as consisting of heightened self-monitoring and intensified processing of internal events, coupled with activation of self-beliefs and appraisal that strains the individual's attentional capacity and reduces the overall efficiency of cognitive functioning (p. 266). By these and other mechanisms, emotion/affect may affect the broad range of attentional functions in ways that impair and/or enhance cognitive functioning.

Complexity of Attentional Systems in the Brain

Given the wide spectrum of cognitive functions associated with attention, it is not surprising that many aspects of brain function seem to be involved. Attention is clearly not a unitary or modular function in the brain; it is not identified specifically with any singular brain structure. As Colby (1991) noted, "Attention is a distributed process . . . subserved by many brain structures" (p. S90).

In a review of findings from neuroimaging studies of the human brain, Posner and Raichle (1994, pp. 154–179) showed evidence of at least three anatomic networks that function separately and together to support various aspects of attention. These interacting networks are 1) an orienting network consisting of parietal, midbrain, and thalamic circuits; 2) an executive attention network including the left lateral frontal areas and the anterior cingulate; and 3) a vigilance network comprising the right frontal and right parietal lobes as well as the locus coeruleus.

Although many researchers rightly emphasize the role of the prefrontal cortex in problems of executive function, working memory, and ADHD, it seems likely that the wide spectrum of impairments associated with inattention will be found to involve many aspects of brain function. Denckla (1991b) emphasized this when she wrote "ADHD . . . exemplifies the need to broaden our differential localization beyond the prefrontal cortex to include neural substrates of activation, orientation, motivation and vigilance as these connect with and influence executive function" (p. x).

Among these neural substrates, which may be especially important in executive function, working memory, and ADDs, are those of the nigrostriatal structures. Crinella et al. (1997) reported findings from animal studies suggesting that nigrostriatal structures contribute essential, superordinate control of functions such as shifting mental set, planning action, and sequencing (i.e., executive functions).

Yet structural localization and dispersion of functions may not be the most important way to understand the impairments associated with inattention. As Pennington and colleagues (1996) pointed out, many developmental disorders may result

> from a general change in some aspect of brain development such as neuronal number, structure, connectivity, neurochemistry, or metabolism . . . such a general change could have a differential impact across different domains of cognition, with more complex aspects of cognition such as executive functions being most vulnerable and other aspects being less vulnerable. (p. 331)

In this same context, Pennington et al. noted that the executive function impairments associated with ADHD and some other developmental disorders may all involve varying degrees of dopamine depletion in the prefrontal cortex and related areas (p. 330).

Neurochemical Contributions to Attentional Impairments

For many years, researchers have suspected that the attentional impairments of ADDs are related to inherited neurochemical deficiencies in the brain. Pliszka et al. (1996) reviewed evidence that ADD symptoms may be related specifically to the catecholamines, a specific set of neurotransmitter chemicals manufactured in the brain. Yet most of the research on the role of catecholamines in ADDs has not differentiated between inattention and hyperactive-impulsive symptoms.

The possibility that attention impairments resulting from ADDs may be closely related to dopamine depletion in certain areas of the brain finds support in the numerous studies that have demonstrated dopaminergic medications (e.g., methylphenidate, dextroamphetamine) to be effective in alleviating a wide variety of inattention symptoms (see Levy 1991). Although noradrenergic medications (e.g., desipramine, nortriptyline) and α_2-agonist medications (e.g., clonidine, guanfacine) have been demonstrated to be effective in alleviating hyperactivity-impulsivity symptoms of ADHD, there is some evidence that these nonstimulant medications are less effective in alleviating inattention symptoms (American Academy of Child and Adolescent Psychiatry 1997; Levy and Hobbes 1988; Spencer et al. 1996).

These findings suggest that a specific neurotransmitter system, the dopaminergic system, may play a particularly important role in inattention symptoms of ADD. Servan-Schreiber et al. (1998) summarized research literature on the impact of dopamine on specific neural networks in human information processing and developed and tested a model demonstrating that dopamine has a direct positive effect on the increase of gain in the activation function of the neural networks underlying attentional processing. Additional evidence for the critical role of dopamine in management of cognitive functions comes from recent laboratory studies summarized by Wickelgren (1997), which indicate that in many species dopamine plays a critical role in mobilizing attention, facilitating learning, and motivating behavior that is critical for adaptation. The role of dopamine in facilitating these functions may be far more broad, subtle, and complex than has previously been thought. Inattention symptoms of ADD may be reflecting impairments resulting primarily from insufficient functioning of aspects of dopaminergic transmission in the human brain.

DIAGNOSTIC ISSUES IN ADD IMPAIRMENTS

Disentangling ADD Inattention From Hyperactivity

As more is learned about the nature and complexity of inattention, it is becoming increasingly clear that the long-held linkage between inattention and hyperactivity in ADD needs to be reconsidered. Recently, both Barkley (1997; Barkley et al. 1996) and Quay (1997) proposed that the predominantly inattentive type of ADD should be considered a disorder separate from the combined type of ADHD. Both argue that combined-type ADHD results from impairment in the behavioral-inhibition system of the brain, whereas the predominantly inattentive type is a very different cluster of problems with a different etiology to which their "impaired capacity to inhibit behavior" models do not apply. They argue that the "hyperactive-impulsive" symptoms associated with the current ADHD diagnosis constitute a cluster of developmental problems with a different cause and different course than those of the predominantly inattentive type, even though both types may respond to the same medications.

For reasons mentioned earlier in this chapter, separating the diagnosis of ADD inattention from the hyperactivity-impulsivity of ADHD may be sensible. DSM-IV has already separated the inattention symptoms of ADHD from the hyperactivity-impulsivity symptoms of ADHD. Currently, sufficient symptoms in either symptom set provide grounds for an ADHD diagnosis. The present confusion rests simply in the persistence of linking both symptom sets within the name of the disorder.

Perhaps a useful next step might be simply to change the labels of these diagnoses to further clarify their independence. What is currently called ADHD, predominantly inattentive type, might be called simply "attention-deficit disorder" without reference to hyperactivity. ADHD, predominantly hyperactive-impulsive type, might be called "hyperactivity-impulsivity disorder." Persons with ADHD, combined type, might be given diagnoses for both ADD and hyperactive-impulsivity disorder.

Regardless of what may eventually be done in refining the official nomenclature for diagnosis, current practice in many clinical and educational settings is to use the official terms for ADHD only for formal diagnosis. The term *attention-deficit disorder* is already commonly used to refer to the attentional impairments of ADHD, regardless of whether they are accompanied by hyperactivity-impulsivity.

DSM-IV and the Diagnosis of ADD Inattention

If diagnosis of the inattention impairments of ADDs can be separated from the hyperactivity-impulsivity symptoms of ADHD, it might be easier for clinicians to be alert to the wide range of cognitive impairments associated with ADDs, especially in adults. In the present diagnostic system, DSM-IV, there is no diagnostic category that picks up the wide range of cognitive impairments associated with the broad spectrum of inattention symptoms of ADHD. The DSM-IV section "Delirium, Dementia, and Amnestic and Other Cognitive Disorders" comprises disorders in which the "predominant disturbance" is a cognitive deficit that represents "a significant change from a previous level of functioning" (American Psychiatric Association 1994, p. 123) (e.g., dementia of the Alzheimer's type or dementias due to vascular insufficiency, head trauma, or neurological disease), but all these disorders relate to impairment of cognitive functions that were once intact. Except for ADD, there is no diagnostic category in DSM-IV for cognitive impairments that are developmentally based, in which the individual of normal intelligence has had these same problems of impairment in organization, inattention, short-term memory, and so forth from early in life. In short, there is in DSM-IV no diagnostic category for developmentally based impairment of executive functions in persons of normal intelligence.

Although psychiatry has diagnostic categories to describe conditions of persons with executive functions that, once adequate, became impaired because of injury or disease, it does not yet have a diagnosis for the condition of those whose executive functioning has been significantly impaired from the outset of life, with or without accompanying hyperactivity-impulsivity. It appears that ADD is currently functioning as a category of diagnosis for many children, adolescents, and adults who have chronic, developmentally based impairments of executive functions and working memory.

In recognizing that the diagnosis of ADD is being used to label impaired executive functions, some might consider inventing a new name for this disorder of cognitive impairments; terms like "executive function disorder," "cognitive management disorder," and "developmental neurocognitive disorder" might be considered for future editions of the diagnostic manual. Yet it is not clear that such a change of terms would yield any greater clarity of understanding. There may be ways to adapt existing diagnostic terms—attention-deficit disorder and hyperactivity-impulsivity disorder—in ways that would preserve some continuity of terms and yet more adequately reflect the newly emerging understanding of these impairments.

ADD as Diagnosis for Developmentally Impaired Executive Function

Following the lead of Douglas (1988), Denckla (1991b, 1993, 1994, 1996), Pennington and Ozonoff (1996), Pennington and Welsh (1995), Pennington et al. (1996), and others, theorists and researchers are increasingly beginning to conceptualize ADD as a diagnostic construct for developmentally impaired executive function and working memory. Tannock and Schachar (1996) observed, "There is growing consensus that the fundamental problems (in ADHD) are in self-regulation and that ADHD is better conceptualized as an impairment of higher-order cognitive processing known as 'executive function'" (p. 129). Castellanos (1999) made a similar observation: "The unifying abstraction that currently best encompasses the faculties principally affected in ADHD has been termed executive function (EF), which is an evolving concept. . . . there is now impressive empirical support for its importance in ADHD" (p. 179).

The notion of "higher order" cognitive processing initially sounds formidably abstract, but it is quite simply illustrated in the situational variability of ADD symptoms. The problem that persons with ADD face is not that they are totally unable to sustain attention, to organize a task, to recall what just happened, and so forth. They are able to exercise all these basic functions quite adequately under certain conditions—for example, in an emergency or when engaged in an activity in which they have a high level of immediate, spontaneous interest. The central problem of persons with ADD is that they are not able to activate and sustain these functions, which they sometimes perform quite well, in many situations when it is necessary or desirable to do so. For example, an individual may be able to "hyperfocus" and sustain intense attention for several hours while playing a sport or using a computer, yet he or she may be unable to sustain attention for more than a few minutes at a time when reading or when sitting in a class or a meeting. The functions—paying attention, organizing, recalling, and so forth—are intact; they are simply not responsive to higher-order processing. That is, the individual is not able readily to activate, deploy, and utilize these functions as needed. They are not readily turned off or on when needed; they are not responsive to "willpower." Executive function is simply a name for those higher-order systems of the brain that activate, integrate, coordinate, and modulate a variety of other cognitive functions.

Tannock and Schachar (1996) also noted the neuropsychological evidence that persons with ADHD tend to show specific impairment in frontal lobe tasks associated with executive function: "The deficits in ADHD appear to be relatively specific to executive function rather than reflecting generalized cognitive impairment[,] because executive dysfunction is evident in ADHD children with above-average IQ and deficient performance is observed on frontal-lobe tasks, but not on measures of temporal lobe functioning or on 'non-executive tasks'" (p. 131). A similar perspective is offered by Seidman (1997b):

> Cognitive deficits, particularly impairments in attention and executive functions, are hypothesized to be a core part of ADHD [Douglas 1972] and are thought to play a major role in the difficult adaptation of children with ADHD. These children exhibit subaverage or relatively weak

> performance on various tasks of vigilance and sustained attention, motoric inhibition, executive functions [such as organization and complex problem solving] and verbal learning and memory [Grodzinsky and Diamond 1992; Barkley et al. 1992; Seidman et al. 1995a, 1995b]. (p. 150)

Seidman makes a very similar report from his study of adults with ADHD: "Unmedicated adults with ADHD performed worse than controls on measures of auditory sustained attention, executive components of verbal learning and arithmetic despite similar levels of education and IQ. These impairments could not be accounted for by age, learning disabilities, psychiatric comorbidity or gender" (Seidman et al. 1998, p. 264).

Impairments of Executive Functions in Cognitive Versus Behavioral ADHD

The formulations of ADHD as impairment in executive function just cited do not distinguish between combined and inattentive types. This is quite different from Barkley's (1997) elaboration of his new theory of ADHD, in which he focuses explicitly on only the combined type and not the inattentive type. Drawing on extensive neuropsychological research, Barkley identifies behavioral inhibition as one of five aspects of executive functioning that he describes as underpinning the impairments of ADHD.

Using a rather elaborate theory extrapolated from Bronowski's formulations about human language, Barkley (1997, p. 108) proposes that behavioral inhibition plays a primary and essential role in the development and proficient performance of four additional executive functions: nonverbal working memory, verbal working memory, self-regulation of affect/arousal, and reconstitution (i.e., capacity to manipulate stored information). He sees combined-type ADHD as a consequence of related impairments in these five aspects of executive function.

Barkley (1997) argues that behavioral inhibition is primary among these executive functions because it "probably assists with the suppression of the observable motor accompaniments associated with each form of executive function, thus facilitating the internalization of behavior" (p. 155). This assumption of the primacy of behavioral inhibition among executive functions is interesting but is thus far not convincingly supported by any empirical data. To the contrary, Barkley's emphasis on behavioral inhibition as the central identifying feature of ADHD has been challenged by Douglas (1999): "Barkley's attempt to establish the primacy of disinhibition differs from my own conceptualization [of ADHD] in which attentional and inhibitory deficits are viewed as different manifestations of an underlying *regulatory control problem*. . . . there is convincing evidence of *both* facilitating (activating) *and* inhibitory problems in ADHD" (p. 108).

I offer a modified view, an alternative to Barkley's theory, as follows: 1) as Barkley and Quay have both argued, impairment of one aspect of executive function, behavioral inhibition, is the core problem in the hyperactive-impulsive type of ADHD but not in the predominantly inattentive type; and 2) other aspects of executive function (e.g., verbal working memory, self-regulation of affect) are impaired in the inattention symptoms of ADD, whether these symptoms appear in the combined type or in the inattentive type.

In this revised formulation, individuals with combined type ADHD would be seen having impairments in a wider range of executive functions—both those that modulate behavioral inhibition and those that modulate the wide variety of cognitive impairments currently listed as inattention symptoms of ADD. Individuals with the predominantly inattentive type of ADD, either primary or after remission of hyperactive-impulsive symptoms, would be seen as having impairment in those aspects of executive function related to the various aspects of inattention.

This understanding could be translated into existing diagnostic terms with a few simple changes of nomenclature. The term *attention-deficit disorder*, without any reference to hyperactivity disorder, could be used to describe the cluster of cognitive impairments described in DSM-IV as inattention symptoms of ADHD. The term *hyperactivity-impulsivity disorder* could be used to describe the cluster of impairments of behavioral control described in DSM-IV as hyperactivity-impulsivity symptoms of ADHD. Persons could be diagnosed as having both disorders so long as the criteria for both disorders are met.

ADD Impairments as Dimensional, Not Categorical

Increasingly, clinicians and researchers are recognizing that ADD impairments occur along a dimension. For example, Levy et al. (1997) reported on a large-scale twin study that yielded genetic evidence that "ADHD is best-viewed as the extreme of a behavior that varies genetically throughout the entire population rather than as a disorder with discrete determinants" (p. 737). This continuum ranges from normal levels of impairments that occur sometimes in virtually everyone to more extreme levels of impairments that occur less frequently and have substantially greater negative impact on the person's life functioning. Put simply, everybody has ADD-type impairments sometimes, but only those who chronically have significant impairment from ADD symptoms should receive an ADD diagnosis. Thus, the ADD diagnosis is analogous to the diagnosis for major depressive disorder; everyone has depressed mood occasionally, but only for those whose depression is persistent and significantly impairing is the diagnosis of major depression considered appropriate. In contrast, pregnancy is not dimensional, but categorical. There are no degrees of pregnancy; either one is pregnant or one is not. There is no defined state in between.

The two main points made by this emphasis on dimensionality of ADD are as follows: 1) The various impairments of cognitive function symptomatic of ADD inattention occur to some degree in virtually everyone. 2) The line between those diagnosed with ADD and those not meeting the diagnostic criteria for ADD is not sharply drawn; the differences between those meeting the criteria on the one side and those almost but not quite meeting the criteria on the other side are not great.

Despite findings that the dimensional view of ADD symptoms yields greater predictive utility for diagnostic purposes than does the categorical view (cf. Fergusson and Horwood 1995), Kagan (1994) and Jensen (1995) remind us that categorical understanding of a disorder like ADD may also be useful. Persons who have a cluster of significant impairments in a particular domain may have qualitatively different experiences than those who have isolated, transient, or less-impairing symptoms. The existing diagnostic criteria for ADHD have led to the identification of groups of people who chronically have a cluster of related impairments that tend to co-occur and to lead to considerable difficulty in a variety of settings.

Regardless of how the diagnostic labels for impairments of ADD may eventually be changed, or of how arbitrary the delineation may be, there will be a continuing need for those involved in diagnosis to determine a cutoff distinguishing the range of ADD impairments that are to be considered "normal" from those of sufficient severity that they can be considered to constitute a "disorder."

Severity Cutoffs for ADD as a Dimensional Disorder

Given that ADD symptoms are dimensional, it becomes clear that making a diagnosis for an ADD requires establishing a cutoff to mark a point beyond which the symptoms are considered to constitute a disorder warranting treatment. DSM-IV appears to establish such a cutoff by its listing of nine symptoms of inattention and nine symptoms of hyperactivity-impulsivity and its stipulation that when six or more of these nine symptoms are present and exclusion criteria are met, the ADHD diagnosis can be appropriately made. Yet counting these symptoms is not like counting cancer cells in a biopsy tissue sample. Careful examination of ADHD symptom lists indicates that each item really encompasses a whole domain of functioning and requires a determination of what constitutes "often," "maladaptive," and "relative to developmental level."

Consider the inattention item: "Is often forgetful in daily activities." This might include forgetting what has been heard or what has been seen, or both, and what has been learned or what has been done, or both. "Often" might mean many times an hour, many times a day, or many times per week. "Developmental level" might mean of the same age, of the same general range of intelligence (IQ above 70), or of the same specific range of intelligence (compared with others with IQs in the superior range).

Many such judgments enter into a clinician's determination of whether any given symptom should or should not be counted toward diagnosis. Similarly, clinical judgment is required for determination of whether any given individual is presenting "clear evidence of clinically significant impairment in social, academic, or occupational functioning" (American Psychiatric Association 1994, p. 84). Making such diagnostic judgments is not always easy; it requires empathic perception, ability to communicate effectively with the patient, a good appreciation of the wide breadth of "normality," and a firm grasp of the multiple varieties in which psychopathology may be manifest. It should be noted that similar clinical judgments are required for diagnosis of virtually every psychiatric disorder, both in differentiating "disorder" from "normality" and in differentiating one disorder from another, especially when they overlap or are concurrent.

COMORBIDITIES WITH ADD

"Dimensions of Impairment" Paradigm for Diagnosis

It is not only for the ADD diagnosis that a dimensional approach to diagnosis of impairments is being recognized. Over recent years researchers and clinicians in both child and adult psychiatry have called attention to the limitations of categorical diagnosis, in which it is assumed that each psychiatric diagnosis is a discrete category with clear boundaries and substantial underlying specificity (Achenbach 1990–1991; Blacker and Tsuang 1992; Caron and

Rutter 1991; Nottelman and Jensen 1995; Skodol and Oldham 1996).

As Skodol and Oldham (1996) noted:

> [P]sychobiological research has led to the discovery of abnormalities in specific neurotransmitter functions in a wide variety of disparately classified disorders. Family studies have demonstrated family aggregation of disorders of apparently different types. Treatment studies have indicated that pharmacological agents, such as antidepressant drugs, can benefit patients with seemingly distinctive types of psychopathology. Thus, the notion that all 200+ DSM-IV categories represent discrete disorders with distinctive etiologies and pathogenetic mechanisms is patently naive, and the search is on for more fundamental psychopathological disturbances. (p. 2)

Many of the diverse discrete categorical diagnoses are increasingly being seen as related in clusters, spectrum, or dimensional groupings, in which the disorders in such groupings are seen as variations of dysfunctions in related functional systems. Examples include schizophrenic spectrum disorders (Bellak 1994), compulsive-impulsive spectrum disorders (Oldham et al. 1996), autistic spectrum disorders (Towbin 1994), and depressive spectrum disorders (Angst and Merikangas 1997).

ADD as a Spectrum Disorder Often Comorbid With Other Disorders

This dimensional, "spectrum" approach to diagnosis seems especially appropriate for ADDs, which, as discussed earlier, appear not to be unitary or categorical. ADDs include many variants of impairments in a wide range of cognitive executive functions. Yet these disparate impairments are related; they often appear concurrently, tend to run in families, and often respond to treatment with the same type of medications.

However, ADD impairments often do not appear alone; they can appear concurrent with a wide variety of other psychiatric disorders and do so with a frequency that greatly exceeds chance. The medical term for this concurrence is *comorbidity*. Comorbidity can apply to the overlap of two or more disorders at the very same moment or, more commonly, to the co-occurrence of two or more disorders in the same lifetime. Generally, it is not the fact of comorbidity itself, but its frequency and causes that are important. It is possible for an individual to have diabetes and influenza (or many other combinations of ailments) at the same time; this would have no special interest unless persons with one of the disorders had an increased risk of having the other, or if the co-occurrence significantly changed the prognosis, course, treatment response, or outcome of either or both disorders.

Studies of the comorbidity of ADD have found extremely elevated rates of co-occurrence between ADD and many other psychiatric disorders (see Angold and Costello 1993; Biederman et al. 1991, 1992; Jensen et al. 1993, 1997). Assessments of comorbidity usually are made by comparing the incidence of two given disorders in the general population and then ascertaining the incidence of one disorder among those persons identified as having the other.

Such comparisons of individuals with ADD and persons without ADD in the general population have yielded markedly higher incidence rates for a wide variety of psychiatric disorders in the ADD samples. For example, the generally reported rate of anxiety disorders in the general population of children is about 5%; among children with ADD the observed rate of anxiety disorders is approximately 25%. Similarly elevated incidences of major depressive disorder, oppositional defiant disorder, conduct disorder, learning disorders, bipolar disorder, Tourette syndrome, substance abuse, and other psychiatric diagnoses have been reported for children and/or adults with ADD (Biederman et al. 1991b, 1993).

Within the present system of diagnostic categories, ADD is very often comorbid with other disorders. Biederman et al. (1992) reported that among the children with ADDs in their sample, 51% met the criteria for at least one other psychiatric diagnosis; among adults with ADDs in this sample, the authors found 77% with at least one comorbid psychiatric diagnosis. These elevated rates of ADD comorbidity are found not only in clinic samples, where one would expect to find individuals with more severe and aggregated problems, but also in community samples, where there has been no selection for those who seek treatment.

Possible Reasons for the High Psychiatric Comorbidity With ADDs

Several proposals have been advanced to explain the high rates of comorbidity of ADD with the wide range of psychiatric disorders. One possible argument is that ADD symptoms may be just one aspect of the comorbid psychiatric disorder. This argument is contradicted by Biederman et al.'s (1992) National Institute of Mental Health family-genetic study of ADHD, in which they presented evidence suggesting that the cognitive impairments observed in the sample of children with ADHD "are caused by the ADHD syndrome itself and do not appear to be accounted for by psychiatric comorbidity" (p. 352). Likewise, in a sample of adults with ADHD, Biederman et al. (1993) reported evidence of ADD cognitive impairments based on neuropsychological measures and unequivocal evidence of school failure, even in those adults whose ADD was not comorbid with any other psychiatric diagnosis in their lifetime.

Children and adults with ADDs who have a comorbid psychiatric disorder, such as depression, anxiety disorder, or conduct disorder, have all the requisite symptoms for the second disorder in addition to the requisite number of symptoms of an ADD. Moreover, ADD can sometimes appear without any comorbid disorder. ADD does not appear to be just another label for other psychiatric diagnoses with which it is comorbid.

Another explanation proffered for the high rates of comorbidity between ADD and other psychiatric disorders is that ADD may not be a single entity. Biederman et al. (1992) argued that ADD may be a name for "a group of conditions with different etiologies and risk factors, as well as different outcomes, rather than a homogenous clinical entity" (p. 339). Conners (1997) made a similar point: "Any effort to find a common mechanism, whether anatomical or purely psychological . . . [, for ADHD] seems doomed to failure as long as we treat the surface symptoms as unitary phenomena instead of the multi-component processes they really are" (p. 9).

From the perspective advanced in this chapter, one might paraphrase and modify Biederman et al.'s argument to say that ADD is a name for a spectrum of impairments of cognitive executive functions that often appear together and often respond to similar treatments, though they may have differing etiologies, risk factors, and outcomes, and are often comorbid with a wide variety of psychiatric disorders, many of which may also be spectrum disorders. This view of ADD as a cluster of attentional/executive impairments that appear and may persist with and without psychiatric comorbidity is consistent with Seidman's findings from neuropsychological assessments of children and adults with ADD (Seidman et al. 1995a, 1995b, 1997a, 1997b, 1998): the impairments of attention/executive function in these individuals tend to be persistent and relatively independent of any comorbid psychiatric disorder that may be present.

Possible Subtypes of ADD Comorbidity

The central question that emerges from recognition of the overlap of ADD with other disorders is, What difference does comorbidity make? In other words, how does the co-occurrence of ADD with another disorder alter the presentation, illness course, or response to treatment of the affected patient? The major purpose of most of the chapters in this volume is to address this important question.

Jensen et al. (1997) recently published a review of 15 years of ADD literature to ascertain the most prevalent patterns of ADD comorbidity and to determine the extent to which specific comorbid patterns may convey unique information about ADHD symptoms, treatment, and outcomes. From this review they derived data that support delineation of two new subclassifications of ADD: ADHD, aggressive subtype, and ADHD, anxious subtype. Data suggest that persons with ADD that is comorbid with conduct disorder tend to have lower IQ, increased learning/reading deficits, and evidence of neuropsychological impairments; also, demonstrably high levels of familiality are evident in this population. Data on those whose ADD is comorbid with anxiety indicate a tendency for this group to demonstrate more inhibition on laboratory measures of attentional processes, decreased impulsivity, and decreased severity of some other associated symptoms (e.g., aggression and conduct disorder symptoms). The authors suggested more research to refine understanding of these two proposed subtypes. At a more general level, Jensen and colleagues suggested, from their review of the data, that clinical course and outcomes of ADD are generally poorer in the presence of comorbid conditions than when there is no comorbidity, whether measured by parent-child interactions, poor school performance, automobile driving behaviors, or risks for later substance abuse and antisocial personality disorder.

Importance of Assessing Comorbidities With ADDs

Clearly the impact of comorbid psychiatric disorders on the course, treatment, and outcomes of ADD is a very important area for further study. Yet, until recently, most researchers of ADD and many other psychiatric disorders have tended to design their studies to focus on individuals who manifested relatively "pure" forms of the disorder without complications of comorbidity. Jensen et al. (1997, p. 1077) strongly suggest that "comorbidity must be more fully considered in the design of future studies of ADHD." They contend that "[r]ather than regard ADHD-associated conditions as 'noise,' that is, as extraneous factors to be controlled for or eliminated," investigators of ADHD should "vigorously study" the nature and impact of comorbidity on ADHD assessment, treatment, and outcome.

The study of the comorbidity of ADD with other psychiatric disorders is important. However, while the needed studies are being designed, carried out, and reported—a process that will take more than a few years—many patients with ADD will be seeking assessment and treatment. It is critically important that those who provide assessment and treatment for these children, adolescents, and adults with ADD learn carefully to take into account the strong likelihood that comorbid disorders may be present with ADD. Likewise, clinicians assessing patients for other psychiatric disorders should seriously consider the possibility that ADD, perhaps masked by other symptoms, may be comorbid with another psychiatric disorder such as a mood disorder, anxiety disorder, conduct disorder, learning disorder, or substance abuse.

In actual practice, clinicians deal with the complications of individual persons, not with simplistic categories of disorder. Often a person, in addition to fully meeting the established diagnostic criteria for one or more disorders, will have some symptoms of other disorders, but not all the symptoms required for diagnosis of those disorders. Good clinicians have long recognized that these more isolated symptoms and "subclinical" forms of disorder need to be taken into account for accurate assessment and effective treatment. Ratey and Johnson (1997) highlighted the importance of these subclinical characteristics, which they have labeled "shadow syndromes."

In any case, adequate assessment and treatment of ADD requires that the clinician take into account not only the wide spectrum of impairments associated with ADD but also the accompanying symptoms of other disorders. Some of the accompanying symptoms may fully meet the diagnostic criteria for specific disorders, whereas others may reflect remission or persistence of the disorder in subclinical form. Sometimes only one comorbid disorder may be present, either actively or in remission. In some cases, the diagnostic criteria for several comorbid disorders may be fully met, with the disorders active at the same time or intermittently.

It should also be noted that generally neither ADD nor comorbid disorders are static in their manifestations. Longitudinal research and clinical experience both indicate that symptom profiles of individuals with ADD often change over time—for example, hyperactive-impulsive symptoms may be lost as a child gets older, and organizational problems may become increasingly evident as an adolescent takes on more adult work and financial responsibilities.

Likewise, symptoms of other psychiatric disorders comorbid with an ADD may remit or exacerbate over time. For example, obsessive-compulsive symptoms may become more or less salient, an adolescent may gradually cease to abuse alcohol or marijuana, and depressive symptoms may lift spontaneously or in response to treatment. The severity of ADD symptoms and their responses to treatment may vary considerably as a function of increased or reduced severity of one of the comorbid disorders or interaction of changes in several comorbid disorders that may be present at a given time.

AREAS FOR FURTHER RESEARCH ON ADD COMORBIDITY

Recognition of ADD as a spectrum of executive impairments comorbid with many other psychiatric disorders raises many questions about the nature, etiology, assessment, course, treatment, and outcome of ADD. These questions apply to ADD both in its relatively uncomplicated forms and when comorbid with various other disorders, singly and in combination. Some areas in which further research might be especially useful are described in the following subsections.

Assessment of ADD Cognitive Impairments Across the Life Span

Although there exists an enormous and continually growing research literature on ADD, most of the reported research thus far has focused primarily on young Caucasian boys with hyperactive-impulsive symptoms. There have been relatively few studies of adolescents and adults with ADD, very few of adolescents and adults with ADD symptoms that did not include hyperactivity, and extremely few of persons with ADD who are female or from ethnic minorities. Moreover, as Jensen et al. (1997) noted, extant research on ADDs has insufficiently studied persons with ADDs that are complicated with comorbidities. The research that has been done on the comorbidities of ADD has focused mainly on varieties of behavioral disorders, especially conduct disorder. Relatively little attention has been paid to other types of comorbidity with ADD.

Since ADD appears to be a highly prevalent developmental disorder that, for at least half of those diagnosed, persists into adulthood, it is extremely important to develop a fuller empirical understanding of how ADD symptoms are manifested in childhood and of how these symptoms persist and/or change over time in the absence and presence of comorbidity.

Some ADHD symptoms may change, for better or worse, in response to developmental learning or advancing brain development. New symptoms may arise as individuals are faced with increasing demands for self-control and independent functioning. Biederman et al. (1998) presented data on the diagnostic continuity of childhood ADHD into adolescence, but far more empirical information is needed on the persistence and changes in the wider range of ADHD symptoms over the life span.

Requirements for increased executive function continue to escalate as development proceeds, from the relatively basic requirements of group activities in day care or kindergarten, to the constantly increasing academic and social challenges of each grade in elementary and high school, to the variegated challenges of preparing to work, eventually moving out of the family nest, getting and functioning in a job, paying one's own bills, managing a household, carrying on multiple social relationships, and, possibly, functioning as a parent. Awareness of these increasing challenges over time to an individual's capacities for executive functions, when coupled with recognition of ADHD as developmentally impaired executive function, may require reassessment of the diagnostic criteria for ADHD pertaining to age at onset and age at impairment. The DSM-IV diagnostic criteria for ADHD specify that at least some of the symptoms of ADHD must have been present prior to age 7 years for the ADHD diagnosis to be used appropriately. Recently, some of those who were involved in establishing those criteria have questioned the validity of the age-at-onset criterion (Applegate et al. 1997). Barkley and Biederman (1997) extended this questioning to argue that the age-at-onset criterion for ADHD should be altogether abandoned or generously broadened.

Persons with various types of ADD and comorbid disorders may experience widely differing levels of impairment and success as they attempt to cope with the ever-changing challenges presented by the demands of changing life circumstances. Some widely circulated popular books offer very useful descriptions of the phenomenology of ADD in adult life (e.g., Hallowell and Ratey 1994; Kelly and Ramundo 1995; Solden 1995). Systematic cross-sectional and longitudinal research is needed to develop adequate empirically based understanding of the developmental course of ADD and how this course may be modified by various comorbid conditions.

One particular need for further research is to develop an empirical basis for diagnostic criteria for ADD in adults. The DSM-IV criteria for the diagnosis of ADD are intended for use with all age groups, but the criteria were developed in field studies that included no adults, only children aged 4 to 17 years. Murphy and Barkley (1996) reported that when the diagnostic cutoffs of DSM-IV are applied to assessment of ADD in adults, only the most severe cases are identified. Their studies of adults not seeking treatment indicate that much lower cutoff points must be utilized to identify adults whose symptoms place them within the 7% of the population most impaired by ADD. To provide adequate criteria for diagnosis of ADD in adults, systematic research is needed to establish the nature, course, and prevalence of symptoms of ADD in late adolescence and throughout adulthood. More systematic research can establish impairment on a more solid foundation than that provided by simply a given percentage of the population or criteria for persistence of impairment derived from studies of samples of children.

Neuropsychological research on ADD impairments of children, adolescents, and adults is particularly important for validating the diagnosis and for developing more adequate diagnostic measures useful for various ages. As Seidman et al. (1997b) observed, cognitive performance measures "are key validating criteria for ADD because they do not share method variance with other measures . . ., directly assess performance . . . and can be given longitudinally to assess (symptom) stability over time" (p. 158). Further research will help to determine the clinical and predictive utility of neuropsychological measures in the assessment and treatment of ADD; it should also lead to development of more effective measures to augment assessment by clinical interview.

Yet there are limits to what can be expected of "objective" measures of executive function impairments of ADD. Rabbit (1997) observed that the usual research strategy of isolating and quantifying one particular variable is not feasible in studying executive function because "an essential property of all 'executive' behavior is that, by nature, it involves the simultaneous management of a variety of different functional processes" (p. 14). Burgess (1997) expressed a similar concern in his review of theory and methodology of executive function research; he cited numerous studies indicating that most current neuropsychological measures of executive function are inadequate because they try to separate interacting aspects of complex integrated functions. To illustrate, he cites Goethe's comment that "dissecting a fly and studying its parts will not tell you how it flies" (p. 99).

Interaction of Genetic and Environmental Factors in ADDs

Numerous studies have demonstrated that ADD impairments are highly familial, linked to genetic factors that apparently have an impact on the functioning of specific neurotransmitter systems (see Chapter 2, this volume, for a review). Yet environmental factors are not without influence on any individual's ADD symptoms. Biederman et al. (1995) replicated the earlier findings of Rutter to demonstrate that psychosocial adversity significantly influences the expression of ADHD symptoms. In this study they found that while no one particular psychosocial stressor increased poor outcome of ADD, the additive effect of multiple stressors (e.g., low socioeconomic class, large family size, parental psychopathology, foster placement) had a significant impact on the level of impairment.

As Mazure and Druss (1995) noted, the relationship between environmental stressors and psychiatric disorders, though not simple, is significant. Several different theories have been advanced to describe the role of stressors and environmental protective factors in contemporary models of psychiatric illness. What these theories have in common is an appreciation of the importance of environmental stressors and supports interacting with genetic vulnerability to psychiatric illness to shape the individual's impairment and development of strengths. Thus far, there has been very little research on the role that environmental stressors and/or supports might play in shaping the course of impairments and development of protection and adaptation in persons with ADD (see Samudra and Cantwell 1999). Yet several workers in developmental psychopathology have reported on studies that may help begin to address these issues.

Rogeness and McClure (1996) reported on the study of environment-neurotransmitter interactions as these shape neural circuits, neurophysiology, and neurochemistry of the brain across development. Likewise, Shore (1996) discussed the role of experience in maturation of the regulatory system in the prefrontal cortex. The perspectives of these researchers suggest a mechanism and a developmental perspective that might be useful in studying these issues with regard to ADHD.

ADD Symptoms Associated With Severe Social/Mental Dysfunction

Many individuals with ADD chronically have difficulties in social relationships with peers, family members, teachers, work supervisors, intimate partners, and others. These difficulties stem from the tendency of these individuals to be chronically inattentive to social communications, especially to subtle verbal and nonverbal cues that often play a critical role in regulating social interaction. Persons with ADD symptoms that include hyperactive-impulsive behavior often have even more social problems because of their tendencies to be impatient, impulsive, and intrusive. Yet, despite such difficulties, most persons with ADD are characterized by relatively normal social development.

Yet ADD inattention symptoms are also found in some children, adolescents, and adults who, despite average or above-average intelligence, are strikingly unusual in their social and emotional development. These individuals with "atypical" characteristics appear qualitatively different from age-mates in the way they relate to other people and/or in the way they express their emotions. In social situations some of these individuals come across as peculiarly detached, showing little evidence of emotional interest or connection to those around them; others in this group relate in uncomfortably intense ways, thrusting themselves on strangers as though they were intimates. Often such children and adolescents impress both peers and adults as "weird" because they appear surprisingly out of touch with even the most basic social expectations.

Emotional expression in these children, adolescents, and adults with atypical characteristics may be very different from that of most other persons, including most others with ADD. They may react to apparently minor frustrations with sudden and sustained "catastrophic" emotions (e.g., inconsolable sobbing or violent, threatening rage). In others of this group, emotional expression is startlingly absent, even in situations where one would expect intense pleasure, sadness, or anger; the individual may simply withdraw or appear totally unaffected.

Some of the children with these atypical characteristics also have stereotyped behavioral mannerisms that make them stand out from other children. They may flap their arms or engage in unusual repetitive hand gestures when excited. These peculiar mannerisms are not tics or flamboyant displays of emotion; they appear more as involuntary movements that occur as unwitting "motoric overflow" in times of excitement (e.g., when the child is frightened or awaiting some pleasure).

Some of these individuals with atypical characteristics are also peculiar in their thought processes. Not only do they have the usual ADD problems of losing focus in conversation, they also tend to "get stuck" on certain topics of conversation and have unusual difficulty in moving on. Sometimes they cannot let go of a particular word, image, or theme; they tend to perseverate in retelling a joke or multiplying fantasies about a situation—for example, describing various ways they could get back at someone who has offended them.

Although these unusual mannerisms of speech, movement, or thought may be quite striking, they often appear as just one more peculiarity of an individual who stands out far more obviously as having impairment in very basic aspects of social interactions and/or emotional expression. These individuals tend to be perceived by peers and elders as awkward, strange, weird, odd, and eccentric. Their social and emotional impairments are not just immature or delayed; they seem outside the usual range of development and quite atypical.

Although some individuals with attention-deficit disorder and these atypical symptoms do not fully meet the diagnostic criteria for another disorder (see Barkley 1990; Guevremont 1993; Rubin and Stewart 1996), some others have persistent emotional detachment that may meet the diagnostic criteria for an autistic spectrum disorder (e.g., Asperger's disorder, pervasive developmental disorder not otherwise specified, or schizoid personality disorder) (Attwood 1998; Klin 1994; Siegel 1996; Towbin 1994; Wolff 1995). Others whose atypicality may manifest more volatile, intense emotional displays may qualify for the diagnosis of borderline personality disorder (Cohen et al. 1983; King and Noshpitz 1991; Lewis 1994; Petti and Vela 1990). Still others who also manifest disordered thinking may meet the criteria for childhood-onset schizophrenia or schizotypal personality disorder (King 1994; Towbin et al. 1993).

Current DSM-IV diagnostic criteria stipulate that the ADHD diagnosis should not be made if symptoms occur "exclusively during the course of a Pervasive Developmental Disorder, Schizophrenia . . . and are not better accounted for by another mental disorder," including a personality disorder (American Psychiatric Association 1994, p. 85). From the point of view described in this chapter, there may be reason to reexamine this stipulation, which is based on a hierarchical model of diagnosis in which the ADD symptoms would be essentially subsumed within the "more severe" diagnosis. From the viewpoint of our emerging conceptualization of an ADD as an impairment in executive function/working memory, ADD inattention symptoms would, it seems, warrant diagnostic attention and possible targeted treatment even if they are present in the context of another, "more severe" disorder.

This viewpoint would be consistent with that of Bellak (1979), who recognized that a significant number of his patients with "schizophrenic spectrum" disorders had "minimal brain dysfunction," the term used at that time for what is now know as ADHD. Subsequently, he more specifically noted an overlap between the schizophrenic syndrome and ADDs (Bellak 1994). More recent research (Green 1996) has noted that the cognitive deficits of schizophrenia with the greatest functional import are not the "positive symptoms" of delusions or hallucinations, but the "negative symptoms" of impairment in information processing involving verbal memory and impaired vigilance. These cognitive impairments in schizophrenic patients, as described by Green (1996), closely resemble the executive function impairments discussed earlier as being central to ADD. Taylor (1995) noted the potential value of further research on the development of attentional impairments in schizophrenia.

Impairments of working memory in persons with schizophrenia have been emphasized by Goldman-Rakic (1991), who argued that "a fundamental problem in schizophrenia is the loss of working memory processes that inexorably lead to a deficit in the regulation of behavior by internalized schemata, symbolic representations, and ideas" (p. 1). She claims that this "singular cognitive operation may account for some cardinal features of the disease" (p. 1). Similarly, Docherty et al. (1996) presented data to support their hypothesis that communication disturbances in schizophrenia reflect specific deficits in working memory and attention. It is not clear how similar or different the impairments of attentional/working memory in persons with schizophrenia may be from those in persons with ADD but no schizophrenia. The findings from one study (Øie and Rund 1999) suggest that ADHD patients have more impairment on some specific measures of attention, verbal memory, and learning, while patients with schizophrenia show more general impairment of brain function.

These observations about possible overlap of ADD and severe autistic or schizophrenic spectrum disorders are of more than theoretical interest; they have important implications for treatment. A recent exchange of letters in a psychiatric journal illustrates the point. One correspondent chided the writer of an earlier article for overlooking the DSM rule that children with autistic disorder should not be diagnosed as having ADHD. The author responded, "Although they may be hyperactive, persons with autistic disorder also may present with executive dysfunction, inattention, impulsivity and distractibility. These individuals may benefit from treatment with methylphenidate or clonidine and have been so treated for many years in the autistic disorder program at Johns Hopkins Hospital" (Harris 1996). Bellak (1994) made a very similar argument for use of stimulant medication in the treatment of a subgroup of patients within the heterogeneity of patients with schizophrenia whom he identified as having "ADD psychosis." He wrote, "It is my experience that people I now consider to be suffering from ADD psychosis respond favorably to dopaminergic medication and poorly to neuroleptics[,] whereas with patients who have been diagnosed with schizophrenic syndrome, the reverse is most often the case" (p. 29). More research is needed to increase understanding of how the executive function/working memory impairments identified here as central to ADDs may be involved in various other psychiatric disorders. Such research may have important implications both for developing more effective treatments and for understanding underlying common features in disorders previously thought to be unrelated.

ADDs and Specific Learning Disorders

Another area in which further research might be especially fruitful concerns the overlap between the executive function/working memory impairments central to ADDs and the domain of specific learning disorders. Although there has been persisting debate about the nature of the relationship between ADD and specific learning disorders, there is considerable evidence of markedly elevated rates of specific learning disorders, such as reading disorder, math disorder, and disorder of written expression, among individuals diagnosed with ADD (Cantwell and Baker 1991). Some have attempted to draw a clear line between these two categories by characterizing ADD as a disorder that may be helped by medication, while viewing specific learning disorders as "hard wired" into the organism and responsive only to alternative instructional techniques. This clear demarcation may be challenged by an alternative view in which impairments of working memory are seen as playing a significant role in both ADDs and learning disorders.

Tannock and Brown (Chapter 7, this volume) note the critical role of working memory in reading, math, and written expression. Reading involves holding in mind and integrating initial portions of a word, phrase, sentence, paragraph, chapter, and so forth long enough to connect these with subsequent portions so that connections can be made and various levels of meanings can be comprehended. Connections must be made between letter shapes and phonemes; diverse associations from elements of long-term memory must be quickly sorted out to select what is appropriate to context and to discard what is not. Smooth execution of these multiple linkages clearly involves not only the learning of phonemes and vocabulary but also ongoing exercise of short-term working memory.

Likewise, most mathematical operations, from the borrowing and carrying of the simplest arithmetic to the intricacies of the most complex calculations for theoretical problem solving, are highly dependent on working memory. Multiple steps must be prioritized and sequenced, and information must be carried from one operation into another. To do arithmetic and mathematics, one needs not only knowledge of specific procedures but also effective working memory. The problem solver's ability to transiently hold "on-line" these various numerical facts and relationships while analyzing problems and invoking appropriate learned procedures is another example of the exercise of working memory.

Similarly, working memory plays an essential role in written expression as one selects and weaves together words and verbal images to convey multiple levels of meaning. In writing, one must hold in mind an overall intention for what is to be communicated in the whole of the phrase, sentence, paragraph, essay, report, chapter, book, and so forth, while simultaneously generating the micro units of words and phrases that will eventually constitute the written work being produced. Complex and rapidly shifting interplay of micro and macro intentions is the essence of creating and self-editing that allows one gradually to shift from the glimmer of an idea, through crude approximations of rough draft, to the greater specificity and polish of a final product in which one has captured in written language what one wants to say. In addition to many more specific skills, the whole process of written expression involves ongoing and often intensive use of working memory.

Research on the differing roles of working memory in the learning and exercise of reading, mathematics, and written expression could be helpful in improving instructional techniques in these skill domains; it could also help in developing more adequate assessment and more effective remediation for those numerous persons whose functioning in one or another of these skills is so impaired that they are identified as having a learning disorder. Existing research suggests that stimulant medication can be effective in improving a wide range of information-processing and working-memory functions for some people with ADDs (e.g., Balthazor et al. 1991). There is need for more intensive research to determine whether treatment with stimulant medications may also be helpful for certain aspects of specific learning disorders, with or without a comorbid ADD.

One would not expect stimulants to cure learning disorders. No medication can establish unlearned skills (e.g., phoneme recognition); this is the work of education. Yet stimulant medications may play a significant role, directly and indirectly, in helping to alleviate chronic executive function/working memory impairments so that persons with both ADD and learning disorder may be enabled to participate in and apply more effectively the remedial education in basic skills that they desperately need (Beitchman and Young 1997).

In addition to the academically based learning disorders of reading, mathematics, and written expression, there is another type of learning disorder that seems often to overlap with the executive function impairments of ADHD: nonverbal learning disorders (NVLDs). Numerous authors (Denckla 1991a, Chapter 8, this volume; Myklebust 1975; Rourke 1985, 1989a, 1989b; Rourke and Fuerst 1991; Semrud-Clikeman and Hynd 1990; Tranel 1987; Voeller 1991; Weintraub and Mesulam 1983) have described this syndrome, which has not yet been adequately studied or conceptualized and is not yet incorporated in the DSM system.

NVLD syndrome has been described as encompassing a wide variety of impairments in cognitive functions required for tactile and visual perception, exploratory behavior in novel situations, pragmatics of social functioning, and ability to shift and integrate visual or conceptual perspectives (Denckla 1991a, Chapter 8, this volume; Rourke 1985, 1989a, 1989b, 1995; Rourke and Fuerst 1991). These impairments may be apparent in a cognitive style characterized by excessively narrow focus and chronic difficulties in grasping the more global, contextual aspects of ideas and situations. Severe impairments of NVLDs are often associated with very severe psychosocial and/or psychiatric problems (Rourke 1989, 1991, 1995; Voeller 1991). Presumably, most NVLD impairments are associated with malfunctions in the right hemisphere of the brain, the functions of which are just beginning to be more clearly understood (see Ornstein 1997).

As Eslinger (1996) noted, current models of executive functions do not yet adequately incorporate the ways in which executive function shapes and impacts social development and functioning. This is an area of learning disorders and executive function in which further theoretical elaboration and empirical research are urgently needed to guide assessment and clinical interventions. Conceptual clarification and empirical research are also needed to illuminate the overlaps between NVLDs and ADHD. Denckla (see Chapter 8, this volume) has suggestsed that distinctions between these two domains of impairment may be simply differences of perspective and vocabulary among academic and clinical disciplines.

ADDs and Developmental Changes in Estrogens

From the perspective taken in this chapter, ADD is a developmental disorder in that affected persons seem generally to be born with the core impairments, manifestations of which gradually emerge over the course of development as the individual is called on to learn and apply an increasingly broad range of functions for behavioral and cognitive self-management. Results from recent studies of adult women with and without ADDs raise another possible understanding of ADD symptoms as "developmental."

Many middle-aged women report that during the course of their menopause, regardless of whether it is naturally occurring or surgically induced, they experience for the first time a constellation of persisting symptoms that closely resembles the inattention symptoms of ADD. They note significant impairment in short-term memory, in ability to screen distractions and to sustain attention, in organization of thoughts and tasks, and so forth (see Warga 1999). Women diagnosed premenopausally with ADD often report significant exacerbation of their long-standing ADD symptoms during the protracted perimenopausal period and thereafter. These reports raise the possibility that ADD symptoms may be exacerbated or developmentally acquired by some women during menopause.

A possible mechanism for such a developmental phenomenon might be the role of estrogen as a facilitator of the release of dopamine. Basic neuroscience research (McEwen 1991; McEwen and Parsons 1982; Mermelstein et al. 1996; Thompson and Moss 1994) suggests that estrogen potentiates and modulates the release of dopamine, especially in brain areas associated with executive function, both genomically and nongenomically, in a variety of complicated ways. If this is so, significant inconsistency or persisting reduction of estrogen levels in a woman's body such as occurs in menopause may contribute substantially to ADD symptom exacerbation in women with ADD and may even produce onset of ADD symptoms in some women who have never previously manifested ADD symptoms in any significant way.

Sherwin (1998; Phillips and Sherwin 1992a, 1992b) has reported research in which she and others demonstrated in controlled studies that administration of estrogen to postmenopausal women enhances verbal memory and maintains the ability to learn new material. Moreover, an MRI study by Shaywitz et al. (1999) demonstrated that administration of estrogen to postmenopausal women increased activation in specific brain regions during verbal and nonverbal working memory tasks.

Much remains to be done before any direct parallels can be inferred between cognitive impairments characteristic of ADD and those often found during menopause. Yet preliminary data are sufficiently suggestive to warrant further investigation of the possible roles of gonadal hormones in the onset, exacerbation, and alleviation of ADD symptoms. If these preliminary findings are confirmed, menopausally induced ADHD symptoms might come to be seen as a form of "secondary ADHD" in the same way that Gerring et al. (1998) proposed to label as "secondary ADHD" the onset and development of ADHD symptoms after closed head injuries.

Longer-Term Treatments for ADDs

Most of the research on treatment of ADDs, thus far, has focused on interventions provided over a relatively short term. The preponderance of the more than 200 studies of medication treatments for ADDs have been of less than 3 months' duration. In 1993 Schachar and Tannock found only 18 studies of psychostimulant studies for ADD with a duration of more than 3 months. Studies of psychosocial interventions have generally been of similarly short duration. Even the recently completed multisite Multimodal Treatment

Study of Attention Deficit Hyperactivity Disorder, the largest and longest-duration controlled study of ADD treatments thus far, provided its medication and psychosocial interventions for only 14 months.

Given this lack of longer-term studies of ADD treatments, it is not surprising that many discussions of ADD treatment recognize the short-term benefits of such treatments but cite the lack of evidence that the treatments provide any long-term benefits. Some have pointed to the few longer-term follow-up studies to argue that individuals treated in childhood do not seem to fare any better than matched control subjects, but this argument carries little weight once it is recognized that the studies on which this argument was based did not continue treatment into adolescence. Trying to determine the long-term effectiveness of a treatment for ADD under such circumstances would be comparable to testing the benefits of wearing eyeglasses by assessing the vision of visually impaired children 10 years after they had been forced to stop wearing their eyeglasses.

The short-term focus of most studies of the treatment of ADDs contrasts sharply with the more long-term, chronic nature of the disorder, of which there has been increasing evidence. It now seems clear that ADD is not a disease that can be cured as one might cure a streptococcal infection with a course of antibiotic treatment. Nor is it usually just a transient affliction of early childhood commonly outgrown. If, as I have argued earlier, ADDs represent a developmental impairment of executive functions of the brain, which for many of those affected appears to have significant negative impact over the life span (Hechtman 1996; see also Chapter 14, this volume), many persons with ADD are likely to need ongoing treatment over a long term, at least through adolescence and possibly well into adulthood.

There will certainly be exceptions—for example, persons with ADDs in childhood who do not need ongoing treatment. Some children do "outgrow" their ADD symptoms as they grow older. Much brain development continues into adolescence and beyond. Fischer and Rose (1994) reviewed research and described the behavioral implications of ongoing brain development (e.g., synaptic growth and pruning) from birth through 30 years of age. For some children, the ADD symptoms appear as a transient "developmental delay," which is eventually fully compensated for by further neurodevelopmental maturation.

For some individuals, some of the problematic ADD symptoms (e.g., hyperactivity) that are present in early childhood may decrease in severity as the individuals mature toward adolescence. Yet, as Hart et al. (1995) and others have reported, other ADD symptoms, especially those in the inattention cluster, tend to persist. Studies are needed to describe empirically which symptoms of impairment tend to persist into adolescence and adulthood, for how long, with what changes, and with what impact on education, work, and social relationships.

Some persons with ADDs may eventually find ways to avoid domains of activity in which their ADD impairments continue to present significant problems. Some specific executive function impairments are more important for certain tasks and settings than others. Boetsch et al. (1996) reported studies showing how some individuals with dyslexia and ADHD, after their schooling ends, self-select, are forced, or wander into areas of work and social relationships that are less demanding and more rewarding for their particular combination of strengths and limitations. Others, perhaps less fortunate or more bold, may attempt to persevere in areas of work, further education, or relationships in which their ADD impairments continue to be more problematic.

Although there are exceptions, longitudinal studies of children with ADD indicate that 50% to 70% or more of persons diagnosed with ADD in childhood continue to meet the diagnostic criteria for ADD at least into later adolescence. Hechtman (1996; see also Chapter 14, this volume) has reviewed research on the variety of outcomes in individuals diagnosed with ADHD in childhood as they emerge into adulthood. These outcomes vary widely, often as a result of not one single factor but according to the additive and interactive impact of multiple protective and deleterious factors within the person and their environments. For the many whose ADD persists in problematic ways into adolescence and adulthood, some sort of continuing treatment is likely to be useful.

Thus far, there is little research to guide longer-term treatment of ADD. The research base for treatment of ADDs is not very different from that for treatment of many other chronic psychiatric disorders. In recent articles, the authors have emphasized this need and suggested guidelines for developing research on interventions designed to sustain treatment effects for the chronic course of: unipolar depression (Nezu et al. 1998), addictive behaviors (Dimeff and Marlatt 1998), eating disorders (Perri 1998), and conduct disorder (Eyberg et al. 1998). Similar research and clinical initiatives are needed for persons with ADDs who may need continuing or intermittent treatment over their life span.

CONCLUSION

This chapter has highlighted the emerging new understandings of attention-deficit disorders as complex, multifaceted clusters of dimensional impairments in the cognitive and behavioral management functions of the brain. Described in this chapter is the emerging shift in paradigm from the old understanding of ADD as a simple disruptive behavior disorder limited to childhood toward a new understanding of ADDs as complex developmental impairments of executive functions in the brain that may cause persisting reverberations of impairment through the life cycle. Yet these understandings are emerging, not fully developed and established. The research base for such models is still fragmentary and suggestive, not complete or definitive. Much work—theoretical and empirical—remains to be done.

The newly emerging perspectives described in this chapter are not consistently incorporated in other chapters of this volume. Some chapter authors have alluded to them, but most of the chapters use the currently orthodox definitions of ADDs provided in DSM-IV. The DSM-IV criteria are the common base of shared understanding on which more adequate conceptualizations and hypotheses can be developed. Despite the amazing progress of the past 10 years, much more research is needed to test, clarify, and enlarge our understanding of how best to conceptualize, assess, and treat these clusters of impairments currently known as ADDs.

In the title of this book and throughout this introductory chapter the plural form ADDs is primarily used to refer to attention-deficit disorders. The purpose of this usage is to highlight the multiplicity of ways in which ADDs present themselves in various individuals at various times. This usage is adopted in an effort to counter those who tend to speak of ADD in simplistic terms as a unitary disorder; it invites recognition of the rich and diverse complexity of these cognitive impairments as they appear sometimes in relatively uncomplicated form and often in comorbid combination with one or more other psychiatric disorders.

Studying the diversity of attentional disorders and their comorbidities offers unparalleled opportunity to appreciate the amazing complexity, resourcefulness, and interconnectedness of the human brain. Hopefully, as clinicians and educators gain increased awareness and understanding of ADDs, they will be better able to dispel the widespread ignorance that unnecessarily increases the frustration and pain of those many children, adolescents, and adults who suffer not only from ADD impairments but also from the blame and criticism of those who continue to believe that ADDs result from lack of willpower rather than from disorders of brain neurochemistry that unfold developmentally in interactions with the individual's environment.

REFERENCES

Achenbach TM: "Comorbidity" in child and adolescent psychiatry: categorical and quantitative perspectives. J Child Adolesc Psychopharmacol 1:271–278, 1990–1991

Achenbach TM, Howell CT, McConaughy SH, et al: Six-year predictors of problems in a national sample, III: transitions to young adult syndromes. J Am Acad Child Adolesc Psychiatry 34:658–669, 1995

American Academy of Child and Adolescent Psychiatry: Practice parameters for the assessment and treatment of children, adolescents, and adults with attention-deficit/hyperactivity disorder. J Am Acad Child Adolesc Psychiatry 36(10, suppl):85S–121S, 1997

American Psychiatric Association: Diagnostic and Statistical Manual of Mental Disorders, 3rd Edition. Washington, DC, American Psychiatric Association, 1980

American Psychiatric Association: Diagnostic and Statistical Manual of Mental Disorders, 3rd Edition, Revised. Washington, DC, American Psychiatric Association, 1987

American Psychiatric Association: Diagnostic and Statistical Manual of Mental Disorders, 4th Edition. Washington, DC, American Psychiatric Association, 1994

Anderson JC, Williams S, McGee R, et al: DSM-III disorders in preadolescent children: prevalence in a large sample from the general population. Arch Gen Psychiatry 44:69–76, 1987

Anderson JR, Bower GH: Human Associative Memory. Washington, DC, Winston, 1973

Angold A, Costello EJ: Depressive comorbidity in children and adolescents: empirical, theoretical, and methodological issues. Am J Psychiatry 150:1779–1791, 1993

Angst J, Merikangas K: The depressive spectrum: diagnostic classification and course. J Affect Disord 45:31–40, 1997

Applegate B, Lahey BB, Hart EL, et al: Validity of the age-of-onset criterion for ADHD: a report from the DSM-IV field trials. J Am Acad Child Adolesc Psychiatry 36: 1211–1221, 1997

Arnold LE: Sex differences in ADHD: conference summary. J Abnorm Child Psychol 24:555–569, 1996

Attwood T: Asperger's Syndrome. London, Jessica Kingsley, 1998

Baddeley A: Working Memory. New York, Oxford University Press, 1986

Balthazor MJ, Wagner RK, Pelham WE: The specificity of the effects of stimulant medication on classroom learning-related measures of cognitive processing for attention deficit disorder children. J Abnorm Child Psychol 19:35–52, 1991

Barkley RA: Attention-Deficit Hyperactivity Disorder: Handbook for Diagnosis and Treatment. New York, Guilford, 1990

Barkley RA: ADHD and the Nature of Self-Control. New York, Guilford, 1997

Barkley RA, Biederman J: Toward a broader definition of the age-of-onset criterion for attention-deficit hyperactivity disorder. J Amer Acad Child Adolesc Psychiatry 36:1204–1210, 1997

Barkley RA, Grodzinsky G, DuPaul G: Frontal lobe functions in attention deficit disorder with and without hyperactivity: a review and research report. J Abnorm Psychol 20:163–188, 1992

Barkley RA, Murphy K, Kwasnik D: Psychological adjustment and adaptive impairments in young adults with ADHD. Journal of Attention Disorders 1:41–54, 1996

Baumgaertel A, Wolraich ML, Dietrich M: Comparison of diagnostic criteria for attention deficit disorders in a German elementary school sample. J Am Acad Child Adolesc Psychiatry 34:629–638, 1995

Beitchman JH, Young AR: Learning disorders with a special emphasis on reading disorders: a review of the past 10 Years. J Am Acad Child Adolesc Psychiatry 36: 1020–1032, 1997

Bellak L: An idiosyncratic overview, in Disorders of the Schizophrenic Spectrum. Edited by Bellak L. New York, Basic Books, 1979, pp 3–22

Bellak L: The schizophrenic syndrome and attention deficit disorder: thesis, antithesis, and synthesis? Am Psychol 49:25–29, 1994

Bhatia MS, Nigam VR, Bohra N, et al: Attention deficit disorder with hyperactivity among pediatric outpatients. J Child Psychol Psychiatry 32:297–306, 1991

Biederman J, Newcorn J, Sprich S: Comorbidity of attention deficit hyperactivity disorder with conduct, depressive, anxiety and other disorders. Am J Psychiatry 148:564–577, 1991

Biederman J, Faraone SV, Lapey K: Comorbidity of diagnosis in attention-deficit disorder, in Attention-Deficit Hyperactivity Disorder. Edited by Weiss G. Philadelphia, PA, WB Saunders, 1992, pp 335–360

Biederman J, Faraone SV, Spencer T, et al: Patterns of psychiatric comorbidity, cognition, and psychosocial functioning in adults with attention deficit disorder. Am J Psychiatry 150:1792–1798, 1993

Biederman J, Millberger S, Faraone S, et al: Family environment risk factors for attention-deficit hyperactivity disorder: a test of Rutter's indicators of adversity. Arch Gen Psychiatry 52:464–470, 1995

Biederman J, Stephen F, Millberger S, et al: Predictors of persistence and remission of ADHD into adolescence: results from a four-year prospective follow-up study. J Am Acad Child Adolesc Psychiatry 35:343–351, 1996b

Biederman J, Faraone SV, Taylor A, et al: Diagnostic continuity between child and adolescent ADHD: findings from a longitudinal clinical sample. J Am Acad Child Adolesc Psychiatry 37:305–313, 1998

Biederman J, Faraone SV, Mick E, et al: Clinical correlates of ADHD in females: findings from a large group of girls ascertained from pediatric and psychiatric referral sources. J Am Acad Child Adolesc Psychiatry 38:966–975, 1999

Bird HR, Canino G, Rubio-Supec M, et al: Estimates of the prevalence of childhood maladjustment in a community survey in Puerto Rico. Arch Gen Psychiatry 45: 1120–1126, 1988

Blacker D, Tsuang MT: Contested boundaries of bipolar disorder and the limits of categorical diagnosis in psychiatry. Am J Psychiatry 149:1473–1483, 1992

Boetsch EA, Green PA, Pennington BF: Psychosocial correlates of dyslexia across the life span. Dev Psychopathol 8:539–562, 1996

Brown TE: Differential diagnosis of ADD vs. ADHD in adults, in A_Comprehensive Guide to Attention Deficit Disorder in Adults. Edited by Nadeau KG. New York, Brunner/Mazel, 1995, pp 93–108

Brown TE: Brown Attention Deficit Disorder Scales. San Antonio, TX, Psychological Corporation, 1996

Burgess PW: Theory and methodology in executive function research, in Methodology of Frontal and Executive Function. Edited by Rabbit P. Hove, East Sussex, UK, Psychology Press, 1997, pp 81–116

Cantwell DP, Baker L: Association between attention deficit-hyperactivity disorder and learning disorders. Journal of Learning Disabilities 24(2):88–95, 1991

Caron C, Rutter M: Comorbidity in child psychopathology: concepts, issues and research strategies. J Child Psychol Psychiatry 32:1063–1080, 1991

Castellanos FX: Psychobiology of attention-deficit/hyperactivity disorder, in Handbook of Disruptive Behavior Disorders. Edited by Quay HC, Hogan AE. New York, Kluwer Academic/Plenum, 1999, pp 179–198

Cohen RA: The Neuropsychology of Attention. New York, Plenum, 1993

Cohen DJ, Shaywitz SE, et al: Borderline syndromes and attention deficit disorders of childhood: clinical and neurochemical perspectives, in The Borderline Child. Edited by Robson KS. New York, McGraw-Hill, 1983, pp 197–221

Colby CL: The neuroanatomy and neurophysiology of attention. J Child Neurol (6, suppl):S90–S118, 1991

Conners CK: Is ADHD a disease? Journal of Attention Disorders 2:3–17, 1997

Cowan N: Attention and Memory: An Integrated Framework. New York, Oxford University Press, 1995

Crinella F, Eghbalieh B, Swanson JM, et al: Nigrostriatal dopaminergic structures and executive functions. Paper presented at the annual convention of the American Psychological Association, Chicago, IL, August 1997

Denckla MB: Academic and extracurricular aspects of non-verbal learning disabilities. Psychiatric Annals 21:717–724, 1991a

Denckla MB: Foreword, in Pennington BF: Diagnosing Learning Disorders: A Neuropsychological Framework. New York, Guilford, 1991b, pp vii–x

Denckla MB: The child with developmental disabilities grown up: adult residua of childhood disorders. Neurol Clin 11:105–125, 1993

Denckla MB: Measurement of executive function, in Frames of Reference for the Assessment of Learning Disabilities. Edited by Lyon GR. Baltimore, MD, Paul H Brookes, 1994, pp 117–142

Denckla MB: Research on executive function in a neurodevelopmental context: application of clinical measures. Developmental Neuropsychology 12:5–15, 1996a

Denckla MB: A theory and model of executive function, in Attention, Memory, and Executive Function. Edited by Lyon GR, Krasnegor NA. Baltimore, MD, Paul H Brookes, 1996b, pp 263–278

Dimeff LA, Marlatt GA: Preventing relapse and maintaining change in addictive behaviors. Clinical Psychology: Science and Practice 5:513–525, 1998

Docherty NM, Hawkins KA, Hoffman RE, et al: Working memory, attention and communication disturbance in schizophrenia. J Abnorm Psychol 105:212–219, 1996

Douglas VI: Stop, look and listen: the problem of sustained attention and impulse control in hyperactive and normal children. Canadian Journal of Behavioral Sciences 4:259–282, 1972

Douglas VI: Cognitive deficits in children with attention deficit disorder with hyperactivity, in Attention Deficit Disorder: Criteria, Cognition, Intervention (supplement to J Child Psychol Psychiatry, no. 5). Edited by Bloomingdale LM, Sergeant J. New York, Pergamon, 1988, pp 65–81

Douglas VI: Cognitive control processes in attention-deficit hyperactivity disorder, in Handbook of Disruptive Behavior Disorders. Edited by Quay HC, Hogan AE. New York, Kluwer Academic/Plenum, 1999, pp 105–138

Eiraldi RB, Power TJ, Nezu CM: Patterns of comorbidity associated with subtypes of attention-deficit/hyperactivity disorder among 6- to 12-year-old children. J Am Acad Child Adolesc Psychiatry 36:503–514, 1997

Eslinger PJ: Conceptualizing, describing, and measuring components of executive function: a summary, in Attention, Memory and Executive Function. Edited by Lyon GR, Krasnegor NA. Baltimore, MD, Paul H Brookes, 1996, pp 367–395

Eyberg SM, Edwards D, et al: Maintaining the treatment effects of parent training. Clinical Psychology: Science and Practice 5:544–554, 1998

Faraone SV, Biederman J, Weber W, et al: Psychiatric, neuropsychological, and psychosocial features of DSM-IV subtypes of attention-deficit/hyperactivity disorder: results from a clinically referred sample. J Am Acad Child Adolesc Psychiatry 37:185–193, 1998

Fergusson DM, Horwood LJ: Predictive validity of categorically and dimensionally scored measures of disruptive childhood behaviors. J Am Acad Child Adolesc Psychiatry 34:477–485, 1995

Fischer KW, Rose SP: Dynamic development of coordination of components in brain and behavior, in Human Behavior and the Developing Brain. Edited by Dawson G, Fischer KW. New York, Guilford, 1994

Gallucci F, Bird HR, Berarni C, et al: Symptoms of attention-deficit hyperactivity disorder in an Italian school sample: findings of a pilot study. J Am Acad Child Adolesc Psychiatry 32:1051–1058, 1993

Gaub M, Carlson CL: Gender differences in ADHD: a meta-analysis and critical review. J Am Acad Child Adolesc Psychiatry 36:1036–1045, 1997

Gerring JP, Brady KD, Chen A, et al: Premorbid prevalence of ADHD and development of secondary ADHD after closed head injury. J Am Acad Child Adolesc Psychiatry 37:647–654, 1998

Goldman LS, Genel M, Bezman R, et al: Diagnosis and treatment of attention-deficit/ hyperactivity disorder in children and adolescents. JAMA 279:1100–1107, 1998

Goldman-Rakic P: Circuitry of the primate prefrontal cortex and the regulation of behavior by representational memory, in Handbook of Physiology, The Nervous System, Higher Functions of the Brain. Edited by Plum F. Bethesda, MD, American Physiological Society, 1987, pp 373–417

Goldman-Rakic PS: Prefrontal cortical dysfunction in schizophrenia: the relevance of working memory, in Psychopathology and the Brain. Edited by Carroll BJ, Barrett JE. New York, Raven, 1991, pp 1–23

Goldman-Rakic PS: Specification of higher cortical functions, in Atypical Cognitive Deficits in Developmental Disorders: Implications for Brain Function. Edited by Broman SH and Grafman J. Hillsdale, NJ, Lawrence Erlbaum, 1994, pp 3–17

Goldman-Rakic PS: Architecture of the prefrontal cortex and the central executive. Ann N Y Acad Sci 769:71–83, 1995

Green MF: What are the functional consequences of neurocognitive deficits in schizophrenia? Am J Psychiatry 153:321–330, 1996

Grodzinsky GM, Diamond R: Frontal lobe functioning in boys with attention deficit hyperactivity disorder. Developmental Neuropsychology 8:427–445, 1992

Guevremont DC: Atypical children: diagnostic and treatment considerations. ADHD Report 1(2):5–6, 1993

Hallowell EM, Ratey JJ: Driven to Distraction: Attention Deficit Disorder in Children and Adults. New York, Pantheon, 1994

Harris JC: Hyperactivity and ADHD (letter). J Am Acad Child Adolesc Psychiatry 34:1262, 1996

Hart EL, Lahey BB, Loeber R, et al: Developmental change in attention-deficit hyperactivity disorder in boys: a four-year longitudinal study. J Abnorm Child Psychol 23:729–749, 1995

Hechtman L (ed): Do They Grow Out of It? Long-Term Outcomes of Childhood Disorders. Washington, DC, American Psychiatric Press, 1996

Jensen PS: Scales vs. categories? Never play against a stacked deck. J Am Acad Child Adolesc Psychiatry 34:485–487, 1995

Jensen PS, Shervette RE, Xenakis SN, et al: Anxiety and depressive disorders in attention deficit disorder with hyperactivity: new findings. Am J Psychiatry 150: 1203–1209, 1993

Jensen PS, Martin D, Cantwell D: Comorbidity in ADHD: implications for research, practice, and DSM-V. J Am Acad Child Adolesc Psychiatry 36:1065–1079, 1997

Kagan J: Galen's Prophecy: Temperament in Human Nature. New York, Basic Books, 1994

Kanbayashi Y, Nakata Y, Fujii K, et al: ADHD-related behavior among non-referred children: parents' ratings of DSM-III-R symptoms. Child Psychiatry Hum Dev 25:13–29, 1994

Kelly K, Ramundo P: You Mean I'm Not Lazy, Stupid or Crazy?! New York, Scribner's, 1995

King RA: Childhood-onset schizophrenia: development and pathogenesis. Child Adolesc Psychiatr Clin N Am 3:1–13, 1994

King RA, Noshpitz JD: Pathways of Growth: Essentials of Child Psychiatry, Vol 2. New York, Wiley, 1991

Klin A: Asperger syndrome. Child Adolesc Psychiatr Clin N Am 3:131–148, 1994

Kosslyn SM, Koenig O: Wet Mind: The New Cognitive Neuroscience. New York, Free Press, 1995

Lahey BB, Carlson CL: Validity of the diagnostic category of attention deficit disorder without hyperactivity: a review of the literature. Journal of Learning Disabilities 24:110–120, 1991

Lahey BB, Applegate B, McBurnett K, et al: DSM-IV field trials for attention deficit hyperactivity disorder in children and adolescents. Am J Psychiatry 151:1673–1685, 1994

LeDoux J: The Emotional Brain. New York, Simon & Schuster, 1996

Leung PWL, Luk SL, Ho TP, et al: The diagnosis and prevalence of hyperactivity in Chinese schoolboys. Br J Psychiatry 168:486–496, 1996

Levy F: The dopamine theory of attention deficit hyperactivity disorder. Aust N Z J Psychiatry 25:277–283, 1991

Levy F, Hobbes G: The action of stimulant medication in attention deficit disorder with hyperactivity: dopaminergic, noradrenergic, or both? J Am Acad Child Adolesc Psychiatry 27:802–805, 1988

Levy F, Hay DA, McStephen M, et al. Attention-deficit hyperactivity disorder: a category or a continuum? Genetic analysis of a large-scale twin study. J Am Acad Child Adolesc Psychiatry 36:734–744, 1997

Lewis M: Borderline disorders in children. Child Adolesc Psychiatr Clin N Am 3:31–42, 1994

Lyon GR, Krasnegor NA (eds): Attention, Memory, and Executive Function. Baltimore, MD, Paul H Brookes, 1996

Mann EM, Ikeda Y, Mueller C, et al: Cross-cultural differences in rating hyperactive-disruptive behaviors in children. Am J Psychiatry 149:1539–1542, 1992

Mazure CM, Druss BG: Historical perspective on stress and psychiatric illness, in Does Stress Cause Psychiatric Illness? Edited by Mazure CM. Washington, DC, American Psychiatric Press, 1995, pp 1–41

McEwen BS: Non-genomic and genomic effects of steroids on neural activity. Trends Pharmacol Sci 12:141–147, 1991

McEwen BS, Parsons B: Gonadal steroid action on the brain: neurochemistry and neuropharmacology. Annu Rev Pharmacol Toxicol 22:555–598, 1982

McGee R, Feehan M: Are girls with problems of attention underrecognized? Journal of Psychopathology and Behavioral Assessment 13:187–198, 1991

Mermelstein PG, Becker JB, Surmeier DJ: Estradiol reduces calcium currents in rat neostriatal neurons via a membrane receptor. J Neurosci 16:595–604, 1996

Miller GA, Galanter E, Pribram KH: Plans and the Structure of Behavior. New York, Holt, Rinehart & Winston, 1960

Millstein RB, Wilens TE, Biederman J, et al. Presenting ADHD symptoms and subtypes in clinically referred adults with AHHD. Journal of Attention Disorders 2:159–166, 1997

Murphy K, Barkley RA: Prevalence of DSM-IV symptoms of ADHD in adult licensed drivers: implications for clinical diagnosis. Journal of Attention Disorders 1:147–162, 1996

Musten LM, Firestone P, Pisterman S, et al: Effects of methylphenidate on preschool children with ADHD: cognitive and behavioral functions. J Am Acad Child Adolesc Psychiatry 36:1407–1415, 1997

Myklebust HR: Nonverbal learning disabilities: assessment and intervention, in Progress in Learning Disabilities, Vol 3. Edited by Myklebust HR. New York, Grune & Stratton, 1975, pp 85–121

Nezu AM, Nezu CM, et al: Treatment maintenance for unipolar depression. Clinical Psychology: Science and Practice 5:496–512, 1998

Nottelman EA, Jensen PS: Comorbidity of disorders in children and adolescents: developmental perspectives, in Advances in Clinical Child Psychology. Edited by Ollendick TH, Prinz RJ. New York, Plenum, 1995, pp 109–155

Øie M, Rund BR: Neuropsychological deficits in adolescent-onset schizophrenia compared with attention deficit hyperactivity disorder. Am J Psychiatry 156:1216–1222, 1999

Oldham JM, Hollander E, Skodol AE (eds): Impulsivity and Compulsivity. Washington, DC, American Psychiatric Press, 1996

Oosterlaan J, Logan GD, Sergeant JA: Response inhibition in AD/HD, CD, comorbid AD/HD+CD, anxious, and control children: a meta-analysis of studies with the stop task. J Child Psychol Psychiatry 39:411–425, 1998

Ornstein R: The Right Mind. New York, Harcourt Brace, 1997

Parasuramen R (ed): The Attentive Brain. Cambridge, MA, MIT Press, 1998

Paternite CE, Loney J, Roberts MA: External validation of oppositional disorder and attention deficit disorder with hyperactivity. J Abnorm Child Psychol 23:453–471, 1995

Pennington BF, Ozonoff S: Executive functions and developmental psychopathology. J Child Psychol Psychiatry 37:51–87, 1996

Pennington BF, Welsh M: Neuropsychology and developmental psychopathology, in Developmental Psychopathology. Edited by Cicchetti D, Cohen DJ. New York, Wiley, 1995, pp 254–290

Pennington BF, Bennetto L, McAleer O, et al: Executive functions and working memory, in Attention, Memory, and Executive Function. Edited by Lyon GR, Krasnegor NA. Baltimore, MD, Paul H Brookes, 1996, pp 327–348

Perri MG: Maintenance of treatment effects in the long-term management of obesity. Clinical Psychology: Science and Practice 5:526–543, 1998

Petti TA, Vela RM: Borderline disorders in childhood: an overview. J Am Acad Child Adolesc Psychiatry 29:327–337, 1990

Phillips SM, Sherwin BB: Effects of estrogen on memory function in surgically menopausal women. Psychoneuroendocrinology 17:485–495, 1992a

Phillips SM, Sherwin BB: Variations in memory function and sex steroid hormones across the menstrual cycle. Psychoneuroendocrinology 17:497–506, 1992b

Pliszka SR, McCracken JT, Maas JW: Catecholamines in attention-deficit hyperactivity disorder: current perspectives. J Am Acad Child Adolesc Psychiatry 35:264–272, 1996

Posner MI, Raichle ME: Images of Mind. New York, Scientific American Library, 1994

Quay HC: Inhibition and attention deficit hyperactivity disorder. J Abnorm Child Psychol 25:7–13, 1997

Rabbit P: Introduction: methodologies and models in the study of executive function, in Methodology of Frontal and Executive Function. Edited by Rabbit P. Hove, East Sussex, UK, Psychology Press, 1997, pp 1–38

Ratey JJ, Johnson C: Shadow Syndromes. New York, Pantheon, 1997

Revelle W: Individual differences in personality and motivation: ©non-cognitive[a] determinants of cognitive performance, in Attention: Selection, Awareness and Control. Edited by Baddeley A, Weiskrantz L. New York, Oxford University Press, 1993, pp 346–373

Richardson JTE: Evolving issues in working memory, in Working Memory and Human Cognition. Edited by Richardson JTE, Engle RW, Hasher L, et al. New York, Oxford University Press, 1996, pp 120–154

Richardson JTE, Engle RW, Hasher L, et al (eds): Working Memory and Human Cognition. New York, Oxford University Press, 1996

Rogeness GA, McClure EB: Development and neurotransmitter-environment interactions. Dev Psychopathol 8:183–199, 1996

Rothbart MK, Posner MI, Hershey KL: Temperament, attention, and developmental psychopathology, in Developmental Psychopathology, Vol I. Edited by Cicchetti D, Cohen DJ. New York, Wiley, 1995, pp 315–340

Rourke BP (ed): Neuropsychology of Learning Disabilities: Essentials of Subtype Analysis. New York, Guilford, 1985

Rourke BP: Non-verbal Learning Disabilities: The Syndrome and the Model. New York, Guilford, 1989

Rourke BP: Syndrome of Nonverbal Learning Disabilities: Neurodevelopmental Manifestations. New York, Guilford, 1995

Rourke BP, Fuerst DR: Learning Disabilities and Psychosocial Functioning: A Neuropsychological Perspective. New York, Guilford, 1991

Rubin KH, Stewart SL: Social withdrawal, in Child Psychopathology. Edited by Mash EJ, Barkley RA. New York, Guilford, 1996, pp 277–307

Samudra K, Cantwell D: Risk factors for attention-deficit/hyperactivity disorder, in Handbook of Disruptive Behavior Disorders. Edited by Quay HC, Hogan AE. New York, Kluwer Academic/Plenum, 1999, pp 199–220

Schachar R, Tannock R: Childhood hyperactivity and psychostimulants: a review of extended treatment studies. J Child Adolesc Psychopharmacol 3:81–97, 1993

Schaughency E, McGee R, Nada Raja S, et al: Self-reported inattention, impulsivity, and hyperactivity at ages 15 and 18 in the general population. J Am Acad Child Adolesc Psychiatry 33:173–184, 1994

Seidman LJ, Benedict K, Biederman J, et al: Performance of ADHD children on the Rey-Osterrieth complex figure: a pilot neuropsychological study. J Child Psychol Psychiatry 36:1459–1473, 1995a

Seidman LJ, Biederman J, Faraone S, et al: Effects of family history and comorbidity on the neuropsychological performance of ADHD children: preliminary findings. J Am Acad Child Adolesc Psychiatry 34:1015–1024, 1995b

Seidman LJ, Biederman J, Faraone SV, et al: A pilot study of neuropsychological function in girls with ADHD. J Am Acad Child Adolesc Psychiatry 36:366–373, 1997a

Seidman LJ, Biederman J, Faraone SV, et al: Toward defining a neuropsychology of attention deficit-hyperactivity disorder: performance of children and adolescents from a large clinically referred sample. J Consult Clin Psychol 65:150–160, 1997b

Seidman LJ, Biederman J, Weber W, et al: Neurological function in adults with attention-deficit hyperactivity disorder. Biol Psychiatry 44:260–268, 1998

Semrud-Clikeman M, Hynd GW: Right hemispheric dysfunction in nonverbal learning disabilities: social, academic, and adaptive functioning in adults and children. Psychol Bull 107:196–209, 1990

Sergeant JA: A theory of attention: an information processing perspective, in Attention, Memory, and Executive Function. Edited by Lyon GR, Krasnegor NA. Baltimore, MD, Paul H Brookes, 1996, pp 57–69

Sergeant JA, Oosterlan J, van der Meere J: Information processing and energetic factors in attention-deficit/hyperactivity disorder, in Handbook of Disruptive Behavior Disorders. Edited by Quay HC, Hogan AE. New York, Kluwer Academic/Plenum, 1999, pp 75–104

Servan-Schreiber D, Carter CS, Bruno RM, et al: Dopamine and the mechanisms of cognition, part II: D-amphetamine effects in human subjects performing a selective attention task. Biol Psychiatry 43:723–729, 1998

Shaywitz SE, Shaywitz BA, et al: Effect of estrogen on brain activation patterns in postmenopausal women during working memory tasks. JAMA 281:1197–1202, 1999

Sherwin BB: Estrogen and cognitive functioning in women. Proc Soc Exp Biol Med 217:17–22, 1998

Shore AN: The experience-dependent maturation of a regulatory system in the orbital prefrontal cortex and the origin of developmental psychopathology. Dev Psychopathol 8:59–87, 1996

Siegel B: The World of the Autistic Child: Understanding and Treating Autistic Spectrum Disorders. New York, Oxford University Press, 1996

Skodol AE, Oldham JM: Phenomenology, differential diagnosis and comorbidity of the impulsive-compulsive spectrum of disorders, in Impulsivity and Compulsivity. Edited by Oldham JM, Hollander E, Skodol AE. Washington, DC, American Psychiatric Press, 1996, pp 1–36

Smith BH, Pelham WE, Gnagy E, et al: Equivalent effects of stimulant treatment for attention-deficit hyperactivity disorder during childhood and adolescence. J Am Acad Child Adolesc Psychiatry 37:314–321, 1998

Solden S: Women With Attention Deficit Disorder. Grass Valley, CA, Underwood, 1995

Spencer T, Biederman J, Wilens T, et al: Is attention-deficit hyperactivity disorder in adults a valid disorder? Harv Rev Psychiatry 1:326–335, 1994

Spencer T, Wilens TE, Biederman J, et al: A double-blind crossover comparison of methylphenidate and placebo in adults with childhood-onset attention-deficit hyperactivity disorder. Arch Gen Psychiatry 52:434–443, 1995

Spencer T, Biederman J, Wilens T, et al: Pharmacotherapy of attention-deficit hyperactivity disorder across the life cycle. J Am Acad Child Adolesc Psychiatry 35:409–432, 1996

Tannock R, Schachar R: Executive dysfunction as an underlying mechanism of behavior and language problems in attention deficit hyperactivity disorder, in Language, Learning, and Behavior Disorders. Edited by Beitchman JH, Cohen NJ, Konstantareas MM, et al. New York, Cambridge University Press, 1996, pp 128–155

Tao KT: Hyperactivity and attention deficit disorder syndromes in China. J Am Acad Child Adolesc Psychiatry 31:1165–1166, 1992

Taylor E: Dysfunctions of attention, in Developmental Psychopathology, Vol II. Edited by Cicchetti D, Cohen DJ. New York, Wiley, 1995, pp 243–273

Taylor GJ, Bagby RM, Parker JDA. Disorders of Affect Regulation: Alexithymia in Medical and Psychiatric Illness. Cambridge, UK, Cambridge University Press, 1997

Thompson TL, Moss RL: Estrogen regulation of dopamine release in the nucleus accumbens: genomic- and nongenomic-mediated effects. J Neurochem 62:1750–1756, 1994

Towbin KE: Pervasive developmental disorder not otherwise specified: a review and guidelines for clinical care. Child Adolesc Psychiatr Clin N Am 3:149–160, 1994

Towbin KE, Dykens EM, Pearson GS, et al: Conceptualizing "borderline syndrome of childhood" and "childhood schizophrenia" as a developmental disorder. J Am Acad Child Adolesc Psychiatry 32:775–782, 1993

Tranel D, Hall LE, Olson S, et al: Evidence for a right-hemisphere developmental learning disability. Developmental Neuropsychology 3:113–127, 1987

Voeller KKS: Social-emotional learning disabilities. Psychiatric Annals 21:735–741, 1991

Warga C: Menopause and the Mind. New York, Free Press, 1999

Weintraub S, Mesulam MM: Developmental learning disabilities of the right hemisphere: emotional, interpersonal, and cognitive components. Arch Neurol 40: 463–468, 1983

Weiss G, Hechtman LT: Hyperactive Children Grown Up: Empirical Findings and Theoretical Considerations. New York, Guilford, 1986

Weiss G, Hechtman LT: Hyperactive Children Grown Up: ADHD in Children, Adolescents and Adults, 2nd Edition. New York, Guilford, 1993

Wells A, Matthews G: Attention and Emotion: A Clinical Perspective. Hillsboro, NJ, Lawrence Erlbaum, 1994

Wender P: Hyperactive Child, Adolescent and Adult: Attention Deficit Disorder Through the Lifespan. New York, Oxford University Press, 1987

Wender PH: Attention-Deficit Hyperactivity Disorder in Adults. New York, Oxford University Press, 1995

Wickelgren I: Getting the brain's attention. Science 278:35–37, 1997

Wilson JM, Marcotte AC: Psychosocial adjustment and educational outcome in adolescents with a childhood diagnosis of attention deficit disorder. J Am Acad Child Adolesc Psychiatry 35:579–587, 1996

Wolff S: Loners: The Life Path of Unusual Children. New York, Routledge, 1995

Wolraich ML, Hannah JN, Pinnock TY, et al: Comparison of diagnostic criteria for attention-deficit hyperactivity disorder in a county-wide sample. J Am Acad Child Adolesc Psychiatry 35:319–324, 1996

2 Genetics of Attention-Deficit/ Hyperactivity Disorder

James J. Hudziak, M.D.

The value of identifying genes that influence the development of attention-deficit/hyperactivity disorder (ADHD) is immense. The prevalence of ADHD is high (between 3% and 7% of the U.S. population) (American Psychiatric Association 1994), the disorder is associated with marked impairment, and in the majority of cases its symptoms are lifelong. For these reasons, the long-term benefits of identifying genes that predict a person's vulnerability to ADHD, and subsequently developing early identification and intervention strategies, are obvious (Hudziak 1997). With advances in molecular genetics, it is likely that we will soon identify a number of genes that place individuals at risk for ADHD. Understanding the genetic contribution to ADHD has become an increasingly important and complicated topic.

Over the past 10 years, tremendous advances have been made, although an ADHD gene, or genes, has not been identified. Many researchers believe that such discoveries are not far off. They have, however, encountered an obstacle to finding genes responsible for ADHD: the need to refine the phenotypic (diagnostic) approach used to identify subjects for molecular genetic studies (Hudziak 1997).

From twin studies, we have learned that the symptoms of ADHD are highly heritable. However, we have also learned of the difficulties of rater bias (Hudziak et al., in press), developmental bias, gender bias (Hudziak et al. 1998), and problems with using DSM categorical approaches. From family studies, we have learned that ADHD is highly familial and associated with a number of comorbid conditions. These studies also have reinforced concerns about informant and gender bias. Finally, molecular genetic studies have provided us with a window on the relationship between genes and at least some cases of ADHD.

CONFOUNDS IN GENETIC STUDIES OF ADHD—CATEGORIES VERSUS CONTINUUM

The classic twin study allows us to estimate genetic and environmental contributions to the development of symptoms of inattention, hyperactivity, and impulsivity (Martin et al. 1997). This is accomplished by using structural equation modeling to compare the correlations of symptoms of ADHD in twin pairs who are monozygotic (genetically identical) with those in twin pairs who are dizygotic (who, on average, share 50% of their genes). The power of studying twins can be diminished by the phenotypic (diagnostic) approach used (Tsuang et al. 1993). Investigators who pursue twin studies of ADHD must decide how to analyze ADHD symptoms. Misclassification is a common problem in psychiatric genetic studies, especially in the study of ADHD. For example, the current system used to classify ADHD is in DSM-IV (American Psychiatric Association 1994). The DSM conceptual framework assumes that ADHD is a discrete categorical entity or subtypes of that entity, such as predominantly inattentive type, predominantly hyperactive-impulsive type, and combined type. As a result, the DSM approach to diagnosing ADHD is often referred to as the "categorical approach," which requires an individual to have a minimum number of symptoms, lasting a specific period of time and causing impairment in at least two areas.

A weakness in the DSM approach that particularly affects genetic studies of ADHD is the lack of quantitative differentiation between individuals (twin pairs or non-twin siblings in family studies). To illustrate, according to DSM-IV criteria, a child with 12 symptoms of ADHD (6 symptoms each of inattention and hyperactivity-impulsivity) is considered to be in the same category as a child with 18 symptoms (9 symptoms from each domain). Furthermore, a child with 10 symptoms of ADHD (5 of 9 symptoms of inattention and 5 of 9 symptoms of hyperactivity-impulsivity, missing the required cutpoint by 1 symptom in each category) does not qualify for an ADHD diagnosis at all. However, a child with 6 symptoms of inattention and 4 symptoms of hyperactivity-impulsivity does qualify for the diagnosis. Of the two children who have 10 symptoms of ADHD, only one child is diagnosed as having ADHD. The DSM approach limits the analysis of twin (and family) studies to categorizing subjects as either having or not having ADHD and ignores the possible variations in the degree to which subjects may manifest the disorder (Hudziak et al. 1996). Thus, in the study of ADHD, investigators are faced with a methodological decision: Should they perform analysis by DSM-III, DSM-III-R, or DSM-IV criteria (American Psychiatric Association 1980, 1987, 1994) or should they use quantitative phenotypic markers of inattention and hyperactivity-impulsivity? For genetic analysis, using DSM-IV diagnostic categories such as those for ADHD will lead to a loss of statistical power if the situation is actually a continuum model in which genetic risk corresponds closely to symptom count. The majority of twin studies of ADHD to date have not used the DSM diagnostic approach.

TWIN STUDIES OF ADHD

It has long been known that quantitative measures of psychopathology confer added statistical power to behavioral genetic research. Many twin studies have been done on the individual symptom domains of ADHD. Willerman (1973) reported on the high heritability (0.77) of "activity" from a questionnaire study of parents of 54 monozygotic and 39 dizygotic pairs. Goodman and Stevenson (1989a, 1989b), using three items from the Rutter Behavioral Questionnaire (RBQ; Rutter 1970), reported an impossibly high heritability estimate (greater than 1.0) for activity. This high estimate was thought to be due to parental rater bias, in which parents overestimate the similarities of monozygotic twins and underestimate the similarities of dizygotic twins. In this study, the correlation reported by parents of dizygotic twins was -0.8, thought to be evidence that parents exaggerate the differences between their dizygotic twins (Levy et al. 1997). Thapar et al. (1995), using the same three items from the RBQ, also reported high heritability estimates for activity and low dizygotic twin correlations. Both studies indicated a parental rater bias, in which the parents either exaggerated differences of dizygotic twins or suggested differential interaction between monozygotic and dizygotic pairs.

Sherman et al. (1997a, 1997b) reported on the heritability of DSM-III and DSM-III-R symptoms of ADHD by using a scale tailored from 40 behavioral items obtained from teachers and mothers. Teacher reports from the Teacher Report Form (Achenbach 1991) and maternal reports from the Diagnostic

Interview for Children and Adolescents (W. Reich 1988) on 194 monozygotic and 94 dizygotic boy pairs were factor analyzed. The results revealed two domains: one for inattention and the other for hyperactivity-impulsivity. Scales representing the two domains were used in genetic analyses. In univariate analysis of the teacher reports, Sherman et al. (1997a) reported that additive genetic influences on symptoms of inattention were 0.30 (with shared environmental effects of 0.39 and nonshared environmental effects of 0.22). These findings were compared with those from maternal reports, which reported additive genetic effects of 0.69, nonshared environmental effects of 0.31, and no effects from shared environment. Higher genetic contributions were reported for hyperactivity-impulsivity than for inattention. Heritability estimates for hyperactivity-impulsivity were 0.69 by teachers and 0.91 by mothers (with mild nonshared environmental and no shared environmental effects) (Sherman et al. 1997a). These data once again support the contention that some type of parental rater bias is at work when ADHD behavioral domains are rated.

In bivariate genetic analyses, cross-twin correlations (e.g., inattention of first twin with hyperactivity-impulsivity of second twin) were examined to determine the genetic and environmental association between these two highly correlated domains (Sherman et al. 1997b). The results suggested that a common genetic factor mediates the association between inattention and hyperactivity-impulsivity. The researchers concluded that the ADHD symptoms of DSM-III and DSM-III-R appeared to be genetically influenced whether the diagnoses were made with reports from teachers or parents. A much higher prevalence of DSM-III or DSM-III-R symptoms was reported by teachers (15%) than parents (6%), with only 3% of symptoms in both reports meeting DSM-III or DSM-III-R criteria, and a lower heritability was reported in teacher (0.73) than in parental (0.89) reports. This study, although involving only boys and using DSM-III and DSM-III-R criteria, was the first to combine information from both teachers and parents. Combined with studies by Goodman and Stevenson (1989a, 1989b) and Thapar et al. (1995), Sherman et al.'s study indicates the need to refine phenotypic strategies to determine the best informants for identifying subjects for molecular genetic studies of ADHD.

In a large-scale twin study of ADHD in Australia, Levy et al. (1997) reported on a cohort of 1,938 families with twins and siblings 4–12 years old, using data obtained from a maternal rating scale of DSM-III-R ADHD criteria. The researchers reported additive genetic effects of 0.75–0.91 across definitions of ADHD, whether considered as part of a continuum or as a disorder with various symptom cutpoints. They concluded that ADHD is best viewed as the extreme of a behavior that varies genetically throughout the entire population rather than as a disorder with discrete genetic determinants. This study, along with the study by Sherman et al. (1997b), has implications in the areas of diagnosis, treatment, and the classification of ADHD and, finally, for the identification of genes for ADHD behavior.

In the Virginia Twin Study of Adolescent Behavioral Development, 1,412 twin pairs, ages 8 through 16, were directly assessed. A fully structured psychiatric interview of each child and the child's mother or father, and other information from parents, teachers, and the child, were used to determine the heritability of DSM-III-R child psychiatric disorders (Hewitt et al. 1997). The researchers performed factor analysis of these data, which indicated that ADHD symptoms are relatively independent of other diagnostic domains but show moderate correlations with conduct disorder, oppositional defiant disorder (ODD), and major depressive disorders. Their results are consistent with the results from a family study by Biederman et al. (1992a). Hewitt and colleagues (1997) also conducted "multitrait-multimethod" confirmatory factor analysis, which revealed large informant-specific influences on the reporting of symptoms in interviews. In a second study from that group, Eaves et al. (1997) indicated that 1) for ADHD, as well as for most measures of adolescent psychopathology, correlations for ratings were generally higher for monozygotic than dizygotic pairs; 2) parents reported higher correlations than children; and 3) higher correlations were reported from questionnaires than from direct interviews. In addition, Eaves and colleagues reported marked sibling contrast effects and rater bias effects on the heritability ratings of ADHD. The results of these studies remind us of the importance of how the type of information, and the type of informant, affect the resulting heritabilities reported in twin studies of ADHD.

Other researchers are studying the heritability of ADHD symptoms to determine the best phenotype for molecular genetic studies. To study DSM-IV ADHD symptoms in girls, Hudziak and colleagues developed the following strategy in their large-scale twin study of 1,629 adolescent female twin pairs in Missouri (Hudziak et al. 1998; J. Hudziak, A. Heath, P. Madden, et al., "Distribution of DSM-IV ADHD Symptoms in General Population Twin Sample," manuscript in preparation; J. Hudziak, A. Heath, P. Madden, et al., "A Twin Study of DSM-IV ADHD in African-American Adolescent Females," submitted for publication). Data on the 18 ADHD symptoms in DSM-IV were collected by maternal reports on consecutive birth cohorts between the ages of 13 and 19 at the time of interview. Additional data on impairment at home and at school and with peer relationships, along with academic performance, school failures, and comorbid conditions, were also collected.

The 18 ADHD symptoms were factor analyzed and then used in latent class analysis to determine 1) if ADHD symptoms could be considered as existing latent liability factors, either as the entire 18-symptom set or as subsets of inattention and hyperactivity-impulsivity, and 2) if the symptoms exist on a continuum distributed throughout the population. Because the data are on twins, the latent classes and factors that emerged from the analyses were subjected to genetic analysis. Thus, the ADHD symptoms were analyzed as individual items, latent class subtypes, and diagnostic categories. The latent classes that emerged from the first set of analyses were exposed to genetic threshold model analyses to determine if individuals with mild, moderate, and severe inattention or hyperactivity-impulsivity, or both, were influenced by the same genetic factors.

The results of these studies are enlightening. First, the categorical analyses support the DSM-IV conceptualization of a predominantly inattentive type of ADHD (4.0%), a combined type (2.0%), and a predominantly hyperactive-impulsive type (0.8%) (Hudziak et al. 1998). The latent class analyses supported considering ADHD not as categorical disorders with discrete cutpoints but rather as separate dimensions that exist on a continuum of severity. For instance, there are three latent classes of inattention problems: mild (or no problem), moderate, and severe. Similarly, there are three latent classes each of the combined type and hyperactive-impulsive type of ADHD. Further supporting the division of symptoms into latent classes of severity was evidence that these classes are associated with different types of impairment. Inattention problems are associated with academic impairment, independent of hyperactivity-impulsivity problems. On the other hand, hyperactivity-impulsivity problems predict more dramatic peer impairment than do inattention problems. The data also dispute the contention that having ADHD precludes a child from academic excellence. Approximately 30% of the children with ADHD of the severe predominantly inattentive, predominantly hyperactive-impulsive, and combined types earned, on average, all A's according to parents' reports (Hudziak 1997).

Genetic analysis revealed that the ADHD domains of inattention and hyperactivity-impulsivity (when considered as symptom counts and categorical subtypes) are highly heritable in girls, influenced by independent and shared genetic factors, and affected by rater contrast. Using categorical subtypes rather than symptom counts led to a loss in statistical power and an inability to identify a zygosity-specific rater contrast effect (Hudziak 1997).

Genetic analysis of the latent classes were performed to determine if the mild, moderate, and severe classes of inattention, hyperactivity-impulsivity, and combined types of ADHD are genetically discrete; for example, such analysis sought to determine if mild, moderate, and severe inattention represent continuous expressions of the same genotype or different genetic subtypes (Hudziak et al. 1998). Each latent class is highly heritable in genetic analyses. Odds ratios and relative risk ratios were calculated to determine if membership in a latent class predicted whether co-twins were members in that same class. The ratios were highly predictive for same-class membership yet did not support a continuum model (e.g., membership in the moderate class of inattention did not translate into an increased risk for the co-twin to be in either the mild or severe classes). The odds ratio and relative risk analyses supported the contention that each class represents discrete subtypes. As further testing of this finding, threshold genetic risk models were fit. None of these models for inattention, hyperactivity-impulsivity, or combined type ADHD were found to fit—an indication of discrete genetic influences on the individual latent classes. Although these findings are preliminary, they suggest that the genetics of moderate inattention differ from the genetics of mild and severe inattention.

To summarize the implications of these papers, Hudziak, Heath, and colleagues reported that DSM-IV ADHD is a highly prevalent and highly heritable set of genetic conditions. DSM-IV ADHD should be considered as existing as separate but highly related domains of inattention and hyperactivity-impulsivity, with each domain associated with different types of impairment. These results agree with those of Sherman et al. (1997a) and Levy et al. (1997) in that they support the contention that liability to ADHD symptoms is distributed throughout the population on severity continua. Hudziak et al. identified rater contrast effects, as did Sherman et al. (1997a), Eaves et al. (1997), and others, but were able to describe a zygosity-specific rater contrast effect in which parents of monozygotic twins overestimated differences between their twins. This is the opposite of the findings reported by Willerman (1973) and Thapar et al. (1995). Finally, a genetic analysis using threshold models and risk ratio analyses indicated that although the latent class and genetic analyses strongly supported the finding that ADHD symptoms are distributed throughout the population, the individual latent classes were not influenced by the same genetic factors. Such findings imply that solving the problem of etiologic heterogeneity—that is, multiple pathogenesis leading to an indistinguishable clinical disorder—remains the primary obstacle to overcome in identifying the gene or genes responsible for ADHD.

The recent work of Eaves, Sherman, Levy, Hudziak, and colleagues supports the need to further refine phenotypic strategies to better understand the genetic liability to the development of symptoms of inattention, hyperactivity, and impulsivity.

FAMILY STUDIES OF ADHD

Family studies suggest that many cases of ADHD are familial. However, because no agreement has been reached on the mode of inheritance for ADHD, further refinement of the phenotype is required. As Rice et al. (1987) pointed out, the first step in a family study is to define an appropriate phenotype (i.e., the observed trait to be studied) and to delineate covariates that mediate the risk of illness. The researchers suggested that etiologic heterogeneity, resulting from multiple pathogenesis leading to an indistinguishable clinical disorder, is one of the main obstacles to classifying and understanding the transmission of common illnesses. Hudziak and Todd (1993) argued that ADHD is an example of such a clinical illness, in which several genetic and nongenetic disorders share a common clinical phenotype.

One approach to solving the dilemma of etiologic heterogeneity in the study of ADHD is to define the phenotype more specifically. Subtyping ADHD with familial aggregation techniques may be a way to further refine the phenotypes of ADHD, thus allowing a more direct assessment by molecular genetic techniques. Studies addressing proband and familial comorbidity of ADHD with anxiety disorders, conduct disorder (CD), affective disorders, and learning disabilities are presented elsewhere in this chapter in the context of the clinical implications of comorbidity. Each is discussed with respect to what we can learn about the heritability of ADHD from comorbidity (Hudziak and Todd 1993).

Subtyping by Comorbidity

Comorbidity with ADHD, or the coexistence of two or more psychiatric disorders in the same patient, is a primary focus of this chapter. Whether the focus of the study is children or adults, comorbidity with ADHD is common (Biederman et al. 1992a). In a comprehensive review of the literature, Hudziak and Todd (1993) cited the following rates of comorbidity in children: ADHD and ODD (35%), CD (50%), mood disorders (15%–75%), anxiety disorders (25%), and learning disabilities (10%–92%). Familial risk analysis, using segregation analysis and genetic models proposed by T. Reich et al. (1972, 1979), is presented by comorbid diagnosis in the following subsections.

Subtyping by Conduct Disorder

Faraone et al. (1991b), in their large family study of boys with ADHD, subtyped probands into groups of children who had ADHD and ODD (45%), ADHD and CD (33%), ADHD without ODD or CD (22%), and control subjects. After subtyping was carried out in this manner, familial risk analysis revealed that the risk for ADHD was highest among first-degree relatives of ADHD/CD probands (38%), moderate among relatives of ADHD/ODD (17%) and ADHD probands (24%), and lowest among relatives of the control subjects (5%). ADHD and CD occurred in the same relative more often than would be expected by chance alone. These findings suggest a multifactorial hypothesis in which ADHD, ADHD/ODD, and ADHD/CD fall along a continuum of increasing levels of severity. Risk analysis of this continuum supports the hypothesis that ADHD/CD may be a distinct genetic subtype of ADHD. In fact, in segregation analyses, there is evidence that the familiality of the ADHD/CD subtype may be due to single gene transmission (Faraone et al. 1992).

After performing a comprehensive review of the ADHD literature, Jensen et al. (1997) concluded that further study of the ADHD-aggressive (conduct) subtype is needed to determine if it reflects a discrete phenotype. Thus, future molecular genetic studies may have to consider ADHD/CD as a marker for a discrete genotype.

Subtyping by Major Depressive Disorder

Family risk analysis has revealed that ADHD and major depressive disorder (MDD) share common familial vulnerabilities (Biederman et al. 1991a). The relatives of ADHD and ADHD/MDD proband subgroups were at a significantly greater risk for ADHD and MDD than the relatives of control subjects. However, ADHD and MDD did not cosegregate in families, suggesting that ADHD and MDD share common vulnerabilities but are not etiologically equivalent. Some have suggested that ADHD with MDD reflects a true comorbid phenotype (i.e., one due to the co-occurrence of two different genetic illnesses). Faraone and Biederman (1997) suggested that ADHD and major depression probably share familial risk factors and that the difference between ADHD patients with and without depression can be attributed to environmental factors. This research points out the need to consider the role of environment in the expression of the familial ADHD phenotype.

Subtyping by Mania

The relationship between ADHD and mania is more complex. Six studies have considered the relationship of ADHD and bipolar disorder in families (Faraone et al. 1997a; Faraone and Biederman 1997). Faraone et al. (1997a) studied 140 ADHD probands, 120 non-ADHD controls, and 822 of their first-degree relatives to determine if there is a familial relationship between

ADHD and bipolar disorder. As Geller and Luby (1997) stated, "The data from that study suggest that comorbid ADHD with bipolar disorder is familially distinct from other forms of ADHD and may be related to what others have termed childhood-onset bipolar disorder. These findings will need to be supplemented by research on the natural course and neurobiology of children with BPD with and without ADHD." Although many criticize these findings, it is important to note, as Geller and Luby stated, that "child psychiatry is in crucial need of research to complete the whole mosaic" for understanding the relationship between ADHD and bipolar disorder. Criticisms include the difficulty of diagnosing mania in children with severe ADHD because of the difficulty in identifying a "discrete change in mood" as specified in DSM-IV. Because of the complex issues involved in understanding the symptom overlap and developmental contributions to mania symptoms in young children, the relationship between mania and ADHD remains unclear. Perhaps only molecular genetic approaches will solve this debate.

Interestingly, some data on the relationship between mania and ADHD are already available. The dopamine transporter gene has been associated with both adult bipolar disorder (Waldman et al. 1997a) and childhood ADHD (Cook et al. 1995; Waldman et al. 1997b) in studies using association techniques such as the transmission disequilibrium test and haplotype risk ratio. These findings, which will be discussed in the section of this chapter on molecular genetics, raise the possibility that the relationship between some forms of childhood ADHD and later bipolar disorder is associated with abnormalities in the dopamine transporter gene. Given the results of the family and molecular genetic structure, future research on the ADHD/bipolar disorder phenotype is needed.

Subtyping by Anxiety Disorder

Family studies of ADHD and anxiety also have been informative. These studies have revealed that relatives of probands with ADHD and anxiety disorders are at increased risk for both disorders. A tendency existed for relatives of ADHD probands who themselves had ADHD to have a higher risk for anxiety disorders than relatives of ADHD probands who did not have ADHD (Biederman et al. 1991c). The familial risk analysis is most consistent with the hypothesis that ADHD and anxiety disorders segregate independently in families (Biederman et al. 1991b). In a separate study, the comorbid relationship between ADHD and overanxious disorder (OAD) was investigated. Children with ADHD/OAD demonstrated less impulsivity, hyperactivity, and CD than children with ADHD alone (Pliszka 1992). These data suggest that

ADHD/OAD may represent a distinct phenotype. Indeed, Jensen et al. (1993, 1997) strongly suggested that ADHD/OAD be considered a separate phenotype for further studies.

In a study of the genetic relationship between the empirically based anxious-depressed scale and attention problems, Hudziak et al. reported that genetic correlations between anxious-depressed syndromes and attention problems are as high as genetic correlations between attention problems and aggressive behavior syndromes (Hudziak et al. 1997; J. Hudziak, D. Boomsma, et al., "Across Syndrome Correlations of Attention, Aggression, and Anxious/Depression in Adolescents and Young Adults," submitted for publication). Although the genetic relationship between ADHD and anxiety remains unclear, studies of this important and interesting phenotype are already under way.

Subtyping by Learning Disability

The comorbidity between learning disability (LD) and ADHD is reported to be between 10% and 92%, depending on the definition of LD (Semrud-Clikeman et al. 1992). Researchers reported a comorbidity rate for ADHD and LD of 17%–38%, based on a liberal versus stringent definition of LD. Faraone et al. (1992) found that the risk for LD was highest among relatives of probands with both ADHD and LD. However, ADHD and LD did not cosegregate in families and there was evidence for assortative mating between spouses with ADHD and LD. These results suggest that ADHD and LD are transmitted independently in families and that their co-occurrence may be a result of nonrandom mating.

These data indicate that LD is a single construct rather than a group of phenotypically and perhaps genotypically discrete disorders. In studies that consider a discrete type of LD, such as reading disorder , the results are quite different. Twin studies of the relationship between ADHD and reading disorder indicate that the majority of covariances between ADHD and reading disorder are due to the same genetic influences (Light et al. 1995). The possibility that certain types of LD are genetically related to ADHD will need to be explored further. The relationship between ADHD and LD is clearly in need of further study—in fact, comorbidity between ADHD and LD is typically underrecognized in clinical settings—yet information on the genetic relatedness between ADHD and a specific LD will almost certainly be forthcoming.

Subtyping by Gender

ADHD is one of only a few conditions that have been studied by gender. DSM-III-R ADHD was reported to be three times more common in boys than in girls (the male-female ratio has not yet been well described for ADHD based on DSM-IV criteria). It is important to investigate the reasons for this profound gender difference. Hudziak et al. (1998) reported a prevalence of DSM-IV ADHD of approximately 8% for their female twin sample derived from the general population. In addition, they reported that ADHD was highly associated with academic, family, and peer impairment. Hudziak et al. also studied ADHD in a minority population of female twins (J. Hudziak, A. Heath, P. Madden, et al., "A Twin Study of DSM-IV ADHD in African-American Adolescent Females," submitted for publication). They reported an increase in ADHD in African American female twins, with heritability estimates similar to those in nonminority populations. In addition, there was evidence of high rates of impairment and lower rates of treatment. Other studies have also demonstrated that ADHD causes significant impairment in females (Faraone et al. 1991a).

The gold-standard study of female ADHD is the family study conducted by Faraone et al. (1991a), which indicated that the relatives of girls with ADHD are at increased risk for ADHD, antisocial disorders, major depression, and anxiety disorders. The higher risk for ADHD could not be accounted for by gender, generation of relative, age of proband, social class, or family intactness. These findings are highly consistent with these researchers' earlier findings on males with ADHD (Biederman et al. 1992a). The results of family studies, combined with the data from twin studies, support the validity of the diagnosis of ADHD in girls and suggest that the sexes share common biological risk factors for ADHD. Faraone et al. (1995) also support the contention that the male-predominated ADHD occurs in boys from families who do not have a history of the disorder. Although not yet validated through empirical data, this finding raises the possibility that boys are at increased risk for environmental insults (e.g., pregnancy, delivery, and infancy complications) that cause nonfamilial phenotypic expression of ADHD.

MOLECULAR GENETIC STUDIES

Because family, twin, and adoption studies indicated that genetic factors may influence many cases of ADHD (Hudziak 1997), many molecular geneticists became interested in ADHD. Although a genetic linkage between ADHD and any gene or genes has not been reported yet, a number of studies have investigated the association between a gene of interest and ADHD. Association studies emphasize the use of "candidate genes," or genes that could play a role in the pathogenesis of ADHD. Principal among the candidate genes in ADHD are the genes of the dopamine receptor system. Pliszka et al. (1996), Levy and Hobbes (1988), and other researchers have long posited that dopamine plays a role in the maintenance of attention. Furthermore, the presence of an abnormal dopamine allele may play a role in dysfunction of the attention system. It is posited that the pathways from the A9/10 nuclei of the ventral tegmentum travel via the mesolimbic dopamine pathways to the shell of the nucleus accumbens (often cited as the site of the reward system of the brain). From there, the fibers travel to the prefrontal cortex (one of the areas of the brain thought to be involved in the maintenance of attention) (Pliszka et al. 1996). According to Levy and Hobbes (1988), "This theory is somewhat supported by clinical experience, where clinicians, patients, and families observe children with ADHD who respond to dopamine agonists such as methylphenidate or dextroamphetamine." Thus, molecular geneticists are well armed to investigate dopamine candidate genes as potential contributors to the pathophysiology of some cases of ADHD. Molecular genetic studies on the association of the dopamine transporter gene (*DAT1*), the dopamine$_2$ receptor gene (*DRD2*), and the dopamine$_4$ receptor gene (*DRD4*) have been conducted.

Comings et al. (1991) reported that 46% of ADHD patients had the abnormal A1 allele of the *Taq*I polymorphism of the D_2 receptor, compared with 20% of control subjects. Thus, if these findings are correct, an abnormal D_2 receptor allele may be responsible for some cases of ADHD. These findings, which are being hotly debated, illustrate the obstacles to identifying genes for ADHD. Hudziak 1997) pointed out that the Comings study did not control for ethnicity, age, gender, or comorbidity—each a major obstacle to identifying discrete phenotypes for molecular genetic studies. To illustrate the impact of ethnic differences, a general population study revealed that as much as 75% of the American Muskoke Indian population have the A1 allele (Barr and Kidd 1993). Even though the significance of the D_2 receptor findings remains unclear, Comings et al.'s study did shed light on the possibility that allelic dysmorphology of one of the dopamine genes may be related to at least some cases of ADHD.

The dopamine transporter gene was the next target for ADHD molecular geneticists because the presumed role of this gene is the reuptake of dopamine from the synapse. The dopamine transporter gene exists in at least two allelic forms: a short form and a long form. Cook et al. (1995), using the haplotype-based haplotype relative risk approach, studied the association between the 480-base-pair dopamine transporter gene allele and ADHD. Using the transmission disequilibrium test, Waldman et al. (1997a) reported a positive relationship between *DAT1* and ADHD, particularly with hyperactive-impulsive symptoms. Gill et al. (1997) also reported a positive association between *DAT1* and ADHD. If these findings are replicated (with larger samples and similar approaches), further molecular analysis of the dopamine transporter gene may identify susceptibility alleles that may be useful in predicting who will have ADHD. According to Cook et al. (1995), "Biochemical analysis of such mutations may lead to the development of more effective therapeutic interventions" (p. 993).

Five studies have investigated *DRD4* and its alleles. LaHoste et al. 1996 reported a positive association between ADHD and *DRD4* and high-risk alleles. Similar findings were reported by Waldman et al. (1997a, 1997b), Swanson et al. (1998), Smalley et al. (1998), and Rowe et al. (1998), who studied associations between ADHD and high-risk alleles of the *DRD4* system. Castellanos et al. (1998) did not find an association between *DRD4* and ADHD. Waldman et al. (1997a) reported that the *DRD4* association is more strongly related to symptoms of inattention than to symptoms of hyperactivity-impulsivity. This finding, combined with the Waldman (1988) report on the relationship between the dopamine transporter gene and hyperactive-impulsive symptoms, raises the possibility that molecular researchers will be able to identify specific mutations for each of the three symptom domains of ADHD. As Swanson et al. (1998) stated, "Speculation hypotheses have suggested that specific alleles of the dopamine genes may alter dopamine transmission in the neural networks implicated in ADHD (e.g., that the ten repeat allele of the DAT1 gene may be associated with hyperactive reuptake of dopamine or that the seven repeat allele of the DRD4 gene may be associated with a subsensitive postsynaptic receptor)." In his McMasters symposium work, Swanson discusses in detail each of the dopamine alleles that are currently being studied in association with ADHD.

Molecular Comorbidity—Using Molecular Genetic Findings to Explain DSM Comorbidity

Perhaps molecular genetic findings will help us solve the perplexing problem of interpreting DSM comorbidity. Currently, there is a great deal of debate on how to understand the relationships between ADHD and anxiety, depression, mania, and substance use disorders. These relationships are difficult to understand because of developmental, gender, informant, and categorical confounds. Molecular genetic analyses of these comorbid conditions may shed light on the relationships between ADHD and other neuropsychiatric disorders.

Waldman et al. (1997a) reported a positive association between the dopamine transporter gene and bipolar disorder. If, as Geller (1997) pointed out, some forms of childhood ADHD may be considered a form of bipolar disorder, identifying children with the dopamine transporter gene allele may serve a dual purpose: first, to identify children who are at risk for ADHD and, second, to identify children with ADHD who are at risk for bipolar disorder. Furthermore, if the Waldman et al. (1997b) findings—that the dopamine transporter gene is more strongly associated with symptoms of hyperactivity-impulsivity than with symptoms of inattention—hold up, diagnosticians will have a phenotypic (symptom-based) approach to differentiating children at risk for combined ADHD/bipolar disorder.

Molecular genetic studies have also presented another interesting example of "molecular comorbidity." The D_4 receptor gene has been associated with nicotine addiction and some forms of depression (Lerman et al. 1998). Specifically, smoking practices were significantly heightened in smokers with depression who were homozygous for the short alleles of *DRD4*. Lerman et al. (1998) concluded that "the rewarding effects of smoking and the beneficial effects of nicotine replacement therapy for depressed smokers may depend , in part, on genetic factors involved in dopamine transmission" (p. 56).

These findings, like those of studies on the relationship between the dopamine transporter gene and ADHD/bipolar disorder, raise interesting questions that cannot be simply explained away. Pomerleau et al. (1995) reported that ADHD subjects were twice as likely to smoke as the general population. Davidson et al. (1997) reported that both childhood ADHD and having taken stimulant medication were risk factors for nicotine dependence. Levin et al. (1996) reported that nicotine (approximately 21 mg/day, administered with a nicotine skin patch) caused an overall significant reduction in reaction time on continuous performance tasks, as well as a significant reduction in inattention measures and clinician-generated clinical global impressions. Because the improvements occurred among nonsmoker ADHD subjects as well, the nicotine effect appears to be not merely a relief of withdrawal symptoms. Levin concluded, "Nicotine deserves further clinical trials with ADHD" (p. 55). Milberger et al. (1996) reported that maternal smoking during pregnancy is a risk factor for ADHD. Thus, molecular genetic evidence for the role of *DRD4* in childhood ADHD and in smoking may provide a way for us to understand the relationships between ADHD, nicotine dependence, and perhaps other psychiatric disorders as well.

Sabol et al. (1999) provided a window on another allele of the dopamine transporter system referred to as SLC6A3-9. In the study, allele 9 of the dopamine transporter gene was seen as possible protection against long-term nicotine addiction. In fact, as Sabol et al. (1999) stated,

> A significant association between the allele 9 and smoking status was confirmed as due to an effect on the cessation rather than initiation. This same allele has been associated with low scores for novelty seeking which was the most significant personality correlate of smoking cessation. It is hypothesized that individuals carrying the A9 polymorphism have altered dopamine transmission which reduces their need for novelty and reward by external stimuli including cigarettes. (p. 7)

This raises the possibility that individuals with allele 9 of the dopamine transporter gene are less likely to have ADHD.

Although each of the findings discussed here must be considered preliminary, they illustrate how far the field has advanced in its approach to the study of ADHD.

Molecular Genetics of ADHD Beyond Dopamine

To date, most molecular genetic analyses of ADHD have focused on the dopaminergic system. Future studies may need to focus on the role of norepinephrine receptors as genetic risk factors for ADHD. As Pliszka et al. (1996) and Levy and Hobbes (1988) pointed out, there is significant evidence that norepinephrine plays a role in both the hyperactive-impulsive and inattentive symptoms of ADHD. Comings et al. (1991) reported that there is an additive effect of three noradrenergic genes—the noradrenergic α_{2A} receptor gene (*ADRA2A*), the noradrenergic α_{2C} receptor gene (*ADRA2C*), and the dopamine β-hydroxylase gene (*DBH*)—on ADHD. The Levy and Hobbes study indicated a significant increase in the number of variant norepinephrine genes progressing from subjects without attention-deficit disorders or learning disorders, to subjects with attention-deficit disorders but not learning disorders, to patients with attention-deficit disorders and learning disorders. In addition, there was no compatible additive effect of dopamine genes in this study. The study by Comings and Hobbes supported an association between norepinephrine genes in ADHD, especially in subjects with learning disorders.

With the development of advanced multiloci molecular genetic techniques, future studies will likely consider the roles of the noradrenergic, serotonergic, muscarinic, and nicotinic receptor systems in the etiology of ADHD.

FUTURE DIRECTIONS

As molecular genetic techniques are refined, many more exciting relationships between genes and ADHD behaviors will doubtlessly be reported. Although, to date, the majority of reports center on the association between genes of the dopaminergic system and ADHD behavior, it is likely that relationships between the noradrenergic system, and the cholinergic (especially nicotinic) system, and ADHD will be reported. Regardless of the number of markers studied and the sophistication of multipoint linkage analyses that are already part of our technology, the primary obstacle to identifying the genetic and environmental contributions to ADHD remains in the area of phenotypic refinement. Until a phenotypic strategy emerges that is developmentally, gender, informant, and quantitatively sensitive and takes into account confounds such as comorbidity, discovery of the genetic etiology of ADHD will be difficult to achieve.

Significant steps have already been made toward clarifying the phenotype. We know that ADHD symptoms are highly heritable in boys and girls. We have preliminary evidence that these symptoms are better conceived as existing on a continuum of attention problems with and without hyperactivity-impulsivity. We also have preliminary evidence of different molecular genetic risk factors for inattention and hyperactivity-impulsivity. We have identified moderate and severe latent classes of inattention problems with and without hyperactivity and know that these classes are influenced by discrete genetic factors. We have evidence that the presentation of individuals with inattention of the moderate latent class does not fulfill DSM diagnostic criteria; hence, clinical cases and true genotypes will not be appropriately identified. We have evidence from family studies that ADHD is familial and that ADHD/CD, ADHD/mood disorder, and ADHD/bipolar disorder comorbid subtypes may be examples of discrete genetic subtypes. We remain curious about what the genetic relationship between ADHD and mania is and how to interpret the role of the dopamine transporter gene in both these disorders.

From twin studies, we have learned that parental reports of ADHD symptoms are highly influenced by a zygosity-specific rater contrast effect, in which parents underestimate the severity of the symptoms in the less affected twin, and that this effect is more profound in monozygotic than in dizygotic twins. This rater contrast leads to inflated heritability estimates and may have a role in hiding the true phenotype. Furthermore, we have learned that teacher reports generally lead to more conservative heritability estimates than parental reports. The impact of rater bias is tremendous in attempting to identify genes for ADHD. Thus, models that include reports from teachers, parents, and the child are currently being tested to determine the best informant, or combination of informants, for phenotypic studies of ADHD.

Twin, family, and molecular genetic studies of ADHD support the contention that genetic factors play an important role in many cases of ADHD. A great deal of work needs to be done to determine the role of environment, development, gender, ethnicity, and parental psychopathology in the etiology of ADHD. Because a tremendous amount of work is already under way, we should know a great deal more about the etiology and treatment of ADHD in the near future.

REFERENCES

Achenbach TM: Integrative Guide for the 1991 CBCL/4–18, YSR, and TRF Profiles. Burlington, University of Vermont, 1991

American Psychiatric Association: Diagnostic and Statistical Manual of Mental Disorders, 3rd Edition. Washington, DC, American Psychiatric Association, 1980

American Psychiatric Association: Diagnostic and Statistical Manual of Mental Disorders, 3rd Edition, Revised. Washington, DC, American Psychiatric Association, 1987

American Psychiatric Association: Diagnostic and Statistical Manual of Mental Disorders, 4th Edition. Washington, DC, American Psychiatric Association, 1994

Barr CL, Kidd KK: Population frequencies of the A1 allele at the dopamine 2 receptor locus. Biol Psychiatry 34:204–209, 1993

Biederman J, Faraone SV, Keenan K, et al: Evidence of familial association between attention deficit disorder and major affective disorders. Arch Gen Psychiatry 148:633–642, 1991a

Biederman J, Faraone SV, Keenan K, et al: Familial association between attention deficit disorder and anxiety disorders. Am J Psychiatry 148:251–256, 1991b

Biederman J, Newcorn J, Sprich S, et al: Comorbidity of attention deficit hyperactivity disorder with conduct, depressive, anxiety, and other disorders. Am J Psychiatry 148:564–577, 1991c

Biederman J, Faraone SV, Lapey K, et al: Comorbidity of diagnosis in attention deficit hyperactivity disorder. Child Adolesc Psychiatr Clin N Am 1:335–360, 1992a

Biederman J, Faraone SV, Keenan K, et al: Further evidence for family-genetic risk factors in attention deficit hyperactivity disorder: patterns of comorbidity in probands and relatives in psychiatrically and pediatrically referred samples. Arch Gen Psychiatry 49:728–738, 1992b

Castellanos FX, Lau E, Tayebi N, et al: Lack of an association between a dopamine-4 receptor polymorphism and attention-deficit/hyperactivity disorder: genetic and brain morphometric analyses. Mol Psychiatry 3:431–434, 1998

Comings DE, Comings BG, Muhleman D, et al: The dopamine D2 receptor locus as a modifying gene in neuropsychiatric disorders. JAMA 266:1793–1800, 1991

Cook EH Jr, Stein MA, Krasowski MD, et al: Association of attention-deficit disorder and the dopamine transporter gene. Am J Hum Genet 56:993–998, 1995

Davidson E, et al: Effects of methylphenidate and tobacco on subsequent drug use. Presentation at the Joint SRNT/CNG, 1997

Eaves LJ, Silberg JL, Meyer JM, et al: Genetics and developmental psychopathology, 2: the main effects of genes and environment on behavioral problems in the Virginia Twin Study of Adolescent Behavioral Development. J Child Psychol Psychiatry 38:965–980, 1997

Faraone SV, Biederman J: Do attention deficit hyperactivity disorder and major depression share familial risk factors? J Nerv Ment Dis 185:533–541, 1997

Faraone SV, Biederman J, Keenan K, et al: A family-genetic study of girls with DSM-III attention deficit disorder. Am J Psychiatry 148:112–117, 1991a

Faraone SV, Biederman J, Keenan K, et al: Separation of DSM-III attention deficit disorder and conduct disorder: evidence from a family-genetic study of American child psychiatric patients. Psychol Med 21: 109–121, 1991b

Faraone SV, Biederman J, Chen WJ, et al: Segregation analysis of attention deficit hyperactivity disorder: evidence for single gene transmission. Psychiatr Genet 2:357–375, 1992

Faraone SV, Biederman J, Chen WJ, et al: Genetic heterogeneity in attention-deficit hyperactivity disorder (ADHD): gender, psychiatric comorbidity, and maternal ADHD. J Abnorm Psychol 104:334–345, 1995

Faraone SV, Biederman J, Mennin D, et al: Attention-deficit hyperactivity disorder with bipolar disorder: a familial subtype? J Am Acad Child Adolesc Psychiatry 36:1378–1387, 1997a

Faraone SV, Biederman J, Wozniak J, et al: Is comorbidity with ADHD a marker for juvenile-onset mania? J Am Acad Child Adolesc Psychiatry 36:1046–1055, 1997b

Gill M, Daly G, Heron S, et al: Confirmation of association between attention deficit hyperactivity disorder and a dopamine transporter polymorphism. Mol Psychiatry 2:311–313, 1997

Goodman R, Stevenson J: A twin study of hyperactivity, I: an examination of hyperactivity scores and categories derived from Rutter teacher and parent questionnaires. J Child Psychol Psychiatry 30:671–689, 1989a

Goodman R, Stevenson J: A twin study of hyperactivity, II: the aetiological role of genes, family relationships and perinatal adversity. J Child Psychol Psychiatry 30: 691–709, 1989b

Hewitt JK, Silberg JL, Rutter M, et al: Genetics and developmental psychopathology, I: phenotypic assessment in the Virginia Twin Study of Adolescent Behavioral Development. J Child Psychol Psychiatry 38:943–963, 1997

Hudziak J: The identification of phenotypes for molecular genetic studies of common childhood psychopathology, in Handbook of Psychiatric Genetics. Edited by Blum K, Noble E. New York, CRC Press, 1997

Hudziak JJ, Geller B: Interethnic psychopharmacologic research in children and adolescents. Psychopharmacol Bull 32:259–263, 1996

Hudziak J, Todd RD: Familial subtyping of ADHD. Curr Opin Psychiatry 6:489, 1993

Hudziak J, Faraone SV, et al: Attention problems (AP): phenotypic marker for genetic studies of attention-deficit/hyperactivity disorder (ADHD). Poster presentation at the annual meeting of the American Academy of Child and Adolescent Psychiatry, Philadelphia, PA, October 1996

Hudziak J, Boomsma D, Koopmans J: Twin study of emotions and behavior using the YASR. Presentation at the annual meeting of the American Academy of Child and Adolescent Psychiatry, Toronto, October 1997

Hudziak JJ, Heath AC, Madden PF, et al: Latent class and factor analysis of DSM-IV ADHD: a twin study of female adolescents. J Am Acad Child Adolesc Psychiatry 37:848–857, 1998

Jensen PS, Shervette RE III, Xenakis SN, et al: Anxiety and depressive disorders in attention deficit disorder with hyperactivity: new findings. Am J Psychiatry 150: 1203–1209, 1993

Jensen PS, Martin D, Cantwell DP: Comorbidity in ADHD: implications for research, practice, and DSM-V. J Am Acad Child Adolesc Psychiatry 36:1065–1079, 1997

LaHoste GJ, Swanson JM, Wigal SB, et al: Dopamine D4 receptor gene polymorphism is associated with attention deficit hyperactivity disorder. Mol Psychiatry 1:121–124, 1996

Lerman C, Caporaso N, Main D, et al: Depression and self-medication with nicotine: the modifying influence of the dopamine D4 receptor gene. Health Psychol 17(1):56–62, 1998

Levin ED, Conners CK, Sparrow E, et al: Nicotine effects on adults with attention-deficit/hyperactivity disorder. Psychopharmacology (Berl) 123:55–63, 1996

Levy F, Hobbes G: The action of stimulant medication in attention deficit disorder with hyperactivity: dopaminergic, noradrenergic, or both? J Am Acad Child Adolesc Psychiatry 27:802–805, 1988

Levy F, Hay DA, McStephen M, et al: Attention-deficit hyperactivity disorder: a category or a continuum? Genetic analysis of a large-scale twin study. J Am Acad Child Adolesc Psychiatry 6:737–744, 1997

Light J, Pennington BF, Gilger JW, et al: Reading disability and hyperactivity disorder: evidence for a common genetic etiology. Dev Neuropsychol 11:323–335, 1995

Martin N, Boomsma D, Machin G, et al: A twin-pronged attack on complex traits. Nat Genet 17:387–392, 1997

Milberger S, Biederman J, Faraone SV, et al: Is maternal smoking during pregnancy a risk factor for attention deficit hyperactivity disorder in children? Am J Psychiatry 153:1138–1142, 1996

Pliszka SR: Comorbidity of attention-deficit hyperactivity disorder and overanxious disorder. J Am Acad Child Adolesc Psychiatry 31:197–203, 1992

Pliszka SR, McCracken JT, Maas JW: Catecholamines in attention-deficit hyperactivity disorder: current perspectives. J Am Acad Child Adolesc Psychiatry 35:264–272, 1996

Pomerleau OF, Downey KK, Stelson FW, et al: Cigarette smoking in adult patients diagnosed with ADHD. J Subst Abuse 7:373–378, 1995

Reich T, James JW, Morris CA: The use of multiple thresholds in determining the mode of transmission of semi-continuous traits. Ann Hum Genet 36:163–184, 1972

Reich T, Rice J, Cloninger CR, et al: The use of multiple thresholds and segregation analysis in analyzing the phenotypic heterogeneity of multifactorial traits. Ann Hum Genet 42:371–390, 1979

Reich W: Diagnostic Interview for Children and Adolescents Revised: DSM-III-R Version (DICA-R). St. Louis, Washington University, 1988

Rice J, Reich T, Andreasen NC, et al: The familial transmission of bipolar illness. Arch Gen Psychiatry 44:441–447, 1987

Rowe DC, Stever C, Giedinghagen LN, et al: Dopamine DRD4 receptor polymorphism and attention deficit hyperactivity disorder. Mol Psychiatry 3:419–426, 1998

Rutter M. A Children's Behavior Questionnaire for Completion by Parent. London, Longman, 1970

Sabol SZ, Nelson ML, Fisher C, et al: A genetic association for cigarette smoking behavior. Health Psychol 18:7–13, 1999

Semrud-Clikeman M, Biederman J, Sprich-Buckminster S, et al: Comorbidity between ADDH and learning disability: a review and report in a clinically referred sample. J Am Acad Child Adolesc Psychiatry 31:439–448, 1992

Sherman DK, Iacono WG, McGue MK: Attention-deficit hyperactivity disorder dimensions: a twin study of inattention and impulsivity-hyperactivity. J Am Acad Child Adolesc Psychiatry 36:745–753, 1997a

Sherman DK, McGue MK, Iacono WG: Twin concordance for attention deficit hyperactivity disorder: a comparison of teachers' and mothers' reports. Am J Psychiatry 154:532–535, 1997b

Smalley SL, Bailey JN, Palmer CG, et al: Evidence that the dopamine D4 receptor is a susceptibility gene in attention deficit hyperactivity disorder. Mol Psychiatry 3:427–430, 1998

Swanson JM, Sunohara GA, Kennedy JL, et al: Association of the dopamine receptor D4 (DRD4) gene with a refined phenotype of attention deficit hyperactivity disorder (ADHD): a family-based approach. Mol Psychiatry 3:38–41, 1998

Thapar A, Hervas A, McGuffin P: Childhood hyperactivity scores are highly heritable and show sibling competition effects: twin study evidence. Behav Genet 25:537–544, 1995

Tsuang MT, Faraone SV, Lyons MJ: Identification of the phenotype in psychiatric genetics. Eur Arch Psychiatr Clin Neurosci 243:131–142, 1993

Waldman ID, Robinson BF, Feigon SA: Linkage disequilibrium between the dopamine transporter gene (DAT1) and bipolar disorder: extending the transmission disequilibrium test (TDT) to examine genetic heterogeneity. Genet Epidemiol 14:699–704, 1997a

Waldman I, et al: The relation of DRD4 and DAT to ADHD. Poster presentation at the World Congress on Psychiatric Genetics, Sante Fe, NM, 1997b

Waldman ID; Rowe DC; Abramowitz A, et al: Association and linkage of the dopamine transporter gene and attention-deficit hyperactivity disorder in children: heterogeneity owing to diagnostic subtype and severity. Am J Hum Genet 63: 1767–1776, 1998

Willerman L: Activity level and hyperactivity in twins. Child Dev 44:288–293, 1973

3 Attention-Deficit/ Hyperactivity Disorder With Mood Disorders

Thomas Spencer, M.D.
Timothy Wilens, M.D.
Joseph Biederman, M.D.
Janet Wozniak, M.D.
Margaret Harding-Crawford, B.A.

In recent years, evidence has been accumulating regarding high levels of comorbidity in individuals with attention-deficit/hyperactivity disorder (ADHD), extending beyond conduct disorders to include mood disorders (Biederman et al. 1991b). This high level of comorbidity has been found in culturally and regionally diverse epidemiological samples (e.g., New Zealand and Puerto Rico) (Anderson et al. 1987; Bird et al. 1988; McGee et al. 1985), as well as in clinical samples (Biederman et al. 1990a), indicating that ADHD comorbid with mood disorders is likely a subtype of a broader ADHD category, with potentially different etiologic and modifying risk factors and different outcomes. Although DSM-IV (American Psychiatric Association 1994) terminology anchors this review, the diagnostic categories are used generically and include other definitions of disorders or dimensions.

CLINICAL FEATURES OF MOOD DISORDERS

Juvenile mood disorders are commonly classified as bipolar or nonbipolar, based on the presence or absence of mania (Table 3–1). These disorders are also classified as major (e.g., if major depression [Table 3–2] or bipolar disorder is present) or minor (e.g., if dysthymic disorder [Table 3–3] or cyclothymia is present). Compared with the more episodic nature typical of adult mood disorders, juvenile mood disorders tend to be chronic (Ryan et al. 1987). Major depression in a child may be apparent from a sad or irritable mood or a persistent loss of interest or pleasure in the child's favorite activities. Other symptoms include physiologic disturbances such as changes in appetite and weight, abnormal sleep patterns, psychomotor abnormalities, fatigue, and diminished ability to think, as well as feelings of worthlessness or guilt and suicidal preoccupation. Some depressed states in children are severe and include psychotic symptoms. Other associated features of depression in children include school difficulties, school refusal, withdrawal, somatic complaints, negativism, aggression, and antisocial behavior. In fact, conduct disorder and substance abuse commonly co-occur with depression in older children and adolescents.

Dysthymia, as it is called in DSM-III-R (American Psychiatric Association 1987), is a low-grade, protracted form of depression and is well described in children, adolescents, and adults. It is the best predictor of future episodes of depression as well as long-term psychosocial difficulty. Psychosocial difficulty and impairments in relationships that occur during episodes of depression or dysthymia may persist despite abatement of symptoms. Kovacs and colleagues, in a seminal study of outpatient children with depressive mood disorders (Kovacs et al. 1984a, 1984b), elegantly described the chronicity and recurrence of childhood mood disorders. The average episode of major depression lasted 7.5 months, and there was a 72% risk of recurrence in 5 years. In 38% of depressed children, these episodes occurred in the context of overlapping, ongoing dysthymia (so-called "double depression"). Dysthymia in children had an average duration of 3.5 years, and these children had a high risk of an episode of major depression (57% in 3 years). In addition, several studies (Strober and Carlson 1982) have reported that an ultimate bipolar outcome occurs in 20%–37% of children first diagnosed as having unipolar depression. The best predictors of the switch to bipolarity are a family history of bipolarity, acute onset, psychomotor retardation, mood-congruent psychosis, or poor or hypomanic response to antidepressants.

Mania in adults is often characterized by euphoria, elation, grandiosity,

Table 3–1. DSM-IV diagnostic criteria for manic episode

A. A distinct period of abnormally and persistently elevated, expansive, or irritable mood, lasting at least 1 week (or any duration if hospitalization is necessary).

B. During the period of mood disturbance, three (or more) of the following symptoms have persisted (four if the mood is only irritable) and have been present to a significant degree:

(1) inflated self-esteem or grandiosity
(2) decreased need for sleep (e.g., feels rested after only 3 hours of sleep)
(3) more talkative than usual or pressure to keep talking
(4) flight of ideas or subjective experience that thoughts are racing
(5) distractibility (i.e., attention too easily drawn to unimportant or irrelevant external stimuli)
(6) increase in goal-directed activity (either socially, at work or school, or sexually) or psychomotor agitation
(7) excessive involvement in pleasurable activities that have a high potential for painful consequences (e.g., engaging in unrestrained buying sprees, sexual indiscretions, or foolish business investments)

C. The symptoms do not meet criteria for a Mixed Episode (see p. 335).

D. The mood disturbance is sufficiently severe to cause marked impairment in occupational functioning or in usual social activities or relationships with others, or to necessitate hospitalization to prevent harm to self or others, or there are psychotic features.

E. The symptoms are not due to the direct physiological effects of a substance (e.g., a drug of abuse, a medication, or other treatment) or a general medical condition (e.g., hyperthyroidism).

Note: Manic-like episodes that are clearly caused by somatic antidepressant treatment (e.g., medication, electroconvulsive therapy, light therapy) should not count toward a diagnosis of bipolar I disorder.

Source. Reprinted from American Psychiatric Association: *Diagnostic and Statistical Manual of Mental Disorders,* 4th Edition. Washington, DC, American Psychiatric Association, 1994. Copyright 1994, American Psychiatric Association. Used with permission.

and increased energy. The condition may progress to delusions with these same grandiose features or even frank paranoia. In children, mania is more commonly manifested by emotional lability that may include an extremely irritable or explosive mood with associated poor psychosocial functioning, which is often devastating to the child and family (Coryell et al. 1993; Goodwin and Redfield Jamison 1990b). In milder cases, additional symptoms include unmodulated high energy such as decreased sleep, overtalkativeness, racing thoughts, or increased goal-directed activity (social, occupational, educational, sexual), as well as an associated manifestation of markedly poor

Table 3–2. DSM-IV diagnostic criteria for major depressive episode

A. Five (or more) of the following symptoms have been present during the same 2-week period and represent a change from previous functioning; at least one of the symptoms is either (1) depressed mood or (2) loss of interest or pleasure.

Note: Do not include symptoms that are clearly due to a general medical condition, or mood-incongruent delusions or hallucinations.

(1) depressed mood most of the day, nearly every day, as indicated by either subjective report (e.g., feels sad or empty) or observation made by others (e.g., appears tearful). **Note:** In children and adolescents, can be irritable mood.

(2) markedly diminished interest or pleasure in all, or almost all, activities most of the day, nearly every day (as indicated by either subjective account or observation made by others)

(3) significant weight loss when not dieting or weight gain (e.g., a change of more than 5% of body weight in a month), or decrease or increase in appetite nearly every day. **Note:** In children, consider failure to make expected weight gains.

(4) insomnia or hypersomnia nearly every day

(5) psychomotor agitation or retardation nearly every day (observable by others, not merely subjective feelings of restlessness or being slowed down)

(6) fatigue or loss of energy nearly every day

(7) feelings of worthlessness or excessive or inappropriate guilt (which may be delusional) nearly every day (not merely self-reproach or guilt about being sick)

(8) diminished ability to think or concentrate, or indecisiveness, nearly every day (either by subjective account or as observed by others)

(9) recurrent thoughts of death (not just fear of dying), recurrent suicidal ideation without a specific plan, or a suicide attempt or a specific plan for committing suicide

B. The symptoms do not meet criteria for a mixed episode (see American Psychiatric Association 1994, p. 335).

C. The symptoms cause clinically significant distress or impairment in social, occupational, or other important areas of functioning.

D. The symptoms are not due to the direct physiological effects of a substance (e.g., a drug of abuse, a medication) or a general medical condition (e.g., hypothyroidism).

E. The symptoms are not better accounted for by bereavement, i.e., after the loss of a loved one, the symptoms persist for longer than 2 months or are characterized by marked functional impairment, morbid preoccupation with worthlessness, suicidal ideation, psychotic symptoms, or psychomotor retardation.

Source. Reprinted from American Psychiatric Association: *Diagnostic and Statistical Manual of Mental Disorders,* 4th Edition. Washington, DC, American Psychiatric Association, 1994. Copyright 1994, American Psychiatric Association. Used with permission.

Table 3–3. DSM-IV diagnostic criteria for dysthymic disorder

A. Depressed mood for most of the day, for more days than not, as indicated either by subjective account or observation by others, for at least 2 years. **Note:** In children and adolescents, mood can be irritable and duration must be at least 1 year.

B. Presence, while depressed, of two (or more) of the following:

(1) poor appetite or overeating
(2) insomnia or hypersomnia
(3) low energy or fatigue
(4) low self-esteem
(5) poor concentration or difficulty making decisions
(6) feelings of hopelessness

C. During the 2-year period (1 year for children or adolescents) of the disturbance, the person has never been without the symptoms in Criteria A and B for more than 2 months at a time.

D. No major depressive episode (see American Psychiatric Association 1994, p. 327) has been present during the first 2 years of the disturbance (1 year for children and adolescents); i.e., the disturbance is not better accounted for by chronic major depressive disorder, or major depressive disorder, in partial remission.

Note: There may have been a previous major depressive episode provided there was a full remission (no significant signs or symptoms for 2 months) before development of the dysthymic disorder. In addition, after the initial 2 years (1 year in children or adolescents) of dysthymic disorder, there may be superimposed episodes of major depressive disorder, in which case both diagnoses may be given when the criteria are met for a major depressive episode.

E. There has never been a Manic Episode (see p. 332), a mixed episode (see American Psychiatric Association 1994, p. 335), or a hypomanic episode (see American Psychiatric Association 1994, p. 338), and criteria have never been met for cyclothymic disorder.

F. The disturbance does not occur exclusively during the course of a chronic psychotic disorder, such as schizophrenia or delusional disorder.

G. The symptoms are not due to the direct physiological effects of a substance (e.g., a drug of abuse, a medication) or a general medical condition (e.g., hypothyroidism).

H. The symptoms cause clinically significant distress or impairment in social, occupational, or other important areas of functioning.

Specify if:

Early onset: if onset is before age 21 years
Late onset: if onset is age 21 years or older

Specify (for most recent 2 years of dysthymic disorder):

With atypical features (see American Psychiatric Association 1994, p. 384)

Source. Reprinted from American Psychiatric Association: *Diagnostic and Statistical Manual of Mental Disorders,* 4th Edition. Washington, DC, American Psychiatric Association, 1994. Copyright 1994, American Psychiatric Association. Used with permission.

judgment such as thrill-seeking or reckless activities. It is often difficult to differentiate juvenile mania from ADHD, conduct disorder, depression, and psychotic disorders, because of overlapping developmental features. In addition, these disorders commonly co-occur with childhood mania. The clinical course of juvenile mania is frequently chronic and commonly mixed with co-occurring manic and depressive features. In adult-onset mania, one may obtain a clearer picture of childhood-onset illnesses such as ADHD, whose symptoms may precede the first manic episode by many years.

Unlike ADHD, which has an onset before age 7 years, the rate of onset of major depression and mania increases with age. Major depression is estimated to affect 0.3% of preschoolers, 1%–2% of elementary school–age children, and 5% of adolescents (Anderson et al. 1987; Kashani and Orvaschel 1988). Gender representation is equal until adolescence, when the adult pattern emerges, with approximately two-thirds of cases affecting females. Although the lifetime expectancy of bipolarity is estimated to be 1%, 15%–30% of those with the disorder have an onset by age 19 (Strober 1992). Family genetic studies of depression and mania reveal that the risk of these mood disorders in family members of probands with either major depression or mania increases inversely with age at onset (Puig-Antich et al. 1989; Strober 1992).

PSYCHIATRIC COMORBIDITY: ADHD AND MOOD DISORDERS

Literature Review

ADHD and mood disorders have been found to co-occur in 15%–75% of cases in both epidemiologic and clinical samples of children and adolescents (Biederman et al. 1991b). Some investigators, however, have not found higher-than-expected rates of mood disorders in children with ADHD (Gittelman et al. 1985; Lahey et al. 1988; Mannuzza et al. 1993; Stewart and Morrison 1973; Weiss and Hechtman 1986). In clinical samples, the association between ADHD and mood disorders has been reported in studies of children with nonbipolar major depression and dysthymia. For example, in an inpatient sample, Alessi and Magen (1988) reported comorbid attention deficit disorder (ADD) in 25% of children with major depressive disorder (MDD) and in 22% of those with dysthymia. Staton and Brumback (1981) reported that 55% of children with depression met the criteria for hyperactivity and that 75% of hyperactive children met the criteria for depression.

Comorbidity of mood disorders and ADHD has also been demonstrated in adolescents with bipolar disorder (Strober et al. 1988) and in children with ADHD (Biederman et al. 1990a; Bohline 1985; Brown et al. 1988; Munir et al. 1987). In a sample of 223 children consecutively referred for educational evaluation, 74% of those with hyperactivity and 63% of those with depression had both disorders (Brumback et al. 1977). Studies of high-risk children whose parents had mood disorders have found high rates of ADHD in these children (Keller et al. 1988; Orvaschel 1989; Orvaschel et al. 1988). In family studies of children with ADHD, the rate of mood disorders in children with ADHD and their first-degree relatives was significantly higher than the rate in control children and their first-degree relatives (Biederman et al. 1987, 1991a). Studies of adopted children with ADHD have shown higher rates of MDD in their biological relatives than in their adoptive relatives and the biological relatives of control subjects (Deutsch et al. 1982). Case reports have described individuals with a childhood history of ADHD who developed major affective disorders in later years (Dvoredsky and Stewart 1981). It is doubtful that the comorbidity between ADHD and mood disorders can be explained by ascertainment bias, because high levels of comorbidity between ADHD and mood disorders have also been found in culturally and regionally diverse population-based epidemiologic samples (Anderson et al. 1987; Bird et al. 1988; McGee et al. 1985).

In a complementary series of studies, investigators examined populations of children with depression for the presence of comorbid ADHD. Angold and Costello (1993) reviewed seven community studies that assessed the prevalence of childhood disorders comorbid with depression. In five of the studies, the rate of ADHD was significantly higher in children who had depression (0%–57%) than in children without depression. In a recent investigation, we examined children (mean age 11) who were consecutively referred to an outpatient psychopharmacological clinic. Of 136 children diagnosed with depression, 103 (76%) had a comorbid diagnosis of ADHD. Of the 66 children who had severe impairment associated with depression, 49 (74%) had a comorbid ADHD disorder (Biederman et al. 1995).

Follow-up studies of children with ADHD and children with MDD (Kovacs et al. 1984a, 1988) strongly suggest that although these disorders are individually associated with significant long-term psychiatric morbidity, their co-occurrence may be associated with a particularly poor outcome. For example, although self-rated depression at the time of follow-up did not differentiate hyperactive young adults and control subjects, Weiss et al. (1985) reported that the hyperactive young adults who had been hyperactive as children made significantly more suicide attempts than control subjects. Weiss and Hechtman (1986, p. 215) described a subgroup of hyperactive young adults who at follow-up had developed very serious depressions with suicide attempts. In a study that evaluated predictors of suicide in adolescents, Brent et al. (1988) reported that adolescents who committed suicide had increased rates of bipolarity and ADHD in comparison with those who attempted suicide. Thus, the co-occurrence of ADHD and a mood disorder suggests a subpopulation of children with ADHD at higher risk for greater psychiatric morbidity and disability (Weinberg et al. 1989), and perhaps at higher risk for suicide, than other children and adolescents who have ADHD without such comorbidity.

Implications of Comorbid Mood Disorders in ADHD

The comorbidity of ADHD with mood disorders can affect research and clinical practice as a result of its influence on diagnosis, prognosis, treatment, and health care delivery (Maser and Cloninger 1990). From a research perspective, patients with ADHD and mood disorders may represent a more homogeneous subgroup. It remains to be determined whether research findings previously reported in samples of children with ADHD are related to the ADHD itself, the existence of comorbid disorders, or a combination of both (Rutter 1989). From a clinical perspective, subgroups of patients with ADHD and mood disorders may respond differentially to specific therapeutic approaches. From a public health perspective, subgroups of patients with ADHD and mood disorders may be at a higher risk for the development of severe psychopathology. Identifying the subgroup of children with ADHD and mood disorders may permit the development of specific early intervention strategies. This is particularly important in light of published follow-up studies of children with ADHD indicating that a subgroup of ADHD control subjects developed very serious depressions with suicide attempts (Weiss and Hechtman 1986). In addition, the phenomenon of kindling may provide a model of mood disorders and their treatment. Stress and, eventually, recurrent illness may lead to a shift at the level of expression of the genome that induces treatment-resistant spontaneous depressions (Post 1992), thereby emphasizing the critical importance of detection and early intervention.

The observation of comorbidity between ADHD and affective disorders has led some authors to speculate that the diagnosis of hyperactivity/ADHD in some children may be a misdiagnosis of an underlying depressive disorder (Brumback 1988). Others suggested that depressive symptoms in hyperactive children with ADHD may be secondary to chronic failure and demoralization associated with ADHD (Weiss and Hechtman 1986, p. 43). Although the causes and determinants for the development of affective disorders in children with ADHD remain unknown, the literature indicates that depressive symptoms and disorders commonly develop among individuals with ADHD in childhood, adolescence, and adulthood and that their manifestation may not be benign. If not recognized and attended to, the combination of depressive symptoms and ADHD may lead to high morbidity and disability with a poor long-term prognosis (Brumback 1988) and, perhaps, increased mortality (Brent et al. 1988).

Impact of Comorbidity on Diagnostic Considerations

Although DSM represents a categorical approach to diagnosis, many investigators support a dimensional or factorial approach to classification. As opposed to the categorical approach, which assumes that there are psychiatric diseases identifiable by a set of discrete diagnostic criteria, the dimensional approach views symptoms as part of a normal continuum and focuses more on defining interindividual variation than on identifying discrete diseases. In this approach, psychopathology is defined as a significant variation from normality and is identified on the basis of cutoff scores on assessment scales, such as the Child Behavior Checklist (CBCL; Achenbach and Edelbrock 1983).

One approach to cross-validate issues of diagnosis and comorbidity within ADHD is to investigate the correspondence between categorical and dimensional approaches to diagnosis in children with ADHD. To this end, we studied the association between a DSM-III-R–based structured diagnostic interview—the Diagnostic Interview for Children and Adolescents—and the dimensional CBCL (Biederman et al. 1993b). We examined the correspondence between CBCL subscales and structured interview–based diagnoses of ADHD in children with and without comorbidity. Excellent convergence was found for several diagnoses and scales, such as between the anxiety/depression scale and the comorbid diagnoses of anxiety disorders. The comorbid diagnosis of depression increased the scores on the anxiety/depression scale, but this increase did not reach statistical significance in part because the scores of children with noncomorbid ADHD on this scale were already statistically elevated over the scores of the control subjects.

Jensen et al. (1993) reported similar findings on the high prevalence of clinically significant depressive symptomatology in a sample of children with nonpsychiatrically ascertained ADHD with a rating scale that was more specific for depressive symptoms than the CBCL anxiety/depression scale. The authors compared 47 pediatrically referred children with ADHD with a matched sample in a psychiatric clinic and with control subjects. They employed a multidisciplinary team to diagnose the disorder and used dimensional symptom-based instruments. Children completed a self-assessment instrument, the Children's Depression Inventory (CDI; Kovacs 1985), and parents completed the CBCL. Comorbid depression was diagnosed in 38% of the pediatrically referred children with ADHD. The mean score on the CDI was as high in the pediatrically referred children with ADHD as in the children in the psychiatric clinic, with both groups having higher mean scores than the control group. A greater portion of children with ADHD had scores that indicated clinically important depressive symptomatology (34% for the pediatrically referred children, 26.8% for the children in the clinic, and 9% for the control group). Similarly, parent-endorsed CBCL internalizing scale scores were as high in the pediatrically referred children with ADHD as in the children in the psychiatric clinic, with both groups having higher scores than the control group. The authors concluded that clinicians might underappreciate the high rate of clinically significant depression in children with ADHD.

These findings provide further support for the argument that hierarchical diagnosis is not appropriate for the diagnosis of ADHD. The hierarchical approach to diagnosis requires clinicians to exclude a diagnosis if another diagnosis appears to be more prominent. Although this approach is not codified in DSM-IV, it is practiced by some clinicians. As the data we reviewed indicate, exclusion of the ADHD diagnosis in the presence of MDD, or vice versa, will lead to underdiagnosis of ADHD in psychiatric populations and underdiagnosis of MDD in pediatric populations. This could lead to nonoptimal treatment and educational recommendations.

ASSOCIATION BETWEEN ADHD AND MOOD DISORDERS

Results From the NIMH Family Genetic Study of ADHD

The high level of comorbidity in ADHD suggests that the disorder may be a group of conditions with different etiologies and risk factors, as well as different outcomes, rather than a homogeneous clinical entity. Therefore, stratification of ADHD patients based on the presence of co-occurring psychiatric disorders, as was done in our family genetic study of ADHD, is a productive way of identifying homogeneous subgroups within ADHD. In a preliminary study, our group at Massachusetts General Hospital (MGH) (Biederman et al. 1991a) reported findings that support the hypothesis that DSM-III ADD and MDD may share common familial vulnerabilities. It is of note that the mean duration of comorbid childhood depression revealed in this study was 81 weeks. Familial risk analyses revealed the following: 1) the risk for MDD among relatives of patients with ADD was significantly higher than the risk for MDD among relatives of normal comparison children; 2) the risk for MDD was the same among relatives of children with and without MDD, and this risk was significantly higher among relatives of children in both groups than among relatives of children in the control group; and 3) the two disorders did not cosegregate within families. These findings are consistent with the hypothesis that ADD and MDD may represent a different expression of the same etiologic factors responsible for the manifestation of ADD. Why the shared genotype may have differing phenotypic expressions such as ADD, MDD, or ADD with comorbid MDD remains unknown.

This investigation was replicated and extended in a family genetic study of ADHD with a larger sample. Details of our methodology are presented elsewhere (Biederman et al. 1992). We studied two groups of index children: 140 children with ADHD and 120 control subjects. These groups had 454 and 368 first-degree relatives, respectively. Two independent sources provided the index children. We selected both psychiatrically and pediatrically referred ADHD patients. Control subjects were chosen from active outpatients at pediatric medical clinics.

All assessments were made using DSM-III-R-based structured interviews. Psychiatric assessments of children and siblings were made with the Kiddie–Schedule for Affective Disorders and Schizophrenia, Epidemiologic Version (K-SADS-E; Orvaschel 1985). To assess childhood diagnoses in the parents, we administered an addition to the Structured Clinical Interview for DSM-III-R (Spitzer et al. 1992), consisting of unmodified modules from the Kiddie-SADS-E covering childhood DSM-III-R diagnoses. All assessments were made by raters who were blind to the child's diagnosis (whether the child was in the group with ADHD or in the control group) and ascertainment site (MGH or HMO). The diagnosis of major depression was made only if the depressive episode was associated with marked impairment.

Within each sample, children with ADHD were significantly more likely to have MDD (Figure 3–1). However, nearly half the children with ADHD had no comorbidity with MDD (Figure 3–2).

Familial risk analysis revealed that relatives of children with ADHD had a clinically and statistically significant increased risk for ADHD and severe

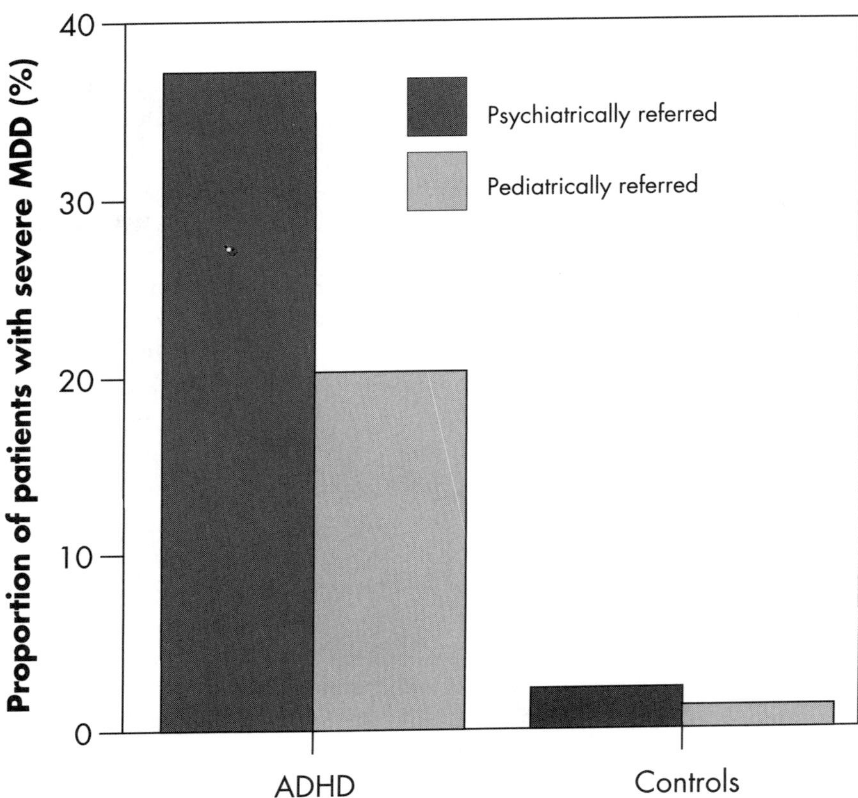

Figure 3–1. Overlap of comorbid major depressive disorder with severe impairment in psychiatrically and pediatrically referred children with ADHD. ADHD = attention-deficit/hyperactivity disorder; MDD = major depressive disorder.
Source. Adapted from Biederman et al. 1992.

MDD (Figure 3–3). To test hypotheses about the nature of the association between ADHD and comorbid disorders in children and relatives, we used models of familial transmission developed by Pauls et al. (1986a, 1986b). In stating these hypotheses, which follow, the expected differences are relative to control subjects and "ADHD + CM" refers to children who have ADHD with the comorbid disorder.

Hypothesis 1. If ADHD and the comorbid disorder are etiologically independent, we would expect to find higher rates of ADHD in relatives of children in both ADHD subgroups than in relatives of control subjects, but an

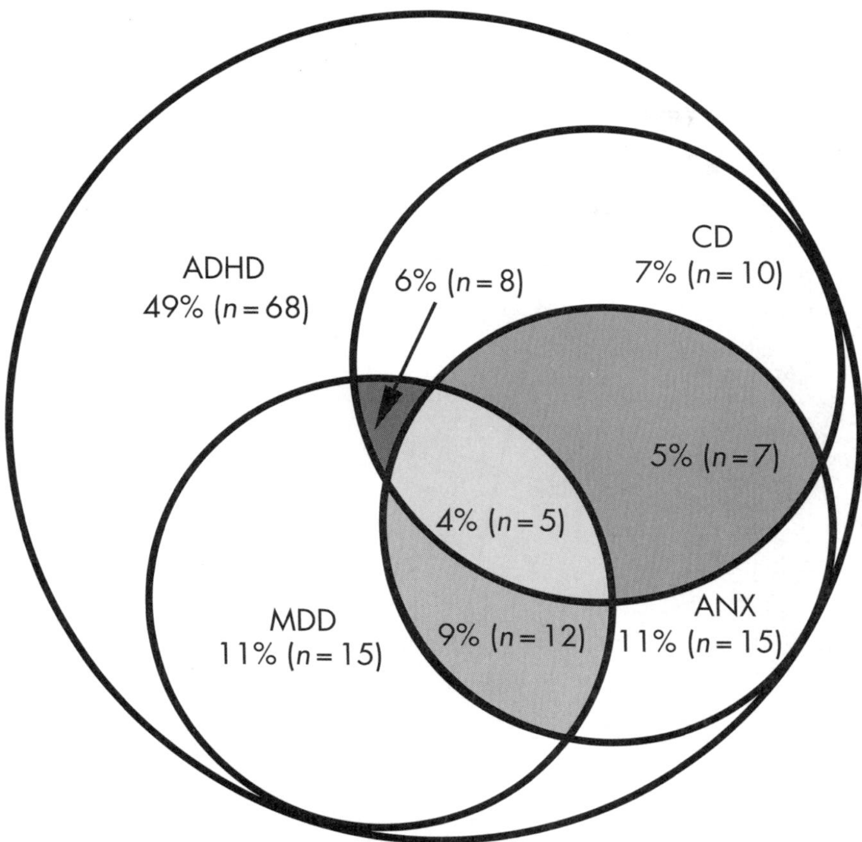

Figure 3–2. Overlap of comorbid disorders in pediatrically and psychiatrically referred children with ADHD. ADHD = attention-deficit/hyperactivity disorder; ANX = multiple anxiety disorders (≥ 2); CD = conduct disorder; MDD = major depressive disorder (severe).
Source. Adapted from Biederman et al. 1992.

increased rate of the comorbid disorder only among relatives of children in the ADHD+CM subgroup.

Hypothesis 2. If ADHD and the comorbid disorder share common familial etiologic factors, we would expect to find higher rates of ADHD and the comorbid disorder in relatives of children in both ADHD subgroups than in relatives of control subjects.

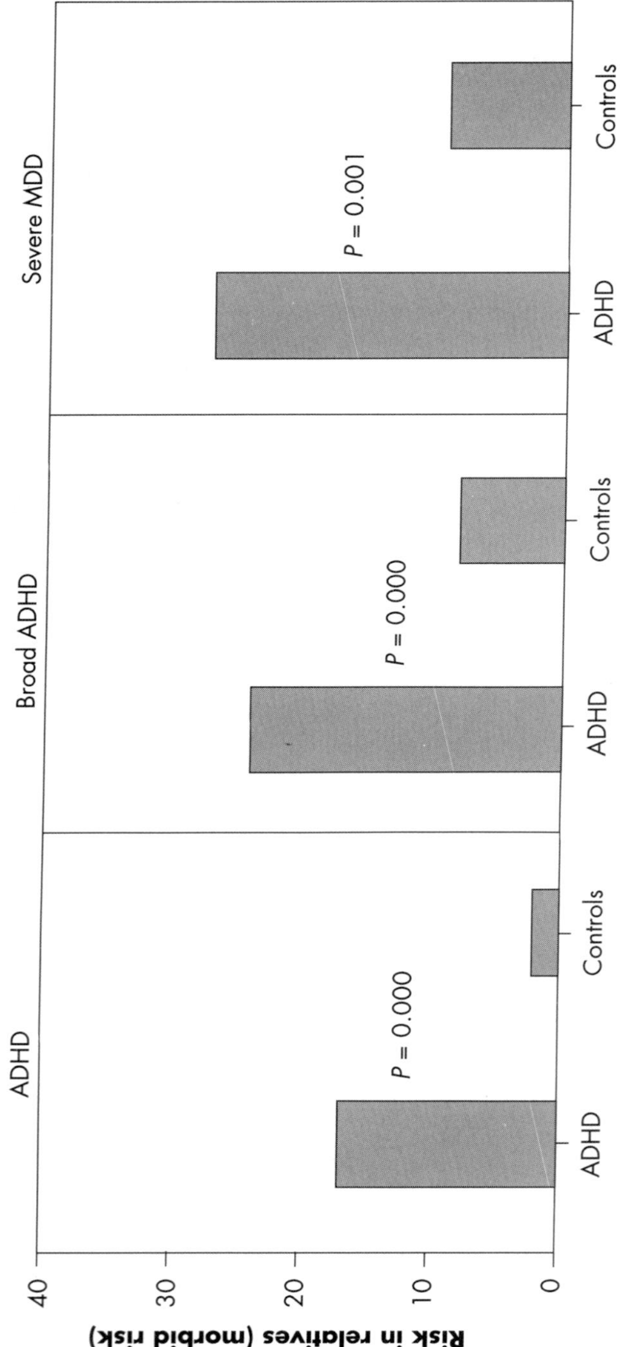

Figure 3–3. Transmission of ADHD and comorbid disorders in families of children with ADHD. Morbid risk represents age-corrected risk. ADHD = attention-deficit/hyperactivity disorder; MDD = major depressive disorder.
Source. Adapted from Biederman et al. 1992.

Hypothesis 3. If ADHD+CM is a distinct familial subtype, we would expect to find higher rates of ADHD in relatives of children in both ADHD subgroups than in relatives of control subjects but high rates of the comorbid disorder only in relatives of ADHD+CM children. In addition, ADHD and the comorbid disorder should cosegregate in these families. We use the term *cosegregate* to indicate that the disorders are transmitted together, not independently (i.e., the degree of comorbidity in relatives is greater than what would be expected by chance).

The risks for ADHD among relatives of children with ADHD+MDD and children who have ADHD without MDD did not differ significantly (21% vs. 14%) but were higher than the risk to relatives of control subjects (3%) (Figure 3–4). The risks for MDD among relatives of children with ADHD+MDD and children who have ADHD without MDD did not differ significantly (20% vs. 15%) but were higher than the risk to relatives of control subjects (9%). Also, ADHD and MDD did not cosegregate among relatives of ADHD+MDD children (i.e., among the relatives of ADHD+MDD children, different relatives accounted for the risks for ADHD and MDD). These findings are most consistent with Hypothesis 2, which postulates that ADHD and MDD share common familial etiologic factors.

MGH Prospective Follow-Up

Using DSM-III-R structured diagnostic interviews and blind raters, we reexamined psychiatric diagnoses at 1- and 4-year follow-ups in children with ADHD and control subjects (average age 15) (Biederman et al. 1996b). Analyses of follow-up findings revealed significant differences between children with ADHD and control subjects in rates of comorbid conduct and mood and anxiety disorders, with these disorders increasing markedly from baseline to follow-up assessment. Lifetime rates of comorbid depression in children with ADHD increased from 29% at baseline to 45% at year 4. These rates continued to be much greater than the rates of 2% and 6%, respectively, in control subjects. Moreover, comorbid disorders at baseline predicted disorder-specific sequelae at follow-up. A baseline diagnosis of conduct disorder predicted conduct disorder and substance use disorders at follow-up, major depression at baseline predicted major depression and bipolar disorder at follow-up, and anxiety disorders at baseline predicted anxiety disorders at follow-up. In addition, depression at baseline predicted lower psychosocial functioning (49 vs. 57; Global Assessment of Functioning Scale) and a higher rate of hospitalization (14% vs. 0%) than in children with noncomorbid ADHD. These results

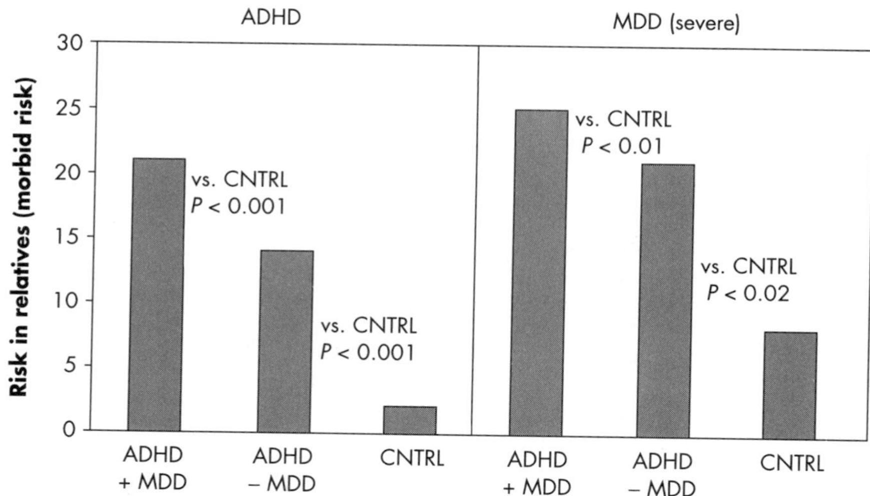

Figure 3–4. Familial transmission of ADHD and comorbid disorders for subtypes of children with ADHD. The risks of ADHD among relatives of children with ADHD plus MDD did not differ significantly from each other, and both were higher than the risk among relatives of control subjects. The risks of MDD among relatives of children with ADHD and MDD and those with ADHD but no MDD did not differ significantly from each other, and both were higher than the risk among relatives of control subjects; ADHD and MDD did not cosegregate. These findings are most consistent with the hypothesis that ADHD and MDD share common vulnerabilities (see text). Morbid risk represents age-corrected risk. ADHD = attention-deficit/hyperactivity disorder; CNTRL = control subjects; MDD = major depressive disorder (severe); cosegregation = comorbidity in relatives is greater than what would be expected by chance.
Source. Adapted from Biederman et al. 1992.

confirmed and extended previous results that indicated that children who have ADHD with mood disorders are at a higher risk for developing a wide range of impairments affecting multiple domains of psychopathology and interpersonal and family functioning.

We examined the predictors of remission and chronicity of depression and ADHD in this longitudinal sample to test whether depression in children with ADHD represented "true" depression or demoralization associated with ADHD (Biederman et al. 1998b). We found that although ADHD was a risk factor for depression, remission from ADHD was not associated with remission from depression. Furthermore, ADHD-related features at baseline, such as ADHD-associated measures of severity and school difficulty, were not associated with either the persistence or remission of depression. In contrast, bipolar disorder and higher indices of interpersonal problems predicted persistence of depression. ADHD and depression had independent and distinct courses, indicating that ADHD-associated depression reflects a "true" depressive disorder and not merely demoralization.

MGH Family Genetic Study of Girls With ADHD

Using a comprehensive methodology identical to the one used in the boys study, we examined clinical correlates in 126 girls with ADHD and 120 girls without ADHD (Biederman et al. 1999). Compared with female control subjects, both pediatrically and psychiatrically referred girls with ADHD were more likely to have conduct, mood, and anxiety disorders. However, in contrast to rates of depression in adult samples, rates of depression in girls with ADHD (mean age 12) were lower than in boys with ADHD (18% vs. 29%). In addition, familial risk analyses revealed findings in girls that were similar to those in boys. Rates of both ADHD and depression were greater in relatives of girls with ADHD than in relatives of girls without ADHD.

Comorbid Depression and School Failure and Cognitive Dysfunction

It is unknown whether school failure in children with ADHD is related to the psychiatric picture of inattention and impulsivity (ADHD), cognitive deficits (learning disorders), a combination of both factors, or perhaps other factors such as social disadvantage or demoralization and consequent decline in motivation (Campbell and Werry 1986). The National Institute of Mental Health (NIMH) family genetic study of ADHD (Biederman et al. 1992) assessed school failure and cognitive functioning in 140 patients and 120 control subjects. Children with ADHD were more likely to have had learning disabilities, to have repeated grades, and to have been placed in special classes and academic tutoring. They also did worse on the Wechsler Intelligence Scale for Children, Revised (WISC-R). ADHD probands with comorbid major depressive disorders ($N = 40$) had higher rates of school placement than ADHD probands without depression ($N = 64$) (53% vs. 20%). However, the comorbid probands did not have higher rates of learning disabilities, repeated grades, and academic tutoring or lower WISC-R scores than the noncomorbid probands. Moreover, the neuropsychological disability of all children with ADHD could not be attributed to comorbid disorders because those without comorbidity had more school failure and lower WISC-R scores than control subjects. Our results are similar to those of Frost et al. (1989), who examined neuropsychological functioning in an unselected cohort of young adolescents. The researchers found evidence of neuropsychological impairment among children with ADHD, but in the absence of comorbid ADHD, children with conduct disorder or depression were similar to control subjects without these disorders. Children with multiple disorders were the most impaired. Further, fine-grained neuropsychological studies are needed to separate deficits that are primary to ADHD from those that may be secondary to its other clinical features.

ADHD and Depression in Adults

Although the systematic evaluation of patterns of comorbidity in adults with ADHD has been limited, the available literature is consistent with findings reported in children with ADHD of high levels of conduct, mood, and anxiety disorders (Biederman et al. 1991b). The use of alternative diagnostic paradigms in adults with ADHD may have obscured the issue of comorbid disorders. For instance, the Utah criteria (Wender et al. 1985) are an alternative diagnostic paradigm commonly employed to aid in the diagnosis of adult ADHD. Although the Utah criteria establish the diagnosis of ADHD in childhood, they employ additional indicators to characterize the adult form of the disorder. The additional indicators are affective lability, hot or explosive temper, stress intolerance, and "dysphoric disorder." Because these symptoms are found in mood and anxiety disorders and are not diagnostic criteria for childhood ADHD, use of the Utah criteria may have incorrectly reinforced the impression that the core symptoms of childhood ADHD were not preserved into adulthood and blurred the distinction that some adults with ADHD have mood disorders and some do not.

As with earlier pediatric studies, clinicians assessing adults with ADHD have often used a hierarchical schema in which only a limited number of diagnoses are permitted. For instance, concentration difficulties are a cardinal feature of many psychiatric disorders including mood and anxiety disorders. Because ADHD in children and adults is frequently comorbid with these disorders (Biederman et al. 1990b), some clinicians rule out the diagnosis of ADHD when the other disorders are present (Wender and Garfinkel 1989). This has prevented researchers from considering the overlap of separate disorders and prevented adult patients with both mood disorders and ADHD from receiving stimulant treatment, even though data suggest that stimulants are helpful to adults with ADHD.

The early studies of ADHD, employing nonblind clinical assessments for diagnoses, consistently reported high rates of comorbidity. Borland and Heckman (1976) reported high rates of antisocial personality, anxiety, and depressive disorders among adults with childhood-only and childhood-onset ADHD. Treatment studies of adults with ADHD also reported psychiatric comorbidity (Gualtieri et al. 1985; Mattes et al. 1984; Spencer et al. 1992; Wender et al. 1981, 1985; Wood et al. 1976). The adults with ADHD in these studies had high rates of substance abuse (27%–46%), antisocial personality disorders (12%–27%), and anxiety disorders (50%). Despite the exclusion of major depressive disorder in many of these studies, investigators reported high rates of dysthymia (67%–81%) (Wender et al. 1981, 1985).

More recently our group (Biederman et al. 1993d) reported that adults with ADHD have high rates of antisocial, anxiety, and mood disorders. We studied 84 referred adult males with a clinical diagnosis of childhood-onset ADHD, confirmed by structured interview. Findings were compared with those from a preexisting sample of referred children with ADHD ($N = 140$), nonreferred ADHD adult relatives of those children ($N = 43$), and adult relatives of children in the control group ($N = 248$). Subjects underwent a comprehensive battery of psychiatric, cognitive, and psychosocial assessments. Referred and nonreferred adults with ADHD were similar to one another but were more disturbed and impaired than non-ADHD control subjects. The rate of major depressive disorder among the adults with ADHD was similar to the rate among children with ADHD: the rate of major depressive disorder in the referred adult ADHD group was 31% ($n = 26$); in the nonreferred ADHD adult relatives of children with ADHD, 17% ($n = 6$); in the referred children with ADHD, 29% ($n = 40$); and in the adults in the control group, 5% ($n = 11$).

In a further analysis, we compared 41 adult females with ADHD with adult males with the disorder for whom there were existing data to determine whether ADHD was expressed differently in male and female adults (Biederman et al. 1994). Gender-specific comparisons with control subjects revealed that adults of both sexes with ADHD had significantly higher rates of major depression, oppositional disorder, and anxiety disorders. However, adult males with ADHD had significantly higher rates of childhood conduct and adult antisocial personality disorder than adult female ADHD patients. Adult female ADHD patients had greater rates of dysthymia and depression than non-ADHD adult females (16% vs. 4% for dysthymia; 36% vs. 6% for depression). The consistency of these findings in juveniles as well as in adults of both sexes further confirms the importance of ADHD as a risk factor for depression through the life cycle.

MANIA AND ADHD

In contrast to a large body of literature on adult bipolar disorder (Goodwin and Jamison 1990) and an emerging literature on childhood major depression (Puig-Antich 1987), much less is known about childhood bipolar disorder. Retrospective surveys of adult patients with bipolar disorder describe a definite but low rate (0.4%) of onset of symptoms before the age of 10 years (Loranger and Levine 1978; Goodwin and Redfield Jamison 1990a). However, case reports and case series in the literature (Campbell 1952; Coll and Bland 1979; Davis 1979; Feinstein 1982; Feinstein and Wolpert 1973; Frommer 1968; Kasanin 1931; McHarg 1954; McKnew et al. 1974; Potter 1983; Poznanski et al. 1984; Reiss 1985; Sadler 1952; Sylvester et al. 1984; Thompson and Schindler 1976; Tomasson and Kuperman 1990; Varanka et al. 1988; Varsamis and MacDonald 1972; Warneke 1975; Weinberg and Brumback 1976; Weller et al. 1986) suggest that juvenile mania may not be uncommon but that it may be difficult to diagnose.

One potential source of diagnostic confusion in prepubertal mania is the symptomatic overlap with ADHD. The symptoms of distractibility, impulsivity, hyperactivity, and emotional lability are characteristic of both ADHD and bipolar disorder (Carlson 1984). The available descriptive literature on manic children notes the frequent overlap of symptoms between the two disorders (Lowe and Cohen 1980; Potter 1983; Reiss 1985; Thompson and Schindler 1976) and documents that some hyperactive children go on to develop manic-depressive illness (Sadler 1952). Moreover, in some cases, ADHD and mania can coexist, and this adds to the diagnostic uncertainties surrounding the diagnosis of juvenile mania.

There are developmental variations in the expression of mania. Although mania in adults may be manifest by a euphoric mood (Bowring and Kovacs 1992; Davis 1979; Warneke 1975; Weinberg and Brumback 1976), the most common mood disturbance in children with mania may be better characterized as extreme irritability, with the occurrence of "affective storms" or prolonged and aggressive temper outbursts (Carlson 1983, 1984; Davis 1979). Young children with bipolar disorder have more irritability, crying, and psychomotor agitation than older children with the disorder, who are more likely to be "classically manic," with euphoria and grandiosity (see Carlson 1983, 1984). Additionally, childhood-onset bipolar disorder tends to be chronic and continuous rather than episodic and acute, as is characteristic of adult-onset bipolar disorder (Carlson 1983, 1984; Feinstein and Wolpert 1973; McGlashan 1988).

ADHD and Bipolar Disorder: Results From the MGH Study

Our group studied children, 12 years or younger, consecutively referred to a pediatric psychopharmacology clinic since 1991 (Wozniak et al. 1993). Of the 183 referrals, 17% (*n* = 32, 72% males) met the criteria for mania and 60% (*n* = 109) met the criteria for ADHD. Of those meeting the criteria for ADHD, 27% (*n* = 29) also met the criteria for mania. In a preexisting sample (Biederman et al. 1992) of prepubertal boys (*n* = 102) evaluated in a family genetic study of DSM-III-R ADHD, 12 also met the criteria for mania. Thus, in all, 44 prepubertal children (32 from the clinic; 12 from the ADHD study sample) with the diagnosis of mania were identified. The mean ages at onset of mania and ADHD were similar in the clinic population and the ADHD study group (4.8 vs. 4.3 years for mania; 2.9 vs. 2.7 years for ADHD).

Mania and ADHD frequently co-occurred. Ninety-one percent (*n* = 29) of children with bipolar disorder in the clinic sample met the full criteria for ADHD. In contrast, only 19% (*n* = 41) of children with ADHD from both the clinic and ADHD study samples met the criteria for mania. Several possibilities can explain the overlap of mania with ADHD: 1) the child with mania plus ADHD has only mania but, because of overlapping symptoms, is misdiagnosed as having ADHD; 2) the child with mania plus ADHD has only ADHD but, because of overlapping symptoms, is misdiagnosed as having mania; or 3) the child with mania plus ADHD has both mania and ADHD.

To explore these possibilities, we examined the extent of symptom overlap between mania and ADHD and whether the diagnoses of these disorders can be maintained after removal of the overlapping symptoms. In addition, we evaluated whether children who satisfy the diagnostic criteria for both ADHD and mania have correlates known to be present in these disorders. For ADHD those correlates include school and cognitive dysfunction and the presence of nonaffective comorbid psychiatric disorders, such as conduct and oppositional disorders. For mania those correlates include a personal history of depressive disorders, a family history of bipolar disorder, and poor global functioning.

We rediagnosed each child after subtracting the overlapping symptoms of mania and ADHD (distractibility, motoric hyperactivity, and talkativeness). Eighty-five percent of children with mania continued to meet full (65%, *n* = 26/40) or subthreshold (20%, *n* = 8/40) criteria for mania. Ninety-seven percent (*n* = 37) of the children with ADHD diagnoses retained full diagnostic status after subtraction of the three overlapping symptoms. This finding is consistent with the findings of a study by Fristad et al. (1992), in which children with mania and children with ADHD received similar scores on the Conners ADHD Rating Scale, whereas children with mania scored significantly higher than children with ADHD on the Mania Rating Scale.

Patients with ADHD comorbid with mania were compared with children and adolescents with ADHD but without mania to examine for the presence of correlates known to be associated with ADHD. Similarities in both groups included age at onset, learning impairment, and cognitive dysfunction measures, as well as patterns of psychiatric comorbidity. The average age at onset of the ADHD in bipolar children was the same as the age at onset of ADHD in the comparison groups of children with ADHD without mania (2.90 vs. 2.85 years, respectively). Rates of school failure (except tutoring) and cognitive dysfunction were similar for ADHD children with and without mania, and these measures significantly differed from those of normal control children. The rate of comorbid conduct, oppositional, and anxiety disorders in bipolar and nonbipolar children with ADHD differed from that in control subjects. The rates of these comorbid disorders were higher among children with both ADHD and bipolar disorder than among children with ADHD but no bipolar disorder.

Patients with ADHD and mania were also examined for evidence of correlates known to be associated with mania. Children with mania had significantly higher rates of major depression (80%, n = 35) than nonbipolar ADHD children (34%, n = 58) and control subjects (4%, n = 3). In the clinic group, the rate of psychosis among children with bipolar disorder was 14% (n = 4) versus 1% (n = 1) among nonbipolar ADHD children. The children with mania for whom this information was available also had significantly higher rates of a positive family history of bipolar disorder (36%, n = 10 than nonbipolar ADHD children (6%, n = 5) and control subjects (8%, n = 6). Furthermore, the children with bipolar disorder had significantly lower mean Global Assessment of Functioning scores (41 ± 6.9) than nonbipolar ADHD children (50 ± 6.0) or control subjects (72 ± 8.6).

Clinical Characteristics and Course of Mania

Our findings indicate that the onset of juvenile mania is usually insidious, manifesting itself in some children at the beginning of life, and that the disorder is usually chronic. These features, as well as the high prevalence of comorbid ADHD, may make identification difficult. Another feature that makes it difficult to diagnose mania in children with ADHD is that the predominant mood is severe irritability rather than euphoria. Although tantrums are common among children with ADHD, the type of irritability observed in prepubertal children with mania in our sample was very severe and included explosive reactions with persistent violence to persons and property. In the absence of euphoria, clinicians may incorrectly attribute irritability in a child to psychosocial factors or conduct disorder rather than to mania. Clinicians are likely to label these children with ADHD as temperamentally difficult or state that their ADHD is due to severe psychosocial stressors. The differential diagnosis of very difficult children with ADHD and mood features should include the possibility of mania.

Our results also showed that prepubertal mania is commonly mixed or dysphoric with symptoms of depression and mania and that prepubertal mania is commonly chronic rather than episodic. Studies in adults with mania emphasize that mixed mania is associated with younger age at onset, suicidality, longer duration of illness, poor outcome, and a higher rate of neuropsychiatric abnormalities (McElroy et al. 1992). Thus, the predominant mood of irritability, mixed presentation with major depression, and chronic course may contribute to the difficulty in diagnosing prepubertal mania in the context of comorbid ADHD.

Although not widely reported in samples of adults, the overlap between mania and ADHD may not be limited to children. A study of early-onset versus late-onset bipolar disorder in adults found comorbid ADHD only in early-onset probands (Sachs et al. 1993). Furthermore, a study of adults with ADHD found a significantly elevated rate of comorbid bipolar disorder in this group (Biederman et al. 1993d). More research of this type can be accomplished only if ADHD is considered in the diagnostic assessment of adult subjects and if patterns of comorbidity are systematically assessed.

MGH Family Genetic Studies of ADHD and Mania

In the same sample (140 children with ADHD and 120 control subjects) described above, we also used DSM-III-R-based structured interviews to examine rates of bipolar disorder in boys with ADHD (Biederman et al. 1996a). Bipolar disorder was detected in 11% of children with ADHD at baseline (mean age 11) and in an additional 12% at 4-year follow-up. In contrast, rates of bipolarity in the control subjects were appropriately low (0% at baseline and 1.8% at follow-up). As in the children with mania ascertained from our clinic, prototypic features of bipolar disorder in the children with ADHD were evident; however, the mood was rarely euphoric but mostly irritable and mixed with depression. Children with ADHD and comorbid bipolar disorder at either baseline or follow-up assessment had other correlates expected in bipolarity, including additional psychopathology, psychiatric hospitalization, and severely impaired psychosocial functioning. Comorbidity between ADHD and bipolar disorder was not simply the result of symptom overlap. Children with

ADHD who developed bipolar disorder at 4-year follow-up had higher initial rates of comorbidity, more symptoms of ADHD, worse scores on the CBCL, and a greater family history of depression than nonbipolar children with ADHD. These findings confirmed previous results documenting that children with ADHD are at increased risk for developing bipolar disorder with its associated severe morbidity, dysfunction, and incapacitation.

After stratification of our ADHD sample into those with and without bipolar disorder, familial risk analyses of 822 first-degree relatives revealed that 1) relatives of both ADHD subgroups were at greater risk for ADHD than relatives of control subjects, but the relatives of the ADHD subgroups did not differ in their risk for ADHD; 2) relatives had an elevated risk for bipolar disorder when probands had ADHD and bipolar disorder but not when probands had ADHD alone; and 3) ADHD and bipolar disorder cosegregated in families. In addition, we did not find significant nonrandom mating between parents with ADHD and those with bipolar disorder (Faraone et al. 1997). Our data suggest that children with ADHD and comorbid bipolar disorder are familially distinct from other children with ADHD and may represent a familial subtype.

We also examined patterns of familial association in a separate sample of clinically ascertained children with bipolar disorder (Wozniak et al. 1995). For comparison, we used a structured interview to examine diagnostic information on the first-degree relatives of children with bipolar disorder, children with ADHD without bipolar disorder, and control children. Our results replicated the familial association analysis of our study of children with ADHD. High rates of both bipolarity and ADHD were found in the first-degree relatives of these children. In addition, ADHD and bipolarity cosegregated among the relatives of children with bipolar disorder. These findings, taken together with those from our study of children with ADHD, provide external validation (family genetic evidence) of bipolar disorder and ADHD when they exist comorbidly in children. Moreover, they suggest that the condition of ADHD with comorbid bipolar disorder may be a distinct nosological entity.

TREATMENT OF MOOD DISORDERS AND ADHD

General Principles

Mood

Suggested pharmacologic approaches for treating children and adolescents with depressive disorders are based on a relatively few controlled studies, available data from adults, and clinical experience. There are four main families of antidepressant medications: the imipramine-like drugs, usually referred to as tricyclic antidepressants (TCAs); fluoxetine-like drugs, usually referred to as selective serotonin reuptake inhibitors (SSRIs); monoamine oxidase inhibitors (MAOIs); and atypical antidepressants such as bupropion. There is increasing evidence that juvenile mood disorders may be more refractory to pharmacologic intervention than adult mood disorders (Geller 1991; Ryan 1990) and that agents with a primarily serotonergic mechanism of action may be more efficacious (Emslie et al. 1997). In adults with depression, bipolarity, atypicality, and psychotic symptoms are associated with poor response to treatment. Antidepressant nonresponders may benefit from treatment strategies that include 1) higher doses of the antidepressant in patients who do not experience adverse effects and who have a relatively low plasma concentration of the drug, 2) a different class of medication, and 3) adjunctive treatment approaches such as combining two antidepressants of a different class, low-dose lithium carbonate, stimulants, thyroid hormone (T3), and antianxiety medications.

For bipolar disorders, manic type, treatment with mood stabilizers is recommended. Mood stabilizers include lithium carbonate and anticonvulsants such as carbamazepine, valproic acid, gabapentin, lamotrigine (not advised in children), and perhaps topiramate, tiagabine, and others. As with juvenile depressive disorders, there is evidence that juvenile-onset mania may be more refractory to pharmacologic intervention than adult disorders (Biederman et al. 1998a; Strober et al. 1988). If there is no response to an adequate trial (in dose and time) of a specific mood stabilizer, or if the patient cannot tolerate the drug, subsequent trials with other mood stabilizers are recommended. In patients with mania who have psychotic symptoms, additional antipsychotic treatment is recommended. There is emerging evidence that atypical antipsychotics that include serotonergic activity (risperidone, olanzapine, clozapine) may be particularly effective in juvenile (Frazier et al. 1999) and adult (Tohen et al. 1999) bipolar disorder. Bipolar disorder with depression, mixed type, requires an aggressive treatment approach combining the therapeutic recommendation outlined earlier for both manic and depressive conditions.

ADHD

Stimulants are the mainstay of pharmacologic treatment for ADHD. There have been more than 100 double-blind controlled studies of stimulants in the treatment of ADHD with an overall response rate of 70% (Spencer et al. 1996). However, there is preliminary evidence suggesting that ADHD patients with certain comorbidities may be somewhat refractory to stimulant treatment. In addition to stimulants, other psychotropics have been evaluated as alternative treatments for ADHD. These include various antidepressants and the α-adrenergic agonists clonidine and guanfacine. TCAs, including imipramine, desipramine, and nortriptyline, have been evaluated for treatment of ADHD. Studies have shown that TCAs are effective in many children with ADHD, even those refractory to stimulants (Biederman et al. 1989; Donnelly et al. 1986; Garfinkel et al. 1983; Greenberg et al. 1975; Rapoport et al. 1974; Waizer et al. 1974; Werry et al. 1980; Winsberg et al. 1972; Yepes et al. 1977). Other antidepressants that have been found to be superior to placebo include the MAOIs and the novel antidepressants bupropion (dopaminergic/noradrenergic) and, possibly, venlafaxine (noradrenergic/serotonergic).

Mood and Comorbid ADHD

Since ADHD is a risk factor for several comorbidities, their existence frequently complicates considerations of pharmacotherapy (Table 3–4). As detailed previously, stimulants are poor treatments for mood disorders, and most antidepressants that treat ADHD are not effective for childhood depression. Similarly, treatments for mania do not treat ADHD and vice versa. The question may arise, "If an individual has a mood disorder, why treat the ADHD? After all ADHD is considered a more benign condition." Additional treatment for ADHD may be needed to address academic, occupational, cognitive, or social dysfunction specific to ADHD symptoms. For example, persistent ADHD may interfere with the psychosocial and educational treatments targeted to the mood disorders themselves, as well as the patient's understanding of the importance of treatment compliance.

Mood disorders with ADHD require an aggressive treatment approach that combines the usual pharmacotherapies for ADHD, the stimulants or α-adrenergic agonists, with antidepressants. Certain classes of antidepressants, including TCAs, MAOIs, and novel antidepressants such as bupropion, have the potential to successfully treat both conditions. Some preliminary evidence indicates that patients with mania and ADHD may be relatively refractory to lithium (McElroy et al. 1992; Ryan and Puig-Antich 1986); therefore, these patients also require an aggressive treatment approach combining the usual pharmacotherapies for ADHD and therapies recommended previously for mania.

Literature Review

With the increasing recognition that ADHD is a heterogeneous disorder, attention has begun to focus on the impact of comorbidity on treatment re-

Table 3–4. Treatment algorithms for ADHD

ADHD simplex	Stimulants TCAs Bupropion Clonidine/guanfacine
ADHD and major depression	Stimulants + SSRIs TCAs/ bupropion ± stimulants
ADHD and anxiety	Stimulants + high-potency BZDs Stimulants + buspirone TCAs Bupropion Stimulants + SSRIs
ADHD and conduct disorder	Clonidine/guanfacine ± stimulants Beta-blockers + stimulants
ADHD and tics	Clonidine/guanfacine TCAs Stimulants + TCAs ± clonidine/guanfacine
ADHD and mania	Lithium/carbamazepine/valproic acid (other anticonvulsants) ± stimulants/ clonidine/TCAs/bupropion
ADHD and multiple comorbidities	Address each comorbidity Prioritize by severity
Treatment-resistant ADHD	Assess for new or old comorbidity Consider alternative pharmacotherapies or combined approaches

Note. Slashes indicate "or." ADHD = attention-deficit/hyperactivity disorder; TCAs = tricyclic antidepressants; SSRIs = selective serotonin reuptake inhibitors. BZDs = benzodiazepines.

sponse. Issues of comorbidity are important in the pharmacologic management of individuals with ADHD because there is evidence that stimulants can induce anxiety (Gittelman and Koplewicz 1986; Swanson et al. 1978) or depression (Barkley 1977, 1990; Gittelman and Koplewicz 1986; Wilens and Biederman 1992) in some patients. In addition, the presence of comorbid mood and anxiety disorders appears to significantly worsen the response of ADHD symptoms to stimulant treatment. There have been five controlled and three open pediatric (N = 450) studies of stimulant treatment in individuals with ADHD and comorbid anxiety or depression. In six of these studies (N = 260 children), investigators reported a lower response of ADHD symptoms to stimulants (DuPaul et al. 1994; Pliszka 1989; Swanson et al. 1978; Tannock et al. 1995; Taylor et al. 1987; Voelker et al. 1983). Consistent with the hypothesis that clinical subtypes might predict differential treatment responses, Garfinkel et al. (1983) reported that for children with ADHD, stimulants were superior for treating symptoms of inattentiveness, while TCAs were superior for treating symptoms of depression. Thus, a comprehensive understanding of drug treatment for children and adults with ADHD requires careful attention to patterns of comorbidity.

The safety and efficacy of combined SSRI and stimulant pharmacotherapy has been addressed in two open studies. Gammon and Brown (1993) reported the successful addition of fluoxetine to stimulants in the management of 32 patients with ADHD and comorbid depressive and anxiety disorders. These children had failed to respond to methylphenidate alone. After the addition of fluoxetine, improvement was noted in both ADHD and depressive symptoms. The combined treatment was well tolerated. Another report detailed the addition of methylphenidate to SSRI treatment (Findling 1996). Twelve children and adults with depression and comorbid ADHD were treated with either fluoxetine or sertraline. While depressive symptoms remitted, ADHD symptoms persisted. Methylphenidate was added and successfully treated the ADHD symptoms, and the combined treatment was well tolerated. With the exception of hypertension in one adult on methylphenidate monotherapy, there were no significant changes in cardiovascular parameters, increased side effects, or emergent aggressiveness or mania.

To clarify the impact of comorbidity on treatment, data from a controlled trial of desipramine (4–5 mg/kg per day) for the treatment of children and adolescents with ADHD were further analyzed (Biederman et al. 1993a) (Figure 3–5). We examined whether comorbidity of ADHD with conduct disorder, major depression, an anxiety disorder, or a family history of ADHD predicted response to desipramine treatment. Contrary to our expectations, neither comorbidity with conduct disorder, depression, or anxiety, nor a family history of ADHD, yielded differential responses to desipramine treatment that could be distinguished from those observed in children without such characteristics. Overall, the response rates of desipramine-treated patients with and without comorbidity or a family history of ADHD were much higher than that of placebo-treated patients, with improvement in characteristic symptoms of ADHD as reported by parents, teachers, and physicians. Moreover, response to desipramine treatment in ADHD patients was not accounted for by the presence of desipramine-responsive comorbidity as indicated by the finding that comorbidity with any of the assessed disorders increased the likelihood of a placebo response but did not change the response to desipramine. Desipramine-treated ADHD patients showed a substantial reduction in depressive symptoms compared with placebo-treated patients (Biederman et al. 1989). Also, the similarly successful treatment outcome observed for mea-

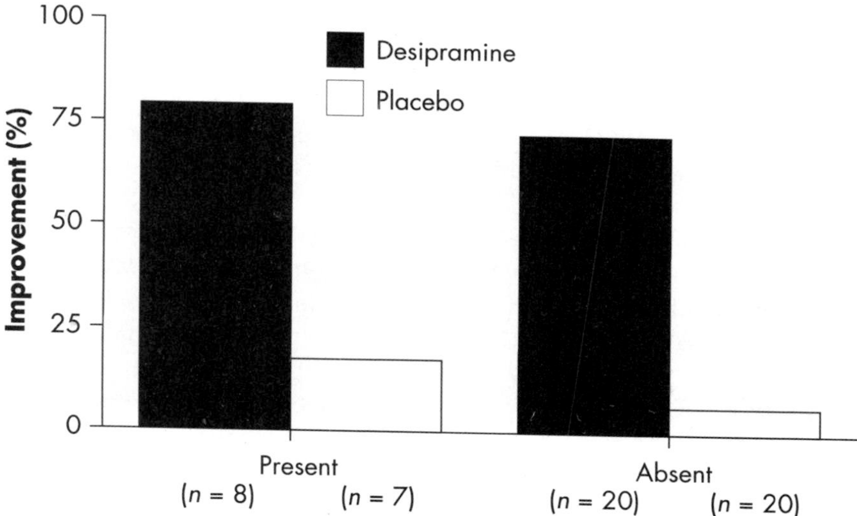

Figure 3–5. Response to desipramine in children with ADHD, with and without comorbid major depressive disorder. Open bars = placebo-treated subjects; shaded bars = desipramine-treated subjects. The response rates of desipramine-treated patients with and without comorbid major depressive disorder were much higher than that of placebo-treated individuals. Comorbidity with major depressive disorder increased the likelihood of a placebo response but did not change the response to desipramine.
Source. Adapted from Biederman et al. 1993a.

sures of ADHD in children with and without comorbid major depression or an anxiety disorder suggests that desipramine may be a particularly appropriate choice of treatment in children with those comorbidities and ADHD. These results provide support for the suggestion that a TCA may be superior to a stimulant in cases of ADHD when depression or anxiety is a prominent comorbidity.

Stimulant Treatment of Adult ADHD and MDD

Despite the increasing recognition of adult ADHD, little is known about the psychopharmacological management of this disorder in adults. In contrast to the more than 100 studies of stimulant efficacy in children and adolescents with ADHD, there are only 6 controlled studies (*N* = 157 subjects) on the efficacy of stimulants in adults with ADHD, and their results have been mixed. For example, of the four previous controlled studies evaluating the efficacy of methylphenidate in adults with ADHD, only one (Wood et al. 1976) reported a robust response to the drug (73%). In contrast, the other three controlled studies reported levels of response ranging from 25% (Mattes et al. 1984) to 57% (Wender et al. 1985). The discrepancies among these studies may be related to low doses, diagnostic uncertainties, and lack of attention to comorbid disorders.

In these studies of stimulant treatment of ADHD, comorbidity has been a prominent factor. For instance, Wender et al. (1981, 1985) and Wood et al. (1976) reported high rates (67%–81%) of minor mood disorders (dysthymia and cyclothymia) in adults with ADHD, even with the exclusion of major mood disorders. Although these investigators reported that stimulants were efficacious in treating adults with ADHD, the effect of such minor mood disorders on treatment outcome was not examined. In a study of clinically referred adults with ADHD, Shekim et al. (1990) also found high rates of mood disorders. Even with the exclusion of major affective disorders in the last 2 years of the study, the authors reported rates of dysthymic disorder of 25% and cyclothymic disorder of 25%; 10% of the subjects in the total sample had a history of major affective disorder. Further, in an open trial of methylphenidate (40 mg/day) in these adults with ADHD, Shekim et al. reported a 70% response with no effect in the presence or absence of mood disorders.

Our group recently conducted a randomized, 7-week, placebo-controlled crossover study of methylphenidate treatment in 23 adult patients with DSM-III-R ADHD, using standardized instruments for diagnosis; separate assessments of ADHD, depressive, and anxiety symptoms; and a robust daily dose of 1.0 mg/kg (Spencer et al. 1995) (Figure 3–6). We found a marked therapeutic response for the methylphenidate treatment of ADHD symptoms that exceeded the placebo response (78% vs. 4%, $P < 0.0001$). We observed only modest improvement in ADHD symptoms with methylphenidate treatment at the daily dose of 0.5 mg/kg attained after the first week of treatment. In contrast, improvement of ADHD symptoms was far more robust at the end of treatment, when higher daily doses of about 1.0 mg/kg were attained. This suggests that the response to methylphenidate in adults with ADHD may be dose dependent. These findings are consistent with pediatric studies in which cognitive, behavioral, and academic improvements occurred in a stepwise manner with increasing doses of methylphenidate (Barkley et al. 1991; Rapport et al. 1987; Wilens and Biederman 1992). Our data strongly suggest that adults, like younger patients, require robust dosing to attain an adequate clinical response.

The positive response to methylphenidate was independent of gender, lifetime history of psychiatric comorbidity with anxiety or moderate depression,

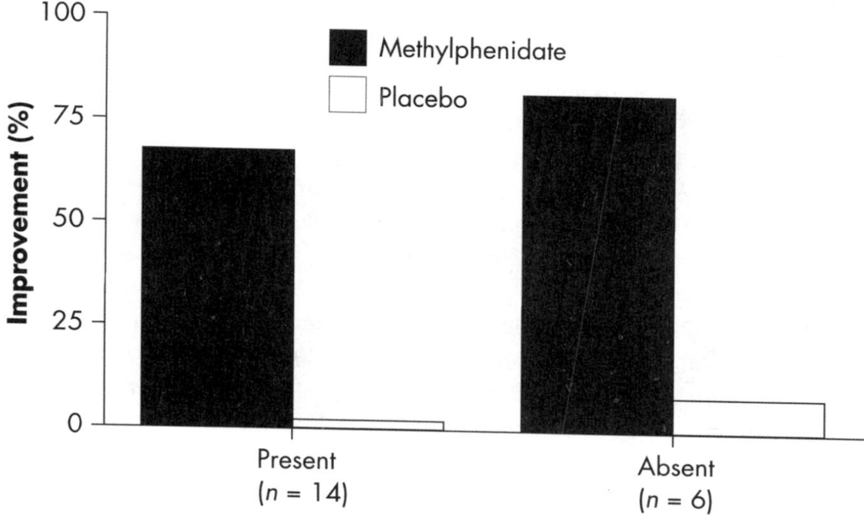

Figure 3–6. Response to methylphenidate in adults who have ADHD with and without comorbid major depressive disorder.
Source. Adapted from Spencer et al. 1995.

and family history of psychiatric disorders, including ADHD, anxiety, and depression. Although our results suggest that methylphenidate response is independent of psychiatric comorbidity when comorbidity is defined in terms of lifetime diagnosis, we could not examine the effects of active, comorbid symptoms because few of our subjects had such symptoms when they started the protocol. These results indicate that robust doses of methylphenidate are effective in the treatment of the symptoms of ADHD in adults with and without a lifetime history of comorbid depression.

Antidepressant Treatment of Adult ADHD and MDD

Despite studies in children and adolescents, there has been little systematic investigation of antidepressants for treatment of adult ADHD. Antidepressants may be particularly helpful for many adults with ADHD who have concurrent anxiety and depressive symptoms for which antidepressants have been shown to be safe, effective, and well tolerated (Baldessarini 1989). As discussed previously, there are several types of antidepressants: TCAs, SSRIs, and novel antidepressants. Although there have been no reports on SSRI treatment in adults with ADHD, the novel antidepressant bupropion was shown in an open study to be moderately helpful in reducing ADHD symptoms in adults (Wender and Reimherr 1990). The novel antidepressant venlafaxine was reported to have a moderate (50%) anti-ADHD effect in four open studies of adults with ADHD (Adler et al. 1995; Findling et al. 1996; Hornig-Rohan and Amsterdam 1995; Reimherr et al. 1995).

TCAs have been shown in controlled investigations to be effective in diminishing ADHD symptoms in children and adolescents. Ratey et al. (1992) reported effective treatment of adult ADHD in an open trial of low-dose desipramine. In a retrospective chart review of TCA treatment for adult ADHD, we also reported that desipramine and nortriptyline were helpful in the management of ADHD (Wilens et al. 1995). Recently, we reported findings from a controlled trial of desipramine at a target daily dose of 200 mg in 41 adult ADHD patients (Wilens et al. 1996). We used standardized structured psychiatric instruments for diagnosis, and as our dependent variables (outcome) we used separate assessments of ADHD, depressive, and anxiety symptoms at baseline and at each biweekly visit. Desipramine was highly effective in treating ADHD symptoms; 68% of subjects treated with the drug, compared with no subjects in the placebo group, were considered to have had a positive response ($P < 0.0001$). Response to desipramine was independent of dose, level, gender, and lifetime psychiatric comorbidity with anxiety or depressive disorders. However, as in our adult methylphenidate study (Spencer et al. 1995), we could not examine the effects of active, comorbid symptoms because few of our subjects had such symptoms when they started the protocol. These results indicate that desipramine is effective in treating symptoms of ADHD in adults with a lifetime history of comorbid depression.

Treatment of Mania and ADHD

To evaluate pharmacological approaches for treating children with ADHD and manic symptoms, we conducted an extensive chart review of 38 patients during multiple visits to assess improvement and prescription patterns (Biederman et al., in press). According to structured diagnostic interviews, the mean duration of manic symptoms prior to treatment at our center was 3.2 ± 2.5 years and the mean age at onset of mania was 5.4 ± 3.9 years. For ADHD, the mean duration of illness was 6.1 ± 3.3 years and the mean age at onset was 2.9 ± 1.9 years. The type and number of each medication prescribed, as well as an indication of improvement in mood and ADHD symptoms, were systematically collected at each follow-up visit from the medical records. The mean number of days of follow-up available for analysis was 617. As previously reported (Biederman et al. 1998a), manic symptoms improved in 34% of the 38 subjects we analyzed after treatment with mood stabilizers. These subjects contributed a total of 330 periods of observation (255 visits before initial reduction of manic symptoms and 75 after initial improvement in manic symptoms). To harvest the maximum information from each medical record, the unit of measurement we used was each visit rather than each subject, which allowed medication and improvement variables to change within subjects. The proportion of visits at which ADHD symptoms were rated as improved after initial improvement in manic-like symptoms was 7.5 times greater than before initial improvement of manic symptoms. The recurrence of manic symptoms after initial stabilization significantly inhibited ADHD response to medication of any type. Stimulants were minimally effective in treating ADHD, even after mood stabilization. Although TCAs significantly increased the probability of ADHD improvement after mood stabilization, there was also a significant association between treatment with TCAs and relapse of manic symptoms. Our results support the hypothesis that mood stabilization is a prerequisite for the successful pharmacological treatment of ADHD in children who have both ADHD and manic-like symptoms. Although TCAs can be helpful in the management of children with ADHD and manic-like symptoms, these drugs should be used with caution because they can also have a destabilizing effect on manic symptoms.

CASE VIGNETTES

Juvenile Major Depression and ADHD

H.R. had been treated with methylphenidate since the age of 8 because he exhibited inattentiveness, impulsivity, and hyperactivity, which resulted in the diagnosis of ADHD. H.R. had additional learning deficits and was in a special class in school. He was viewed as a happy child—he was succeeding in school, was socially accepted, and had no behavioral problems. At age 11 his ability to function began to deteriorate. At times he was angry, irritable, and oppositional. At other times he was withdrawn and not interested in playing with friends. Despite stimulant treatment, he could no longer concentrate on schoolwork and had no energy for the sports he used to love. Family history was significant for major depression and ADHD; his mother had depression, which had also begun in childhood, and her brother had ADHD.

During our evaluation, the diagnosis of major depression was made and methylphenidate treatment was discontinued. Treatment with the TCA desipramine was initiated along with supportive psychotherapy. After 3 weeks of combined treatment, H.R. was markedly improved. During a 1-year follow-up period, he continued to remain euthymic. The desipramine continued to successfully treat H.R.'s attention deficits until seventh grade, when academic demands increased. Reintroduction of methylphenidate, along with desipramine, improved his attentional abilities in a dramatic manner without untoward side effects.

With the new onset of depression, H.R. presented with sadness, irritability, withdrawal, anhedonia, decline in functioning, and agitation that was uncharacteristic of his early childhood. Because his mother had major depression and the clinical picture was so clear and unambiguous, the diagnosis of major depression in H.R. could be easily made despite an early history of ADHD and learning disabilities. Stimulants and academic remediation adequately managed the early clinical picture. The onset of H.R.'s severe depression was not related to major life events or to his ADHD—it was spontaneous and unpredictable. Although the pharmacotherapy of major depression includes antidepressant drugs, the use of a TCA can also ameliorate the additional disorder of ADHD. After 2 years of successful pharmacotherapy, the antidepressant is being slowly discontinued to obtain a new baseline and to evaluate the need for continued treatment.

Juvenile Bipolar Disorder

L.M. was initially evaluated at age 3 because of severe behavioral problems. L.M.'s symptom picture included excessive motor activity, inattentiveness, distractibility, moodiness, irritability, severe insomnia, and low frustration tolerance with aggressive-assaultive outbursts and extreme oppositionalism. His interpersonal approach was marked by total disregard for others to the point that parents described his interactions as "animal-like." The onset of symptoms was dated to infancy, and they were manifest at the time of evaluation in all settings—at home, in the nursery school, and at the clinician's office—and when interacting with peers. L.M.'s father had a history of similar symptoms of inattentiveness, excessive motor activity, and impulsivity in childhood, which have persisted to some extent through his adult life. L.M.'s mother had a history of a lithium-responsive bipolar disorder. Because of the pervasive psychiatric picture, L.M. required multiple school placements. He received individual psychotherapy and parental counseling for several years without much improvement. Methylphenidate treatment was helpful and L.M. was able to comply with a strict behavioral program; however, he remained moody and aggressive when frustrated.

At the age of 12, L.M.'s severe mood instability worsened. He had alternating episodes of depressive and expansive mood swings, with associated behavioral difficulties and deficits in psychosocial functioning. The mood swings, lasting hours to days, were characterized by expansive mood, irritability, pressured speech, grandiose ideation, poor judgment, and wildly agitated behaviors. During the depressive mood swings, he was sad, withdrawn, anhedonic, and fatigued from disturbed sleep and appetite.

L.M.'s symptom picture was compatible with the diagnosis of bipolar disorder with mixed presentation, in which severe mood disturbances of a depressive and manic nature present simultaneously in a continuous, alternating manner. Treatment with sodium valproate along with methylphenidate was initiated. Reports by family members and school personnel indicated that L.M. was more cooperative and less distraught. Several attempts to discontinue valproate treatment resulted in rapidly deteriorating behaviors as a result of emerging manic-like symptoms. After several months, the antidepressant bupropion was added to valproate therapy, targeted to relieve the residual depressive picture. L.M. responded very well to this treatment approach; his depressive symptoms disappeared, and he gained control of the manic symptoms. He was judged by all caretakers as dramatically improved.

Although L.M.'s diagnosis of a bipolar disorder was clear-cut, adequate consideration to the depressive picture in the treatment plan resulted in a better outcome and improved compliance. At 1-year follow-up, L.M. remains stable and more fully functional in academics, behavior, and social settings.

Adult Major Depression and ADHD

A.T., a 42-year-old male, was referred by his long-term psychotherapist to an adult outpatient psychiatric clinic. He had a history of intermittent substance use disorder, with the last episode occurring after the multiple stressors of job loss and a second divorce. A.T.'s therapist noticed that sadness, lack of energy, withdrawal from friends, and sleep disturbance persisted, despite the fact that A.T. remained sober for 5 months. In addition, A.T.'s son had been evaluated for school failure and diagnosed with ADHD. Despite normal intelligence, A.T. had also experienced multiple academic and career failures when he was not depressed and not drinking. A.T., who had outgrown his earlier symptoms of hyperactivity, recognized that he had the same symptoms of inattention and impulsivity as his son.

A.T. was diagnosed with long-standing dysthymia, recurrent major depression, inattentive type ADHD (8 of 9 symptoms of inattention since childhood), along with substance use disorder in remission. Treatment was initiated with the SSRI paroxetine. A.T.'s depressive symptoms improved dramatically, but his difficulties with inattention persisted. The addition of methylphenidate greatly improved his poor attention. With pharmacotherapy, A.T. not only became less depressed, more organized, and able to remain sober but also remained gainfully employed and was able to maintain friendships in a manner previously impossible to achieve. In this case, a stimulant was required to improve his attention. In general, clinicians must be careful in prescribing a stimulant to adults with a history of substance abuse and ADHD; however, in many patients, success with this treatment is an aid to sobriety.

CONCLUSION

There is increasing recognition that ADHD is a heterogeneous disorder with considerable and varied comorbidity. Although the causes of comorbid depressive disorders in ADHD subjects remain unknown, the weight of the available literature indicates that depressive symptoms and disorders may develop in childhood, adolescence, or adulthood and that their manifestation may not be benign. If not recognized and attended to, the combination of comorbid depressive symptoms and ADHD may lead to high morbidity and disability with poor long-term prognosis. For example, follow-up data on children with depressive disorders (Kovacs et al. 1984a, 1988) strongly indicate that juvenile mood disorders are associated with significant long-term psychiatric morbidity, which can add to the known long-term morbidity associated with ADHD. Current research findings have begun to suggest that subgroups might be delineated based on patterns of comorbidity. Recent family genetic data suggest that ADHD and major depression may share common familial vulnerabilities.

Our findings indicate that children with early-onset mania more often than not have comorbid ADHD. Although mania and ADHD have overlapping symptoms, our work identifying correlates of mania and ADHD in these children suggests that both conditions coexist. More work needs to be done to further evaluate the overlap between ADHD and mania in prepubertal children to determine the implications of the comorbid condition for clinical work and research. Such developmentally sensitive research can help identify potentially meaningful forms of ADHD with bipolar disorder and improve efforts aimed at early identification of affected individuals.

These subgroups of ADHD patients may have different risk factors, clinical course, neurobiology, and pharmacological responses; therefore, their proper identification may lead to refinements in prevention and treatment strategies. Although the high level of comorbidity within ADHD may lead to problems in differential diagnosis, these difficulties do not invalidate the diagnosis of the disorder. Rather, further examination of the patterns and structure of observed comorbidity could help revise and improve existing methods of classification.

REFERENCES

Achenbach T, Edelbrock C: Manual for the Child Behavior Checklist and Revised Child Behavior Profile. Burlington, VT, Department of Psychiatry, University of Vermont, 1983

Adler L, Resnick S, Kunz M, et al: Open-label trial of venlafaxine in attention deficit disorder. Orlando, FL, New Clinical Drug Evaluation Unit Program, 1995

Alessi NE, Magen J: Comorbidity of other psychiatric disturbances in depressed, psychiatrically hospitalized children. Am J Psychiatry 145:1582–1584, 1988

American Psychiatric Association: Diagnostic and Statistical Manual of Mental Disorders, 3rd Edition, Revised. Washington, DC, American Psychiatric Association, 1987

American Psychiatric Association: Diagnostic and Statistical Manual of Mental Disorders, 4th Edition. Washington, DC, American Psychiatric Association, 1994

Anderson JC, Williams S, McGee R, et al: DSM-III disorders in preadolescent children: prevalence in a large sample from the general population. Arch Gen Psychiatry 44:69–76, 1987

Angold A, Costello EJ. Depressive comorbidity in children and adolescents: empirical, theoretical, and methodological issues. Am J Psychiatry 150:1779–1791, 1993

Baldessarini RJ: Current status of antidepressants: clinical pharmacology and therapy. J Clin Psychiatry 50:117–126, 1989

Barkley RA: A review of stimulant drug research with hyperactive children. J Child Psychol Psychiatry 18:137–165, 1977

Barkley RA (ed): Attention Deficit Hyperactivity Disorder: A Handbook for Diagnosis and Treatment. New York, Guilford, 1990

Barkley R, DuPaul G, McMurray M: Attention deficit disorder with and without hyperactivity: clinical response to three dose levels of methylphenidate. Pediatrics 87:519–531, 1991

Biederman J, Munir K, Knee D, et al: High rate of affective disorders in probands with attention deficit disorder and in their relatives: a controlled family study. Am J Psychiatry 144:330–333, 1987

Biederman J, Baldessarini RJ, Wright V, et al: A double-blind placebo controlled study of desipramine in the treatment of ADD, I: efficacy. J Am Acad Child Adolesc Psychiatry 28:777–784, 1989

Biederman J, Faraone SV, Keenan K, et al: Family genetic and psychosocial risk factors in DSM-III attention deficit disorder. J Am Acad Child Adolesc Psychiatry 29:526–533, 1990a

Biederman J, Newcorn J, Sprich S: Comorbidity in attention deficit hyperactivity disorder, in Source Book for DSM-IV. Edited by the Task Force on DSM-IV. Washington, DC, American Psychiatric Association, 1990b, pp 145–162

Biederman J, Faraone SV, Keenan K, et al: Evidence of familial association between attention deficit disorder and major affective disorders. Arch Gen Psychiatry 48: 633–642, 1991a

Biederman J, Newcorn J, Sprich S: Comorbidity of attention deficit hyperactivity disorder with conduct, depressive, anxiety, and other disorders. Am J Psychiatry 148:564–577, 1991b

Biederman J, Faraone SV, Keenan K, et al: Further evidence for family-genetic risk factors in attention deficit hyperactivity disorder: patterns of comorbidity in probands and relatives in psychiatrically and pediatrically referred samples. Arch Gen Psychiatry 49:728–738, 1992

Biederman J, Baldessarini RJ, Wright V, et al: A double-blind placebo controlled study of desipramine in the treatment of ADD, III: lack of impact of comorbidity and family history factors on clinical response. J Am Acad Child Adolesc Psychiatry 32:199–204, 1993a

Biederman J, Faraone SV, Doyle A, et al: Convergence of the Child Behavior Checklist with structured interview-based psychiatric diagnoses of ADHD children with and without comorbidity. J Child Psychol Psychiaty 34:1241–1251, 1993b

Biederman J, Faraone SV, Spencer T, et al: Gender differences in a sample of adults with attention deficit hyperactivity disorder. Psychiatry Res 53:13–29, 1994

Biederman J, Faraone SV, Spencer T, et al: Patterns of psychiatric comorbidity, cognition, and psychosocial functioning in adults with attention deficit hyperactivity disorder. Am J Psychiatry 150:1792–1798, 1993d

Biederman J, Faraone S, Mick E, et al: Psychiatric comorbidity among referred juveniles with major depression: fact or artifact? J Am Acad Child Adolesc Psychiatry 4:579–590, 1995

Biederman J, Faraone SV, Mick E, et al: Attention deficit hyperactivity disorder and juvenile mania: an overlooked comorbidity? J Am Acad Child Adolesc Psychiatry 35:997–1008, 1996a

Biederman J, Faraone S, Milberger S, et al: A prospective 4-year follow-up study of attention-deficit hyperactivity and related disorders. Arch Gen Psychiatry 53: 437–446, 1996b

Biederman J, Mick E, Bostic JQ, et al: The naturalistic course of pharmacologic treatment of children with maniclike symptoms: a systematic chart review. J Clin Psychiatry 59:628–637, 1998a

Biederman J, Mick E, Faraone SV: Depression in attention deficit hyperactivity disorder (ADHD) children: "true" depression or demoralization? J Affect Disord 47:113–122, 1998b

Biederman J, Faraone S, Mick E, et al: Clinical correlates of attention deficit hyperactivity disorder in females: findings from a large group of pediatrically and psychiatrically referred girls. J Am Acad Child Adolesc Psychiatry 38:966–975, 1999

Biederman J, Mick E, Prince J, et al: Systematic chart review of the pharmacologic treatment of comorbid ADHD in youth with bipolar disorder. J Child Adolesc Psychopharmacol (in press)

Bird HR, Canino G, Rubio-Stipec M, et al: Estimates of the prevalence of childhood maladjustment in a community survey in Puerto Rico. Arch Gen Psychiatry 45:1120–1126, 1988

Bohline DS: Intellectual and affective characteristics of attention deficit disordered children. J Learn Disabil 18:604–608, 1985

Borland BL, Heckman HK: Hyperactive boys and their brothers: a 25-year follow-up study. Arch Gen Psychiatry 33:669–675, 1976

Bowring MA, Kovacs M: Difficulties in diagnosing manic disorders among children and adolescents. J Am Acad Child Adolesc Psychiatry 31:611–614, 1992

Brent DA, Perper JA, Goldstein CE, et al: Risk factors for adolescent suicide: a comparison of adolescent suicide victims with suicidal inpatients. Arch Gen Psychiatry 45:581–588, 1988

Brown RT, Borden KA, Clingerman SR, et al: Depression in attention deficit–disordered and normal children and their parents. Child Psychiatry Hum Dev 18: 119–132, 1988

Brumback RA: Childhood depression and medically treatable learning disability, in Brain Lateralization in Children. Edited by Molfese DL, Segalowitz SJ. New York, Guilford, 1988, pp 463–505

Brumback RA, Dietz-Schmidt SG, Weinberg WA: Depression in children referred to an educational diagnostic center: diagnosis and treatment and analysis of criteria and literature review. Diseases of the Nervous System 38:529–535, 1977

Campbell J: Manic depressive psychosis in children: report of 18 cases. J Nerv Ment Dis 116:424–439, 1952

Campbell SB, Werry JS: Attention deficit disorder (hyperactivity), in Psychopathologic Disorders of Childhood. Edited by Quay HC, Werry JS. New York, Wiley, 1986, pp 1–35

Carlson GA: Bipolar affective disorders in childhood and adolescence, in Affective Disorders in Childhood and Adolescence. Edited by Cantwell DP, Carlson GA. New York, Spectrum Publications, 1983, pp 61–83

Carlson GA: Classification issues of bipolar disorders in childhood. Psychiatric Developments 2:273–285, 1984

Coll PG, Bland R: Manic depressive illness in adolescence and childhood: review and case report. Can J Psychiatry 24:255–263, 1979

Coryell W, Scheftner W, Keller M, et al: The enduring psychosocial consequences of mania and depression. Am J Psychiatry 150:720–727, 1993

Davis RE: Manic-depressive variant syndrome of childhood: a preliminary report. Am J Psychiatry 136:702–706, 1979

Deutsch CK, Swanson JM, Bruell JH, et al: Overrepresentation of adoptees in children with the attention deficit disorder. Behavioral Genetics 12:231–238, 1982

Donnelly M, Zametkin AJ, Rapoport JL, et al: Treatment of childhood hyperactivity with desipramine: plasma drug concentration, cardiovascular effects, plasma and urinary catecholamine levels, and clinical response. Clin Pharmacol Ther 39: 72–81, 1986

DuPaul G, Barkley R, McMurray M: Response of children with ADHD to methylphenidate: interaction with internalizing symptoms. J Am Acad Child Adolesc Psychiatry 33:894–903, 1994

Dvoredsky A, Stewart M. Hyperactivity followed by manic depressive disorder: two case reports. J Clin Psychiatry 42:212–214, 1981

Emslie GJ, Rush AJ, Weinberg WA, et al: A double-blind, randomized, placebo-controlled trial of fluoxetine in children and adolescents with depression. Arch Gen Psychiatry 54:1031–1037, 1997

Faraone SV, Biederman J, Mennin D, et al: Attention deficit hyperactivity disorder with bipolar disorder: a familial subtype? J Am Acad Child Adolesc Psychiatry 36: 1378–1387, 1997

Feinstein SC: Manic-depressive disorder in children and adolescents. Adolescent Psychiatry 10:256–272, 1982

Feinstein SC, Wolpert EA: Juvenile manic-depressive illness: clinical and therapeutic considerations. J Am Acad Child Adolesc Psychiatry 12:123–136, 1973

Findling RL: Open-label treatment of comorbid depression and attentional disorders with co-administration of serotonin reuptake inhibitors and psychostimulants in children, adolescents, and adults: a case series. J Child Adolesc Psychopharmacol 6:165–175, 1996

Findling R, Schwartz M, Flannery D, et al: Venlafaxine in adults with ADHD: an open trial. J Clin Psychiatry 57:184–189, 1996

Frazier J, Meyer M, Biederman J, et al: Risperidone treatment for juvenile bipolar disorder: a retrospective chart review. J Am Acad Child Adolesc Psychiatry 38: 960–965, 1999

Fristad MA, Weller EB, Weller RA: The Mania Rating Scale: can it be used in children? A preliminary report. J Am Acad Child Adolesc Psychiatry 31:252–257, 1992

Frommer E: Recent developments in affective disorders. Br J Psychiatry 2:117–136, 1968

Frost LA, Moffitt TE, McGee R: Neuropsychological correlates of psychopathology in an unselected cohort of young adolescents. J Abnorm Psychol 98:307–313, 1989

Gammon GD, Brown TE: Fluoxetine and methylphenidate in combination for treatment of attention deficit disorder and comorbid depressive disorder. J Child Adolesc Psychopharmacol 3:1–10, 1993

Garfinkel BD, Wender PH, Sloman L, et al: Tricyclic antidepressant and methylphenidate treatment of attention deficit disorder in children. J Am Acad Child Adolesc Psychiatry 22:343–348, 1983

Geller B: Psychopharmacology of children and adolsecents: pharmacokinetics and relationships of plasma/serum levels to response. Psychopharmacol Bull 27: 401–409, 1991

Gittelman RA, Koplewicz HS: Pharmacotherapy of childhood anxiety disorders, in Anxiety Disorders of Childhood. Edited by Gittelman RA. New York, Guilford, 1986, pp 188–203

Gittelman R, Mannuzza S, Shenker R, et al: Hyperactive boys almost grown up, I: psychiatric status. Arch Gen Psychiatry 42:937–947, 1985

Goodwin F, Jamison K: Manic-Depressive Illness. New York, Oxford University Press, 1990

Goodwin F, Redfield Jamison K: Childhood and adolescence, in Manic-Depressive Illness. Edited by Goodwin F, Redfield Jamison K. New York, Oxford University Press, 1990a, pp 186–209

Goodwin FK, Redfield Jamison K: Suicide, in Manic-Depressive Illness. Edited by Goodwin FK, Redfield Jamison K. New York, Oxford University Press, 1990b, pp 227–246

Greenberg L, Yellin A, Spring C, et al: Clinical effects of imipramine and methylphenidate in hyperactive children. International Journal of Mental Health 4:144–156, 1975

Gualtieri CT, Ondrusek MG, Finley C: Attention deficit disorders in adults. Clin Neuropharmacol 8:343–356, 1985

Hornig-Rohan M, Amsterdam J: Venlafaxine vs. stimulant therapy in patients with dual diagnoses of ADHD and depression. Orlando, FL, New Clinical Drug Evaluation Unit Program, 1995

Jensen P, Shervette R III, Xenakis S, et al: Anxiety and depressive disorders in attention deficit disorder with hyperactivity: new findings. Am J Psychiatry 150:1203–1209, 1993

Kasanin J: The affective psychoses in children. Am J Psychiatry 10:897–926, 1931

Kashani JH, Orvaschel H: Anxiety disorders in mid-adolescence: a community sample. Am J Psychiatry 145:960–964, 1988

Keller MB, Beardslee W, Lavori PW, et al: Course of major depression in non-referred adolescents: a retrospective study. J Aff Disorders 15:235–243, 1988

Kovacs M: The Children's Depression Inventory (CDI). Psychopharmacol Bull 21:995–998, 1985

Kovacs M, Feinberg TL, Crouse-Novak M, et al: Depressive disorders in childhood, I: a longitudinal prospective study of characteristics and recovery. Arch Gen Psychiatry 41:229–237, 1984a

Kovacs M, Feinberg T, Crouse-Novak M, et al: Depressive disorders in childhood, II: a longitudinal study of the risk for a subsequent major depression. Arch Gen Psychiatry 41:643–649, 1984b

Kovacs M, Paulauskas S, Gatsonis C, et al: Depressive disorders in childhood, III: a longitudinal study of comorbidity with and risk for conduct disorders. J Aff Disorders 15:205–217, 1988

Lahey BB, Pelham WE, Schaughency EA, et al: Dimensions and types of attention deficit disorder. J Am Acad Child Adolesc Psychiatry 27:330–335, 1988

Loranger A, Levine P: Age at onset of bipolar affective illness. Arch Gen Psychiatry 35:1345–1348, 1978

Lowe TL, Cohen DJ: Mania in childhood and adolescence, in Mania: An Evolving Concept. Edited by Belmaker RH, van Praag HM. Jamaica, NY, Spectrum Publications, 1980, pp 111–117

Mannuzza S, Klein RG, Bessler A, et al: Adult outcome of hyperactive boys: educational achievement, occupational rank, and psychiatric status. Arch Gen Psychiatry 50:565–576, 1993

Maser JD, Cloninger CR: Comorbidity of anxiety and mood disorders: introduction and overview, in Comorbidity of Mood and Anxiety Disorders. Edited by Maser JD, Cloninger CR. Washington, DC, American Psychiatric Press, 1990, pp 1–12

Mattes JA, Boswell L, Oliver H: Methylphenidate effects on symptoms of attention deficit disorder in adults. Arch Gen Psychiatry 41:1059–1063, 1984

McElroy SL, Keck PE Jr, Pope HG Jr, et al: Clinical and research implications of the diagnosis of dysphoric or mixed mania or hypomania. Am J Psychiatry 149:1633–1644, 1992

McGee R, Williams S, Silva PH: Factor structure and correlates of ratings of inattention, hyperactivity, and antisocial behavior in a large sample of 9-year-old children from the general population. J Consult Clin Psychol 53:480–490, 1985

McGlashan T: Adolescent versus adult onset of mania. Am J Psychiatry 145:221–223, 1988

McHarg JF. Mania in childhood. Archives of Neurology 72:531–539, 1954

McKnew D, Cytryn L, White I: Clinical and biochemical correlates of hypomania in a child. J Am Acad Child Adolesc Psychiatry 13:576–584, 1974

Munir K, Biederman J, Knee D: Psychiatric comorbidity in patients with attention deficit disorder: a controlled study. J Am Acad Child Adolesc Psychiatry 26:844–848, 1987

Orvaschel H: Psychiatric interviews suitable for use in research with children and adolescents. Psychopharmacol Bull 21:737–745, 1985

Orvaschel H: Comorbidity of attention deficit disorder and depression. Paper presented at the World Federation of Societies of Biological Psychiatry Regional Meeting, Jerusalem, Israel, 1989

Orvaschel H, Walsh-Allis G, Ye W. Psychopathology in children of parents with recurrent depression. J Abnorm Child Psychol 16:17–28, 1988

Pauls DL, Hurst CR, Kruger SD, et al: Gilles de la Tourette's syndrome and attention deficit disorder with hyperactivity: evidence against a genetic relationship. Arch Gen Psychiatry 43:1177–1179, 1986a

Pauls DL, Towbin KE, Leckman JF, et al: Gilles de la Tourette's syndrome and obsessive-compulsive disorder: evidence supporting a genetic relationship. Arch Gen Psychiatry 43:1180–1182, 1986b

Pliszka SR: Effect of anxiety on cognition, behavior, and stimulant response in ADHD. J Am Acad Child Adolesc Psychiatry 28:882–887, 1989

Post RM. Transduction of psychosocial stress into the neurobiology of recurrent affective disorder. Am J Psychiatry 149:999–1010, 1992

Potter RL: Manic-depressive variant syndrome of childhood: diagnostic and therapeutic considerations. Clin Pediatr 22:495–499, 1983

Poznanski E, Israel M, Grossman J: Hypomania in a four-year-old. J Am Acad Child Adolesc Psychiatry 23:105–110, 1984

Puig-Antich J: Affective disorders in children and adolescents: diagnostic validity and psychobiology, in Psychopharmacology: The Third Generation of Progress. Edited by Meltzer HY. New York, Raven, 1987, pp 843–859

Puig-Antich J, Goetz D, Davies M, et al: A controlled family history study of prepubertal major depressive disorder. Arch Gen Psychiatry 46:406–418, 1989

Rapoport JL, Quinn P, Bradbard G, et al: Imipramine and methylphenidate treatment of hyperactive boys: a double-blind comparison. Arch Gen Psychiatry 30:789–793, 1974

Rapport MD, Jones JT, DuPaul GJ, et al: Attention deficit disorder and methylphenidate: group and single-subject analyses of dose effects on attention in clinic and classroom settings. J Clin Child Psychol 16:329–338, 1987

Ratey J, Greenberg M, Bemporad J, et al:. Unrecognized attention-deficit hyperactivity disorder in adults presenting for outpatient psychotherapy. J Child Adolesc Psychopharmacol 2:267–275, 1992

Reimherr F, Hedges D, Strong R, et al: An open trial of venlaxine in adult patients with attention deficit hyperactivity disorder. Orlando, FL, New Clinical Drug Evaluation Unit Program, 1995

Reiss AL: Developmental manifestations in a boy with prepubertal bipolar disorder. J Clin Psychiatry 46:441–443, 1985

Rutter M. Isle of Wight revisited: twenty-five years of child psychiatric epidemiology. J Am Acad Child Adolesc Psychiatry 28:633–653, 1989

Ryan ND: Pharmacotherapy of adolescent major depression: beyond TCAs. Psychopharmacol Bull 26:75–79, 1990

Ryan ND, Puig-Antich J: Affective illness in adolescence, in American Psychiatric Association Annual Review. Edited by Frances AJ, Hales RE. Washington, DC, American Psychiatric Press, 1986, pp 420–450

Ryan ND, Puig-Antich J, Ambrosini P, et al: The clinical picture of major depression in children and adolescents. Arch Gen Psychiatry 44:854–861, 1987

Sachs GS, Conklin A, Lafer B, et al: Psychopathology in children of late vs. early onset bipolar probands. Proceedings, American Academy of Child and Adolescent Psychiatry Annual Meeting, San Antonio, TX, 1993

Sadler W: Juvenile manic activity. Nervous Child 9:363–368, 1952

Shekim WO, Asarnow RF, Hess E, et al: A clinical and demographic profile of a sample of adults with attention deficit hyperactivity disorder, residual state. Compr Psychiatry 31:416–425, 1990

Spencer TJ, Biederman J, Wilens T, et al: Methylphenidate treatment in adults with childhood onset attention deficit hyperactivity disorder, in Scientific Proceedings of the American Academy of Child and Adolescent Psychiatry Annual Meeting, Washington, DC, 1992

Spencer T, Wilens TE, Biederman J, et al: A double-blind, crossover comparison of methylphenidate and placebo in adults with childhood-onset attention-deficit hyperactivity disorder. Arch Gen Psychiatry 52:434–443, 1995

Spencer T, Biederman J, Wilens T, et al: Pharmacotherapy of attention-deficit hyperactivity disorder across the life cycle. J Am Acad Child Adolesc Psychiatry 35:409–432, 1996

Spitzer RL, Williams JBW, Gibbon M, et al: The Structured Clinical Interview for DSM-III-R (SCID). Arch Gen Psychiatry 49:624–629, 1992

Staton RD, Brumback RA: Non-specificity of motor hyperactivity as a diagnostic criterion. Percept Mot Skills 52:323–332, 1981

Stewart MA, Morrison JR: Affective disorders among the relatives of hyperactive children. J Child Psychol Psychiatry 14:209–212, 1973

Strober M: Relevance of early age-of-onset in genetic studies of bipolar affective disorder. J Am Acad Child Adolesc Psychiatry 31:606–610, 1992

Strober M, Carlson G: Predictors of bipolar illness in adolescents with major depression: a follow-up investigation. Journal of Adolescent Psychiatry 10:299–319, 1982

Strober M, Morrell W, Burroughs J, et al: A family study of bipolar I disorder in adolescence: early onset of symptoms linked to increased familial loading and lithium resistance. J Aff Disorders 15:255–268, 1988

Swanson J, Kinsbourne M, Roberts W, et al: Time-response analysis of the effect of stimulant medication on the learning ability of children referred for hyperactivity. Pediatrics 61:21–24, 1978

Sylvester CE, Burke PM, McCauley EA, et al: Manic psychosis in childhood: report of two cases. J Nerv Ment Dis 172:12–15, 1984

Tannock R, Ickowicz A, Schachar R: Differential effects of methylphenidate on working memory in ADHD children with and without comorbid anxiety. J Am Acad Child Adolesc Psychiatry 34:886–896, 1995

Taylor E, Schachar R, Thorley G, et al: Which boys respond to stimulant medication? A controlled trial of methylphenidate in boys with disruptive behaviour. Psychol Med 17:121–143, 1987

Thompson R, Schindler F: Embryonic mania. Child Psychiatry Hum Dev 6:149–154, 1976

Tohen M, Sanger TM, McElroy SL, et al: Olanzapine versus placebo in the treatment of acute mania: Olanzapine HGEH Study Group. Am J Psychiatry 156:702–709, 1999

Tomasson K, Kuperman S: Bipolar disorder in a prepubescent child. J Am Acad Child Adolesc Psychiatry 29:308–310, 1990

Varanka TM, Weller RA, Weller EB, et al: Lithium treatment of manic episodes with psychotic features in prepubertal children. Am J Psychiatry 145:1557–1559, 1988

Varsamis J, MacDonald SM: Manic depressive disease in childhood: a case report. Journal of the Canadian Psychiatric Association 17:279–281, 1972

Voelker SL, Lachar D, Gdowski LL: The personality inventory for children and response to methylphenidate: preliminary evidence for predictive validity. J Pediatr Psychol 8:161–169, 1983

Waizer J, Hoffman SP, Polizos P, et al: Outpatient treatment of hyperactive school children with imipramine. Am J Psychiatry 131:587–591, 1974

Warneke L: A case of manic-depressive illness in childhood. Journal of the Canadian Psychiatric Association 20:195–200, 1975

Weinberg WA, Brumback RA: Mania in childhood. American Journal of Diseases of Children 130:380–385, 1976

Weinberg WA, McLean A, Snider RL, et al: Depression, learning disability, and school behavior problems. Psychological Reports 64:275–283, 1989

Weiss G, Hechtman LT: Hyperactive Children Grown Up. New York, Guilford, 1986

Weiss G, Hechtman L, Milroy T, et al: Psychiatric status of hyperactives as adults: a controlled prospective 15-year follow-up of 63 hyperactive children. J Am Acad Child Psychiatry 24:211–220, 1985

Weller RA, Weller EB, Tucker SG, et al: Mania in prepubertal children: has it been underdiagnosed? J Affect Disord 11:151–154, 1986

Wender PH, Garfinkel BD: Attention-deficit hyperactivity disorder: adult manifestations, in Comprehensive Textbook of Psychiatry. Edited by Sadock HI, Kaplan BJ. Baltimore, MD, Williams and Wilkins, 1989, pp 1837–1841

Wender PH, Reimherr FW: Bupropion treatment of attention-deficit hyperactivity disorder in adults. Am J Psychiatry 147:1018–1020, 1990

Wender PH, Reimherr FW, Wood DR. Attention deficit disorder ("minimal brain dysfunction") in adults: a replication study of diagnosis and drug treatment. Arch Gen Psychiatry 38:449–456, 1981

Wender PH, Reimherr FW, Wood DR, et al: A controlled study of methylphenidate in the treatment of attention deficit disorder, residual type, in adults. Am J Psychiatry 142:547–552, 1985

Werry JS, Aman MG, Diamond E: Imipramine and methylphenidate in hyperactive children. J Child Psychol Psychiatry 21:27–35, 1980

Wilens T, Biederman J: The stimulants, in Psychiatric Clinics of North America. Edited by Schaffer D. Philadelphia, PA, WB Saunders, 1992, 191–222

Wilens TE, Biederman J, Mick E, et al: A systematic assessment of tricyclic antidepressants in the treatment of adult attention-deficit hyperactivity disorder. J Nerv Ment Dis 183:48–50, 1995

Wilens TE, Biederman J, Prince J, et al: Six-week, double-blind, placebo-controlled study of desipramine for adult attention deficit hyperactivity disorder. Am J Psychiatry 153:1147–1153, 1996

Winsberg BG, Bialer I, Kupietz S, et al: Effects of imipramine and dextroamphetamine on behavior of neuropsychiatrically impaired children. Am J Psychiatry 128:1425–1431, 1972

Wood DR, Reimherr FW, Wender PH, et al: Diagnosis and treatment of minimal brain dysfunction in adults: a preliminary report. Arch Gen Psychiatry 33:1453–1460, 1976

Wozniak J, Biederman J, Kiely K, et al: Prepubertal mania revisited, in Scientific Proceedings of the American Academy of Child and Adolescent Psychiatry Annual Meeting, San Antonio, TX, 1993

Wozniak J, Biederman J, Mundy E, et al: A pilot family study of childhood-onset mania. J Am Acad Child Adolesc Psychiatry 34:1577–1583, 1995

Yepes LE, Balka EB, Winsberg BG, et al: Amitriptyline and methylphenidate treatment of behaviorally disordered children. J Child Psychol Psychiatry 18:39–52, 1977

4 Attention-Deficit/ Hyperactivity Disorder With Anxiety Disorders

Rosemary Tannock, Ph.D.

Attention-deficit/hyperactivity disorder (ADHD) and anxiety disorders are the most prevalent psychiatric problems in childhood and adolescence, as demonstrated by recent epidemiological studies (e.g., Anderson et al. 1987; Bird et al. 1988). Moreover, these two disorders frequently occur in the same individual: ADHD and anxiety disorders occur together in approximately 25% of cases in both epidemiological and clinical samples (Biederman et al. 1991b). This finding challenges the clinical tradition of differentiating ADHD and anxiety disorders along the polarized dimensions of externalizing and internalizing disorders, respectively, and poses problems for nosology, clinical practice, and research. For example, the comorbid pattern of ADHD and anxiety disorders presents clinicians with diagnostic and therapeutic challenges. Do children who meet diagnostic criteria for both disorders exhibit 1) attention difficulties that are secondary to anxiety (i.e., a "masked" anxiety disorder); 2) anxiety problems that occur as a result of persistent demoralization from the problems associated with ADHD (i.e., "complex"

This work was supported in part by a Scientist Award from the Medical Research Council of Canada and a grant from the National Institutes of Health (RO1 HD31714). The author thanks Drs. Ickowicz, Manassis, Bradley, and Schachar, in the Department of Psychiatry at The Hospital for Sick Children, Toronto, for their helpful comments on this chapter. Special thanks to Dr. Ickowicz and to Patricia Fulford for their clinical and research help with the children with ADHD and anxiety.

ADHD); 3) two disorders, each with its distinct etiology and treatment response; or 4) a heretofore unclassified disorder with an etiology, course, and treatment response that is distinct from those of both ADHD and anxiety disorders? Should clinicians treat the ADHD symptoms, the anxiety symptoms, or both sets of symptoms? Does the presence of anxiety disorder alter the indications for treatment of the ADHD?

My primary objective in this chapter is to review the literature to determine whether the presence of concurrent anxiety disorders alters the meaning of ADHD in terms of its clinical presentation, correlates and risk factors, clinical course, and response to treatment. I then discuss the implications for diagnostic assessment and treatment of anxious children with ADHD. However, before I embark on the body of the review of the comorbidity between ADHD and anxiety disorders, a few comments are warranted on the classification, prevalence, and correlates of anxiety disorders in childhood. (Comprehensive reviews of childhood anxiety disorders can be found in numerous articles [Bernstein and Borchardt 1991; Biederman 1990; Kashani et al. 1991; Rapoport 1991; Werry 1991] and texts [Gittelman 1986; Husain and Kashani 1991; Klein and Last 1989; Last 1988; March 1995].)

ANXIETY DISORDERS IN CHILDREN: A SYNOPSIS

Many children experience fears and anxieties in childhood and adolescence that are transitory or specific to a stage of development (Bell-Dolan et al. 1990). These fears and anxieties are considered to reflect normal development. By contrast, some anxieties or fears are persistent, accompanied by impairments in social function, and may meet the diagnostic criteria for a clinically meaningful disorder.

Classification

DSM-III-R (American Psychiatric Association 1987) delineated three anxiety disorders that are specific to children and adolescents and other anxiety disorders that can be assigned throughout the age span (Table 4–1). However, of the three disorders specific to childhood or adolescence, only separation anxiety disorder was preserved in DSM-IV (American Psychiatric Asociation 1994), and the duration criterion for the disorder was increased from 2 weeks to 4 weeks. Overanxious disorder was subsumed under generalized anxiety disorder, and avoidant disorder was subsumed under social phobia.

Table 4–1. Diagnostic taxonomies for anxiety disorders

DSM-III-R[a]	DSM-IV[b]
Anxiety disorders of childhood or adolescence	**Anxiety disorders of childhood or adolescence**
Separation anxiety disorder	Separation anxiety disorder
Overanxious disorder	
Avoidant disorder	
Adult anxiety disorders	**Anxiety disorders[c]**
Panic disorder (with and without agoraphobia)	Panic disorder (with and without agoraphobia)
Agoraphobia (with and without panic disorder)	Agoraphobia (with history of panic disorder)
Social phobia	Social phobia (social anxiety disorder)
Simple phobia	Specific phobia
Obsessive-compulsive disorder	Obsessive-compulsive disorder
Posttraumatic stress disorder	Posttraumatic stress disorder
Generalized anxiety disorder	Acute stress disorder
Anxiety disorder not otherwise specified	Generalized anxiety disorder[d]
Adjustment disorder	
Adjustment disorder with anxious mood	

[a]American Psychiatric Association 1987.
[b]American Psychiatric Association 1994.
[c]Child, adolescent, and adult.
[d]Includes overanxious disorder of childhood.

Overanxious disorder was defined as generalized, persistent anxiety that had lasted at least 6 months and that was not related to a specific situation, person, object, or recent stressor. As shown in Table 4–2, the DSM-III-R and the DSM-IV diagnostic criteria for this type of childhood anxiety disorder differ substantially. Also, DSM-IV poses an additional requirement that the anxiety, worry, or physical symptoms cause clinically significant distress or impairment in social, occupational, or other important areas of functioning. The implication of these proposed changes on the pattern of comorbidity between ADHD and anxiety disorders is unknown, but the increase in overlapping features of generalized anxiety disorder and ADHD (e.g., restlessness, difficulty concentrating, irritability, sleep disturbance) may result in an apparent increase in their comorbidity. The advantage of the nosological change

Table 4–2. Diagnostic criteria for overanxious disorder (DSM-III-R) and generalized anxiety disorder (DSM-IV) in childhood

Overanxious disorder	**Generalized anxiety disorder**
A. Excessive anxiety or worry for at least 6 months, indicated by at least 4 symptoms:	A. Excessive anxiety or worry more days than not for at least 6 months about a number of events and activities
1. Worry about future events	B. Difficult to control the worry
2. Worry about past behavior	C. Anxiety and worry associated with at least one of the following symptoms:
3. Concern about competence	
4. Somatic complaints	1. Restlessness
5. Masked self-consciousness	2. Easily fatigued
6. Continual need for reassurance	3. Difficulty concentrating/mind goes blank
7. Tense/unable to relax	4. Irritability
B. Focus of symptoms are not confined to another Axis I disorder	5. Muscle tension
C. If 18 years or older, does not meet the criteria for generalized anxiety disorder	6. Sleep disturbance (difficulty falling or staying asleep, or restless, unsatisfying sleep)
D. Occurrence not exclusively during course of pervasive developmental disorder, schizophrenia, or other psychotic disorder	D. Focus of anxiety or worry not confined to features of of Axis I disorder
	E. Anxiety, worry, or physical symptoms cause significant impairment
	F. Disturbance not due to the direct physiological effects of substance or medical condition, nor occurs exclusively during mood disorder, psychotic disorder, or pervasive developmental disorder

Source. Criteria adapted from DSM-III-R (American Psychiatric Association 1987) and DSM-IV (American Psychiatric Association 1994), which subsumes overanxious disorder under generalized anxiety disorder.

is the implicit recognition that anxiety disorders in childhood may be continuous with those in adulthood, although the nature of the association between anxiety disorders in childhood and adulthood is unclear. The disadvantage is that little is known in children about the anxiety disorders listed in the "adult" section of DSM-IV, because most of the available studies of anxiety disorders in children and the comorbid condition of ADHD and anxiety disorder have focused primarily on the anxiety disorders specific to childhood.

Epidemiology

In contrast to clinical beliefs that anxiety disorders in childhood are uncommon, transient, and benign (e.g., Graham and Rutter 1973; Robins 1984), subsequent epidemiological work suggests not only that anxiety disorders are the most common problems of childhood but also that their prevalence increases through adolescence. Prevalence figures for the anxiety disorders, as well as those for ADHD, are shown in Table 4–3 (see also Table 3 in Angold et al. 1999). However, one major problem in obtaining a composite picture of the epidemiology of anxiety disorders is the use of different approaches to combining information from different informants, such as the child, parent, and teacher (Bernstein and Borchardt 1991). Systematic investigations of methods for aggregating information from multiple informants indicate the following:

1. Prevalence rates of anxiety disorders that are based on child interview alone are much higher than those based on parent interview alone.
2. There is little overlap between parent and child report of the child's anxiety symptoms; children who report anxiety disorders are generally not the children whose parents report anxiety disorders in their children.
3. There is marked disagreement about anxiety symptoms and level of impairment even among adult informants, such as parents, teachers, and clinicians (e.g., Benjamin et al. 1990; Bird et al. 1992; Costello et al. 1988).

Comorbidity

Approximately one-third of children with anxiety disorders meet the criteria for two or more anxiety disorders (Kashani and Orvaschel 1990; Strauss and Last 1993; for a recent critical review of this comorbidity, see Angold et al. 1999). Also, comorbidity with depression and with ADHD is common (e.g., Angold and Costello 1993; Benjamin et al. 1990; Biederman et al. 1991b; Kashani and Orvaschel 1988; Last et al. 1992; McGee et al. 1990). Thus, a complex pattern of ADHD with comorbid anxiety disorders and depression may be expected (see Anderson et al. 1989; Jensen et al. 1993; Livingston et al. 1990; McClellan et al. 1990; Rende 1993).

Correlates and Risk Factors

A number of family and child variables have been identified as possible correlates and risk factors of anxiety disorder. These include the following:

Table 4–3. Prevalence of childhood anxiety disorders and attention-deficit disorders

				Proportion of sample (%)							ADHD + ANX	
Location	***N***	**Age (years)**	**Informant**[a]	**OAD**	**SAD**	**SiPh**	**SoPh**	**OCD**	**ANX (any)**[b]	**ADHD**[b]	**% ADHD with ANX**	**% ANX with ADHD**
Canada 1 (Offord et al. 1987)	2,679	4–16	C,P,T	—	—	—	—	—	7.9 (M) 11.9 (F)	8.9 (M) 3.3 (F)	—	—
Canada 2 (Bowen et al. 1990)	1,299	12–16	C	3.6	2.4	—	—	—	—	—	22.6	21.2
Israel (Zohar et al. 1992)	562	16–17	C	—	—	—	—	3.6	—	3.9	—	—
New Zealand 1 (Anderson et al. 1987)	792	11	C,P,T	2.9	3.5	2.4	0.9	—	7.5	6.7	26	24
New Zealand 2[c] (McGee et al. 1990, 1992)	750	11 15	C,P C,P	2.5 5.2	1.9 1.7	1.7 3.1	0.4 1.3	— —	10.7	1.7 1.2	20	6
New Zealand 3 (Fergusson et al. 1993)	986	15	P C	0.6 2.1	0.1 0.5	0.7 1.7	1.3 5.1	— —	3.9 10.8	3.0 2.8	— —	— —
Puerto Rico (Bird et al. 1988)	386	4–16	C,P	—	4.7	2.6	—	—	6.6	9.5	8	18

United States												
New York State (Velez et al. 1989)	766	9–12[d]	C,P	19.1	25.6	—	—	—	—	16.6	—	—
		13–18[d]	C,P	12.7	6.8	—	—	—	—	9.9		
		11–14[e]	C,P	9.7	15.3	—	—	—	—	12.8		
		15–20	C,P	8.6	4.4	—	—	—	—	6.8		
Missouri (Kashani et al. 1987)	150	14–16	C,P	7.3	0.7	4.7	—	—	8.7	2.0	—	—
Pittsburgh (PA) (Benjamin et al. 1990; Costello et al. 1988)	789	7–11	P	2.8	0.4	3.0	0	—	6.6	1.6	—	22.4
			C	2.0	4.1	6.7	1.0	—	10.5	0.6		
			P/C	4.6	4.1	9.2	1.0	—	—	2.2		

Note. OAD = overanxious disorder; SAD = separation anxiety disorder; SiPh = simple phobia; SoPh = social phobia; OCD = obsessive-compulsive disorder; ANX = anxiety disorders; ADHD = attention-deficit disorder or attention-deficit hyperactivity disorder. Dashes indicate not reported.

[a]C = child; P = parent; T = teacher.

[b]M = male; F = female.

[c]Prospective follow-up study of the 1987 (New Zealand 1) cohort; children reassessed every 2 years.

[d]ANX defined as "emotional disorder."

[e]Follow-up study of the two preceding age cohorts.

1. Familial patterns of anxiety (e.g., Benjamin et al. 1990; Crowe et al. 1983; Last et al. 1987; Rende 1993; Sylvester et al. 1987; Turner et al. 1987; Weissman et al. 1984)
2. Problems in pregnancy (Velez et al. 1989)
3. Specific temperamental traits in infancy and early childhood, such as high emotionality in infancy (Rende 1993) or excessive and persistent shyness and withdrawal in unfamiliar situations throughout infancy and early childhood (Biederman et al. 1990b, 1993c; Hirshfeld et al. 1992; Rosenbaum et al. 1988)
4. A high frequency of stressful life events (Benjamin et al. 1990; Bernstein et al. 1989; Kashani et al. 1990)
5. Low self-esteem (Anderson et al. 1989) and impaired social and academic function that is perceived by teachers (but not by parents) to be as problematic as the impairment associated with externalizing, disruptive behavior disorders (Benjamin et al. 1990; Bowen et al. 1990)

The pattern of risk factors may differ for boys and girls (Rende 1993). However, caution is required when interpreting these research findings, because few of the studies demonstrated that the correlates and risk factors differentiate anxiety disorders from other psychiatric disorders or controlled for comorbid disorders. Thus, these correlates and risk factors may not be specific to anxiety disorders (Links et al. 1990).

Clinical Course

Childhood anxiety disorders are not transient and benign, nor do they appear to remit spontaneously as often as believed (e.g., Robins 1984). Their persistent course is indicated by both cross-sectional and longitudinal follow-up studies, although the relative persistence of internalizing versus externalizing disorders remains an ongoing source of controversy (e.g., compare Esser et al. 1990; Verhulst and van der Ende 1992). Lifetime estimates predicted that 46% of children with untreated anxiety disorders would be likely to remain ill for at least 8 years (Keller et al. 1992). Prospective studies of community samples suggest that clinicians can expect untreated anxiety disorders (and other internalizing disorders) to persist for at least 4–6 years in approximately 25%–33% of cases (Feehan et al. 1993; McGee et al. 1992; Offord et al. 1992; Verhulst and van der Ende 1992).

Advances in the knowledge of the prevalence, protracted course, and severity of anxiety disorders in children and adolescents (e.g., Keller et al. 1992;

Last et al. 1992; Benjamin et al. 1990) have challenged the common beliefs that these disorders are uncommon, transient, and innocuous (e.g., Robins 1984). In the next section I review the literature on the impact of comorbid anxiety on ADHD, while considering, reciprocally, the impact of comorbid ADHD on anxiety disorders.

ADHD WITH COMORBID ANXIETY DISORDERS

Epidemiology

About one in four children with ADHD is likely to present with one or more concurrent anxiety disorders according to recent epidemiological work. As shown in Table 4–3, the high level of comorbidity between ADHD and anxiety disorders has been found in culturally and regionally diverse epidemiological samples, as well as in clinically referred samples of children with ADHD and children with anxiety disorders. As might be expected, higher rates of comorbidity are found in clinical samples (Berkson 1946). As shown in Table 4–4, 30%–40% of the ADHD children referred to clinics are likely to meet the diagnostic criteria for one or more anxiety disorders. Conversely, studies of clinically referred children with anxiety disorders indicate that 15%–30% of these children meet the diagnostic criteria for ADHD (Table 4–4).

No specific links have been found between the various types of anxiety disorders and ADHD, but a study by Last and colleagues (1992) suggested that ADHD was more strongly linked with overanxious disorder or separation anxiety disorder than with phobia. For example, the rates of lifetime disruptive behavior disorders (ADHD, oppositional defiant disorder, conduct disorder) ranged from a low of 8% for social phobia, to 15% for avoidant disorder, to highs of 20% for overanxious disorder and 27% for separation anxiety disorder. Moreover, although cases of ADHD with comorbid obsessive-compulsive disorder (OCD) have been reported (e.g., Bussing and Levin 1993; Last et al. 1992), there is no evidence that ADHD is significantly elevated among individuals with OCD relative to population rates (Zohar et al. 1992). Since the rate of ADHD is elevated among individuals with Tourette syndrome (Walkup et al. 1999), and the rate of Tourette syndrome is elevated among individuals with OCD (Zohar et al. 1992), the co-occurrence of ADHD and OCD may be mediated by the links between each disorder and Tourette syndrome (Pauls and Leckman 1986). Reciprocally, no specific links have been found between subtypes of ADHD and anxiety disorders. Some studies have suggested a specific link between one subtype of attention-deficit disorder (attention-deficit

Table 4–4. Prevalence of comorbid ADHD and anxiety disorders in clinical studies

Study	ANX with ADHD	ADHD with ANX	ADHD + ANX
Studies of anxiety disorders			
Last et al. 1987	20%–27%		
Last et al. 1992	17%–18%		
Strauss et al. 1988	35% (<12 years) 9% (≥12 years)		
Studies of ADHD			
Biederman et al. 1991[b]		30%	
Biederman et al. 1999		34%[a]	
Jensen et al. 1993		27%	
Lahey et al. 1987		43% (ADD/–H) 10% (ADD/+H)	
Livingston et al. 1990		40% (ANX/MOOD)	
Munir et al. 1987		27%	
Pliszka 1989		28%	
Risk studies (for anxiety disorders and/or depression)			
Keller et al. 1992			16%[a]
McClellan et al. 1990			32%[b]
Other studies			
Woolston et al. 1989			38%[b] 23%[c]

Note. ANX = anxiety disorders; ADHD = attention-deficit hyperactivity disorder; ADHD + ANX = comorbid attention-deficit hyperactivity disorder and anxiety disorders; ADD/–H = attention-deficit disorder without hyperactivity; ADD/+H = attention-deficit disorder with hyperactivity; ANX/MOOD = anxiety and/or mood disorders; PD = panic disorder.
[a]Proportion of females with ADHD who also had one or more anxiety disorders; study restricted to females. [b]Proportion of children with anxiety disorders who also had ADHD. [c]Proportion of children with ADHD who also had anxiety disorders.

disorder without hyperactivity) and anxiety disorders (Lahey et al. 1984, 1987), but others have not found differential rates of anxiety disorders among children with this subtype (Barkley et al. 1990a; Edelbrock et al. 1984; Hynd et al. 1989).

The observed rate of association between ADHD and anxiety disorders is greater than would be expected by chance alone, given the base rates of each disorder in the community. Thus, the comorbidity of ADHD with anxiety disorders is not simply an artifact of the detection method. For example, estimates based on epidemiological studies report prevalence figures ranging from 6% to 10% for ADHD and from 2% to 9% for any anxiety disorder (Table 4–3). The expected association at chance levels would range from 0.5% to 1.0% (product of the probability levels for each disorder alone), which is substantially lower than the observed association of 8%–25%. (When based on pooled diagnostic groupings [e.g., all anxiety disorders were combined], the rate of comorbidity may be underestimated [Caron and Rutter 1991].) This high rate of overlap between ADHD and anxiety disorder, particularly in clinically referred samples, indicates the need for clinicians routinely to assess the emotional functioning of children with ADHD rather than focusing exclusively on the more salient and disruptive behavioral symptoms.

Clinical Description

Children with comorbid ADHD and anxiety disorders are "worriers." In striking contrast to nonanxious children with ADHD, those with comorbid ADHD and anxiety disorders worry about their competency and performance in the areas of academics, athletics, and social situations. They even worry about their behavior. They also worry about future events, such as appointments with doctors or dentists, tests at school, and new activities. These children may not voice their worries spontaneously, but they are remarkably forthright and open when asked to complete self-ratings of anxiety or to respond to specific probes for anxiety during diagnostic interviews. In addition, many children who receive a diagnosis of ADHD and an anxiety disorder(s) manifest overt signs and symptoms of anxiety. For example, during formal assessment (e.g., diagnostic, psychoeducational, or neuropsychological), children with comorbid ADHD and anxiety disorders ask frequently for reassurance about their accuracy and competency (e.g., "Is this the right answer?" "Am I doing OK?" "Did other kids do better than me?"). Some may show reluctance to leave their parents or make frequent requests or excuses to go and see their parents at a level that is inappropriate for their age.

Anxiety Profile

An examination of the specific nature, frequency, and severity of anxiety symptoms suggests that the anxiety profile in the comorbid condition closely resembles that found in children with "pure" manifestations of a specific anxiety disorder. For example, as shown in Figure 4–1, the most common symptoms endorsed by at least 80% of parents of children with ADHD and comorbid overanxious disorder were 1) overconcern about competence in a

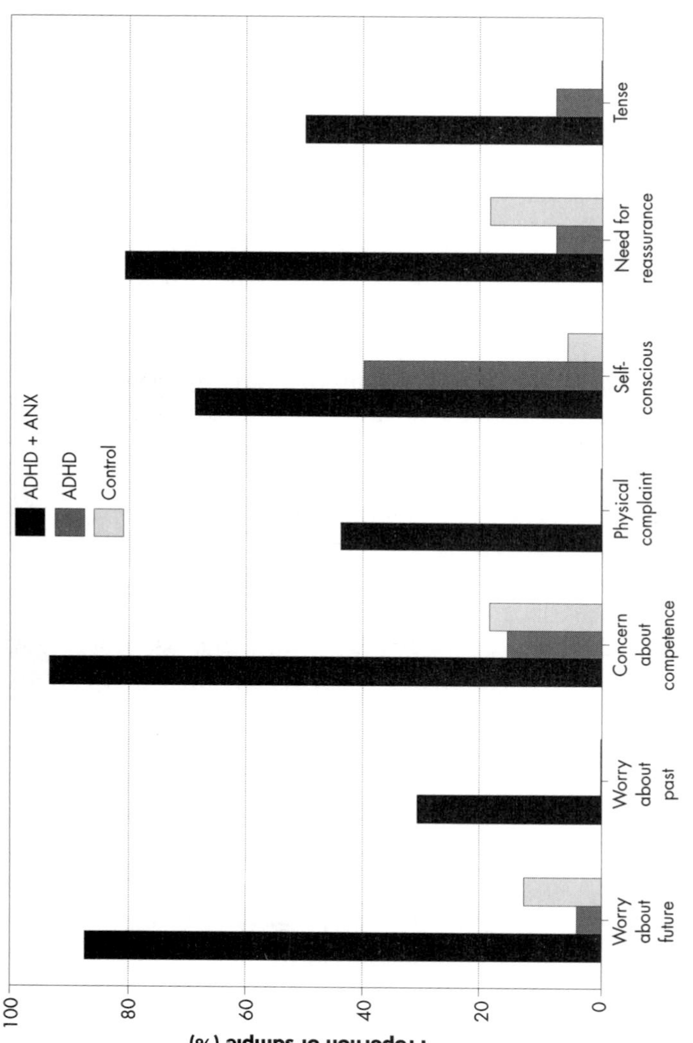

Figure 4–1. Frequency of overanxious symptoms (DSM-III-R criteria) in children with ADHD with (ADHD + ANX) and without (ADHD) comorbid anxiety disorders and control children, matched for age and IQ score.
Source. Data from an unpublished study by R. Tannock and R. J. Schachar, presented in a symposium at the 39th annual meeting of the American Academy of Child and Adolescent Psychiatry, Washington, DC, October 1992.

variety of areas, 2) unrealistic worry about future events, and 3) excessive need for reassurance (Tannock and Schachar, unpublished data, 1992). The most common symptoms manifested by children with "pure" overanxious disorder are 1) unrealistic worry about future events, 2) preoccupation with appropriateness of the individual's behavior in the past, 3) overconcern about competence in a variety of areas, 4) somatic complaints, and 5) marked self-consciousness or susceptibility to embarrassment or humiliation (Keller et al. 1992; Strauss et al. 1988). Direct comparison of the anxiety profile of comorbid ADHD and anxiety disorders with that of anxiety disorders is required to confirm the apparent similarity of the anxiety profiles in comorbid and pure conditions.

ADHD Profile

Despite their worries about their performance and behavior, children with comorbid ADHD and anxiety disorders also exhibit marked ADHD symptoms. Parents typically report a developmental history of short attention span and restless, impulsive behavior. They also describe presenting problems that include restless, fidgety, and off-task behavior, with difficulty concentrating on and completing the task at hand. In other words, these children clearly meet the DSM-III-R or DSM-IV diagnostic criteria for ADHD, as well as for one or more anxiety disorders, even when structured and semistructured diagnostic interviews are used (e.g., Pliszka 1992; Pliszka et al. 1993; Tannock et al. 1995b).

There is some evidence that the presence of concurrent anxiety disorder may alter the ADHD symptoms, but it is unclear in what way, because the research findings are inconsistent. One strand of research based on DSM-III criteria linked attention-deficit disorder without hyperactivity with anxiety disorders (e.g., Barkley 1990, pp. 74–105; Lahey et al. 1987). Other studies based on DSM-III-R criteria produced inconsistent findings. For example, Pliszka (1989, 1992) found that children with comorbid ADHD and anxiety disorders were rated as less inattentive and overactive by teachers and exhibited fewer behavioral symptoms of ADHD (e.g., off-task behavior, fidgeting, playing with objects, out of seat) during structured activities in laboratory settings, compared with nonanxious children with ADHD (Pliszka 1989, 1992). In contrast, Livingston et al. (1990) found that teachers rated boys with attention-deficit disorder and anxiety/mood disorders as more inattentive, hyperactive, and aggressive than those with attention-deficit disorder alone. Others have found no differences in ADHD symptoms between children with ADHD and comorbid anxiety disorders and those with ADHD alone (Pliszka et al. 1993, 1997). More recent studies based on DSM-IV criteria have also yielded inconsistent findings (e.g., Eiraldi et al. 1997; Faraone et al. 1998; Gaub and Carlson 1997; Morgan et al. 1996). The discrepant findings may reflect sampling biases, variation in diagnostic criteria and/or diagnostic procedures, or differences in other comorbid disorders (e.g., conduct disorder, learning disabilities) rather than systematic differences that are attributable to the impact of comorbid anxiety disorders on ADHD.

To summarize, the current data suggest that clinicians should not expect the presenting symptoms of ADHD or anxiety disorders to provide a clue to the comorbidity in terms of the distinction between primary and secondary diagnoses (i.e., whether the anxiety symptoms are secondary to ADHD or vice versa). Investigations of symptom expression in comorbid ADHD and anxiety disorders versus ADHD have provided little evidence to date that the presence of an anxiety disorder alters the clinical presentation of ADHD in a systematic way. Comparisons of children with "pure" anxiety disorders and those with comorbid ADHD and anxiety disorders are required before we can conclude that the presence of comorbid ADHD does not alter the anxious symptoms in anxiety disorders.

Correlates and Risk Factors

Potential predictors and correlates of the early emergence and persistence of ADHD include familial history of ADHD, perinatal complications, and overactivity and demandingness in infancy (e.g., Barkley et al. 1990a; Hartsough and Lambert 1985; Nichols and Chen 1981). These variables stand in apparent contrast to several of the predictors and correlates associated with anxiety disorders that were described previously (e.g., family history of anxiety disorders, shy and inhibited behavior in infancy, and a high frequency of stressful life events).

Investigations of the correlates and risk factors associated with comorbid ADHD and anxiety disorders, although few in number, provide an opportunity to examine competing hypotheses for the overlap between ADHD and anxiety disorders. For example, evidence that the correlates of the comorbid group resemble those of one of the pure groups (e.g., anxiety disorder) would support the interpretation of a primary disorder (i.e., anxiety disorder in this example) that leads to a phenocopy of the other disorder (e.g., ADHD), which would thus be deemed secondary.

Psychosocial Correlates

A limited number of studies provide information about family history, perinatal complications, early temperament, life stresses, adaptive functioning, and self-esteem in children with comorbid ADHD and anxiety disorders versus ADHD alone, but comparisons with anxiety disorders are not yet available. Recent family genetic studies indicate not only a familial association between attention-deficit disorder and anxiety disorders but also differences in the pattern for ADHD children with and without comorbid anxiety disorders (Biederman et al. 1990a, 1991a; Sylvester et al. 1987). A central finding was that first-degree relatives (i.e., parents and siblings) of children with comorbid attention-deficit disorder and anxiety disorders had a similar risk for attention-deficit disorder but a much greater risk (twice as high) for anxiety disorders than did relatives of nonanxious children with attention-deficit disorder (Biederman et al. 1991a). More specifically, the relatives of children with comorbid ADHD and anxiety disorders had significantly higher risks for overanxious, panic, and phobic disorders, but not for separation anxiety disorder, avoidant disorder, agoraphobia, or OCD. Also, relatives of children with attention-deficit disorder who themselves had attention-deficit disorder tended to have a higher risk for anxiety disorders than those without attention-deficit disorder, but there was no evidence for assortative mating (Biederman et al. 1991a). From these findings, Biederman et al. (1991a) concluded that attention-deficit disorder and anxiety disorders may be transmitted independently in families.

Perinatal complications (e.g., problems during pregnancy, delivery, and the neonatal period) are likely to be more common in children with ADHD and comorbid anxiety disorders. Mothers of children with comorbid ADHD and anxiety disorders reported a higher frequency of perinatal problems and developmental delays than mothers of nonanxious children with ADHD and those of control subjects (Tannock and Schachar, unpublished data, 1992). Also, Sprich-Buckminster et al. (1993) found that the association between ADHD and perinatal complications was strongest for children with ADHD and a comorbid disorder (anxiety, major depressive, or conduct disorder), especially those without a familial history of ADHD. The sample size did not permit further analysis by specific type of comorbidity, but the data suggest that perinatal complications may be risk factors for comorbid disorders in general rather than ADHD or comorbid ADHD and anxiety disorders in particular. It should be noted that both studies used retrospective reporting and therefore were subject to potential recall bias.

Preliminary findings from an ongoing study provide not only information about several correlates (e.g., infant temperament, life stress, academic achievement, self-esteem) in ADHD versus comorbid ADHD and anxiety disorders but also the opportunity to investigate potential differences between children with comorbid ADHD and anxiety disorders based on whether the anxiety was reported by the child or the parent (M. Heung, R. Schachar, R. Tannock, unpublished data; Urman et al. 1995). The data presented here were derived from three groups of children with ADHD who were identified in a larger, clinically referred sample participating in a longer-term treatment study: 1) children whose presenting picture, as reported by either parent or child, did not meet the diagnostic criteria for an anxiety disorder; 2) those with concurrent anxiety as ascertained by child report only; and 3) those with concurrent anxiety as ascertained by parent report only. The three groups did not differ in age or IQ or in severity of ADHD, as estimated by the number of symptoms endorsed during diagnostic clinical interviews with the child's parents and teacher. None of the children had been treated previously with medication. As shown in Table 4–5, there was no evidence that the two groups with ADHD and anxiety and the group with ADHD only differed in terms of being overactive in infancy. In contrast, children in both of the groups with ADHD and anxiety were more likely to be described as aggressive in the toddler and preschool years than were children in the ADHD-only group. This differential pattern of aggressiveness appears to have persisted into middle childhood, because only the children with ADHD and anxiety (i.e., none of the children with ADHD) met the DSM-III-R diagnostic criteria for conduct disorder.

Stressful events in the child's life (e.g., parental separation or divorce; multiple parenting figures; exposure to violence, abuse, or psychiatric problems within the family) were much more common among both of the groups with comorbid ADHD and anxiety than among the ADHD group (Table 4–5). These findings are consistent with data reported by Jensen et al. (1993) showing that ADHD children with either depressive and/or anxiety disorders experienced more stressful events than children with ADHD alone. The finding that stress in the child's life, reported by parents, was associated with the child's self-rating of anxiety (Jensen et al. 1993; Tannock et al. 1992) suggests that the link between stress and anxiety is not simply an artifact of information source (Benjamin et al. 1990). The stress-anxiety link has also been reported in studies of childhood anxiety (e.g., Bernstein et al. 1989; Costello et al. 1988; Kashani et al. 1990), but since neither of the two studies on ADHD with and without anxiety included a group of children with "pure" anxiety, it is not known whether the association between stress and anxiety in the comorbid ADHD and anxiety group is comparable to that in the anxiety group.

One important finding from a clinical perspective is that children's ratings of self-esteem differentiated children with ADHD and child-reported anxiety from those with ADHD and parent-reported anxiety (Table 4–5). Not only were the self-esteem scores of the child-reported anxiety ADHD group significantly lower than those of the other two groups, but they also were suffi-

Table 4–5. Diagnostic characteristics and psychosocial correlates in children with ADHD and child-reported anxiety, parent-reported anxiety, or no anxiety

	ADHD groups			
	1 Child-ANX	**2 Parent-ANX**	**3 No ANX**	**Findings**
N	15	16	25	
Age (years)	8.4	8.2	7.9	NS
IQ score (WISC-R)	102.4	114.1	110.2	NS
No. of ADHD symptoms				
Parent interview	11.5	12.0	11.4	NS
Teacher interview	10.1	10.8	10.2	NS
No. of ANX symptoms				
OAD	1.3	3.9	1.2	2 > 1,3
SAD	1.1	1.9	0.6	2 > 1,3
RCMAS (T score)	66.3	44.4	41.9	1 > 2,3
Additional diagnoses (% sample)				
ODD	27	44	64	
Conduct disorder	40	38	0	
RLD	80	50	68	
ALD	80	19	56	
Correlates				
Infant characteristics[a] (% sample)				
Overactive	47.0	62.0	52.0	
Aggressive	40.0	56.0	24.0	
Child stress[b] (% sample)	60.0	62.0	28.3	
Self-esteem[c]				
Scholastic	13.3	16.3	16.3	1 < 3
Social	13.1	16.3	18.0	1 < 3
Athletic	15.9	18.8	20.0	1 < 3
Physical appearance	16.7	19.1	20.2	1 < 3

(continued)

Table 4–5. Diagnostic characteristics and psychosocial correlates in children with ADHD and child-reported anxiety, parent-reported anxiety, or no anxiety *(continued)*

	ADHD groups			
	1 Child-ANX	**2 Parent-ANX**	**3 No ANX**	**Findings**
Self-esteem[c] *(continued)*				
Behavior	13.5	14.1	15.7	NS
Global self-worth	15.9	20.9	18.9	1 < 2

Note. ADHD = attention-deficit/hyperactivity disorder; ANX = anxiety symptoms, based on parent interview; MLD = learning disorder in mathematics, defined as WRAT-R arithmetic score ≤ 90; NS = nonsignificant; OAD = overanxious disorder; ODD = oppositional defiant disorder; RCMAS = Revised Children's Manifest Anxiety Scale (Reynolds and Richmond 1978); RLD = learning disorder in reading, defined as WRAT-R reading score ≤ 90; SAD = separation anxiety disorder; Wechsler Intelligence Scale for Children—Revised (Wechsler 1974); WRAT-R = Wide Range Achievement Test—Revised (Jastak and Wilkinson 1984). All diagnoses DSM-III-R.

[a]Infant temperament reported by parents; overactive in infancy, aggressive in toddler/preschool years.

[b]Proportion of parents reporting stressful events in child's life (e.g., parental separation or divorce, multiple parenting figures, exposure to violence or abuse).

[c]Self-Perception Profile for Children (Harter 1985); higher scores indicate better self-esteem.

ciently low to be of clinical concern. By contrast, the scores of the other two groups did not exceed clinical cutoffs. The results suggest that children with ADHD and self-reported anxiety that is not recognized by the parents may be a group at high risk for not receiving treatment for concurrent anxiety that is causing significant impairment. Moreover, the findings highlight the importance of obtaining the child's self-report of internalizing problems: anxiety problems and poor self-esteem in children with ADHD may be overlooked by clinicians as well as parents.

Finally, children with comorbid ADHD and anxiety disorders have been found to exhibit greater impairments in adaptive functioning in school, spare-time activities, peer relations, and home life than children with ADHD only (Biederman et al. 1993b). It is important to note that children with ADHD and other comorbid disorders (depression, conduct disorder) also exhibited greater impairments relative to the group with ADHD only, but they did not differ from the group with comorbid ADHD and anxiety disorders. These findings indicate that any psychiatric comorbidity in ADHD, rather than a specific comorbidity (e.g., anxiety), may confer an increased risk for psychosocial dysfunction.

Cognitive Correlates

A small set of studies have compared children with ADHD with and without comorbid anxiety on various laboratory measures of cognitive function to determine whether anxiety alters the cognitive profile associated with ADHD. The findings from these studies are summarized in Table 4–6. The children with comorbid ADHD and anxiety disorders showed more impairment on some tasks (e.g., the serial addition task, Trailmaking Test B, complex display of memory scanning task), but less impairment on others (e.g., continuous performance test, stop signal paradigm), than the nonanxious children with ADHD.

It is important to note that the tasks on which the children with comorbid ADHD and anxiety disorders were found to have more impairment are cognitively complex and place demands on short-term or working memory—a system that is concerned with both active processing and the transient storage of information (Baddeley 1986). In contrast, tasks such as the continuous performance test (Rosvold et al. 1956), Gordon's (1979) Differential Reinforcement of Low Response Rates task, and the Stop Signal paradigm (Logan et al. 1984) are all reaction-time tasks that require response inhibition but do not require any appreciable retention of information.

Thus, these few studies yield a remarkably consistent pattern of findings and suggest that one effect of comorbid anxiety is to increase the difficulties of children with ADHD in performing tasks with high demands for working memory and effortful processing. It is unclear from these studies whether the comorbid anxiety serves to enhance performance of children with ADHD on sustained reaction time tasks in general, to counteract the inhibitory control deficits associated with ADHD (e.g., Schachar and Logan 1990; Schachar et al. 1993), or to produce both effects. Nor is it known whether the impact on cognitive function is attributable primarily to a specific cluster of anxiety symptoms (i.e., as in overanxious disorder and separation anxiety disorder) or to heightened levels of anxiety in general.

What could account for this pattern of findings? One explanation may be found in theories that account for the effects of anxiety on performance (Eysenck and Calvo 1992; Humphreys and Revelle 1984). According to these theories, the worry about task performance that results from anxiety has two main effects: 1) it serves to preempt some of the processing and storage resources of the working memory system, and 2) it has a motivational function that leads to the allocation of additional processing resources (i.e., effort) and the initiation of alternative processes (e.g., strategies) designed to improve performance. Theoretically, the motivational effect of worry may reduce or

Table 4–6. Findings of studies comparing cognitive function in anxious and nonanxious children with ADHD

Study	Sample size (*n*) and diagnoses	Diagnostic method for ANX	Measures	Findings
Pliszka 1989	57 ADHD 22 ADHD + OAD	Child report; clinical interview	Memory Scanning Test	ADHD + OAD children: slower performance only on most complex display, indicating impairment in effortful mental processing
Livingston et al. 1990	61 ADD 29 ADD + ODD/CD 21 ADD + ANX/MOOD 27 ADD + ODD/CD + ANX/MOOD	Child report; structured interview	Trail Making Test Coding Test DRLRR Timed arithmetic	ADD children with internalizing-type diagnoses: lower arithmetic and verbal IQ scores; poorer performance on Trail Making Test B and on Coding Test.
Pliszka 1992	58 ADHD 34 ADHD + OAD 12 healthy control	Child report; structured interview	CPT, Inhibition Version	ADHD + OAD children: Fewer commission errors, indicating better inhibition and less impulsiveness
Tannock et al. 1995b	22 ADHD 18 ADHD + ANX[a]	Parent and/or child report; semistructured interview with parent; child self-rating (RCMAS, STAIC)	CHIPASAT	ADHD + ANX children: Poorer performance only at the slowest rate of presentation, indicating impairment in working memory
Pliszka et al. 1993	26 ADHD 17 ADHD + OAD 8 ADHD + CD 31 healthy control 18 psychiatric control	Child report; structured interview	Stop Signal paradigm	ADHD + OAD children: Less impairment in inhibitory control than in children with ADHD or psychiatric control subjects

Note. ADD = attention deficit disorder (DSM-III-R); ADHD = attention-deficit hyperactivity disorder (DSM-III-R); ANX = anxiety disorder; ANX/MOOD = anxiety disorder or mood disorder; CD = conduct disorder; CHIPASAT = Children's Paced Auditory Serial Addition Task; CPT = continuous performance test; DRLRR = Differential Reinforcement Low Response Rates; OAD = overanxious disorder (DSM-III-R); ODD/CD = oppositional defiant disorder or conduct disorder; RCMAS = Revised Children's Manifest Anxiety Scale; STAIC = State-Trait Anxiety Inventory for Children.
[a]Mainly OAD.

eliminate the negative effects of anxiety on simple reaction time tasks by promoting the application of additional effort, but it may not counteract the negative effects on performance on tasks with heavy demands on both storage and processing resources of the working memory system (Eysenck and Calvo 1992; Humphreys and Revelle 1984). Thus, this theory predicts that anxious children with ADHD will have more impairment on working memory tasks than will nonanxious children with ADHD but less impairment on reaction time tasks—precisely the pattern of findings shown in Table 4–6.

Psychophysiological Correlates

Theoretically, ADHD and anxiety disorders are dimensionally on opposite poles in terms of neurophysiological models of behavior and childhood mental disorders (Gray 1982; Quay 1988). According to these models, two neurophysiological systems are central in controlling the individual's response to signals related to impending reward (behavioral activation system) or punishment (behavioral inhibition system). The behavioral inhibition system is believed to be controlled primarily by noradrenergic and serotonergic systems (Gray 1982). Children with anxiety are expected to show increased noradrenergic function and increased activity in the behavioral inhibition system and, thus, to be more sensitive to signals of punishment. Conversely, children with ADHD are expected to show decreased noradrenergic function and decreased activity in the behavioral inhibition system and, therefore, to be less responsive to punishment signals. In a recent test of this theory, children with ADHD, comorbid ADHD and anxiety disorders, and control subjects were compared on a classical conditioning paradigm (Pliszka et al. 1993). Skin conductance and cardiac measures (interbeat interval) were used to index psychophysiological response to a conditioned stimulus that had been paired with an aversive unconditioned stimulus. There was no evidence that comorbid anxiety altered the psychophysiological response in the children with ADHD, which in turn did not differ from that of the control children (Pliszka et al. 1993).

The limited data available suggest that children with comorbid ADHD and anxiety disorders share some of the correlates and risk factors found for nonanxious children with ADHD (e.g., family history of ADHD, overactivity in infancy). On the other hand, many of the variables that discriminated between comorbid ADHD and anxiety disorders and ADHD alone (e.g., family history of anxiety disorders; life stresses; cognitive function) have been identified as potential correlates and risk factors for anxiety disorders. Direct comparisons between ADHD, anxiety disorders, and comorbid ADHD and anxiety disorders are required to support the hypothesis that the comorbid group shares the correlates and risk factors of both of the groups with "pure" disorders.

The psychosocial and cognitive correlates of comorbid ADHD and anxiety disorders are of clinical concern for several reasons. Most academic tasks (e.g., reading, problem solving) involve working memory and effortful processing (Baddeley 1986), which are those aspects of cognitive functioning that are particularly compromised in children with ADHD who have concurrent anxiety. Moreover, many children with comorbid ADHD and anxiety disorders are also likely to have very low self-esteem (Tannock et al. 1992). Thus, clinicians should anticipate that children presenting with both ADHD and one or more anxiety disorders may have very low self-esteem that is continuously fuelled by major problems with academic and social functioning at school. Moreover, it is important to recall that in many cases the parents may be unaware of the child's anxiety (and most likely of the child's low self-esteem) and may themselves have anxiety disorders. These findings should alert clinicians to the need to obtain the child's self-report of anxiety symptoms and to assess and monitor self-esteem and academic functioning in highly anxious children with ADHD (particularly when the parents do not endorse the high levels of anxiety reported by their children). Also, the data suggest the need for clinicians to probe and address the discrepancy between the child's and parent's perceptions or awareness of the child's problems and to utilize a family systems approach in formulating a treatment/management plan.

Clinical Course

There are no systematic studies of the clinical course of comorbid ADHD and anxiety disorders. However, several prospective follow-up studies indicate a chronic course for both ADHD and anxiety disorders alone, as well as persisting overlap between internalizing and externalizing symptoms in ADHD from childhood to adolescence (e.g., Biederman et al. 1996; Feehan et al. 1993; Fischer et al. 1993). The majority of children with ADHD (over 80%) continue to have the disorder in adolescence. Moreover, problems with behavior in general, and with ADHD symptoms specifically, persist into adulthood in 50%–60% of cases. Furthermore, according to one prospective 4-year follow-up study of a large group of boys with ADHD, the rates of comorbid mood and anxiety disorders increased across this follow-up period (Biederman et al. 1996).

The relative salience of the ADHD and the anxious symptoms and associated impairments is likely to change from childhood to adolescence and adulthood. Specifically, among the ADHD symptoms, hyperactivity problems decline, but difficulties with attention and self-regulation persist into adulthood (Barkley et al. 1990b; Fischer et al. 1993). In contrast, anxiety symptoms may wax and wane from childhood to adolescence or evolve into other anxiety or depressive disorders (e.g., Last et al. 1992; Reinherz et al. 1993; Strauss et al. 1988). Thus, ADHD symptoms (along with any concurrent symptoms of oppositional defiant disorder or conduct disorder) are typically the major concerns of the parents and school personnel during the early and middle childhood years (Barkley 1990, pp. 106–129). In contrast, poor achievement in schoolwork, problems with authority figures, and low self-esteem tend to be the major concerns in adolescence, and internalizing problems (e.g., anxiety, sadness, somatic problems) and concerns about underachievement predominate in adulthood (Weiss and Hechtman 1986).

Treatment

Numerous strategies have been used in the treatment of children with ADHD, including parent training and counseling, behavioral and cognitive-behavioral therapy, educational management, psychotherapy, and a range of pharmacological interventions (e.g., psychostimulants, tricyclic antidepressants, specific serotonergic antidepressants, clonidine) (for review, see Barkley 1990; Schachar and Tannock 1993; Schachar et al. 1996). Stimulant medication (primarily methylphenidate) is not only the most common treatment used in North America (Safer and Krager 1988) but also often the sole treatment received (Wolraich et al. 1990), despite strong recommendations for multimodal treatment (e.g., Shaywitz and Shaywitz 1991). Psychosocial treatments are recommended and applied less often in the United States (Barkley et al. 1990b; Wolraich et al. 1990).

Psychostimulants

Treatment with psychostimulants typically produces immediate (and often dramatic) improvements in the behavioral symptoms of ADHD, as well as in cognitive function, academic performance, and social functioning. These short-term benefits of stimulant treatment for children with ADHD have been documented in an extensive number of well-controlled trials (e.g., for reviews, see Gadow 1986; Jacobvitz et al. 1990; Rapport and Kelly 1991). (It should be noted that long-term benefits from stimulant treatment are less clear, primarily because of the limited number of well-controlled trials; for reviews, see Jacobvitz et al. 1990; Schachar and Tannock 1993.)

In contrast, psychostimulants may be less helpful for children with comorbid ADHD and anxiety disorders. The results from several controlled studies suggest that the presence of high levels of anxiety in children with ADHD may impede their response to stimulant treatment (DuPaul et al. 1994; Ickowicz et al. 1993; Pliszka 1989; Tannock et al. 1995a, 1995b; Taylor et al. 1987), although findings are not always consistent (cf. Diamond et al. 1999; Livingston et al. 1992). For example, Livingston et al. (1992) found no evidence that children with attention-deficit disorder and comorbid emotional disorders (i.e., anxiety and/or depressive disorders) responded less well than other children with ADHD. Rather, these investigators suggested that children with attention-deficit disorder with both anxiety/depression and oppositional defiant disorder/conduct disorder diagnoses may need higher doses to obtain therapeutic benefit (e.g., 0.6 mg/kg rather than 0.3 mg/kg), than children with attention-deficit disorder with either anxiety disorders/depression or oppositional defiant disorder/conduct disorder. This study employed a parallel group design (as opposed to a crossover design), and no placebo control was used. Therefore, the authors could not investigate the possibility of a placebo response, nor could they rule out the possibility that initial group differences (e.g., in severity of symptoms) may have accounted for the differential dose response in the comorbid groups.

According to one study, higher levels of concurrent "emotional problems" (i.e., anxiety and depressive symptoms) in children with antisocial, disruptive, or overactive behavior predicted a poorer behavioral response to stimulants (Taylor et al. 1987). Another study found that children with ADHD and comorbid overanxious disorder showed only modest and nonsignificant improvement in teacher ratings of inattentive/overactive behavior with methylphenidate, compared with the improvements exhibited by the group with ADHD only (Pliszka 1989). There was no evidence that the behavior of the comorbid group worsened with stimulants, but many of the children exhibited a placebo response (i.e., they did as well when taking a placebo as when taking a stimulant).

Results of yet another study indicated that methylphenidate failed to improve working memory in children with ADHD and comorbid anxiety disorders, but it did improve working memory in nonanxious children with ADHD (Tannock et al. 1995b). This finding is particularly worrisome because children with comorbid ADHD and anxiety disorders are likely to exhibit greater deficits in working memory than nonanxious children with ADHD (see discussion of cognitive correlates earlier in this chapter). Also, although the two groups of children did not differ in heart rate in an unmedicated state and methylphenidate increased heart rate in all children, a low dose (0.3 mg/kg) produced more dramatic increases in heart rate in the children with comorbid ADHD and anxiety disorders (comparable to those produced by the higher doses), particularly 1 hour after its administration. This pattern of findings is consistent with the predictions of theories that relate anxiety, arousal, and cognitive performance—namely, that increases in arousal (in this case, induced experimentally by methylphenidate) do not counteract deficits in working memory that result from heightened levels of anxiety (Eysenck and Calvo 1992; Humphreys and Revelle 1984). It should be noted that methylphenidate was demonstrated to improve overt restlessness in both groups—a finding that is inconsistent with what was demonstrated in Pliszka's (1989) study.

Not only may children with comorbid ADHD and anxiety disorders gain less benefit from psychostimulants, they also may experience more intolerable side effects. According to one study, approximately two-thirds of a clinically referred sample of children with ADHD exhibited repetitive, abnormal movements (e.g., facial tics, oral dystonia); one-third exhibited obsessive-compulsive behaviors (e.g., morbid preoccupations and meticulous, perseverative play); and two-thirds exhibited dysphoria (Ickowicz et al. 1993; Tannock and Schachar 1992). A central finding of that study was that the majority of children who exhibited obsessive-compulsive symptoms or dysphoria (i.e., 70% and 75%, respectively) had comorbid anxiety disorders. Abnormal movements were equally distributed between the anxious and nonanxious children with ADHD.

Collectively, the preceding findings suggest that the presence of comorbid anxiety in ADHD may alter the therapeutic cost-benefit ratio of stimulant treatment, at least in the short term. Not surprisingly, several investigators have reported that fewer children with comorbid ADHD and anxiety disorders were classified as "responders" compared with the nonanxious children with ADHD (e.g., 30% vs. 80%) (Pliszka 1989), and fewer were recommended to continue stimulant treatment (e.g., 30% vs. 60%) (Ickowicz et al. 1993).

Since psychostimulants are typically prescribed for several years rather than several days or weeks as in the preceding studies, a critical question is whether similar results would be found with prolonged stimulant treatment. Preliminary findings from two recent randomized controlled studies (4-month and 14-month course of stimulant treatment, respectively), in which dose was titrated as in standard clinical practice and monitored carefully with ongoing adjustments permitted, suggest that the answer is likely to be "no" (Conners et al. 1998; Diamond et al. 1999). Specifically, these studies found no evidence of differential response to stimulant medication between ADHD alone and comorbid ADHD and anxiety disorders in terms of either the behavioral response or the side effects. Both studies included an assessment of behavioral and side effects in the natural setting rather than a laboratory setting as in most (but not all) of the acute challenge studies. These findings suggest that perhaps acute challenges generate a differential drug response in children with comorbid ADHD and anxiety only in the short term. From a clinical perspective, the available evidence suggests that stimulant medication should still be considered as the drug of first choice for children with comorbid ADHD and anxiety disorders but that the medication should be titrated and monitored carefully, consistently, and continuously.

Antidepressants

Tricyclic antidepressants (TCAs), such as desipramine and imipramine, have been proposed as alternatives for children with comorbid ADHD and anxiety disorders who fail to respond to stimulants (Pliszka 1987). However, the sole study to date that has addressed this issue found no evidence of specificity of desipramine for children with comorbid ADHD and anxiety disorders (Biederman et al. 1993a). Also, the findings suggested that desipramine acted to reduce primarily the ADHD rather than the anxiety disorder symptoms, and this suggests that there was only partial coverage of symptoms in children with this comorbidity. Moreover, the potential cardiac effects of some TCAs, including reports of four sudden deaths (Abramowicz 1990; Riddle et al. 1991b, 1993), have caused clinicians to question the use of TCAs as a first-line intervention for children with ADHD.

Other antidepressants, such as fluoxetine (a selective serotonin reuptake inhibitor), have been used alone and in combination with stimulants to treat children with ADHD, particularly those children with comorbid anxiety/depression (Barrickman et al. 1991; Bussing and Levin 1993; Gammon and Brown 1993). The limited data available are of importance because they highlight the need for careful monitoring of medication effects on more than one disorder in cases of comorbid disorders. For example, as noted previously, fluoxetine is an effective treatment for OCD, but it may aggravate motor symptoms (e.g., restlessness, sleep disturbance), particularly in those children with comorbid ADHD (Bussing and Levin 1993; Riddle et al. 1991a, 1992).

Two reports of the use of psychostimulants in combination with fluoxetine for the treatment of ADHD with comorbid anxiety/depressive disorders highlight the importance of monitoring a broad spectrum of symptoms when polypharmacy is deemed necessary. A case report by Bussing and Levin (1993) indicated that fluoxetine alleviated the obsessive-compulsive symptoms in a child with OCD, major depression, and a history indicative of ADHD, but this medication aggravated or elicited the ADHD symptoms. The addition of a stimulant ameliorated the ADHD symptoms, and the child was successfully maintained on the combined treatment regimen. Conversely, in the second report, Gammon and Brown (1993) addressed the addition of fluoxetine to methylphenidate to produce a more complete response in children and adolescents with ADHD and comorbid anxiety/depression. Methylphenidate was only partially effective in ameliorating the behavioral symptoms and was ineffective for the affective symptoms exhibited by these youngsters. The gradual addition of small doses of fluoxetine to augment the methylphenidate treatment was reported to resolve the affective symptoms, which included depressed or anxious mood, chronic irritability, and obsessive/perseverative tendencies.

Clonidine

Clonidine, an α_2-adrenergic receptor agonist that is commonly used as an antihypertensive agent, is worth considering as a viable alternative for highly anxious children with ADHD. In child psychiatry clonidine is used to treat Tourette syndrome (Cohen et al. 1980; Leckman et al. 1991; Steingard et al. 1993) and ADHD (Hunt et al. 1985, 1990), autism (Fankhauser et al. 1992), and aggressiveness (Hunt et al. 1990; Kemph et al. 1993).

Clonidine inhibits firing of the locus coeruleus, thereby suppressing central noradrenergic activity. It may, therefore, be particularly effective in reducing arousal and anxiety mediated by heightened noradrenergic activity (for review, see Shenker 1992). From the point of view of a functional model, ADHD and anxiety disorders have each been associated with increased noradrenergic activity (Gray 1982; Mefford and Potter 1989; Quay 1988). Thus, clonidine might be particularly effective for the subgroup of patients with comorbid ADHD and anxiety disorders, who are at risk for heightened noradrenergic activity and hyperarousal. Also, from a clinical perspective, clonidine has been found to have acute anxiolytic and sedative properties as well as analgesic properties (Carabine et al. 1991; Maze 1988). Moreover, it is reported to be particularly useful for ADHD children with high levels of emotional reactivity or those who have exhibited a poor response to stimulants (Hunt et al. 1990). But there is a paucity of well-controlled trials of clonidine in the treatment of ADHD, and there are no systematic empirical investigations of its use in patients with comorbid ADHD and anxiety disorders. Thus, the clinical usefulness of clonidine for comorbid ADHD and anxiety disorders is unknown.

To summarize, the collective findings from these treatment studies suggest not only that children with comorbid ADHD and anxiety disorders may exhibit a less robust behavioral response to the most commonly used treatment for ADHD (i.e., psychostimulants), but also that their deficits in effortful cognitive processing may not be ameliorated by this treatment. Moreover, these children may be more vulnerable to the cardiovascular effects of stimulant treatment and at risk for intolerable treatment-emergent side effects. These findings should be interpreted to suggest not that stimulants should never be used in the treatment of children with comorbid ADHD and anxiety disorders, but rather that stimulant treatment may be ineffective with many of these children or that high levels of anxiety may alter the risk-benefit ratio of stimulant treatment. The effect of comorbid anxiety on the response of children with ADHD to behavioral treatments is unknown: it will be important to investigate this issue in future treatment studies. However, the differential response to stimulant treatment in children with comorbid ADHD and anxiety disorders versus ADHD alone provides additional support for the hypothesis that ADHD comorbid with anxiety disorders represents a distinct etiological subtype of ADHD (see Jensen et al. 1997).

The search for pharmacological treatments that are safe and effective for children with comorbid ADHD and anxiety disorders is a primary clinical concern, given the prevalence of this comorbid pattern, the prominence of these children's difficulties, and their frequent lack of responsiveness to stimulant medication. Two approaches are evident in the literature: 1) use of a different class of medication, alone; and 2) augmentation of stimulants with a different class of medication (i.e., copharmacy). There is no empirical evidence to date for a different class of medication that provides full coverage for the wide range of behavioral and affective problems exhibited by children with comorbid ADHD and anxiety disorders. Combined medication may be useful for some, but copharmacy is still controversial (see Wilens 1994 and Chapter 16, this volume; see also Green 1991, p. 23; Werry and Aman 1993, p. 18). (Polypharmacy refers to the simultaneous use of two or more similar drugs, usually from the same class; copharmacy is the simultaneous use of drugs from different classes; see Green 1991, p. 23.) The wide range of impairments exhibited by children with comorbid ADHD and anxiety disorders indicates the need for multimodal treatment in which pharmacological treatment is one component.

IMPLICATIONS FOR ASSESSMENT AND TREATMENT

The diagnosis of one or more anxiety disorders (or a high level of anxiety symptoms that do not meet the criteria for a specific DSM-III-R or DSM-IV anxiety disorder) in a child with ADHD complicates clinical management.

This chapter is not intended to provide details about the clinical management of ADHD or anxiety disorders per se. Comprehensive information about the clinical management of ADHD is provided in other texts (e.g., Barkley 1998; Goldstein and Goldstein 1998; Rubin 1998; Silver 1991). Information about the management of anxiety disorders can be found in works by March (1995), Allen et al. (1995), and Bernstein et al. (1996). Also, see the guidelines for assessment and treatment of ADHD and those for assessment and treatment of anxiety disorders published by the American Academy of Child and Adolescent Psychiatry (AACAP) (AACAP 1997a for anxiety disorders; AACAP 1997b for ADHD). Nonetheless, this synthesis of the literature suggests several guidelines for assessment and treatment of ADHD with possible comorbid anxiety in clinical practice and research settings.

Assessment Guidelines

1. Recognize the high rate and clinical significance of anxiety disorders among children with ADHD and the high comorbidity of anxiety disorders and depression, particularly among clinically referred children. *Routinely* screen for and assess the emotional functioning of children with ADHD in terms of both anxiety and depressive symptoms.
2. Recall there are no specific measures or tests (e.g., blood tests, brain scans, heart rate, blood pressure, neuropsychological tests) that can provide reliable and valid diagnosis of either ADHD or anxiety disorders. Diagnosis of both ADHD and anxiety disorders is made by compiling information obtained from a detailed history of the presenting problems, developmental history, past medical history, school history, and family history of psychiatric disorders:

    a. Probe the child's developmental and family history during the clinical interview with parents for correlates and risk factors associated with anxiety disorders (e.g., familial history of anxiety disorders, behavioral inhibition or high levels of emotionality/reactivity in infancy, stressful experiences in the child's life such as parental divorce, separation, or exposure to violence or abuse).

    b. Obtain parent ratings and child's self-ratings of the child's symptoms of anxiety. Suggested rating scales are listed at the end of this subsection.

    c. Note overt signs of anxiety in the child during the assessment, including separation difficulty, motor tension, autonomic hyperactivity (e.g., sweaty palms; dry mouth resulting in frequent lip licking or "clicking sound" while speaking; flushing), variations in speech (e.g., quavering voice, loss of voicing, whispering, rapid or cluttered speech, frequent dysfluencies), and nervous mannerisms (e.g., nail biting, leg jiggling, breath holding or gulping).

d. Investigate positive indicators for anxiety systematically in clinical interviews to confirm the diagnosis of one or more concurrent anxiety disorders or to document high levels of anxiety that may not fulfill the criteria for a specific disorder but that require consideration in the clinical management.

3. Recognize that parents and teachers are better informants than children about children's externally observable behavior associated with ADHD but that children are better informants about their own internalizing symptoms. Parents and teachers may not be aware of children's internalizing symptoms:

    a. Obtain the child's self-reports of anxiety and depressive symptoms and self-assessment of impairment. Structured diagnostic interviews designed for children that include or focus exclusively on anxiety are listed at the end of this subsection.

    b. If the child's report of symptom severity and degree of impairment warrants, make a diagnosis of anxiety disorder on the basis of the child's report alone (i.e., even when the child's anxiety is not endorsed by the parents or teacher).

Children's self-report rating scales of anxiety include the Multidimensional Anxiety Scale for Children (March and Sullivan 1999; March et al. 1997), the Revised Children's Manifest Anxiety Scales (Reynolds and Richmond 1978), the State-Trait Anxiety Inventory for Children (Spielberger 1973), and the Revised Fear Survey Schedule for Children (Ollendick 1983). The Children's Depression Inventory (Kovaacs 1989) is commonly used to obtain children's self-report of depressive symptoms.

Parent rating scales that contain an evaluation of anxiety and/or depression include the Child Behavior Checklist (Achenbach 1991), the Revised Conners' Parent Rating Scales (Conners 1997), the Strengths and Difficulties Questionnaire (Goodman 1997, 1999; Goodman and Scott 1999; Goodman et al. 1998), and the Revised Ontario Child Health Scale (Boyle et al. 1993), which is an adaptation of the Child Behavior Checklist that permits the assessment of a range of DSM-III-R diagnoses. Teacher versions of the parent scales are also available. These rating scales are quick to administer (approximately 10–20 minutes for any single instrument) and score; most have normative data and provide clinical cutoff scores to aid interpretation.

A number of structured interviews that are available for use with children include an assessment of anxiety: Diagnostic Interview for Children and Adolescents—Revised (Herjanic and Reich 1982; Reich and Welner 1990a, 1990b), Diagnostic Interview Schedule for Children—Version 2.3 (Schaffer et al. 1996), and Schedule for Affective Disorders and Schizophrenia for School-Aged Children (Ambrosini and Dixon 1996; Chambers et al. 1985; Kaufman et al. 1997). Other interviews focus exclusively on anxiety disorders: Anxiety Disorders Interview Schedule for Children (Silverman and Nelles 1988; Silverman and Eisen 1992) and the Child Interview for Overanxious Disorder (Pliszka 1992). Several of these instruments have parallel versions for parents (e.g., Diagnostic Interview for Children and Adolescents, Diagnostic Interview Schedule for Children, and Anxiety Disorders Interview Schedule for Children).

Treatment Guidelines

1. Recognize that parents, teachers, or primary care physicians may not be aware of children's anxiety. Educate parents and other caregivers about the symptoms, clinical course, treatment options, and prognosis and consult with school personnel and primary care physician as appropriate. An awareness that the child's worries and fears may contribute to or exacerbate the behavioral problems may help parents and teachers to better understand and help the child.
2. Consider both disorders (i.e., ADHD and anxiety disorder) in the treatment plan and monitor treatment effects on both disorders. The course of the disorders is variable, and each may require short-term, intermittent, or long-term treatment and follow-up:
    a. Involve the child and the child's teacher as well as the parents in identifying which problem areas are to be given first priority for treatment (e.g., from the child's perspective, anxiety rather than ADHD may be the primary concern).
    b. Determine whether the treatment selected for ADHD produces the expected beneficial effects in the presence of comorbid anxiety; whether treatment of the ADHD produces any effects (i.e., symptom reduction or exacerbation or no effects) in the comorbid anxiety disorder; and, conversely, whether treatment of the anxiety has any impact on the ADHD symptoms.
3. Recognize that treatment response may vary across different domains of functioning (e.g., behavioral, cognitive, academic, affective, psycho-

social). Include measures from each domain in the evaluation of treatment response.

4. Consider a range of treatment modalities—including counseling/educational, pharmacological, behavioral, cognitive-behavioral, family systems, and psychoanalytic approaches—to suit the needs of the individual child and family.
5. Modify extant behavioral and cognitive-behavioral treatment programs designed for ADHD to include techniques used in the treatment of anxiety disorders to deal with excessive worries and concerns about competence (e.g., systematic desensitization, exposure and response prevention, extinction, counterconditioning, modeling, operant techniques).
6. If the severity of symptoms warrants, consider pharmacological approaches. Establish the response of *both* disorders to single medications (e.g., methylphenidate, tricyclic antidepressants, benzodiazepines, clonidine) before using polypharmacy:
   a. Recognize that methylphenidate (Ritalin) may not retain its effectiveness when coexisting anxiety is present and that comorbid anxiety may increase the risk for intolerable side effects, such as dysphoria.
   b. Consider another stimulant (e.g., dextroamphetamine) before moving to other classes of medication (Elia and Rapoport 1991).
   c. The database for the efficacy of other medications (e.g., TCAs, benzodiazepines, clonidine) for the treatment of either ADHD or anxiety disorders is limited: the efficacy of these agents for treating comorbid ADHD and anxiety disorders is unknown. Consult existing guidelines for the use of these alternative medications (e.g., Coffey 1990; Green 1991; Hunt et al. 1990; Ryan 1990; Werry and Aman 1993).

CASE VIGNETTES

Two case reports are presented to illustrate how comorbid anxiety complicates the clinical management of ADHD. The first case describes how establishing the response of the two disorders (ADHD, anxiety disorder) to methylphenidate and clonidine, respectively, led to the successful use of these medications in combination within a multimodal treatment approach. The second illustrates the risks and benefits of pharmacological treatment of an anxious child with ADHD and the resultant compromises that may have to be considered.

B.G. is a 7-year-old boy who was referred by a psychologist for evaluation of severe hyperactivity, impulsiveness, poor concentration, and poor social behavior that was interfering with his learning and social functioning at school and home. His developmental history revealed overactivity and difficult-to-manage behavior since 1 year of age, which became worse when he started kindergarten. At that time B.G. also developed a moderate to severe stutter. Family history was significant for "gifted and ADHD" in an older male sibling.

B.G. comes from an intact, well-functioning family. Clinical diagnostic interviews confirmed the following DSM-III-R diagnoses: ADHD (severe and pervasive), oppositional defiant disorder, separation and anxiety disorder, as well as severe stuttering and other anxiety traits (overanxious, phobic, obsessive-compulsive). B.G. scored in the superior range in intellectual abilities, but his academic achievement scores were well below average. The parents' primary concerns were the ADHD symptoms, poor social relations, and stuttering, but they had not thought of B.G. as anxious: the child was worried about his family, problems at school, and lack of friends.

Treatment included counseling and educating the family about anxiety and ADHD, referral to an on-site group program for parents for help with behavioral management strategies, and systematic crossover trials of methylphenidate (0.3 mg/kg/dose twice daily titrated up over 3 weeks), placebo (2 weeks), and clonidine (3.5 µg/kg/day, titrated slowly over 3 weeks, then tapered off to zero). B.G. did not tolerate a higher dose of clonidine because of excessive sedation.

Methylphenidate improved B.G.'s behavior and academic performance and his stuttering (relative to baseline and placebo) but had no impact on anxiety. It also resulted in mild dysphoria as well as marked rebound effects at the end of the day. Clonidine had little effect on either the ADHD or the anxiety symptoms, and the stuttering continued to be problematic. But there was no dysphoria or rebound. Based on the results of this trial, treatment with methylphenidate (7.5 mg A.M. and 5 mg noon) was initiated. Teachers reported remarkable improvements in classroom behavior, completion of academic tasks, and ability to sustain attention. However, B.G. began to experience poor appetite, moderate rebound phenomena in the early evening, and insomnia. The addition of clonidine (25 µg 6:00 P.M. and 25 µg at bedtime) allowed B.G. to maintain the behavioral and academic gains while eliminating the dysphoria and rebound as well as normalizing sleep patterns. Prior to the pharmacological intervention, B.G.'s school placement in a special program for gifted children had been considered in jeopardy; but in a recent meeting, his parents were advised that given B.G.'s improvement in behavior and academic performance, the placement was no longer in question.

T.J. first presented for evaluation and treatment at age 6 years. He was described as having been very active and impulsive since his toddler years, with his difficulties becoming more prominent at age 4 years, when the family emigrated to Canada. Teachers reported that from kindergarten through first grade, he fidgeted constantly, was unable to stay seated, often disrupted and annoyed his classmates, and did not respond to usual disciplinary methods. This resulted in his spending a great deal of time in the principal's office. Also, parents indicated that although T.J. had always been a sensible child, he had had a lot of trouble sleeping and still woke up several times each night. They reported that he also showed great anxiety during transient separations from parents and seemed to be worrying about something the whole time. T.J. confirmed experiencing "terrible bad dreams" and worrying about the fighting and arguing taking place at home, and he also expressed a sense that no one liked him. Psychoeducational assessment was attempted but was considered unreliable because of the child's extreme overactivity and distractibility.

Clinical and structured interviews confirmed the diagnosis of ADHD, separation anxiety disorder, and some overanxious traits. He was scheduled to participate in an acute placebo-controlled trial with methylphenidate, but after a single 7.5-mg dose (0.3 mg/kg), T.J. experienced a marked dysphoric reaction that led to an early termination of the trial and consideration of alternative treatment with a TCA.

T.J. was followed for the next 3 years by a psychiatrist in an ambulatory care clinic. The family attended regular visits, and T.J. received imipramine 50 mg/day. T.J. made excellent progress in social adjustment and language development, but he continued to exhibit severe academic problems. Formal psychoeducational assessment at age 9 revealed that he was still unable to read or spell and that his arithmetic skills were at the first-grade level. Attendance at a summer camp for children with learning disabilities resulted in remarkable gains in self-competence, but attention and learning remained problematic. Imipramine was discontinued during the summer.

When T.J. was 10 years old, his father requested another evaluation.

T.J. was now attending a special education program. Gains in the areas of communication were confirmed, but he remained overactive, disinhibited, and rambunctious. An open trial with methylphenidate was conducted, starting at 5 mg bid and increasing to 10 mg bid (0.3 mg/kg/dose). The lower dose had virtually no effect, but the moderate dose produced remarkable improvements in T.J.'s attention span, activity level, and disinhibition. Moreover, for the first time, he showed tangible progress in reading, writing, and spelling ("a 2-year leap in 8 weeks" according to the teacher). The price for this improvement was witnessing T.J. become somber, subdued, solemn, and somewhat less interested in social contact. His academic progress over the next 2 months continued above expectations, but he remained somber and subdued while on the medication. Despite this, the family has preferred to continue with the stimulant in view of the academic progress.

CONCLUSION

The literature suggests that presence of comorbid anxiety disorders alters the meaning of ADHD in clinically significant ways: ADHD alone and comorbid ADHD and anxiety disorders may have different etiologies and correlates, be associated with different cognitive styles, and have different responses to treatment. In the absence of unequivocal evidence to support either the belief that the comorbidity between ADHD and anxiety disorders is a "masked" anxiety disorder (i.e, ADHD symptoms are secondary to a primary anxiety disorder) or the belief that it is "complex" ADHD (i.e., the anxiety is secondary to ADHD), concurrent anxiety disorder should be interpreted as a comorbid disorder.

REFERENCES

Abramowicz H: Sudden death in children treated with a tricyclic antidepressant. Med Lett Drugs Ther 32:53, 1990

Achenbach TM: Manual for the Child Behavior Checklist/4–18 and 1991 Profile. Burlington, VT, TM Achenbach, 1991

Ambrosini P, Dixon D: The Schedule for Affective Disorders and Schizophrenia for School-Age Children, 4th Version, Revised (K-SADS-IVR). Unpublished, Medical College of Pennsylvania and Hahnemann University, Philadelphia

American Academy of Child and Adolescent Psychiatry: Practice parameters for the assessment and treatment of children and adolescents with anxiety disorders. J Am Acad Child Adolesc Psychiatry 36 (10, suppl):69S–84S, 1997a

American Academy of Child and Adolescent Psychiatry: Practice parameters for the assessment and treatment of children, adolescents, and adults with attention-deficit/hyperactivity disorder. J Am Acad Child Adolesc Psychiatry 36(10, suppl): 85S–121S, 1997b

American Psychiatric Association: Diagnostic and Statistical Manual of Mental Disorders, 3rd Edition, Revised. Washington, DC, American Psychiatric Association, 1987

American Psychiatric Association: Diagnostic and Statistical Manual of Mental Disorders, 4th Edition. Washington, DC, American Psychiatric Association, 1994

Anderson JC, Williams S, McGee R, et al: DSM-III-R disorders in preadolescent children: prevalence in a large sample from the general population. Arch Gen Psychiatry 44:69–76, 1987

Anderson JC, Williams S, McGee R, et al: Cognitive and social correlates of DSM-III disorders in preadolescent children. J Am Acad Child Adolesc Psychiatry 28:842–846, 1989

Angold A, Costello EJ: Depressive comorbidity in children and adolescents. Am J Psychiatry 150:1779–1791, 1993

Angold A, Costello EJ, Erkanli A: Comorbidity. J Child Psychol Psychiatry 40:57–87, 1999

Baddeley AD: Working Memory. Oxford, UK, Clarendon Press, 1986

Barkley RA (ed): Attention Deficit Hyperactivity Disorder: A Handbook for Diagnosis and Treatment, 2nd Edition. New York, Guilford, 1998

Barkley RA, DuPaul GJ, McMurray MB: Comprehensive evaluation of attention deficit disorder with and without hyperactivity as defined by research criteria. J Consult Clin Psychol 58:775–789, 1990a

Barkley RA, Fischer M, Edelbrock CS, et al: The adolescent outcome of hyperactive children diagnosed by research criteria, I: an 8-year prospective follow-up study. J Am Acad Child Adolesc Psychiatry 29:546–557, 1990b

Barrickman L, Noyes R, Kuperman S, et al: Treatment of ADHD with fluoxetine: a preliminary trial. J Am Acad Child Adolesc Psychiatry 30:762–767, 1991

Bell-Dolan DJ, Last CG, Strauss CC: Symptoms of anxiety in normal children. J Am Acad Child Adolesc Psychiatry 29:759–765, 1990

Benjamin RS, Costello EJ, Warren M: Anxiety disorders in a pediatric sample. J Anxiety Disord 4:293–316, 1990

Berkson J: Limitations of the application of fourfold table analysis to hospital data. Biometrics Bull 2:47–52, 1946

Bernstein GA, Borchardt CM: Anxiety disorders of childhood: a critical review. J Am Acad Child Adolesc Psychiatry 30:519–532, 1991

Bernstein GA, Borchardt CM, Perwien AR: Anxiety disorders in children and adolescents: a review of the past 10 years. J Am Acad Child Adolesc Psychiatry 35:1110–1119, 1996

Bernstein GA, Garfinkel BD, Hoberman HM: Self-reported anxiety in adolescents. Am J Psychiatry 146:384–386, 1989

Biederman J: The diagnosis and treatment of adolescent anxiety disorders. J Clin Psychiatry 51 (no 5, suppl):20–26, 1990

Biederman J, Faraone SV, Keenan K, et al: Family genetic and psychosocial risk factors in DSM-III attention deficit disorder. J Am Acad Child Adolesc Psychiatry 29:526–533, 1990a

Biederman J, Rosenbaum JF, Hirshfeld DR, et al: Psychiatric correlates of behavioral inhibition in young children of parents with and without psychiatric disorders. Arch Gen Psychiatry 47:21–26, 1990b

Biederman J, Faraone SV, Keenan K, et al: Familial association between attention deficit disorder and anxiety disorder. Am J Psychiatry 148:251–256, 1991a

Biederman J, Newcorn J, Sprich S: Comorbidity of attention deficit hyperactivity disorder with conduct, depressive, anxiety, and other disorders. Am J Psychiatry 148:564–577, 1991b

Biederman J, Baldessarini RJ, Wright V, et al: A double-blind placebo controlled study of desipramine in the treatment of ADD, III: lack of impact of comorbidity and family history factors on clinical response. J Am Acad Child Adolesc Psychiatry 32:199–204, 1993a

Biederman J, Faraone SV, Chen WJ: Social Adjustment Inventory for Children and Adolescents: concurrent validity in ADHD children. J Am Acad Child Adolesc Psychiatry 32:1059–1064, 1993b

Biederman J, Rosenbaum JF, Bolduc-Murphy EA, et al: A 3-year follow-up of children with and without behavioral inhibition. J Am Acad Child Adolesc Psychiatry 32:814–821, 1993c

Biederman J, Faraone SV, Milberger S, et al: A prospective 4-year follow-up study of attention-deficit hyperactivity and related disorders. Arch Gen Psychiatry 53: 437–446, 1996

Bird HR, Canino G, Rubio-Stipec M, et al: Estimates of the prevalence of childhood maladjustment in a community survey in Puerto Rico. Arch Gen Psychiatry 45:1120–1126, 1988

Bird HR, Gould MS, Staghezza B: Aggregating data from multiple informants in child psychiatry epidemiological research. J Am Acad Child Adolesc Psychiatry 31:78–85, 1992

Bowen RC, Offord DR, Boyle MH: The prevalence of overanxious disorder and separation anxiety disorder: results from the Ontario Child Health Survey. J Am Acad Child Adolesc Psychiatry 29:753–758, 1990

Boyle MH, Offord DR, Racine Y, et al: Evaluation of the Revised Ontario Child Health Study Scales. J Child Psychol Psychiatry 43:189–213, 1993

Bussing R, Levin GM: Methamphetamine and fluoxetine treatment of a child with attention-deficit hyperactivity disorder and obsessive-compulsive disorder. J Child Adolesc Psychopharmacol 3:53–58, 1993

Carabine UA, Milligan KR, Moore JA: Adrenergic modulation of preoperative anxiety: a comparison of temazepam, clonidine and timolol. Anesth Analg 73:633–637, 1991

Caron C, Rutter M: Comorbidity in child psychopathology: concepts, issues and research strategies. J Child Psychol Psychiatry 32:1063–1080, 1991

Chambers W, Puig-Antich J, Hirsch M, et al: The assessment of affective disorders in children and adolescents by semi-structured interview: test-retest reliability of the Schedule for Affective Disorders and Schizophrenia for School-Age Children, Present Episode Version. Arch Gen Psychiatry 42:696–702, 1985

Coffey BJ: Anxiolytics for children and adolescents: traditional and new drugs. J Child Adolesc Psychopharmacol 1:57–83, 1990

Cohen DJ, Detlor J, Young JG, et al: Clonidine ameliorates Gilles de la Tourette syndrome. Arch Gen Psychiatry 37:1350–1354, 1980

Conners CK: Manual for Conners' Rating Scales—Revised. New York, Multi-Health Systems, 1997

Conners CK, Hechtman L, Arnold LE, et al: Fourteen-month outcomes from the Multimodal Treatment Study of ADHD: first report. Paper presented at the 45th annual meeting of the American Academy of Child and Adolescent Psychiatry, Anaheim, CA, October 27–November 1, 1998

Costello EJ, Costello AJ, Edelbrock C, et al: Psychiatric disorders in pediatric primary care: prevalence and risk factors. Arch Gen Psychiatry 45:1107–1116, 1988

Crowe RR, Noyes R, Pauls DL, et al: A family study of panic disorder. Arch Gen Psychiatry 40:1065–1069, 1983

Diamond IR, Tannock R, Schachar RJ: Response to methylphenidate in children with ADHD and comorbid anxiety. J Am Acad Child Adolesc Psychiatry 38:402–409, 1999

DuPaul GJ, Barkley RA, McMurray MB: Response of children with ADHD to methylphenidate: interaction with internalizing symptoms. J Am Acad Child Adolesc Psychiatry 33:894–903, 1994

Edelbrock CS, Costello AJ, Kessler MD: Empirical corroboration of attention deficit disorder. Journal of the American Academy of Child Psychiatry 23:285–290, 1984

Eiraldi RB, Power TJ, Nezu CM: Patterns of comorbidity associated with subtypes of attention-deficit/hyperactivity disorder among 6- to 12-year-old children. J Am Acad Child Adolesc Psychiatry 36:503–514, 1997

Elia J, Rapoport JL: Ritalin versus dextroamphetamines in ADHD: both should be tried, in Ritalin: Theory and Patient Management. Edited by Greenhill LL, Osman BB. New York, Mary Ann Liebert, 1991, pp 69–74

Esser G, Schmidt MH, Woerner W: Epidemiology and course of psychiatric disorders in school-age children—results of a longitudinal study. J Child Psychol Psychiatry 31:243–263, 1990

Eysenck MW, Calvo MG: Anxiety and performance: the processing efficiency theory. Cognition and Emotion 6:409–434, 1992

Fankhauser MP, Karumanchi VC, German ML, et al: A double-blind, placebo-controlled study of the efficacy of transdermal clonidine in autism. J Clin Psychiatry 53:77–82, 1992

Faraone SV, Biederman J, Weber W, et al: Psychiatric, neuropsychological, and psychosocial features of DSM-IV subtypes of attention-deficit/hyperactivity disorder: results from a clinically referred sample. J Am Acad Child Adolesc Psychiatry 37:185–193, 1998

Feehan M, McGee R, Williams SM: Mental health disorders from age 15 to age 18 years. J Am Acad Child Adolesc Psychiatry 32:1118–1126, 1993

Fergusson DM, Horwood LJ, Lynskey MT: Prevalence and comorbidity of DSM-III-R diagnoses in a birth cohort of 15 year olds. J Am Acad Child Adolesc Psychiatry 32:1127–1134, 1993

Fischer M, Barkley RA, Fletcher KE, et al: The stability of dimensions of behavior in ADHD and normal children over an 8-year followup. J Abnorm Child Psychol 21:315–337, 1993

Gadow KD: Hyperactivity, in Children on Medication, Vol 1: Hyperactivity, Learning Disabilities, and Mental Retardation. Edited by Gadow KD. Boston, MA, Little, Brown, 1986, pp 31–95

Gammon GD, Brown TE: Fluoxetine and methylphenidate in combination for treatment of attention deficit disorder and comorbid depressive disorder. J Child Adolesc Psychopharmacol 3:1–10, 1993

Gaub M, Carlson CL: Behavioral characteristics of DSM-IV ADHD subtypes in a school-based population. J Abnorm Child Psychol 25:103–111, 1997

Gittelman R (ed): Anxiety Disorders of Childhood. New York, Guilford, 1986

Goldstein S, Goldstein M: Managing Attention Disorders in Children: A Guide for Practitioners, 2nd Edition. New York, Wiley, 1998

Goodman R: The Strengths and Difficulties Questionnaire: a research note. J Child Psychol Psychiatry 38:581–586, 1997

Goodman R: The extended version of the Strengths and Difficulties Questionnaire as a guide to child psychiatric caseness. J Child Psychol Psychiatry 40:791–799, 1999

Goodman R, Scott S: Comparing the Strengths and Difficulties Questionnaire and the Child Behavior Checklist: is small beautiful? J Abnorm Child Psychol 27:17–24, 1999

Goodman R, Meltzer H, Bailey V: The Strengths and Difficulties Questionnaire: a pilot study on the validity of the self-report version. Eur Child Adolesc Psychiatry 7:125–130, 1998

Gordon M: The assessment of impulsivity and mediating behaviors in hyperactive and nonhyperactive boys. J Abnorm Child Psychol 6:221–236, 1979

Graham P, Rutter M: Psychiatric disorder in the young adolescent: a follow-up study. Proceedings of the Royal Society of Med 66:1226–1229, 1973

Gray JA: The Neuropsychology of Anxiety. New York, Oxford University Press, 1982

Green WH: Child and Adolescent Clinical Psychopharmacology. Baltimore, MD, Williams & Wilkins, 1991

Harter S: Manual for the Self-Perception Profile for Children [revision of the Perceived Competence Scale for Children]. Denver, CO, University of Denver, 1985

Hartsough CS, Lambert NM: Medical factors in hyperactive and normal children: prenatal, developmental, and health history findings. Am J Orthopsychiatry 55: 190–210, 1985

Herjanic B, Reich W: Development of a structured interview for children, Part 1: agreement between child and parent on individual symptoms. J Abnorm Child Psychol 10:307–324, 1982

Hirshfeld DR, Rosenbaum JF, Biederman J, et al: Stable behavioral inhibition and its association with anxiety disorder. J Am Acad Child Adolesc Psychiatry 31: 103–111, 1992

Humphreys MS, Revelle W: Personality, motivation, and performance: a theory of the relationship between individual differences and information processing. Psychol Rev 91:153–184, 1984

Hunt RD, Mindera RB, Cohen DJ: Clonidine benefits children with attention deficit disorder and hyperactivity: report of a double-blind placebo-controlled crossover study. J Am Acad Child Adolesc Psychiatry 24:617–629, 1985

Hunt RD, Capper L, O'Connell P: Clonidine in child and adolescent psychiatry. J Child Adolesc Psychopharmacol 1:87–102, 1990

Husain SA, Kashani JH: Anxiety Disorders in Children and Adolescents. Washington, DC, American Psychiatric Press, 1991

Hynd GW, Nieves N, Connor RT, et al: Attention deficit disorder with and without hyperactivity: reaction time and speed of cognitive processing. J Learning Disabil 22:573–580, 1989

Ickowicz A, Tannock R, Fulford P, et al: Transient tics and compulsive behaviors following methylphenidate: evidence from a placebo controlled double blind clinical trial (abstract). J Am Acad Child Adolesc Psychiatry 32:885, 1993

Jacobvitz D, Sroufe A, Stewart M, et al: Treatment of attentional and hyperactivity problems in children with sympathomimetic drugs: a comprehensive review. J Am Acad Child Adolesc Psychiatry 29:677–688, 1990

Jastak S, Wilkinson GS: The Wide Range Achievement Test—Revised: Administration Manual. Wilmington, DE, Jastak Associates, 1986

Jensen PS, Shervette RE, Xenakis SN, et al: Anxiety and depressive disorders in attention deficit disorder with hyperactivity: new findings. Am J Psychiatry 150:1203–1209, 1993

Jensen PS, Martin D, Cantwell D: Comorbidity in ADHD: implications for research, practice, and DSM-V. J Am Acad Child Adolesc Psychiatry 36:1065–1079, 1997

Kashani JH, Orvaschel H: Anxiety disorders in mid-adolescence: a community sample. Am J Psychiatry 145:960–964, 1988

Kashani JH, Orvaschel H: A community study of anxiety in children and adolescents. Am J Psychiatry 147:313–318, 1990

Kashani JH, Vaidya AF, Soltys SM, et al: Correlates of anxiety in psychiatrically hospitalized children and their parents. Am J Psychiatry 147:319–323, 1990

Kashani JH, Dandoy AC, Orvaschel H: Current perspectives on anxiety disorders in children and adolescents: an overview. Compr Psychiatry 32:481–495, 1991

Kaufman J, Birmaher B, Brent D, et al: Schedule for Affective Disorders and Schizophrenia for School-Age Children—Present and Lifetime Version (K-SADS-PL): initial reliability and validity data. J Am Acad Child Adolesc Psychiatry 36:980–988, 1997

Keller MB, Lavori PW, Wunder J, et al: Chronic course of anxiety disorders in children and adolescents. J Am Acad Child Adolesc Psychiatry 31:595–599, 1992

Kemph JP, DeVane CL, Levin GM, et al: Treatment of aggressive children with clonidine: results of an open pilot study. J Am Acad Child Adolesc Psychiatry 32:577–581, 1993

Klein RG, Last CG: Anxiety Disorders in Children. Newbury Park, CA, Sage, 1989

Kovaacs M: Children's Depression Inventory Manual. New York, Multi-Health Systems, 1989

Lahey BB, Schaughency EA, Strauss CC, et al: Are attention deficit disorders with and without hyperactivity similar or dissimilar? J Am Acad Child Adolesc Psychiatry 23:302–309, 1984

Lahey BB, Schaughency EA, Hynd GW, et al: Attention deficit disorder with and without hyperactivity: comparison of behavioral characteristics of clinic-referred children. J Am Acad Child Adolesc Psychiatry 26:718–723, 1987

Last CG: Anxiety disorders in childhood and adolescence, in Handbook of Anxiety Disorders. Edited by Last CG, Hersen M. New York, Pergamon, 1988, pp 531–540

Last CG, Phillips JE, Statfeld A: Childhood anxiety disorders in mothers and their children. Child Psychiatry Hum Dev 18:103–112, 1987

Last CG, Perrin S, Hersen M, et al: DSM-III-R anxiety disorders in children: sociodemographic and clinical characteristics. J Am Acad Child Adolesc Psychiatry 31:1070–1076, 1992

Leckman JF, Hardin MT, Riddle MA, et al: Clonidine treatment of Gilles de la Tourette's syndrome. Arch Gen Psychiatry 48:324–328, 1991

Links PS, Offord DR, Boyle MH: Correlates of emotional disorder from a community survey. Can J Psychiatry 35:419–425, 1990

Livingston RL, Dykman RA, Ackerman PT: The frequency and significance of additional self-reported psychiatric diagnoses in children with attention deficit hyperactivity disorder. J Abnorm Child Psychol 18:465–478, 1990

Livingston RL, Dykman RA, Ackerman PT: Psychiatric comorbidity and response to two doses of methylphenidate in children with attention deficit disorder. J Child Adolesc Psychopharmacol 2:115–122, 1992

Logan GD, Cowan WB, Davis KA: On the ability to inhibit simple and choice reaction time responses: a model and a method. J Exp Psychol: Hum Percept Perform 10:276–291, 1984

March JS: Anxiety Disorders in Children and Adolescents. New York, Guilford, 1995

March JS, Sullivan K: Test-retest reliability of the Multidimensional Anxiety Scale for Children. J Anxiety Disord 13:349–358, 1999

March JS, Parker JD, Sullivan K, et al: The Multidimensional Anxiety Scale for Children (MASC): factor structure, reliability, and validity. J Am Acad Child Adolesc Psychiatry 36:554–565, 1997

Maze M, Segal I, Bloor B: Clonidine and other alpha-2 adrenergic agonists: strategies for the rational use of these novel anesthetic agents. J Clin Anesth 1:146–157, 1988

McClellan JM, Rubert MP, Reichler RJ, et al: Attention deficit disorder in children at risk for anxiety and depression. J Am Acad Child Adolesc Psychiatry 29:534–539, 1990

McGee R, Feehan M, Williams S, et al: DSM-II disorders in a large sample of adolesents. J Am Acad Child Adolesc Psychiatry 29:611–619, 1990

McGee R, Feehan M, Williams S, et al: DSM-III disorders from age 11 to age 15 years. J Am Acad Child Adolesc Psychiatry 31:50–59, 1992

Mefford IN, Potter WZ: A neuroanatomical and biochemical basis of attention deficit disorder with hyperactivity in children: a defect in tonic adrenaline mediated inhibition of locus coeruleus stimulation. Med Hypotheses 29:33–42, 1989

Morgan AE, Hynd GW, Riccio CA, et al: Validity of DSM-IV ADHD predominantly inattentive and combined types: relationship to previous DSM diagnoses/subtype differences. J Am Acad Child Adolesc Psychiatry 35:325–333, 1996

Munir K, Biederman J, Knee D: Psychiatric comorbidities in patients with attention deficit disorder: a controlled study. J Am Acad Child Adolesc Psychiatry 26:844–888, 1987

Nichols PL, Chen TC: Minimal Brain Dysfunction: A Prospective Study. Hillsdale, NJ, Erlbaum, 1981

Offord DR, Boyle MH, Szatmari P, et al: Ontario Health Study: six-month prevalence of disorder and rates of service utilization. Arch Gen Psychiatry 44:832–836, 1987

Offord DR, Boyle MH, Racine YA, et al: Outcome, prognosis, and risk in a longitudinal follow-up study. J Am Acad Child Adolesc Psychiatry 31:916–923, 1992

Ollendick TH: Reliability and validity of the Revised Fear Survey Schedule for Children (FSSC-R). Behav Res Ther 21:685–692, 1983

Pauls DL, Leckman JF: The inheritance of Gilles de la Tourette's syndrome and associated behaviors: evidence for autosomal dominant transmission. N Engl J Med 315:993–997, 1986

Pliszka SR: Tricyclic antidepressants in the treatment of children with attention deficit disorder. J Am Acad Child Adolesc Psychiatry 26:127–132, 1987

Pliszka SR: Effect of anxiety on cognition, behavior, and stimulant response in ADHD. J Am Acad Child Adolesc Psychiatry 28:882–887, 1989

Pliszka SR: Comorbidity of attention-deficit hyperactivity disorder and overanxious disorder. J Am Acad Child Adolesc Psychiatry 31:197–203, 1992

Pliszka SR, Hatch JP, Borcherding SH, et al: Classical conditioning in children with attention deficit hyperactivity disorder (ADHD) and anxiety disorders: a test of Quay's model. J Abnorm Child Psychol 21:411–423, 1993

Pliszka SR, Borcherding SH, Spratley K, Leon S, et al: Measuring inhibitory control in children. J Dev Behav Pediatr 18:254–259, 1997

Quay HC: The behavioral reward and inhibition systems in childhood behavior disorders, in Attention Deficit Disorder, Vol 3. Edited by Bloomingdale LM. Oxford, UK, Pergamon, 1988, pp 176–186

Rapoport JL: Recent advances in obsessive-compulsive disorder. Neuropharmacology 5:1–10, 1991

Rapport MD, Kelly KL: Psychostimulant effects on learning and cognitive function: findings and implications for children with attention deficit hyperactivity disorder. Clin Psychol Rev 11:61–92, 1991

Reich W, Welner Z: Diagnostic Interview for Children and Adolescents—Revised, Adolescent Version. St Louis, MO, Washington University, Division of Child Psychiatry, 1990a

Reich W, Welner Z: Diagnostic Interview for Children and Adolescents—Revised, Child Version. St Louis, MO, Washington University, Division of Child Psychiatry, 1990b

Reich W, Welner Z: Diagnostic Interview for Children and Adolescents—Revised, Parent Version. St Louis, MO, Washington University, Division of Child Psychiatry, 1990c

Reich W, Herjanic B, Welner Z: Development of a structured psychiatric interview for children, Part 2: agreement on diagnosis comparing child and parent interviews. J Abnorm Child Psychol 10:325–336, 1982

Reinherz HZ, Giaconia RM, Pakiz B, et al: Psychosocial risks for major depression in late adolescence: a longitudinal community study. J Am Acad Child Adolesc Psychiatry 32:1155–1163, 1993

Rende RD: Longitudinal relations between temperament traits and behavioral syndromes in middle childhood. J Am Acad Child Adolesc Psychiatry 32:287–290, 1993

Reynolds CR, Richmond BO: What I Think and Feel: a revised measure of children's manifest anxiety. J Abnorm Child Psychol 6:271–280, 1978

Riddle MA, King RA, Hardin MT, et al: Behavioral side effects of fluoxetine in children and adolescents. J Child Adolesc Psychopharmacol 1:193–198, 1991a

Riddle MA, Nelson JC, Kleinman CS, et al: Sudden death in children receiving Norpramin: a review of three reported cases and commentary. J Am Acad Child Adolesc Psychiatry 30:104–108, 1991b

Riddle MA, Scahill L, King RA, et al: Double-blind crossover trial of fluoxetine and placebo in children and adolescents with obsessive-compulsive disorder. J Am Acad Child Adolesc Psychiatry 31:1062–1069, 1992

Riddle MA, Geller B, Ryan N: Case study: another sudden death in a child treated with desipramine. J Am Acad Child Adolesc Psychiatry 32:792–797, 1993

Robin AL: ADHD in Adolescents: Diagnosis and Treatment. New York, Guilford, 1998

Robins LN: Deviant Children Grown Up. Baltimore, MD, Williams & Wilkins, 1984

Rosenbaum JF, Biederman J, Gersten M, et al: Behavioral inhibition in children of parents with panic disorder and agoraphobia: a controlled study. Arch Gen Psychiatry 45:463–470, 1988

Rosvold HE, Mirsky AF, Sarason I, et al: A continuous performance test of brain damage. Journal of Consulting Psychology 20:343–350, 1956

Ryan ND: Pharmacotherapy of adolescent depression: beyond TCAs. Psychopharmacol Bull 26:75–79, 1990

Safer DJ, Krager JM: A survey of medication treatment for hyperactive-inattentive students. JAMA 260:2256–2258, 1988

Schachar RJ, Logan GD: Impulsivity and inhibitory control in normal development and childhood psychopathology. Dev Psychol 26:710–720, 1990

Schachar R, Tannock R: Childhood hyperactivity and psychostimulants: a review of extended treatment studies. J Child Adolesc Psychopharmacol 3:81–97, 1993

Schachar R, Tannock R, Logan G: Inhibitory control, impulsiveness and attention deficit hyperactivity disorder. Clin Psychol Rev 13:721–739, 1993

Schachar R, Tannock R, Cunningham C: Treatment of childhood hyperactivity, in Hyperactive Disorders. Edited by Sandberg S. Cambridge, UK, Cambridge University Press, 1996, pp 433–476

Shaffer D, Fisher P, Dulcan MK, et al: The NIMH Diagnostic Interview Schedule for Children Version 2.3 (DISC-2.3): description, acceptability, prevalence rates, and performance in the MECA Study. Methods for the Epidemiology of Child and Adolescent Mental Disorders Study. J Am Acad Child Adolesc Psychiatry 35:865–877, 1996

Shaywitz SE, Shaywitz BA: Attention deficit disorder: diagnosis and role of Ritlain in management, in Ritalin: Theory and Patient Management. Edited by Greenhill LL, Osman BB. New York, Mary Ann Liebert, 1991, pp 45–67

Shenker A: The mechanism of action of drugs used to treat attention-deficit hyperactivity disorder: focus on catecholamine receptor pharmacology. Adv Pediatr 39:337–382, 1992

Silver LB: Attention-Deficit Hyperactivity Disorder: A Clinical Guide to Diagnosis and Treatment. Washington, DC, American Psychiatric Press, 1991

Silverman WK, Eisen AR: Age differences in the reliability of parent and child reports of child anxious symptomatology using a structured interview. J Am Acad Child Adolesc Psychiatry 31:117–124, 1992

Silverman WK, Nelles WB: The Anxiety Disorders Interview Schedule for Children. J Am Acad Child Adolesc Psychiatry 27:772–778, 1988

Spielberger CD: Manual for the State-Trait Anxiety Inventory for Children. Palo Alto, CA, Consulting Psychologists Press, 1973

Sprich-Buckminster S, Biederman J, Milberger S, et al: Are perinatal complications relevant to the manifestation of ADD? Issues of comorbidity and familiality. J Am Acad Child Adolesc Psychiatry 32:1032–1037, 1993

Steingard R, Biederman J, Spencer T, et al: Comparison of clonidine response in the treatment of attention deficit hyperactivity disorder with and without comorbid tic disorders. J Am Acad Child Adolesc Psychiatry 32:350–353, 1993

Strauss CC, Last CG: Social and simple phobias in children. J Anxiety Disord 7: 141–152, 1993

Strauss CC, Lease CA, Last CG, et al: Overanxious disorder: an examination of developmental differences. J Abnorm Child Psychol 16:433–443, 1988

Sylvester CE, Hyde TS, Reichler RJ: The Diagnostic Interview for Children and Personality Inventory for Children in studies of children at risk for anxiety disorders or depression. J Am Acad Child Adolesc Psychiatry 26:668–675, 1987

Tannock R, Schachar R: Is ADHD with comorbid overanxious disorder different from ADHD? Presentation in "Comorbidity of ADHD: Discriminating Features and Methodologic Problems" (Newcorn J, Chair). Symposium held at the 39th annual meeting of the American Academy of Child and Adolescent Psychiatry, Washington, DC, October 1992

Tannock R, Fulford P, Purvis K, et al: Longer-term effects of stimulant treatment of attention deficit hyperactivity disorder: a continuous 12-month follow-up study. Poster presented at the annual meeting of the Canadian Academy of Child Psychiatry, Montreal, Quebec, September 1992

Tannock R, Fine J, Heintz T, et al: A linguistic approach detects stimulant effects in two children with attention deficit hyperactivity disorder. J Child Adolesc Psychopharmacol 5:177–189, 1995a

Tannock R, Ickowicz A, Schachar R: Differential effects of methylphenidate on working memory in ADHD children with and without comorbid anxiety. J Am Acad Child Adolesc Psychiatry 34:886–896, 1995b

Taylor E, Schachar R, Thorley G, et al: Which boys respond to stimulant medication? A controlled trial of methylphenidate in boys with disruptive behaviour. Psychol Med 17:121–143, 1987

Turner SM, Beidel DC, Costello AJ: Psychopathology in the offspring of anxiety disorders patients. J Consult Clin Psychol 55:229–235, 1987

Urman R, Ickowicz A, Fulford P, et al: An exaggerated cardiovascular response to methylphenidate in ADHD children with anxiety. J Child Adolesc Psychopharmacol 5:29–37, 1995

Velez CN, Johnson J, Cohen P: A longitudinal analysis of selected risk factors of childhood psychopathology. J Am Acad Child Adolesc Psychiatry 28:861–864, 1989

Verhulst FC, van der Ende J: Six-year developmental course of internalizing and externalizing problem behaviors. J Am Acad Child Adolesc Psychiatry 31:924–931, 1992

Walkup JT, Khan S, Schuerholz, et al: Phenomenology and natural history of tic-related ADHD and learning disabilities, in Tourette's Syndrome: Tics, Obsessions, Compulsions. Edited by Leckman JF, Cohen DJ. New York, Wiley, 1999, pp 63–79

Wechsler D: The Wechsler Intelligence Scale for Children—Revised. New York, Psychological Corporation, 1974

Weiss G, Hechtman L: Hyperactive Children Grown Up. New York, Guilford, 1986

Weissman MM, Leckman JF, Merikangas KR, et al: Depression and anxiety disorders in parents and children. Arch Gen Psychiatry 44:847–853, 1984

Werry JS: Overanxious disorder: a review of its taxonomic properties. J Am Acad Child Adolesc Psychiatry 30:533–544, 1991

Werry JS, Aman MG: Practitioner's Guide to Psychoactive Drugs for Children and Adolescents. New York, Plenum, 1993

Wolraich ML, Lindgren S, Stromquist A, et al: Stimulant medication use by primary care physicians in the treatment of attention deficit hyperactivity disorder. Pediatrics 86:95–101, 1990

Woolston JL, Rosenthal SL, Riddle MA, et al: Childhood comorbidity of anxiety/affective disorders and behavior disorders. J Am Acad Child Adolesc Psychiatry 28:707–713, 1989

Zohar AH, Ratzoni G, Pauls DL, et al: An epidemiological study of obsessive-compulsive disorder and related disorders in Israeli adolescents. J Am Acad Child Adolesc Psychiatry 31:1057–1061, 1992

5 Attention-Deficit Disorders With Oppositionality and Aggression

Jeffrey H. Newcorn, M.D.
Jeffrey M. Halperin, Ph.D.

Comorbidity with conduct problems, including oppositional behavior, defiance, aggression, and delinquency, accounts for the majority of reported comorbidity in children with attention-deficit/hyperactivity disorder (ADHD). The term *conduct problems,* as used in this chapter, applies to the spectrum of behavior that includes oppositionality, defiance, verbal and physical aggression, and frank delinquency. These behaviors may be classified under two different disruptive behavior disorder diagnoses in DSM-IV (American Psychiatric Association 1994): oppositional defiant disorder (ODD) and conduct disorder (CD). Also, they may occur at the subthreshold level (i.e., when the criteria for either diagnosis are not met). Symptoms of ODD include defiance of authority, failure to comply with adult requests, bullying, blaming others, and performing other behaviors that constitute minor violations of age-appropriate societal norms. In contrast, CD describes children with aggressive and delinquent behaviors that represent major violations of age-appropriate societal norms. CD symptoms may be either aggressive (e.g., initiating fights, carrying weapons, or committing assault) or nonaggressive (e.g., lying, committing truancy, running away, or stealing without confronting the victim).

ODD, CD, and aggression are often interrelated; therefore, they are frequently discussed together in the research literature. It is reasonable to consider these conditions as a spectrum because approximately 90% of children with CD also have ODD (Lahey et al. 1994) and there is a developmental progression from ODD to CD with increasing age (Loeber 1988; Loeber et al. 1993). Nevertheless, despite their similarities, these conditions may differ in important and predictable ways. In this regard, it is noteworthy that not all children with ODD progress to CD (Rey 1993).

Several epidemiological studies (Anderson et al. 1987; Bird et al. 1988; Szatmari et al. 1989b) indicate that ODD and CD are present in 40%–70% of children with ADHD, although some of these children also have comorbid internalizing disorders. These comorbidity figures are not unidirectional. Among children with ODD and/or CD in these studies, 40%–60% were estimated to also have ADHD. In addition, if one goes beyond the boundaries of categorical diagnoses and considers the full spectrum of oppositional behavior, aggression, and conduct problems (i.e., some clinically significant problems are present but the full diagnosis is not met), the percentage of children with ADHD who present with this pattern of comorbidity is greater still.

The prevalence of comorbid ODD, CD, and aggression among children with ADHD in clinical populations is probably even higher than it is in epidemiological samples, since the co-occurrence of these conditions is likely to generate substantial impairment and would be expected to result in increased referrals for mental health treatment. However, the frequency of comorbid conduct problems in children with ADHD is also likely to vary considerably across clinical settings. This is particularly relevant for understanding differences between children with ADHD who present to psychiatrists and those who present to pediatricians or other professionals and, therefore, for understanding how these different professionals are likely to view ADHD. For example, children with ADHD seen in psychiatric settings are more likely to evidence greater impairment and be more disruptive than those seen in pediatric settings. This difference is largely accounted for by the increased representation of comorbidity with conduct problems among children with ADHD in psychiatric settings (Epstein et al. 1991; Shaywitz and Shaywitz 1991).

Despite the frequency with which ADHD and conduct problems co-occur, the two major systems of psychiatric classification—DSM-IV and ICD-10 (World Health Organization 1992)—handle the phenomenon differently. ICD-10 generally follows the rule of "medical parsimony," which emphasizes identification of the single diagnostic formulation that best accounts for the presenting clinical situation. In contrast, DSM-IV more freely encourages the use of multiple diagnoses within a single individual, on the assumption that it is often not possible to identify a formulation that adequately accounts for all aspects of a clinical situation. To a large extent, these apparent differences are more stylistic than real. ICD provides a separate diagnostic category—

hyperkinetic conduct disorder—to describe children with mixed pathology. However, a study that compared diagnostic practices in the United States with those in the United Kingdom (Prendergast et al. 1988) found that most British psychiatrists diagnosed CD, rather than hyperkinetic disorder or hyperkinetic conduct disorder, when both ADHD and conduct problems were present. As a result, the latter two diagnoses were used much less frequently in the United Kingdom than in the United States, even though the actual prevalence of these disorders was similar in the two countries.

Disagreements on how comorbidity is best handled in DSM-IV and ICD-10 highlight two central questions regarding comorbidity of ADHD and other disruptive disorders: How are we to understand these extremely high prevalence figures? What are the implications regarding the validity and distinctiveness of these disorders? Critics of the DSM model argue that there are numerous ways estimates of comorbidity may be inflated (Achenbach 1990–1991; Caron and Rutter 1991). Potential confounds in ascertaining clinical status that could lead to artifactually high comorbidity figures include 1) inaccuracies in reported information caused by different individuals' understanding of what is normal or abnormal (informant bias); 2) the fact that certain target behaviors may be more prominent in one setting than another (and therefore may vary considerably across raters); and 3) halo effects on standardized rating instruments (i.e., disruptive children may be identified as inattentive and hyperactive when they are not). Inflated estimates of comorbidity could also result from categories that are either too broadly or too narrowly defined, either by increasing the degree of overlap of two individual disorders or by restricting the definition of one of the disorders to a group that is almost certain to be comorbid. Finally, spurious comorbidity could also result from excluding important information from diagnostic algorithms, which would result in decreasing the distinctiveness of a disorder and, therefore, increasing the likelihood that it will overlap with another condition. For example, attentional testing, which is not part of the ADHD algorithm, might be helpful in determining which disruptive children who are *rated* inattentive are *truly* inattentive (comorbid group) and which are not (artifact secondary to halo effect).

It is reasonable, therefore, to conclude that estimates of the extent of comorbidity between ADHD and other disruptive behavior disorders may be somewhat inflated because of artifact and measurement error. However, it is equally important to note that the rate with which this comorbidity occurs greatly exceeds what would be predicted based on probability estimates derived from the prevalence of each disorder alone, and that the figures have been replicated across numerous epidemiological and clinical samples

(Biederman et al. 1991; Costello 1992; Szatmari et al. 1989b). Thus, there can be little doubt that this phenomenon is real and has considerable clinical significance.

The high degree of comorbidity between ADHD and conduct problems raises several important conceptual and operational questions:

- Are ADHD, ODD, and CD distinct psychiatric conditions, or are they different aspects of the same general phenomenon?
- Why is comorbidity with ODD, CD, and/or aggression so common in children with ADHD?
- Does the presence of comorbid conduct problems alter the clinical presentation of children with ADHD?
- Does the comorbid configuration of ADHD and CD represent a distinct subtype?
- How does understanding the comorbidity of ADHD with conduct problems affect clinical decision making?
- Are additional or different treatments required for children with ADHD and comorbid conduct problems?

In this chapter we address these questions in order to review the complex relationship between ADHD and conduct problems and to develop a strategy for clinical decision making when these conditions are thought to co-occur. Clinical material is used to illustrate various points. For simplicity, we discuss ODD, CD, and aggression together, even though they may differ in important and predictable ways (Rey 1993). Our focus in this chapter is on comorbidity of ADHD and conduct problems in children and adolescents, and not in adults. The majority of published studies examining this phenomenon have been conducted in children and adolescents, and data indicate that comorbidity profiles in adults with ADHD do not differ appreciably from those in youth (Biederman et al. 1993c). Nevertheless, we do consider longitudinal course.

ARE ADHD, ODD, AND CD DISTINCT PSYCHIATRIC CONDITIONS OR DIFFERENT ASPECTS OF THE SAME GENERAL PHENOMENON?

This question has been the topic of considerable debate in the literature for more than 20 years, with findings supporting both positions (see Hinshaw

1987). Careful examination of the diagnostic criteria for ADHD, ODD, and CD indicates that there is very little overlap in the symptoms used to define these disorders. However, the frequent co-occurrence of inattention, hyperactivity, impulsivity, oppositionality, and aggression within individuals suggests that these symptom domains are very closely related, which makes them difficult to disentangle both heuristically and in clinical practice. This is particularly problematic because it is essential that two conditions be shown to be distinct before it is possible to even discuss their comorbid occurrence.

Several studies (Conners 1969, 1970; Trites and Laprade 1983; Werry et al. 1975) have used factor-analytic methods to assess whether the domain of hyperactivity is distinct from that of conduct problems and aggression. This method examines the intercorrelations among symptoms and groups together those symptoms that are highly interrelated. Factor-analytic studies have generally identified a robust conduct problems factor, which accounts for the largest percentage of variance in disruptive behavior. Symptoms of inattention and hyperactivity sometimes load with conduct problem symptoms and sometimes load on a separate factor. However, even when these symptoms load on separate factors, they often have been highly intercorrelated. Therefore, the findings from factor-analytic studies have not been persuasive in proving that hyperactivity and conduct problems are distinct.

Werry et al. (1987b) and Reeves et al. (1987) examined the descriptive and associated features of nonpsychotic children with a range of psychiatric problems and those of children with ADHD and CD. The researchers concluded that there was little basis on which to distinguish one diagnostic group from another. In addition, several early investigations that used objective laboratory measures failed to find meaningful differences between ADHD and other nonpsychotic disorders, including ADHD with comorbid CD (Koriath et al. 1985; Shapiro and Garfinkel 1986; Werry et al. 1987a).

In contrast, other studies have indicated that it is possible to distinguish symptoms of ADHD from those of aggression by using a variety of descriptive, psychosocial, developmental, and laboratory measures. This line of research has been greatly facilitated by the use of rating instruments that can more clearly distinguish symptoms of inattention-overactivity from symptoms of aggression. One such instrument, the IOWA Conners (Loney and Milich 1982), contains five empirically derived items from the larger Conners Teacher Rating Scale (Goyette et al. 1978) that were found to be specific to children described as inattentive and overactive but not aggressive, and five items that were found to be divergently valid for aggression but not hyperactivity. This 10-item scale continues to represent a quick method for differentially assessing symptoms of ADHD and aggression in clinical practice, although the aggression subscale more accurately describes defiance and oppositional behavior than actual physical aggression. Published norms are available (Pelham et al. 1989).

The distinctiveness of ADHD and CD has been demonstrated in several epidemiologically derived samples (McGee et al. 1984; Moffit 1990; Szatmari et al. 1989a). These researchers examined differential correlates of the two conditions. Children with ADHD were generally characterized by a persistent pattern of developmental problems and cognitive impairments, whereas children with CD were characterized as having lower socioeconomic status and experiencing higher levels of psychosocial adversity, including increased family problems. Psychopathology was not present more often in parents of children who had ADHD without CD than it was in parents of control subjects (Lahey et al. 1988; Schachar and Wachsmuth 1990). It is important to note that epidemiological and clinical studies (Schachar and Tannock 1993; Szatmari et al. 1989a) indicated that children who were comorbid for ADHD and CD presented with the risk factors and associated features characteristic of both disorders. The findings from these and other studies are consistent with the hypothesis that CD may be a more environmentally driven condition than ADHD, although they do not preclude genetic-neurobiological contributions to the pathogenesis of CD, as well as the role of psychosocial mechanisms in ADHD. Biederman et al. (1995a, 1995b) highlighted the importance of psychosocial adversity in ADHD. The finding that children with ADHD and CD present with the risk factors and associated features of both disorders is also consistent with the findings of Walker et al. (1987) and Moffit (1990), which indicate that comorbid CD accounts for the poorest outcome among children with ADHD and, conversely, that comorbid ADHD confers increased risk for poor outcome in children with CD.

The distinctiveness of ADHD and CD has also been demonstrated in studies using objective laboratory measures. The Structured Observation Assessment in Playroom Setting (SOAPS; Roberts 1990) provides an in vitro observation method that accurately classifies children with ADHD, CD, and ADHD with comorbid CD according to their performance on free play and restricted academic tasks. The comorbid group performs worst on this measure. Children with CD only are indistinguishable from control subjects, whereas children with ADHD alone have scores that fall between those of the comorbid and control groups.

Studies using computerized continuous performance tests (CPTs) (Halperin et al. 1988, 1991; Rosvold et al. 1956) and acceleration-sensitive actigraphs (Reichenbach et al. 1992; Teicher et al. 1996) have also shown that children who have ADHD without comorbidity can be distinguished from children who have ODD or CD without ADHD (Halperin et al. 1993). The children with ADHD in the Halperin et al. (1993) study made significantly more inattention and impulsivity errors on the CPT measures than did the children with ODD and/or CD, children with anxiety disorders but no disruptive disorders, and control subjects. In contrast, the non-ADHD groups did not differ from control subjects and from one another on the CPT measures. Children with ADHD also showed a trend for higher motor activity during the CPT, as measured by an actigraph. It is noteworthy that children with ADHD were found to differ from children without ADHD and control subjects when "relatively pure" groups were studied (e.g., comorbidity within a single diagnostic grouping was permitted so that children with multiple anxiety disorders were included in the anxiety disorder group) but not when comorbid groups were examined (Halperin et al. 1992).

In summary, although there is still considerable overlap and diagnostic imprecision, recent research indicates that ADHD and conduct problems do not represent variations on a single theme. Children with these conditions without comorbidity present with different core symptoms, have different patterns of psychosocial correlates, and perform differently on objective measures of ADHD symptoms. Children with comorbidity present with the symptoms and psychosocial correlates of both disorders and account for the poorest outcome within each group. The failure to demonstrate a distinction between ADHD and conduct problems in earlier studies is likely related to the use of rating scales rather than direct observational and/or objective assessment measures, as well as to the failure to separate the comorbid group in data analysis.

WHY IS COMORBIDITY WITH ODD, CD, AND/OR AGGRESSION COMMON IN CHILDREN WITH ADHD?

If ADHD is distinct from conduct problems, why do 50%–70% of children with ADHD also present with comorbid ODD or CD? Clearly, there must be some interactions among these conditions that can account for the especially high rate of comorbidity (see Caron and Rutter 1991; Rutter 1989). Possible explanations include the following:

- One disorder represents a developmental precursor to another.
- One disorder represents a risk factor for the subsequent development of the other disorder.

- The disorders share the same or related risk factors.
- There is a common underlying symptomatic basis for one or more of these disorders.

To a certain extent, all these explanations are at least partially correct, although no one explanation is sufficient to explain the phenomenon.

There is little evidence that ADHD represents a developmental precursor to CD. This explanation more frequently has been advanced with respect to ODD and CD. However, children with ADHD and comorbid ODD or CD characteristically present with early onset of aggression, and data from numerous studies indicate that this group is at increased risk for persistent aggression and antisocial disturbance in later childhood and adolescence. In contrast to early-onset CD, late-onset CD first emerges after the age of 10, is much less often characterized by aggressive behavior, and is generally not associated with a premorbid history of ADHD (Lahey et al. 1994; Loeber 1990; Robins 1991). However, the question of whether ADHD represents a developmental precursor to CD hinges on whether children who have ADHD without an early presentation of aggression or comorbidity with ODD and/or CD are also at increased risk for development of the latter conditions. In other words, is the increased risk for antisocial behavior among children with ADHD when they reach adolescence entirely accounted for by comorbid conduct problems in childhood, or can this outcome occur independently of comorbidity with conduct problems?

This question has been the subject of several investigations, although the data have been somewhat contradictory and therefore difficult to interpret. MacDonald and Achenbach (1996), in a 6-year study of dimensional ratings on the Child Behavior Checklist (CBCL) and Youth Self-Report questionnaires, found that antisocial outcomes among children with ADHD followed into adolescence were entirely predicted by the coexistence of ADHD and aggression in childhood. However, in a carefully evaluated sample drawn from an epidemiological sample of 6- and 7-year-old schoolchildren, Taylor et al. (1996) found that the risk for CD was elevated as a function of the severity of hyperactivity in childhood, independent of comorbidity. Biederman et al. (1996b) also found that comorbidity with CD was higher in children with persistent ADHD. The researchers, however, did not follow their sample far enough into adolescence and young adulthood to ascertain the incidence of antisocial personality. In addition, comorbidity with disorders other than ODD or CD was equally likely to be associated with the persistence of ADHD in this study, which indicates that the association of ADHD with ODD and CD is not specific.

A related, but more moderate, hypothesis is that although ADHD and CD are not part and parcel of the same general phenomenon, ADHD may represent a risk factor for the subsequent development of CD. This hypothesis, which has been developed by Loeber and colleagues (Loeber 1988, 1993; Loeber et al. 1992), posits a developmental progression of pathology within the disruptive disorders, which proceeds in a stepwise manner. Although these studies deal more specifically with the incremental worsening of symptoms of ODD and CD than they do with ADHD, data indicate that coexistent ADHD may speed the transition through these various steps and therefore contribute to increased risk for CD. Additional data supporting this contention includes the findings that ADHD represents a risk factor for poor outcome among children with CD (Walker et al. 1987) and that the development of antisocial personality in adults who formerly had ADHD is much greater when ADHD symptoms are severe and persistent (Barkley et al. 1990; Mannuzza et al. 1993). The findings from the Taylor et al. (1996) study—that risk for CD was increased by severe hyperactivity in early childhood, independent of comorbidity with CD—might also be seen as supporting this hypothesis. However, the findings from two different follow-up studies do not support this hypothesis. Loney et al. (1981) found that nonaggressive children with ADHD present with anxiety symptoms and learning problems in adolescence but not conduct problems, antisocial behavior, or substance abuse. Biederman et al. (1997) reported that adolescents with and without ADHD had similar risk for substance abuse and that this risk was mediated by the presence of CD and/or bipolar disorder but not ADHD alone.

The notion that ADHD and CD share common risk factors has been the subject of several studies, whose findings indicate the need to reexamine existing theories. Psychosocial adversity, including parental psychopathology, low socioeconomic status, family discord, and exposure to peer antisocial behavior, has often been associated with high risk for aggression and CD but not ADHD. However, more recent studies by Biederman and colleagues (Biederman et al. 1995a, 1995b) indicated that although no single psychosocial adversity factor is specifically associated with ADHD, the accumulation of several adversity factors—including parental conflict, diminished family cohesion, and parental psychopathology—is associated with increased risk for ADHD.

Similarly, risk factors associated with ADHD may also confer an increased risk for CD. For example, having a parent with ADHD could increase a child's risk for CD as well as ADHD, since the likelihood of exposure to family discord and inconsistent parental discipline (known risk factors for CD) may also be higher in families in which one parent has ADHD. In this example, a risk factor for ADHD (e.g., parental ADHD) could lead to the development of risk factors for CD (e.g., family discord and/or aggression), which then could contribute to the development of CD in offspring. Thus, although the risk factors for ADHD and CD may be distinct (e.g., genetic loading for ADHD as a risk factor for ADHD, and exposure to family discord and erratic and inconsistent parenting as risk factors for CD), in some situations they may interact to produce additive risk.

Data are also emerging that support the contention that ADHD and CD share an underlying symptomatic basis, although the symptoms may present differently in the two conditions. Data from the Mount Sinai Hospital outpatient clinic indicate that objectively measured impulsivity is present not only in children with ADHD but also in children who fight but do not have ADHD (Halperin et al. 1995). This finding held up even when children with subthreshold ADHD were removed from the aggressive group. Indeed, the main effects were greater for aggression than for ADHD. These data are consistent with the hypothesis that individuals with ADHD and/or aggression share an underlying impulsive personality style and suggest a mechanism by which ADHD could represent a risk factor for aggression. However, it is not known whether the basic nature and neurobiological determinants of impulsivity are the same in children with ADHD, children with CD, and children with ADHD and comorbid CD.

These studies suggest that children with ADHD, particularly those with severe and persistent ADHD symptoms, are at increased risk for the development of conduct problems, including ODD and CD. Children with ADHD who have early onset of aggression are at greatest risk. When specific risk factors for CD are not present, the likelihood for CD to develop is low, even when ADHD is present. However, when risk factors and early clinical warning signs for CD are present, the simultaneous presence of ADHD may escalate the development of aggression into full-blown CD.

DOES THE PRESENCE OF COMORBID CONDUCT PROBLEMS ALTER THE CLINICAL PRESENTATION OF CHILDREN WITH ADHD?

Several important questions can be asked about the clinical presentation of children with ADHD and comorbid conduct problems: Do these children have the same core ADHD symptoms as those with ADHD who do not have this comorbid presentation or those with ADHD and other comorbid conditions? In other words, are children with ADHD and comorbid conduct problems equally inattentive, impulsive, and hyperactive, or is one or more of these symptom domains accentuated, diminished, or otherwise altered in this group? Finally, are there differences in the severity or age at onset of the presenting symptoms in children with ADHD and comorbid conduct problems?

Case Vignette

Peter, a 5-year-old boy, was referred by his parents for evaluation regarding the appropriateness of medication treatment. The oldest of two children, Peter lives with his parents and younger sister in an upper-middle-class urban community. He was first diagnosed with ADHD several months ago during a psychological evaluation. Peter was always extremely overactive, often to the point of being uncontrollable. He would fidget constantly and touched other people and objects frequently. He was a climber, and his climbing had already resulted in several accidents. He was also very impulsive, frequently picking up something nearby and throwing it without thinking. His attention span was variable. Sometimes he could sit still and look at a book with his parents, but this usually was not the case. However, he was often able to watch TV calmly for extended periods of time.

Peter had been seen by a social worker therapist for about a year but was referred for a more extensive workup and possible change in treatment plan because of escalating aggression. Peter was very difficult to manage in nursery school, aggressive with peers, and frequently unresponsive to limits. He did relatively better when he had one-to-one supervision at home and at school. Fortunately, he was often able to receive this level of care. However, recent increases in the level of aggression both at home (he was frequently aggressive with his younger sister) and at school (as a result of this behavior, he had almost no friends), as well as his inability to meet the increased demands for self-regulation and on-task behavior at school, were becoming serious problems. The school was threatening to place Peter in a special education class or to hold him back in kindergarten. His parents were becoming exasperated and found themselves losing patience with him more frequently. All involved with the case recognized that the situation was escalating out of control.

This case illustrates several problems that are frequently observed in children with ADHD and comorbid conduct problems. The age at onset is very early, with very high levels of activity almost always present. Attention may or may not be disturbed but is usually very difficult to evaluate because of the high activity level. There is a persistent pattern of impulsive behavior, which may lead to injury to themselves or others. As a result of the early presentation of severe and disruptive behaviors, referral for treatment is often made during preschool or in the early school years. Frequently, there are significant problems in peer relationships and parent-child interactions. Psychosocial and behavioral interventions alone (in this case, use of a generic, supportive, child-centered psychotherapy, as well as one-to-one observation) may not be sufficient, and evaluation for possible pharmacotherapy is often requested.

There are some empirical data in the literature that support these clinical impressions of children with ADHD and comorbid conduct problems. However, many aspects of this profile remain unsubstantiated. There is general agreement regarding the existence of two partially distinct groups of children with ADHD, whose conditions have been variably described as cognitive and behavioral (August and Garfinkel 1989), inattentive and noninattentive (Halperin et al. 1990a), or nonaggressive and aggressive (Halperin et al. 1990b, 1994; Matier et al. 1992) subtypes. Children in the cognitively impaired/inattentive/nonaggressive group are characterized by one or more of the following: inattention, absence of aggressive behavior, presence of learning disabilities or academic underachievement, and comorbidity with mood or anxiety disorders. These children have been shown to make many inattention errors (i.e., omission errors and some types of commission errors) on CPTs. In contrast, children in the behaviorally impaired/noninattentive/aggressive group are characterized by higher levels of motor activity and impulsivity, with or without high levels of objectively measured inattention, and have a greater likelihood of being aggressive. Similar distinctions in comorbidity profiles have also been described in children who have attention-deficit disorders with and without hyperactivity (Lahey et al. 1987). Children who have attention-deficit disorders *without* hyperactivity are more likely to present with internalizing and/or cognitive disorders; children who have attention-deficit disorders *with* hyperactivity are more likely to demonstrate comorbid externalizing disorders.

No published studies have examined the nature and distribution of ADHD symptoms in children with ADHD and comorbid ODD or CD with objective measures, although some such data have been presented (Newcorn et al. 1992; Newcorn 1993; Schachar and Tannock 1993). Data collected at the Mount Sinai Hospital outpatient clinic examined CPT performance and actigraph-measured motor activity during a structured psychometric testing session. Forty children with ADHD were identified with a best-estimate procedure:

23 (54%) had comorbid ODD or CD, and 17 (42%) did not. The children in the comorbid group were older than those in the noncomorbid group (10.0 versus 8.5 years), but the groups did not differ in intellectual capacity or academic performance (the data were therefore age-controlled). The two groups did not differ significantly on any of the objective measures. Both groups scored higher than control subjects on the CPT inattention and actigraph measures. Both groups also scored higher than control subjects on the CPT impulsivity measures, although significance at the $P < 0.05$ level was achieved in the comorbid group only (Halperin and Newcorn 1998; Newcorn et al. 1992).

These findings indicate that the nature of ADHD symptoms is similar in children with ADHD and comorbid ODD/CD/aggression and in those without this comorbidity. However, consistent with clinical impressions, children in the comorbid group may be somewhat more impulsive. These findings are particularly noteworthy in the context of a parallel analysis that examined these same CPT and actigraph variables as a function of ADHD with and without comorbid anxiety (Halperin and Newcorn 1998; Newcorn et al. 1992). Interestingly, only children with ADHD who did not have comorbid anxiety disorders scored higher than control subjects on CPT impulsivity; those with comorbid anxiety disorders were indistinguishable from control subjects on this measure. Most important, few of the children with ADHD and comorbid anxiety disorders were diagnosed as having only these two disorders; the majority also were diagnosed with ODD or CD. This suggests that the simultaneous presence of anxiety disorders in children with ADHD and comorbid conduct problems may mitigate the otherwise high level of impulsive behavior. Therefore, it is important in clinical practice to determine whether children with ADHD and comorbid conduct problems also present with an anxiety disorder, since the additional presence of anxiety may serve as a protective factor against the high level of impulsivity usually seen in children with ADHD and comorbid conduct problems.

DOES THE COMORBID CONFIGURATION OF ADHD AND CD REPRESENT A DISTINCT SUBTYPE?

Of the many comorbid configurations of ADHD, comorbidity of ADHD and CD has the most data sustantiating its consideration as a distinct subtype. These data include 1) results of family studies, which indicate that transmission of the comorbid condition has a strong familial component; 2) results of longitudinal studies, which suggest that children with ADHD and comorbid CD are at increased risk for poor outcome, including the development of antisocial behavior and substance abuse in adolescence and adulthood; and 3) findings from studies using peripheral and central measures of neurotransmitter function, as well as response to pharmacological challenge, which point to differences in the neurobiological basis of ADHD with and without aggression. The most robust findings have come from family genetic and longitudinal studies.

Biederman and colleagues (1992a, 1992b) conducted extensive double-blind controlled studies on the prevalence of psychiatric disorders in first-degree relatives of ADHD probands. Several psychiatric disorders, including major depression, anxiety disorders, ODD, and CD, were found to be increased in these pedigrees. However, in the case of ADHD and CD, the disorders cosegregated such that the increased prevalence of CD in first-degree relatives was entirely accounted for in the pedigrees of ADHD with comorbid CD probands (Faraone et al. 1991). The risk of antisocial disorders in relatives of children with ADHD and comorbid ODD was also higher than in relatives of probands who had ADHD only but was lower than in relatives of children with ADHD and comorbid CD (Biederman et al. 1992a, 1992b). These findings are consistent with the hypotheses that ADHD with comorbid CD represents a different or more virulent presentation of ADHD, which is characterized by familial transmission, and that ODD may be a less severe variant of CD. However, these findings do not resolve several important "nature versus nurture" questions regarding ADHD and comorbid CD, because the findings could be accounted for by familial, nongenetic contributions to the development of CD and by individuals with a nongenetic etiology for their ADHD (Faraone and Biederman 1994). Answering these questions requires further testing, with use of more extensive clinical assessment and genetic mapping techniques.

Findings from several longitudinal studies also point to the distinctiveness of ADHD and CD, although there are some noteworthy discrepancies in the findings. All the major follow-up studies (Barkley et al. 1990; Gittelman et al. 1985; Hechtman et al. 1984; Klein and Mannuzza 1991; Loney et al. 1981; Mannuzza et al. 1993; Weiss and Hechtman 1993; Weiss et al. 1985) indicate that children with comorbid ADHD and CD are at increased risk for antisocial behavior in adolescence and adulthood. Moreover, the preponderance of poor behavioral outcome in children with ADHD seems to be accounted for by this comorbidity. In addition, persistence of ADHD over time seems to be related to the overall presence of comorbidity, although this presence is not restricted to comorbidity with CD (Biederman et al. 1996b). Loney et al.

(1981) found that prepubertal children with ADHD who did not have comorbid aggression were at increased risk for developing cognitive impairment and anxiety symptoms in adolescence, but not antisocial behavior. Barkley et al. (1991), in a follow-up of children with ADHD into adolescence, found that comorbidity with ODD at the time of follow-up accounted for the preponderance of negative family interaction, ratings of home conflict, and maternal psychological distress. However, Hechtman and Offord (1994) and Hechtman et al. (1984) cautioned that although early aggressive behavior constitutes a risk for poor outcome, a variety of other factors, including individual personality characteristics, family psychopathology, socioeconomic status, and intelligence, may also play a role.

There is somewhat more disagreement regarding the development of substance abuse in children with ADHD who are followed into adolescence and adulthood, and its relationship to comorbid conduct problems in childhood. Follow-up studies by Loney et al. (1981) and Weiss and Hechtman (1993) did not indicate an increase in adolescent substance abuse among children with ADHD. This finding has sometimes been interpreted to mean that psychostimulant treatment does not lead to the development of substance abuse, because the majority of the children in these studies received at least some stimulant treatment. In contrast, Klein and Mannuzza (1991), Mannuzza et al. (1993), and Barkley et al. (1990), in follow-up studies of children with ADHD, did indicate an increased risk for the development of substance abuse into adolescence and, to a lesser extent, adulthood. This outcome occurred primarily in individuals who also had antisocial personality or CD. Most important, Gittelman et al. (1985), Klein and Mannuzza (1991), and Mannuzza et al. (1993) found that continuation of ADHD symptoms into adolescence and adulthood represents the most important risk factor for the subsequent development of CD, suggesting an interaction between these conditions. The conclusion that the principal risk for substance abuse among children with ADHD is carried by those who develop CD or antisocial personality is further supported by data from Halikas et al. (1990), who used regression analyses to demonstrate that aggressivity, but not ADHD, predicted substance abuse in a sample of adolescent juvenile offenders.

A preponderance of evidence indicates that the risk for substance abuse among children with ADHD is high only among those who progress to antisocial personality. Both the severity and duration of ADHD symptoms and the early onset of aggressive behavior have been shown to increase the likelihood of this outcome. It therefore stands to reason that children with ADHD and comorbid CD in early childhood are at highest risk for the development of antisocial behavior and substance abuse in adulthood.

Data on the neurobiological distinctiveness of ADHD with and without aggression are also emerging. However, there are few studies, and their meaning is still open to debate. A variety of methodologies have been used, including measures of peripheral neurotransmitter levels, direct and indirect measures of central neurotransmitter activity, and pharmacological trials. In our clinic, Matier et al. (1992) gave a 5-mg challenge dose of methylphenidate to aggressive and nonaggressive children with ADHD to assess the differential response of individual ADHD symptom domains (and thereby determine whether the neurobiological basis of these conditions is the same). Children with ADHD were tested twice, once on medication, 1 hour after the medication was administered, and once off medication. Control subjects, who were not given medication, were also tested twice. The aggressive group and the nonaggressive group of children with ADHD, both of which were initially found to have inattention, showed a reduction in CPT-measured inattention following medication, which was then equal to the level in control subjects. Impulsivity, as measured by the CPT, was elevated only in the group with aggressive ADHD, and this was not affected by the 5-mg methylphenidate dose. Activity level was initially elevated in both aggressive and nonaggressive groups, but only the nonaggressive group showed a decrease in motor activity following medication. These findings are consistent with the hypothesis that activity level is mediated through different neurobiological mechanisms in aggressive and nonaggressive children with ADHD, although differential response to the low methylphenidate dose cannot be ruled out.

Findings from studies examining peripheral and central measures of neurotransmitter function also point to differences in the neurobiologic basis of ADHD and aggression. However, it is not yet known whether children who have ADHD and aggression, ADHD without aggression, and aggression without ADHD are distinct. These studies have focused primarily on measures of catecholaminergic and serotonergic function. Among studies that have examined peripheral measures in children with ADHD and comorbid CD, noteworthy findings include the following: 1) low levels of the enzyme dopamine β-hydroxylase (which converts dopamine to norepinephrine) were found in the plasma of children with aggressive CD and children with CD and comorbid ADHD (Rogeness et al. 1984, 1986), and 2) platelet imipramine binding, a measure of presynaptic serotonin (5-HT; 5-hydroxytryptamine) function, is inversely correlated with externalizing (disruptive) symptoms in children, including children with ADHD and comorbid CD (Birmaher et al. 1990; Bowden et al. 1988; Cook et al. 1995). Thus, both noradrenergic and serotonergic mechanisms are implicated.

More recent studies have focused on central measures of serotonergic activity. Consistent with a sizable literature on animals and adults with aggression, cerebrospinal fluid (CSF) 5-hydroxyindoleacetic acid (5-HIAA), a metabolite of 5-HT, was found to be lower in a group of aggressive children and adolescents (Kruesi et al. 1990), approximately two-thirds of whom had ADHD. Moreover, low 5-HT function at the time of initial assessment predicted conduct problems at 2-year follow-up (Kruesi et al. 1992). However, a second study from the same laboratory found an increase, rather than a decrease, in 5-HT among aggressive children (Castellanos et al. 1994). Interestingly, when the two cohorts were compared, the sample used by Castellanos and colleagues, in which CSF 5-HIAA was found to be elevated in aggressive children, had a greater preponderance of comorbid ADHD, were less aggressive, and were younger. These findings are consistent with the hypothesis that neurobiological mechanisms in aggressive children with and without ADHD are different.

Results of studies using the prolactin response to acute administration of the serotonergic releaser/reuptake blocker fenfluramine as an indirect measure of central serotonergic activity also point to the distinctiveness of ADHD with and without aggression. However, interpretation of findings has been complicated by differences across samples and probable developmental influences. Data from adult studies have generally indicated that prolactin response to fenfluramine is blunted in impulsive-aggressive adults with mood and personality disorders (Coccaro et al. 1989; O'Keane et al. 1992). In children, the prolactin response to fenfluramine administration was found to be higher in aggressive children with ADHD than in nonaggressive children with ADHD (Halperin et al. 1994) and also in the siblings of boys convicted of crimes, who were at risk for aggression but who were not necessarily aggressive themselves (Pine et al. 1996). However, the finding of elevated serotonergic activity in childhood aggression was not replicated by Halperin et al. (1997b) in a second study. Indeed, when the two samples studied by Halperin and colleagues were merged to form a single, larger data set, several known risk factors for the persistence of aggression—such as severity of aggression, pervasiveness of aggression, positive family history of aggression, and high levels of emotional reactivity—were found to be associated with decreased prolactin response to fenfluramine (Halperin et al. 1997a; McKay et al. 1996; Newcorn et al. 1996).

Integrating these heterogeneous neurobiological findings into a unitary hypothesis is challenging. The data presented indicate that both serotonergic and noradrenergic mechanisms are implicated in aggression and that the neurobiologic basis of aggression in the presence of ADHD may be different from that in aggression alone. In contrast, the leading hypotheses regarding neurochemical function in ADHD involve noradrenergic and dopaminergic mechanisms (Arnsten et al. 1996; Pliszka et al. 1996). It is therefore reasonable to assume that children with comorbid pathology have abnormalities in both catecholaminergic and serotonergic systems. However, it remains unknown whether the neurochemical dysfunction in children with ADHD and aggression represents a combination of findings from studies of children with ADHD and aggression alone, or whether the neurochemistry is distinct in children in the comorbid group. Inconsistencies in the serotonergic findings both within and across studies are consistent with this latter hypothesis. The fact that aggressive children may have either high or low serotonergic function suggests that there are differences in serotonergic function in different groups of aggressive children. Comorbidity with ADHD is one of the possible explanations that has been advanced thus far. However, potential confounds related to age and severity of aggression cannot be ruled out. Clearly, more extensive study is required before any conclusions can be reached.

There are considerable data indicating that identification of the comorbid configuration ADHD and CD is of great clinical and prognostic significance and that children with this comorbidity may be different from other children with ADHD in important associated features (e.g., family history, longitudinal course, and neurochemical function). However, in our opinion, the substantial degree of evidence required to establish comorbidity of ADHD and CD as a distinct subtype of ADHD has not yet been reached.

HOW DOES UNDERSTANDING THE COMORBIDITY OF ADHD WITH CONDUCT PROBLEMS AFFECT CLINICAL DECISION MAKING?

There are several ways in which understanding the frequency, clinical presentation, and treatment response of children with ADHD and comorbid conduct problems influences clinical decisions. First and foremost, this understanding removes some of the burden from the clinician to determine whether a child has ADHD, ODD, or CD when features of multiple conditions are present, and facilitates a less polarized approach to differential diagnosis and treatment planning. Identification of all aspects of a clinical case is required for optimal treatment planning. To accomplish this, the clinician must aggressively look for features of less obvious problems. Clinicians who are not comfortable with the concept of comorbidity are more likely to miss important, coexistent problems and, therefore, to offer an incorrect or less comprehensive treatment plan (i.e., interventions targeting the comorbid conditions might not be represented).

Of course, when aggression is present, it is almost always identified. However, the reverse is not true. Comorbid ADHD could easily be missed in a child who exhibits obvious disruptive and aggressive behavior. This is especially true if the child is older or female, because motor overactivity is present less often in these ADHD patients. From a therapeutic vantage point, identifying comorbid ADHD in children with ODD, CD, or aggression is beneficial because it widens the scope of treatments that may be brought to bear on disruptive behavior. For example, children who exhibit disruptive behavior and who also are diagnosed with comorbid ADHD might be seen as candidates for treatment with psychostimulant medications, antidepressants, and/or α-adrenergic agents. Identifying this pattern of comorbidity might also offer an added dimension for understanding the child's impulsive behavior and indicate the need for additional psychosocial treatment strategies and behavioral targets. Similarly, in ADHD patients, identifying comorbidity with ODD or CD might help clinicians be better informed regarding the regulation of medication dose.

Several other "clinical pearls" may follow from the clinician's understanding of the comorbidity of ADHD and conduct problems. The majority of children with ADHD and comorbid internalizing disorders are also likely to have comorbid externalizing disorders; conversely, a significant proportion of children who have ADHD with comorbid disruptive disorders may demonstrate internalizing symptoms as well. It is, therefore, important to look for comorbid internalizing symptoms in children with ADHD and comorbid conduct problems. Girls with ADHD should be carefully evaluated for the presence of ODD or CD. This comorbid configuration is frequently underdiagnosed in girls, despite the fact that ODD or CD may actually be present in a higher percentage of girls with ADHD than of boys with ADHD (Szatmari et al. 1989a). Most important, children with ADHD who present with early aggression should receive the most intensive intervention, because they are at highest risk for poor outcome.

WHAT IS THE EFFECT OF COMORBIDITY ON TREATMENTS FOR CHILDREN WITH ADHD AND COMORBID CONDUCT PROBLEMS?

Despite the high prevalence of comorbidity in children with ADHD, this phenomenon has been poorly accounted for in the majority of treatment studies.

However, several investigations have examined 1) the impact of comorbid ODD/CD/aggression on psychostimulant treatment of ADHD symptoms, 2) the effects of stimulant treatment on comorbid aggression in children with ADHD, and 3) differential effects of comorbidity on stimulant dose response in children with ADHD. There also are data on the use of nonstimulant medications, such as tricyclic antidepressants and α-adrenergic agents, in the treatment of ADHD and comorbid aggression. Finally, there is a growing, but often anecdotal, literature on a variety of other medications used to treat aggressive children, which may have relevance for treating children with ADHD and comorbid conduct problems. It also should be noted that little research has been done on the impact of comorbidity on psychosocial treatment of children with ADHD, although enhanced efficacy from combined pharmacological and psychosocial treatments has been presumed.

In studies using dimensional rather than categorical assessment measures, Barkley et al. (1989) and Klorman et al. (1988) found that children with ADHD and comorbid aggression responded as well to treatment with methylphenidate (i.e., ADHD symptoms were reduced) as children with ADHD only. This finding was replicated in the recently completed multicenter Multimodal Treatment Study of Children With ADHD (MTA) (MTA Cooperative Group, in press). Barkley and colleagues further reported that children with ADHD and comorbid aggression had a better response to stimulant medication—perhaps as a function of having a greater opportunity for clinical improvement with treatment because they were more impaired before treatment than children with ADHD only. Taylor et al. (1987) also found that children with ADHD and comorbid CD were the most responsive to stimulant medication. Amery et al. (1984) and Kaplan et al. (1990) further suggested that stimulant medication may reduce aggression as well as ADHD symptoms in children with ADHD and comorbid aggression. There also is evidence that covert symptoms of behavior disturbance (i.e., those that are less overtly disruptive and do not involve direct confrontation with another person, such as stealing and lying) may also be decreased by stimulant treatment (Hinshaw et al. 1992). Interestingly, one such covert behavior, cheating on exams, increased in the latter study, perhaps as a function of increased on-task behavior following treatment.

An important question for the clinician is whether comorbidity of ADHD with conduct problems alters the required stimulant dose in patients treated with medication. A related question is whether there is a dissociation of cognitive and behavioral effects of stimulant medication, which could have important implications for the treatment of comorbid groups. These two questions remain largely unanswered. One study (Sprague and Sleator 1977) found that optimal cognitive performance was achieved at low doses (i.e., 0.3 mg/kg), whereas optimal behavioral function was achieved at high doses (i.e., 1.0 mg/kg). Cognitive function declined at the optimal behavioral dose in this study, but this finding has not been replicated. Other studies (Pelham et al. 1985) have reported a linear rather than a curvilinear dose-response curve but did not test high enough doses to formulate any conclusion regarding the existence of a "descending limb" relative to cognitive function.

Livingston et al. (1992) examined whether stimulant dose varies as a function of comorbidity by giving two doses of methylphenidate (0.3 mg/kg and 0.6 mg/kg) in an ADHD sample stratified according to the presence of comorbid internalizing and/or externalizing disorders. The study indicated that the low dose was effective for both the group with comorbid internalizing disorders and the group with comorbid externalizing disorders alone. However, children with ADHD who had both comorbid internalizing and externalizing disorders responded only at the higher dose. This study points to the importance of testing multiple doses of medication and determining the full extent of comorbidity in arriving at the optimal stimulant dose.

Nonstimulant medications have also been studied. The noradrenergic tricyclic antidepressants, principally imipramine and desipramine, have received the most attention. The most rigorous of these studies (Biederman et al. 1989a, 1989b) used a double-blind, placebo-controlled methodology; doses up to 5 mg/kg/day were evaluated. When the data were analyzed as a function of comorbidity, it was found that no single comorbid group responded better or worse to the medication treatment (Biederman et al. 1993b). The decision to prescribe tricyclics for children with ADHD must be made with the knowledge that several sudden deaths have been reported in children taking desipramine (Popper and Elliott 1990; Riddle et al. 1991). Biederman and colleagues (Biederman 1991; Biederman et al. 1989b; Biederman et al. 1993a) have argued that data from their research do not support the conclusion that tricyclics have a high degree of cardiovascular toxicity in children. Nevertheless, proper informed consent should be obtained and careful baseline assessments should be undertaken before proceeding with treatment. It also should be noted that neither imipramine nor desipramine is approved by the U.S. Food and Drug Administration (FDA) for the treatment of children with ADHD.

Alpha-adrenergic agents, such as clonidine (Hunt et al. 1985, 1991) and guanfacine (Chappell et al. 1995; Hunt et al. 1995), have also been the subject of several investigations. These medications, originally marketed as antihypertensive agents, work by enhancing α_2-receptor activity in the prefrontal cortex and/or the locus coeruleus (Arnsten et al. 1996; Pliszka et al. 1996).

Clonidine is reportedly most effective in treating symptoms of hyperactivity, impulsivity, and aggression in children with ADHD; therefore, it seems ideally suited for use in children who have ADHD with comorbid CD or aggression. However, it has been less effective in improving attentional function. Guanfacine may present several potential advantages over clonidine, although more study is required. It is somewhat longer acting, less sedating, and perhaps better for regulation of attention. Improvement in attentional function may be attributable to the fact that guanfacine is a more specific α_2-adrenergic agent (Arnsten et al. 1996). Both clonidine and guanfacine have been shown to be useful in treating ADHD patients who either have diagnosed tic disorders (Chappell et al. 1995; Steingard et al. 1993) or are at increased risk for developing these disorders, such as children with a positive family history of tics. This is particularly important because as many as 40%–60% of patients with Tourette syndrome seen in psychiatric settings have ADHD (Biederman et al. 1991) and many of these individuals have significant behavior problems.

The α-adrenergic agents have been used alone or in combination with stimulants. Although there are no usage data related to comorbidity, it is our impression that the combined treatment has been used most often in children with ADHD and comorbid conduct problems. However, combined stimulant-clonidine administration should be approached with caution because of the potential for untoward cardiovascular events. Several sudden deaths have been reported, although it remains uncertain whether these deaths were directly attributable to the medication combination (Fenichel 1995; Popper 1995; Walkup 1995). Because clonidine is not FDA approved for use in ADHD, informed consent should clearly indicate that this is an "off-label" treatment.

A variety of other psychopharmacological agents have been used to treat children with ADHD, aggression, or episodic dyscontrol and may be considered for treating children with ADHD and aggression who do not respond to more traditional therapies. However, the majority of these medications have not been systematically studied, and there are few data specific to the group of children with ADHD and comorbid CD or aggression. Therefore, efficacy can only be inferred from the mechanisms of action of these medications and from the results of the few studies conducted in children with either ADHD or CD alone.

Two open studies have described the utility of fluoxetine in treating children with ADHD. Although it is not clear how comorbidity with ODD, CD, or aggression would affect this medication response, the use of selective serotonin reuptake inhibitors (SSRIs) may be of interest in treating the comorbid group in light of recent findings implicating serotonergic mechanisms in aggression. In an open study by Barrickman et al. (1991), fluoxetine was administered to 19 children and adolescents with ADHD, 8 of whom had either comorbid ODD or CD. There was a favorable medication response in 60% of the cases, although the results were not analyzed as a function of comorbidity. Gammon and Brown (1993) used fluoxetine and methylphenidate in combination in an open study of 32 children with ADHD, principally directed at the treatment of comorbid depression (78% of their sample). The children studied were reported to have an inadequate response to methylphenidate alone. Interestingly, almost 60% of these children also had comorbid ODD, and 13% had CD. Because virtually all the children (30 of 32) improved on this combined treatment, at least some children with comorbid conduct problems were successfully treated. In contrast, findings from an open study examining the use of SSRIs in children with aggression have been disappointing, with even a suggestion that the medication made verbal aggression worse (Constantino et al. 1997).

Lithium has been the best studied medication used for treating aggression or episodic dyscontrol in children. Its efficacy has been demonstrated in well-designed studies of aggressive children (Campbell et al. 1984) and impulsive-aggressive adolescents and young adults who demonstrated delinquent behavior (Sheard et al. 1976). However, there are no data specific to the group with ADHD and aggression. Licamele and Goldberg (1989) reported the successful use of methylphenidate and lithium administered in combination to a child with ADHD and atypical CD and affective symptoms whose symptoms could not be adequately controlled with methylphenidate alone. Carbamazepine has also been used clinically, but few studies have been done. Data supporting the utility of this treatment for children with ADHD were reviewed (Silva et al. 1996), but the review draws mostly on literature published outside the United States. Lithium and other mood-stabilizing agents are of particular interest in the treatment of aggressive children with ADHD because of reports indicating a high degree of comorbidity between ADHD and bipolar disorder (Biederman et al. 1996a) and the recognition that aggression is a frequent presenting symptom in these patients. In pilot studies, propranolol has also been reported to be effective in children with aggression and episodic dyscontrol (Stewart et al. 1990; Williams et al. 1982), although this medication is often reserved for those with organic syndromes. Because the aforementioned treatments have not been systematically studied in children with ADHD as well as aggression, they should be considered only as a last resort in treating this group.

A variety of psychosocial treatments have also been demonstrated to be effective in treating children with ADHD (see Pelham and Murphy 1986) and should certainly be considered for treating children with ADHD and comorbid conduct problems. However, there has been little systematic study that specifically accounts for comorbidity. Therefore, recommendations regarding the use of these interventions as part of a comprehensive treatment plan can only be extrapolated from efficacy data collected in groups with noncomorbid ADHD and groups with behavior disorders (Abikoff and Klein 1992). Treatment has principally involved behavioral intervention, including parent management training, use of a daily report card to monitor behavior at home and at school, contingency reward programs, anger control, and cognitive behavioral therapy. Although the latter treatment has not been shown to be effective in treating children with ADHD, findings do suggest its efficacy in treating children with CD. Thus, this treatment may be considered for treating children with ADHD and comorbid CD (Abikoff and Klein 1992).

ARE ADDITIONAL OR DIFFERENT TREATMENTS REQUIRED FOR CHILDREN WITH ADHD AND COMORBID CONDUCT PROBLEMS?

Multimodal treatment strategies, usually consisting of simultaneous administration of pharmacological and nonpharmacological treatments, have considerable face validity for treating children with comorbidity given that multiple problems are present. Yet their efficacy has not been conclusively demonstrated in systematic clinical trials. Satterfield and colleagues (1979, 1981) studied the combined use of a variety of individually tailored pharmacological and nonpharmacological treatments over an extended period. The researchers reported improved symptomatic response and greater sustained benefit over time. However, studies that have attempted to replicate these findings with rigorously applied, systematic interventions have found only modest or no improvement in the multimodal group (Abikoff 1991; Abikoff and Klein 1992; Horn et al. 1991; Ialongo et al. 1993). It may be that less effective psychosocial treatments were chosen in these latter studies or that longer-term intervention is required to demonstrate improvement.

To better compare the possible role of multimodal treatments with monomodal treatments, the National Institute of Mental Health funded a large-scale multicenter study (Arnold et al. 1997; Greenhill et al. 1996; National Institute of Mental Health 1992; Richters et al. 1995). For this study, 579 children with ADHD from six sites were recruited and treated for 14 months with either medication, behavioral treatment, or the combination.

Comorbidity was carefully assessed at baseline and over the course of treatment. This study should therefore be able to describe the impact of comorbid conduct problems in children with ADHD and to ascertain whether this comorbid group responds better to any of the interventions studied, and particularly whether there is any advantage for combined treatment. At present, the most appropriate clinical recommendation is to target each problem recorded on the "problem list" in children with ADHD and comorbid conduct problems with an appropriate clinical intervention and to try treatments with demonstrated efficacy in children who have ADHD without comorbidity in the comorbid group.

Case Vignette

George, who had always been described as an extremely overactive boy, was the only child of an intact but troubled two-parent family. George's behavior was always extremely difficult to regulate, and he was diagnosed with ADHD very early in childhood. George was frequently aggressive and had very few friends. He also had impaired academic function. At the age of 8, after undergoing several years of treatment with stimulant medication given by his pediatrician, George's family consulted a child psychiatrist. At the time, George was taking 40 mg of short-acting methylphenidate twice daily. (Note: This total daily dose exceeds the FDA recommended ceiling of 60 mg.) However, there was concern that this dose was excessive and should be reduced. In addition, the medication was effective for only approximately 2 hours following administration, there was evidence of behavioral rebound, and there were significant behavior problems at home. George and his mother were in constant conflict. She would often yell at him or hit him when he did not listen to her. He, in turn, was assaultive toward her. There was also considerable marital discord. When George's mother attempted to discipline him, her authority was frequently undermined by his father and paternal grandmother, and there was open conflict between the parents about his care.

George's methylphenidate dose was reduced and spread more evenly over the day. However, he continued to show behavioral problems, including frequent defiance and physical aggression toward his mother. Therefore, a series of medication trials with other agents was undertaken. George was given a trial of dextroamphetamine and then a trial of pemoline. Although each of these stimulants yielded moderate improvement, there were considerable residual symptoms. A tricyclic trial was undertaken but was not effective. It was decided that of the medications tried, George responded best to methylphenidate, with the optimal dose being 20 mg, given three times daily. Because there was still considerable room for improvement, clonidine was added to further target overactivity and aggression. This provided additional improvement in behavioral control.

A variety of psychosocial interventions with George and his family were also undertaken. George received individual therapy, emphasizing response to limits and development of improved self-control. Work with George's parents was aimed at decreasing family discord and teaching principles of behavioral management. These interventions were helpful, although there was still considerable room for improvement. As a result, additional services were requested from the relevant educational and social service systems. The local board of education provided a paraprofessional aid in the classroom to work with George. A social service agency agreed to provide a homemaker for several hours a day to assist the mother and help regulate George's behavior at home after school. Substantial additional improvement resulted from these systemic and behavioral interventions.

When reports surfaced of sudden death in several children on combined stimulant-clonidine treatment, it was decided to discontinue the combined pharmacological treatment and return to the methylphenidate alone. This decision was based on the recognition that multiple psychosocial interventions, which were not part of the treatment plan at the time of initial medication trials, were now in place. In conjunction with these interventions, the stimulant medication alone proved to be successful. However, it seemed to become less effective over time. Dose adjustments were not successful in reestablishing behavioral control. Therefore, clonidine treatment was reinstituted, this time alone, resulting in substantial improvement in impulsive and aggressive behavior. However, this medication wore off after several hours, there was intermittent sedation, and attentional function was noted to be less satisfactory than it had been when stimulant treatment was effective and well controlled. Therefore, a trial of guanfacine was recommended.

Although George and his family continued to demonstrate considerable symptoms over the course of treatment, this very difficult case was able to be managed in the home and at school as a result of combined use of intensive pharmacological and nonpharmacological interventions. This case highlights many of the problems encountered in treatment planning for children with

ADHD and comorbid ODD, CD, and aggression. These important issues include 1) the presence of multiple developmental and psychosocial risk factors, which often produce severe symptoms; 2) the possibility that even somewhat effective medication treatment may not provide sufficient stabilization; 3) the occasional need for relatively high doses of stimulants, administered three times a day; and 4) the need for combined pharmacological and psychosocial treatment. This case also highlights the fact that pharmacological intervention, which may be viewed as inadequate when given alone, may be sufficient in the context of a broader multimodal plan. Most important, the introduction of discrete treatments targeting each presenting problem is essential.

CONCLUSION

Comorbidity of ADHD with ODD, CD, and aggression is a significant clinical and public health problem. This comorbidity is seen in as many as half of all children with ADHD, making it more common than most noncomorbid psychiatric disorders. Most important, it accounts for the majority of poor behavioral outcome among children with ADHD, as well as among those with CD. Although it has often been difficult to distinguish ADHD and CD, the two conditions have recently been shown to be distinct. However, they may share an underlying symptomatic basis (i.e., impulsivity) and seem to interact in important and somewhat predictable ways. Findings from studies examining the family genetic patterns, longitudinal course, and neurobiological basis of ADHD with comorbid conduct problems are consistent with the hypothesis that this comorbid configuration represents a distinct subtype or a more virulent presentation of ADHD. Furthermore, emerging data are consistent with the hypothesis that ADHD is a risk factor for the development of CD.

Treatment studies in children with ADHD and comorbid conduct problems lag behind descriptive studies. Therefore, treatment recommendations for children in the comorbid group are best extrapolated from strategies with demonstrated efficacy in treating each individual disorder, regardless of comorbidity. There is one noteworthy exception to this: there is ample evidence suggesting that psychostimulant medication can have an important role in the treatment of children with ADHD and comorbid ODD, CD, or aggression. However, the multitude of problems with which these children present suggests that no single treatment intervention will be sufficient. The combined use of pharmacotherapy and psychosocial interventions is promising in this regard but awaits further testing in well-controlled clinical trials.

REFERENCES

Abikoff H: Interaction of Ritalin and multimodal therapy in the treatment of attention deficit hyperactive behavior disorder, in Ritalin: Theory and Patient Management. Edited by Greenhill LL, Osman BB. New York, Mary Ann Liebert, 1991, pp 147–154

Abikoff H, Klein RG: Attention-deficit hyperactivity and conduct disorder: comorbidity and implications for treatment. J Consult Clin Psychol 60:881–892, 1992

Achenbach TM: "Comorbidity" in child and adolescent psychiatry: categorical and quantitative perspectives. J Child Adolesc Psychopharmacol 1:271–278, 1990–1991

American Psychiatric Association, Diagnostic and Statistical Manual of Mental Disorders, 4th Edition. Washington, DC, American Psychiatric Association, 1994

Amery B, Minichiello MD, Brown GL: Aggression in hyperactive boys: response to d-amphetamine. J Am Acad Child Psychiatry 23:291–294, 1984

Anderson JC, Williams S, McGee R, et al: DSM-III disorders in preadolescent children: prevalence in a large sample from the general population. Arch Gen Psychiatry 44:69–76, 1987

Arnold LE, Abikoff HB, Cantwell, DP, et al: National Institute of Mental Health Collaborative Multimodal Treatment Study of Children With ADHD (the MTA): design challenges and choices. Arch Gen Psychiatry 54:865–870, 1997

Arnsten AF, Steere JC, Hunt RD: The contribution of alpha-2 noradrenergic mechanisms to prefrontal cortical cognitive function. Arch Gen Psychiatry 53:448–455, 1996

August GJ, Garfinkel BD: Behavioral and cognitive subtypes of ADHD. J Am Acad Child Adolesc Psychiatry 28:739–748, 1989

Barkley RA, McMurray MB, Edelbrock CS, et al: The response of aggressive and nonaggressive ADHD children to two doses of methylphenidate. J Am Acad Child Adolesc Psychiatry 28:873–881, 1989 (published erratum appears in J Am Acad Child Adolesc Psychiatry 29:670, 1990)

Barkley RA, Fischer M, Edelbrock CS, et al: The adolescent outcome of hyperactive children diagnosed by research criteria, I: an 8-year prospective follow-up study. J Am Acad Child Adolesc Psychiatry 29:546–557, 1990

Barkley RA, Fischer M, Edelbrock C, et al: The adolescent outcome of hyperactive children diagnosed by research criteria, III: mother-child interactions, family conflicts and maternal psychopathology. J Child Psychol Psychiatry 32:233–255, 1991

Barrickman L, Noyes R, Kuperman S, et al: Treatment of ADHD with fluoxetine: a preliminary trial. J Am Acad Child Adolesc Psychiatry 30:762–767, 1991

Biederman J: Sudden death in children treated with a tricyclic antidepressant (commentary). J Am Acad Child Adolesc Psychiatry 30:495–498, 1991

Biederman J, Baldessarini RJ, Wright V, et al: A double-blind placebo controlled study of desipramine in the treatment of ADD, I: efficacy. J Am Acad Child Adolesc Psychiatry 28:777–784, 1989a

Biederman J, Baldessarini RJ, Wright V, et al: A double-blind placebo controlled study of desipramine in the treatment of ADD, II: serum drug levels and cardiovascular findings. J Am Acad Child Adolesc Psychiatry 28:903–911, 1989b

Biederman J, Newcorn J, Sprich, S: Comorbidity of attention deficit hyperactivity disorder with conduct, depressive, anxiety, and other disorders. Am J Psychiatry 148:564–577, 1991

Biederman J, Faraone SV, Keenan K, et al.: Further evidence for family-genetic risk factors in attention deficit hyperactivity disorder: patterns of comorbidity in probands and relatives in psychiatrically and pediatrically referred samples. Arch Gen Psychiatry 49:728–738, 1992a

Biederman J, Faraone SV, Lapey K: Comorbidity of diagnosis in attention-deficit hyperactivity disorder. Child Adolesc Psychiatr Clin N Am 1:335, 1992b

Biederman J, Baldessarini RJ, Goldblatt A, et al: A naturalistic study of 24-hour electroencephalographic recordings and echocardiographic findings in children and adolescents treated with desipramine. J Am Acad Child Adolesc Psychiatry 32:805–813, 1993a

Biederman J, Baldessarini RJ, Wright V, et al: A double-blind placebo controlled study of desipramine in the treatment of ADD, III: lack of impact of comorbidity and family history factors on clinical response. J Am Acad Child Adolesc Psychiatry 32:199–204, 1993b

Biederman J, Faraone S, Spencer T, et al: Patterns of psychiatric comorbidity, cognition and psychosocial functioning in adults with attention deficit hyperactivity disorder. Am J Psychiatry 150:1792–1798, 1993c

Biederman J, Milberger S, Faraone S, et al. Family environment risk factors for ADHD: a test of Rutter's indicators of adversity. Arch Gen Psychiatry 52:464–470, 1995a

Biederman J, Milberger S, Faraone S, et al. Impact of adversity on functioning and comorbidity in children with attention-deficit hyperactivity disorder. J Am Acad Child Adolesc Psychiatry 34:1495–1503, 1995b

Biederman J, Faraone S, Mick E, et al: Attention-deficit hyperactivity disorder and juvenile mania: an overlooked comorbidity? J Am Acad Child Adolesc Psychiatry, 35:997–1008, 1996a

Biederman J, Faraone S, Milberger S, et al: Predictors of persistence and remission of ADHD into adolescence: results from a four-year prospective follow-up study. J Am Acad Child Adolesc Psychiatry 35:343–351, 1996b

Biederman J, Wilens T, Mick E, et al: Is ADHD a risk factor for psychoactive substance use disorders? Findings from a four-year prospective follow-up study. J Am Acad Child Adolesc Psychiatry 36:21–29, 1997

Bird HR, Canino G, Rubio-Stipec M, et al: Estimates of the prevalence of childhood maladjustment in a community survey in Puerto Rico: the use of combined measures. Arch Gen Psychiatry 45:1120–1126, 1988

Birmaher B, Stanley M, Greenhill L, et al: Platelet imipramine binding in children and adolescents with impulsive behavior. J Am Acad Child Adolesc Psychiatry 29: 914–918, 1990

Bowden CL, Deutsch CK, Swanson JM: Plasma dopamine-beta-hydroxylase and platelet monoamine oxidase in attention deficit disorder and conduct disorder. J Am Acad Child Adolesc Psychiatry 27:171–174, 1988

Campbell M, Small AM, Green WH, et al: Behavioral efficacy of haloperidol and lithium carbonate. Arch Gen Psychiatry 41:650–656, 1984

Caron C, Rutter M: Comorbidity in child psychopathology: concepts, issues and research strategies. J Child Psychol Psychiatry 32:1063–1080, 1991

Castellanos FX, Elia J, Kruesi MJ, et al: Cerebrospinal fluid monoamine metabolites in boys with attention-deficit hyperactivity disorder. Psychiatry Res 52:305–316, 1994

Chappell PB, Riddle MA, Scahill L, et al: Guanfacine treatment of comorbid attention-deficit hyperactivity disorder and Tourette's syndrome: preliminary clinical experience. J Am Acad Child Adolesc Psychiatry 34:1140–1146, 1995

Coccaro EF, Siever LJ, Klar HM, et al: Serotonergic studies in patients with affective and personality disorders: correlates with suicidal and impulsive aggressive behavior. Arch Gen Psychiatry 46:587—599, 1989 (published erratum appears in Arch Gen Psychiatry 47:124, 1990)

Conners CK: A teacher rating scale for use in drug studies with children. Am J Psychiatry 126:884–888, 1969

Conners CK: Symptom patterns in hyperkinetic, neurotic, and normal children. Child Dev 41:667–682, 1970

Constantino JN, Liberman M, Kincaid M: Effects of serotonin reuptake inhibitors on aggressive behavior in psychiatrically hospitalized adolescents: results of an open trial. J Child Adolesc Psychopharmacol 7:31–44, 1997

Cook EH, Stein MA, Ellison T, et al: Attention deficit hyperactivity disorder and whole blood serotonin level: effects of comorbidity. Psychiatry Res 57:13–20, 1995

Costello EJ: Comorbidity in epidemiologic samples. Paper presented at the annual meeting of the American Academy of Child and Adolescent Psychiatry, Washington, DC, October 1992.

Epstein MA, Shaywitz SE, Shaywitz BA , et al: The boundaries of attention deficit disorder. J Learn Disabil 24(2):78–86, 1991

Faraone S, Biederman J: Is attention deficit hyperactivity disorder familial? Harv Rev Psychiatry 1:271–287, 1994

Faraone SV, Biederman J, Keenan K, et al: Separation of DSM-III attention deficit disorder and conduct disorder: evidence from a family-genetic study of American child psychiatric patients. Psychol Med 21:109–121, 1991

Fenichel RR: Combining methylphenidate and clonidine: the role of post-marketing surveillance. J Child Adolesc Psychopharmacol 5:155–156, 1995

Gammon GD, Brown TE: Fluoxetine and methylphenidate in combination for treatment of attention deficit disorder and comorbid depressive disorder. J Child Adolesc Psychopharmacol 3:1–10, 1993

Gittelman R, Mannuzza S, Shenker R, et al: Hyperactive boys almost grown up, I: psychiatric status. Arch Gen Psychiatry 42:937–947, 1985

Goyette CH, Conners CK, Ulrich RF: Normative data on revised Conners parent and teacher rating scales. J Abnorm Child Psychol 6:221–236, 1978

Greenhill LL, Abikoff HB, Arnold LE, et al: Medication treatment strategies in the MTA: relevance to clinicians and researchers. J Am Acad Child Adolesc Psychiatry 35:1304–1313, 1996

Halikas JA, Meller J, Morse C, et al: Predicting substance abuse in juvenile offenders: attention deficit disorder versus aggressivity. Child Psychiatry Hum Dev 21:49–55, 1990

Halperin JM, Newcorn JH: Impulsivity and aggression in children with ADHD, in Neurobiology and Clinical Views on Aggression and Impulsivity. Edited by Maes M, Coccaro EF. Chichester, West Sussex, England, Wiley, 1998, pp 47–61

Halperin JM, Wolf LE, Pascualvaca DP, et al: Differential assessment of attention and impulsivity in children. J Am Acad Child Adolesc Psychiatry 27:326–329, 1988

Halperin JM, Newcorn JH, Sharma V, et al.: Inattentive and noninattentive ADHD children: do they constitute a unitary group? J Abnorm Child Psychol 18:437–449, 1990a

Halperin JM, O'Brien JD, Newcorn JH, et al: Validation of hyperactive, aggressive, and mixed hyperactive/aggressive childhood disorders: a research note. J Child Psychol Psychiatry 31:455–459, 1990b

Halperin JM, Sharma V, Greenblatt E, et al: Assessment of the continuous performance test: reliability and validity in a non-referred sample. J Consult Clin Psychol 3:603–608, 1991

Halperin JM, Matier K, Bedi G, et al: Specificity of inattention, impulsivity, and hyperactivity to the diagnosis of attention-deficit hyperactivity disorder. J Am Acad Child Adolesc Psychiatry 31:190–196, 1992

Halperin JM, Newcorn JH, Matier K, et al: Discriminant validity of attention-deficit hyperactivity disorder. J Am Acad Child Adolesc Psychiatry 32:1038–1043, 1993

Halperin JM, Sharma V, Siever LJ, et al: Serotonergic function in aggressive and nonaggressive boys with attention-deficit hyperactivity disorder. Am J Psychiatry 151:243–248, 1994

Halperin JM, Newcorn JH, Matier K, et al: Impulsivity and the initiation of fights in children with disruptive behavior disorders. J Child Psychol Psychiatry 36:1199–1211, 1995

Halperin JM, Newcorn JH, Kopstein I, et al: Serotonin, aggression, and parental psychopathology in children with attention-deficit hyperactivity disorder. J Am Acad Child Adolesc Psychiatry 36:1391–1398, 1997a

Halperin JM, Newcorn JH, Schwartz ST, et al: Age-related changes in the association between serotonergic function and aggression in boys with ADHD. Biol Psychiatry 41:682–689, 1997b

Hechtman L, Offord DR: Long-term outcome of disruptive disorders. Child Adolesc Psychiatr Clin N Am 3:379–404, 1994

Hechtman L, Weiss G, Perlman T, et al: Hyperactives as young adults: initial predictors of adult outcome. J Am Acad Child Adolesc Psychiatry 23:250–260, 1984

Hinshaw, SP: On the distinction between attentional deficits/hyperactivity and conduct problems/aggression in child psychopathology. Psychol Bull 101:443–463, 1987

Hinshaw SP, Heller T, McHale JP: Covert antisocial behavior in boys with attention-deficit hyperactivity disorder: external validation and effects of methylphenidate. J Consult Clin Psychol 60:274–281, 1992

Horn WF, Ialongo NS, Pascoe JM, et al: Additive effects of psychostimulants, parent training, and self-control therapy with ADHD children. J Am Acad Child Adolesc Psychiatry 30:233–240, 1991

Hunt RD, Minderaa RB, Cohen DJ: The therapeutic effect of clonidine in attention deficit disorder with hyperactivity: report of a double-blind placebo-controlled crossover study. J Am Acad Child Psychiatry 24:617–629, 1985

Hunt RD, Lau S, Ryu J: Alternative therapies for ADHD, in Ritalin: Theory and Patient Management. Edited by Greenhill LL, Osman BB. New York, Mary Ann Liebert, 1991, pp 75–95

Hunt RD, Arnsten AF, Asbell MD: An open trial of guanfacine in the treatment of attention-deficit hyperactivity disorder. J Am Acad Child Adolesc Psychiatry 34:50–54, 1995

Ialongo NS, Horn WF, Pascoe JM, et al: The effects of a multimodal intervention with attention-deficit hyperactivity disorder children: a 9-month follow-up. J Am Acad Child Adolesc Psychiatry 32:182–189, 1993

Kaplan SL, Busner J, Kupietz S, et al: Effects of methylphenidate on adolescents with aggressive conduct disorder and ADDH: a preliminary report. J Am Acad Child Adolesc Psychiatry 29:719–723, 1990

Klein RG, Mannuzza S: Long-term outcome of hyperactive children: a review. J Am Acad Child Adolesc Psychiatry 30:383–387, 1991

Klorman R, Brumaghim JT, Salzman LF, et al: Effects of methylphenidate on attention-deficit hyperactivity disorder with and without aggressive/noncompliant features. J Abnorm Psychol 97:413–422, 1988

Koriath U, Gualtieri CT, Van Bourgondien ME, et al: Construct validity of clinical diagnosis in pediatric psychiatry: relationship among measures. J Am Acad Child Psychiatry 24:429–436 , 1985

Kruesi MJ, Rapoport JL, Hamburger S, et al.: Cerebrospinal fluid monoamine metabolites, aggression, and impulsivity in disruptive behavior disorders of children and adolescents. Arch Gen Psychiatry, 47:419–426, 1990

Kruesi MJ, Hibbs ED, Zahn TP, et al: A 2-year prospective follow-up study of children and adolescents with disruptive behavior disorders: prediction by cerebrospinal fluid 5-hydroxyindoleacetic acid, homovanillic acid, and autonomic measures? Arch Gen Psychiatry 49:429–435, 1992

Lahey BB, Schaughency EA, Hynd GW, et al: Attention deficit disorder with and without hyperactivity: comparison of behavioral characteristics of clinic-referred children. J Am Acad Child Adolesc Psychiatry 26:718–723, 1987

Lahey BB, Piacentini JC, McBurnett K, et al.: Psychopathology in the parents of children with conduct disorder and hyperactivity. J Am Acad Child Adolesc Psychiatry 27:163–170, 1988 (published erratum appears in J Am Acad Child Adolesc Psychiatry 27:516, 1988)

Lahey BB, Applegate B, Barkley RA, et al. DSM-IV field trials for oppositional defiant disorder and conduct disorder in children and adolescents. Am J Psychiatry 151:1163–1171, 1994

Licamele WL, Goldberg RL: The concurrent use of lithium and methylphenidate in a child. J Am Acad Child Adolesc Psychiatry 28:785–787, 1989

Livingston RL, Dykman RA, Ackerman PT: Psychiatric comorbidity and response to two doses of methylphenidate in children with attention deficit disorder. J Child Adolesc Psychopharmocol 2:115–122, 1992

Loeber R: Natural histories of conduct problems, delinquency, and associated substance use: evidence for developmental progressions, in Advances in Clinical Child Psychology, Vol. 11. Edited by Lahey BB and Kazdin AE. New York, Plenum, 1988, pp 73–124

Loeber R: Development and risk factors of juvenile antisocial behavior and delinquency. Clin Psychol Rev 10:1–41, 1990

Loeber R, Green SM, Lahey BB, et al: Developmental sequences in the age of onset of disruptive child behaviors. Journal of Child and Family Studies 1:21–41, 1992

Loeber R, Wung P, Keenan K, et al: Developmental pathways in disruptive child behavior. Dev Psychopathol 5:103–133, 1993

Loney J, Milich R: Hyperactivity, inattention, and aggression in clinical practice. Advances in Developmental and Behavioral Pediatrics 3:113–147, 1982

Loney J, Kramer J, Milich RS: The hyperactive child grows up: predictors of symptoms, delinquency and achievement of follow-up, in Psychosocial Aspects of Drug Treatment for Hyperactivity. Edited by Gadow KD, Loney J. Boulder, CO, Westview, 1981, pp 381–416

MacDonald VM, Achenbach TM.: Attention problems versus conduct problems as six-year predictors of problem scores in a national sample. J Am Acad Child Adolesc Psychiatry 35:1237–1246, 1996

Mannuzza S, Klein RG, Bessler A, et al: Adult outcome of hyperactive boys: educational achievement, occupational rank, and psychiatric status. Arch Gen Psychiatry 50:565–576, 1993

Matier K, Halperin JM, Sharma V, et al: Methylphenidate response in aggressive and nonaggressive ADHD children: distinctions on laboratory measures of symptoms. J Am Acad Child Adolesc Psychiatry 31:219–225, 1992

McGee R, Williams S, Silva PA: Behavioral and developmental characteristics of aggressive, hyperactive and aggressive-hyperactive boys. J Am Acad Child Adolesc Psychiatry 23:270–279, 1984

McKay K, Newcorn JH, Halperin JM: Situationally vs. pervasively aggressive boys: behavioral, cognitive and neurochemical differences, in Scientific Proceedings, American Academy of Child and Adolescent Psychiatry Annual Meeting, Vol XII, Philadelphia, PA, October 1996, p 102

Moffit TE: Juvenile delinquency and attention deficit disorder: Boys' developmental trajectories from age 3 to age 15. Child Dev 61:893, 1990

MTA Cooperative Group: Moderators and mediators of treatment response for children with attention-deficit hyperactivity disorder. Arch Gen Psychiatry 56: 1088–1096, 1999

National Institute of Mental Health: Cooperative Agreement for a Multi-Site Multimodal Treatment Study of Attention-Deficit Hyperactivity Disorder (ADHD)/ Attention Deficit Disorder (ADD), MH-92-03. Washington DC, National Institute of Mental Health, 1992

Newcorn JH: Comorbidity of attention deficit disorders with oppositional behavior and aggression. Paper presented at the American Academy of Child and Adolescent Psychiatry Annual Meeting, San Antonio, TX, October 31, 1993

Newcorn JH, Sharma V, Matier K, et al: Comorbidity of ADHD: differential effect of oppositional/conduct and anxiety disorders in individual symptom domains. Poster presented at Society for Research in Child and Adolescent Psychopathology Annual Meeting, Sarasota, FL, February 1992

Newcorn JH, McKay K, Loeber R, et al: Emotionality and serotonergic function in aggressive and non-aggressive ADHD children, in Scientific Proceedings of the American Academy of Child and Adolescent Psychiatry (AACAP) Annual Meeting, Vol XII. AACAP, October 1996, p 94

O'Keane V, Moloney E, O'Neil H, et al: Blunted prolactin responses to d-fenfluramine in sociopathy: evidence for subsensitivity of central serotonergic function. Br J Psychiatry 160:643–646, 1992

Pelham WE, Murphy HA: Attention deficit and conduct disorders, in Pharmacological and Behavioral Treatments: An Integrative Approach. Edited by Hersen M. New York, Wiley, 1986, pp 108–148

Pelham WE, Bender ME, Caddell JM, et al: Methylphenidate and children with attention deficit disorder: dose effects on classroom academic and social behavior. Arch Gen Psychiatry 42:948–952, 1985

Pelham WE, Milich R, Murphy DA, et al: Normative data on the IOWA Conners' Teacher Rating Scale. J Clin Child Psychol 3:259–262, 1989

Pine DS, Wasserman GA, Coplan J, et al: Platelet serotonin 2A (5-HT2A) receptor characteristics and parenting factors in boys at risk for delinquency—a preliminary report. Am J Psychiatry 153:538–544, 1996

Pliszka SR, McCracken JT, Maas JW: Catecholamines in attention deficit disorder: current perspectives. J Am Acad Child Adolesc Psychiatry 35:264–272, 1996

Popper CW: Combining methylphenidate and clonidine: pharmacologic questions and news reports about sudden death. J Child Adolesc Psychopharmacol 5:157–166, 1995

Popper CW, Elliott GR: Sudden death and tricyclic antidepressants: clinical considerations for children. J Child Adolesc Psychopharmacol 1:125–132, 1990

Prendergast M, Taylor E, Rapoport JL, et al: The diagnosis of childhood hyperactivity: a U.S.-U.K. cross-national study of DSM-III and ICD-9. J. Child Psychol Psychiatry 29: 289–300, 1988

Reeves JC, Werry JS, Elkind GS, et al: Attention deficit, conduct, oppositional, and anxiety disorders in children, II: clinical characteristics. J Am Acad Child Adolesc Psychiatry 26:144–155, 1987

Reichenbach L, Halperin JM, Sharma V, et al: Children's motor activity: reliability and relationship to attention and behavior. Developmental Neuropsychology 8: 87–97, 1992

Rey JM: Oppositional defiant disorder. Am J Psychiatry 150:1769–1778, 1993

Richters JE, Arnold LE, Jensen PS, et al: NIMH collaborative multisite multimodal treatment study of children with ADHD, I: background and rationale. J Am Acad Child Adolesc Psychiatry 34:987–1000, 1995

Riddle MA, Nelson JC, Kleinman CS, et al: Sudden death in children receiving Norpramin: a review of three reported cases and commentary. J Am Acad Child Adolesc Psychiatry 30:104–108, 1991

Roberts MA: A behavioral observation method for differentiating hyperactive and aggressive boys. J Abnorm Child Psychol 18:131–142, 1990

Robins LN: Conduct disorder. J Child Psychol Psychiatry 32:193–212, 1991

Rogeness GA, Hernandez JM, Macedo CA, et al: Clinical characteristics of emotionally disturbed boys with very low activities of dopamine-beta-hydroxylase. J Am Acad Child Adolesc Psychiatry 23:203–208, 1984

Rogeness GA, Hernandez JM, Macedo CA, et al: Near-zero plasma dopamine-beta-hydroxylase and conduct disorder in emotionally disturbed boys. J Am Acad Child Psychiatry 25:521–527, 1986

Rosvold HE, Mirsky AF, Sarason I, et al: A continuous performance test of brain damage. J Consult Psychol 20:343–350, 1956

Rutter M: Isle of Wight revisited: twenty-five years of child psychiatric epidemiology. J Am Acad Child Adolesc Psychiatry 28:633–653, 1989

Satterfield JH, Cantwell DP, Satterfield BT: Multimodality treatment: a one-year follow-up of 84 hyperactive boys. Arch Gen Psychiatry 36:965–974, 1979

Satterfield JH, Satterfield BT, Cantwell DP: Three-year multimodality treatment study of 100 hyperactive boys. J Pediatr 98:650–655, 1981

Schachar R, Tannock R: Distinction between ADHD and ADHD+CD: cognitive, psychosocial and developmental risk, in Scientific Proceedings of the American Academy of Child and Adolescent Psychiatry, Vol IX, San Antonio, TX, October 1993, pp 42–43

Schachar R, Wachsmuth R: Hyperactivity and parental psychopathology. J Child Psychol Psychiatry 31:381–392, 1990

Shapiro SK, Garfinkel HD: The occurrence of behavior disorders in children: the interdependence of attention deficit disorder and conduct disorder. J Am Acad Child Psychiatry 25:809–819, 1986

Shaywitz BA, Shaywitz SE: Comorbidity: a critical issue in attention deficit disorder. J Child Neurol 6(suppl):S13–S22, 1991

Sheard MH, Marini JL, Bridges CI, et al: The effect of lithium on impulsive aggressive behavior in man. Am J Psychiatry 133:1409–1413, 1976

Silva RR, Munoz DM, Alpert M: Carbamazepine use in children and adolescents with features of attention-deficit hyperactivity disorder: a meta-analysis. J Am Acad Child Adolesc Psychiatry 35:352–358, 1996

Sprague RL, Sleator EK: Methylphenidate in hyperkinetic children: differences in dose effects on learning and social behavior. Science 198:1274–1276, 1977

Steingard R, Biederman J, Spencer T, et al: comparison of clonidine response in the treatment of attention-deficit hyperactivity disorder with and without comorbid tics. J Am Acad Child Adolesc Psychiatry 32:350–353, 1993

Stewart JT, Myers WC, Burket RC, et al: A review of the pharmacotherapy of aggression in children and adolescents. J Am Acad Child Adolesc Psychiatry 29:269–277, 1990

Szatmari P, Boyle M, Offord DR: ADDH and conduct disorder: degree of diagnostic overlap and differences among correlates. J Am Acad Child Adolesc Psychiatry 28:865–872, 1989a

Szatmari P, Offord DR, Boyle MH: Ontario Child Health Study: prevalence of attention deficit disorder with hyperactivity. J Child Psychol Psychiatry 30:219–230, 1989b

Taylor E, Schachar R, Thorley G, et al: Which boys respond to stimulant medication? A controlled trial of methylphenidate in boys with disruptive behaviour. Psychol Med 17:121–143, 1987

Taylor E, Chadwick O, Heptinstall E, et al: Hyperactivity and conduct problems as risk factors for adolescent development. J Am Acad Child Adolesc Psychiatry 35: 1213–1226, 1996

Teicher MH, Ito Y, Glod CA, et al: Objective measurement of hyperactivity and attentional problems in ADHD. J Am Acad Child Adolesc Psychiatry 35:334–342, 1996

Trites RL, Laprade K: Evidence for an independent syndrome of hyperactivity. J Child Psychol Psychiatry 24:573–586, 1983

Walker JL, Lahey BB, Hynd GW, et al: Comparison of specific patterns of antisocial behavior in children with conduct disorder with or without coexisting hyperactivity. J Consult Clin Psychol 55:910–913, 1987

Walkup J: Methylphenidate and clonidine. AACAP News, September-October 1995, p 11

Weiss G, Hechtman L: Hyperactive Children Grown Up. New York, Guilford, 1993

Weiss G, Hechtman L, Milroy T, et al: Psychiatric status of hyperactives as adults: a controlled prospective 15-year follow-up of 63 hyperactive children. J Am Acad Child Psychiatry 24:211–220, 1985

Werry JS, Sprague RL, Cohen MN: Conners' Teacher Rating Scale for use in drug studies with children—an empirical study. J Abnorm Child Psychol 3:217–299, 1975

Werry JS, Elkind GS, Reeves JC: Attention deficit, conduct, oppositional, and anxiety disorders in children, III: laboratory differences. J Abnorm Child Psychol 15:409–428, 1987a

Werry JS, Reeves JC, Elkind GS: Attention deficit, conduct, oppositional, and anxiety disorders in children, I: a review of research on differentiating characteristics. J Am Acad Child Adolesc Psychiatry 26:133–143, 1987b

Williams DT, Mehl R, Yudofsky S, et al.: The effect of propranolol on uncontrolled rage outbursts in children and adolescents with organic brain dysfunction. J Am Acad Child Psychiatry 21:129–135, 1982

World Health Organization: International Classification of Diseases, 10th Revision. Geneva, World Health Organization, 1992

6 Attention-Deficit Disorders With Obsessive-Compulsive Disorder

Thomas E. Brown, Ph.D.

This chapter begins with a discussion of the nature of obsessions and compulsions in normal development and a description of how these differ from the diagnosis known as obsessive-compulsive disorder (OCD). The characteristics, epidemiology, causes, and outcome of OCD are considered. Some factors that may contribute to the overlap of attention-deficit disorders (ADDs) with OCD are then addressed. The chapter ends with a discussion of how patients with ADDs and comorbid OCD can be recognized and effectively treated.

NORMAL OBSESSIONS AND COMPULSIONS

At some times in their lives most people find themselves "stuck" in repeated thinking about certain worries or disturbing images that they consider excessive or unreasonable but about which, for a time, they are unable to make themselves forget. Examples might be ruminating over possible health problems one might encounter or images of how a loved one who is traveling might get injured in an auto accident.

The author is grateful to John S. March, M.D., for his helpful comments on an earlier draft of this chapter.

Likewise, virtually everyone has engaged in some superstitious or repetitive behaviors that they themselves consider unnecessary or foolish and yet feel they must do anyway, otherwise they just cannot relax or do not feel "right." These behaviors might include repeating special phrases to say "take care and be safe" to a family member who is leaving on a trip, repeatedly checking whether a door has been locked, or engaging in special gestures or routines to "bring good luck" before going to bat in a baseball game.

For most people such thoughts and behaviors consume very little time or effort and are, at most, only transiently disturbing. Yet for some individuals these, or any of a myriad of other such disturbing thoughts or repetitive behaviors, become very persistent and repeatedly intrusive such that they cause chronic distress or significantly disrupt the person's functioning.

DIAGNOSTIC CONSTRUCT

Obsessive-compulsive disorder is the DSM-IV (American Psychiatric Association 1994) diagnosis used to describe the disorder in children, adolescents, or adults who have recurrent disturbing thoughts (obsessions) or persistent, chronic repetitive behaviors that they feel compelled to perform (compulsions) and that result in their having significant impairment in their daily functioning.

Obsessions are characterized in DSM-IV as persistent ideas, thoughts, impulses, or images that are experienced as intrusive and inappropriate and that cause marked anxiety or distress. These might include unwarranted, persistent fears that one has become contaminated by touching someone, or chronic worries that one has left a stove burner on and that a fire may result, or recurrent, vivid mental images of doing embarrassing or horrible acts, such as shouting obscenities in church or hurting one's child.

Although most obsessions involve specific ideas, thoughts, impulses, or images that recurrently intrude in the individual's conscious thought processes, obsessions can be variable. Some persons with OCD repeatedly get "stuck" in obsessional ruminations over various aspects of whatever they are reading, writing, discussing, or thinking. They are unable to shift focus to continue the flow of their efforts. They have significant chronic difficulties in disengaging their attention from one specific focus to move on and complete tasks. They have recurrent disruptions in the flow of their attention and thought, often immobilized by their feeling a need to complete a specific behavior in a manner "just so" (King et al. 1999).

In reading a text, these individuals may become fixated on a particular question or concept and be unable to continue their reading until considerable time has been spent in excessive ruminations about that one specific idea or issue, which may be relatively unimportant. While writing, they may become perseveratively stuck in trying to find just the right words for one particular sentence, unable to set that portion aside, even temporarily, to continue writing other portions of the text for which they do have ideas and words. The whole essay may remain unfinished or have to be handed in quite beyond the deadline because of excessive obsessional ruminations about how to complete a specific sentence or paragraph in a way that will seem to them "just right."

In this sort of obsession, there may not be a single persistent obsessional idea or image; instead, the time-consuming impairment may be in recurrently getting stuck in excessive ruminations about an ever-changing variety of ideas, images, or tasks encountered. This "variable-focus" type of obsessional thinking is very similar to what was described by Kinsbourne (1991/1999) as "overfocusing," wherein the individual demonstrates "a sticky perseveration of mental set and task orientation." This overfocused, perseverative obsessional thinking can be fully as impairing as obsessional fixation on any single idea or image. It is often linked to compulsive behaviors that can be very time-consuming.

Compulsions are defined by DSM-IV as repetitive behaviors, such as hand washing, ordering, or checking, or mental acts, such as repetitive counting, compulsively praying, or repeating words silently, whose goal is to reduce the distress associated with an intrusive obsession or to prevent some dreaded event or situation (American Psychiatric Association 1994, p. 418). Sometimes compulsive behaviors are preceded by a subjective feeling that something in the environment is not "just right" (see King et al. 1999).

To meet the diagnostic criteria for OCD, the obsessions and/or compulsions must cause the individual marked distress, be time-consuming (more than 1 hour per day), or significantly interfere with the individual's normal routine, occupational functioning or with his or her usual social activities or relationships with others (American Psychiatric Association 1994, p. 419).

Examples of impairment might be a child worriedly asking parents and teachers 30 to 100 times each day, "I thought about something naughty, is that OK?" or an adult often feeling compelled to drive back home just after arriving at work to be certain that she has turned off the stove, or while driving often turning back to circle the block to verify that he has not unwittingly injured some pedestrian standing at the curb. OCD impairments can severely disrupt academic, social, and family functioning (Leonard et al. 1993).

EPIDEMIOLOGY, ETIOLOGY, AND COURSE OF OCD

Epidemiology

Although the symptoms of OCD have been rather consistently described for more than 100 years, until the mid-1980s OCD was thought to be a rare disorder with a poor prognosis (Rasmussen and Eisen 1990). Epidemiological studies published in 1985 and 1988 contradicted this view with data indicating that OCD was almost twice as prevalent in the general population as panic disorder or schizophrenia, with lifetime prevalence rates of 2.5%–3% (Bland et al. 1988; Robins et al. 1984).

Lifetime incidence of OCD in the general population has been estimated at 2.5% (American Psychiatric Association 1994), while epidemiological studies have reported incidence among children and adolescents to be 2%–4% in the United States, Israel, New Zealand, and Denmark (Geller et al. 1998). In children, OCD occurs in both genders but is more common in boys (male-to-female ratio 2:1). In adolescents and adults, the gender ratio is 1:1 (March 1998b, p. 549).

Among adults with OCD, the average age at onset has been reported as 19.8 years (± 9.6 years). In about 65% of cases symptoms develop before age 25 years; among adults with OCD one-third to one-half report having developed the disorder during childhood (Rasmussen and Eisen 1990). Studies of OCD in children at the National Institute of Mental Health (NIMH) found a modal age at onset of 7 years and a mean age at onset of 10.2 years. Boys were more likely to have a prepubertal onset; girls were more likely to experience onset of OCD symptoms during adolescence (March and Leonard 1996).

A more recent study by the Harvard group suggests that OCD of childhood onset may be a somewhat different variant of OCD than that of late-adolescent or adult onset. Geller et al. (1998) reviewed 43 studies of juvenile OCD and found that the mean age at onset ranged from 7.5 years to 12.5 years, with a mean of 10.3 years. On average, the studies reported assessment at age 13.2 years, usually about 2.5 years after onset. In these studies most children had both obsessions and compulsions, but compulsions without obsessions were more common during childhood. There were indications that 38%–54% of the juvenile cases appeared to have their onset in response to some psychosocial stressor, and there tended to be high rates of comorbidity among the children with OCD—not only with mood and anxiety disorders common in adults with OCD but also with disruptive behavior disorders, including ADHD, and specific developmental or learning disorders.

The main point made by Geller et al. (1998) on the basis of their literature review was that onset of OCD appears to have a bimodal distribution, with one peak in childhood and another in adulthood, and that these two groups tend to have rather different characteristics. Childhood-onset OCD tends to be characterized not only by prepubertal onset but also by male-dominant distribution, strong family aggregation, and higher rates of comorbidity with a wider range of other disorders, particularly ADDs. These factors combine to suggest that childhood-onset OCD may indicate a much more complicated course than adult-onset OCD.

Etiology

Causes

Until the late 1980s, OCD was generally considered a "neurotic" or psychologically based disorder. Freud discussed this syndrome as being a result of unconscious conflicts and defenses against unrecognized, unacceptable wishes (Freud 1913). In contrast, theorists and therapists with a behavioral orientation conceptualize OCD in terms of learning theory, which suggests that the symptoms result from environmental conditioning of behaviors intended to reduce anxiety (Baer and Minichiello 1990).

Still another perspective is suggested by the work of Kagan (1994), who presented data to argue that temperamental factors may play an important role in the etiology of anxiety disorders; this perspective was supported by research of Biederman et al. (1993), who demonstrated that behavioral inhibition is a temperamental risk factor for a wide variety of anxiety disorders. OCD was not explicitly addressed in the Kagan or Biederman et al. studies, but their data clearly indicate that about 2 of 10 individuals are born with a physiological makeup that predisposes them from infancy to a relatively inhibited behavioral style and, in turn, to one or more disorders of anxiety.

Whatever the etiology of OCD may be, there are clearly some important physiological processes underlying this disorder. These are summarized by March and Leonard (1998).

Neuroimaging studies of OCD patients have generally shown hyperfrontality during resting or provoked states and changes in frontal lobe activity (usually decreased hyperfrontality) following treatment (Cottraux and Gerard 1998). Some, but not all, imaging studies of OCD have noted abnormalities in the striatum, orbital cortex, and cingulate areas of the brain that are presumed associated with the wide variety of OCD symptoms (Baxter et al. 1990).

A model proposed by Brody and Saxena (1996) suggests that two specific pathways may be involved in OCD: one pathway projects from the cortex to the striatum, through the globus pallidus and thalamus, then back to the cortex; another, indirect pathway goes from the cortex to the striatum, then from the striatum to the subthalamic nucleus via the external segment of the globus pallidus, and then returns to the globus pallidus, the thalamus, and the cortex. According to Cottraux and Gerard (1998), this dual-route model posits that OCD results from an imbalance between serotonin, dopamine, and acetylcholine in these two pathways.

Rosenberg and Keshavan (1998) have proposed a neurodevelopmental model of OCD that builds on the fact that 80% of individuals with OCD have onset of the disorder in childhood or adolescence. In their magnetic resonance imaging studies, these authors identified volumetric abnormalities in ventral prefrontal cortical and striatal regions of the brains of children with OCD. These abnormalities led them to posit a developmentally mediated network dysplasia in ventral prefrontal cortical circuits that may disrupt brain functions that mediate purposive behaviors and may cause development of OCD symptoms. Rosenberg and Keshavan also have argued that the developmentally mediated changes in serotonin and dopamine ratios in the brain may have an impact on development of ADD and OCD symptoms.

Although precise details regarding involvement of various brain structures in OCD are not yet fully elaborated in research, considerable evidence indicates that OCD symptoms often respond to treatment with medications of a very specific type: those that increase the availability of the neurotransmitter serotonin in the neural synapse. There is also some evidence to suggest that the neurotransmitter dopamine may play some role in OCD (Billett et al. 1998; McDougal 1994).

Thus far, only those medications that are potent inhibitors of the reuptake of serotonin at the synapse (e.g., clomipramine, fluoxetine, sertraline, paroxetine, fluvoxamine) have been found to be generally and consistently effective in controlling obsessional symptoms in adults (Insel and Winslow 1990) or in children (March and Leonard 1996). These findings suggest that impaired serotonergic function plays a critical role in the development of OCD symptoms.

A Spectrum Model of OCD

OCD has long been categorized as an anxiety disorder and remains so in DSM-IV. Hollander (1993) explained this classification as stemming from the anxiety-provoking character of obsessions and the anxiety-reducing nature of compulsions. Hollander proposed an alternative understanding of OCD as one of a group of disorders identified as representing the impulsive-compulsive spectrum; he described the hallmark of these disorders as the "inability to delay or inhibit repetitive behaviors" (Hollander and Cohen 1996, p. 145).

Disorders on the compulsive end in Hollander's model of the impulsive-compulsive spectrum include OCD, hypochondriasis, body dysmorphic disorder, anorexia nervosa, and depersonalization. The impulsive end of the spectrum includes borderline personality disorder and antisocial personality disorder. Hollander recognizes as mixed compulsive-impulsive disorders Tourette syndrome, trichotillomania, pathological gambling, and sexual compulsions (Hollander and Cohen 1996, p. 144). Further elaboration of this OCD spectrum model has been offered by Goldsmith et al. (1998).

Hollander asserts that disorders on the impulsive-compulsive spectrum have significant overlap in clinical symptoms, associated features (e.g., age at onset, comorbidity, course of illness), family history, and possibly preferential response of serotonin reuptake inhibitors and specific forms of behavior therapy (Hollander and Cohen 1996, p. 143). He notes that all these disorders tend to involve disruption of aspects of the serotonergic system and that all often respond favorably to serotonin reuptake inhibitors.

Genetics

Family and twin studies provide considerable evidence of the heritability of OCD (for review, see Billett et al. 1998). The monozygotic-to-dizygotic ratio of 2.19:1 found by Billett et al. (1998) in their review of the 14 published twin studies on OCD is very close to what is usually taken as evidence of a single susceptibility gene rather than the combined effects of multiple genes. They noted that this ratio constitutes stronger evidence of single-gene etiology for OCD than exists for schizophrenia or bipolar disorder. Family studies give further support to the notion that OCD is inherited. The reported rate of OCD and OCD behavior in relatives of persons with OCD ranges from 17% to 35%; the fact that this rate is markedly higher than the 2%–3% lifetime prevalence of OCD strongly supports the heritability of OCD.

Course

Although it was once thought that OCD in adults always ran a chronic, deteriorating course, evidence speaks to the contrary. Goodwin et al. (1969) reviewed the follow-up studies on OCD and found that most yielded results consistent with three course categories: 1) unremitting and chronic; 2) phasic, with periods of complete remission; and 3) episodic, with incomplete remission that generally permitted normal social functioning. Most of the studies reviewed found that in the majority of cases the course was episodic, with only about 10% of patients diagnosed with OCD characterized as having progressive deterioration.

Studies of children and adolescents with OCD indicate that, as in adults, OCD is generally chronic, although the severity of symptoms tends to wax and wane over time, often in response to stress (March and Leonard 1996). In an NIMH study of 54 patients in a clinical setting followed for as long as 7 years, Leonard et al. (1993) found that 43% still met the full diagnostic criteria for OCD, whereas only 11% were totally free of OCD symptoms. In contrast, Bolton et al. (1995) reported a recovery rate of 57% after 9–14 years in a sample of 14 individuals treated vigorously for OCD during their adolescence.

COMORBIDITY OF OCD WITH ADDS

OCD has been found to be comorbid with many other psychiatric disorders. Although many studies of OCD in children did not address comorbidity with ADDs, either because they simply did not assess for them or because they explicitly excluded persons with ADDs from their samples, children and adolescents with OCD have been found to have high rates of comorbidity with Tourette syndrome, mood disorders, anxiety disorders, and disruptive behavior disorders (Curry and Murphy 1995; Geller et al. 1996).

In those studies of children and adolescents with OCD that did assess for ADDs, the percentages of those found to meet the diagnostic criteria for ADDs have varied, but the variability may be related to methodological and selection differences between the studies. Toro et al. (1992) reported a 6% overlap between OCD and attention-deficit/hyperactivity disorder (ADHD), while other investigators found overlaps of 10% (Riddle et al. 1990; Swedo et al. 1989), 16% (Hanna 1995), and 32% and 33% (Geller et al. 1995 and 1996, respectively). Thus far, there have been no published reports of the incidence of OCD in adults with ADDs or of ADDs in adults with OCD, but Weiss et al. (1999) have provided case descriptions of this overlap.

Familial Patterns in Anxiety Disorders and ADDs

As discussed earlier, OCD and other anxiety disorders, like ADDs, tend to run in families. Biederman and colleagues have studied the overlap of ADDs and anxiety disorders in relatives of persons with ADDs (Biederman et al. 1991). They reported that the overall risk of anxiety disorders is markedly elevated among relatives of patients with ADDs compared with relatives of comparison subjects without ADDs. The relatives of patients with both an ADD and an anxiety disorder were found to have twice the risk of anxiety disorders as the relatives of persons with an ADD and no anxiety disorder. Biederman et al. concluded from this finding that ADDs and anxiety disorders are separately inherited, even though individuals with ADDs are at significantly higher risk of inheriting an anxiety disorder than are those without ADDs (Biederman et al. 1991).

Cognitive Deficits in OCD and ADDs

Patients with OCD have been shown to have a variety of cognitive deficits associated with frontal and/or striatal functions. Schmidtke et al. (1998) found that, relative to control subjects, OCD patients have selective deficits in tasks involving controlled attentional processing and self-guided, spontaneous behavior. Purcell et al. (1998) reported that OCD patients, compared with control subjects, demonstrated specific cognitive deficits on tasks of executive and visual memory function. These neuropsychological findings are not directly linked to the obsessions or compulsions that are the diagnostic criteria symptoms of OCD, but they are closely related to cognitive impairments associated with diagnostic criteria for ADHD. It may be that these studies of cognitive impairments in OCD patients are actually offering evidence of ADD impairments often found in patients with OCD who have unrecognized comorbid ADDs. Neither of these two studies reported assessing for ADHD.

Screening for Possible Comorbidity of OCD With ADDs

Patients with comorbid OCD and an ADD often seek treatment without being aware of their having both disorders. Those who are aware of having attention problems may attribute these difficulties solely to their having an ADD and may not be aware that their ongoing obsessional worries or compulsive behaviors are related to an altogether different disorder. Or, they may suspect that they have both an ADD and "something else" but may not be ready to discuss with the evaluating clinician any symptoms other than those recognized as being related to the ADD.

Many persons with OCD are embarrassed about their private obsessions and/or compulsions. Realizing that the thoughts or behaviors are irrational in intensity, content, or both, yet seemingly unavoidable, they may fear others' thinking of them as immature, weak-willed, "perverted," or "crazy." Such fears cause some individuals to avoid mentioning their OCD symptoms during their initial evaluation, especially if they are not specifically asked about such difficulties. They may hope that an ADD diagnosis and the associated treatment will rid them of their OCD symptoms as well. Or they may simply prefer to present initially to the evaluating clinician their less embarrassing ADD symptoms, deferring discussion of OCD impairments until after they have had an opportunity to become acquainted and to build a more trusting relationship with the clinician.

Some individuals seek treatment for recognized OCD symptoms without being aware that some of their concentration problems may be more related to an ADD. Their route to seeking evaluation may be referral from a relative with diagnosed OCD, having read an article or book on OCD, or having seen a television show describing OCD and its treatment. If such patients have symptoms that actually meet the diagnostic criteria for OCD, treatment for those symptoms probably is a sensible first intervention. Additional treatment for their ADD symptoms can be offered later if it seems desirable. If, on the other hand, such a patient does not have OCD but does meet the diagnostic criteria for ADD, then the focus of the evaluation ought to be shifted, with appropriate explanations about the similarities and differences between the two disorders.

A careful evaluation for possible ADDs should include some screening questions to probe for OCD and for other possible psychiatric or learning disorders that may be concurrent with the ADD symptoms or that may have been problematic in the past and may potentially be problematic in the present if ADD treatment is undertaken. Guidelines for a comprehensive evaluation for ADDs are provided elsewhere in this volume (see Chapter 15).

For the present, suffice it to say that during an initial evaluation for ADDs, the clinician should query the patient about whether he or she currently has or in the past has had excessive worries or fears, panic attacks, disturbing thoughts that are hard to keep out of one's mind, or repetitious behaviors that he or she feels compelled to do even though they may not make very much sense. It is important to ask explicitly not only about anxiety manifest in excessive worries, nervousness, or panic attacks but also about obsessions and compulsions. Four common symptom factors in OCD are obsessions and checking, symmetry and order, cleaning and washing, and hoarding (Leckman et al. 1997). It may be useful if the clinician mentions at least these specific types when inquiring about obsessions and compulsions.

Kinsbourne (1991/1999) has provided descriptors that can help to differentiate persons whose chronic attentional problems are related to "overfocusing" in an obsessional-perseverative mode from those with more traditional inattention problems. He notes that persons with attention deficits who are overfocused are unlike the more usual underfocusers, who fail to finish tasks because they too quickly jump from one incomplete task to another; overfocusers tend to sustain their attention on one aspect of one task to excess. These overfocusers rarely act before thinking; they tend to obsess excessively before acting and may not act at all. They hate to be wrong and would rather not do a task at all, rather than risk doing it incorrectly. They prefer to focus on just one thing at a time, and they tend strenuously to resist shifting attention of changing activities on someone else's timetable. Many characteristics included in Kinsbourne's profile overlap with descriptions of children with Asperger's syndrome (Klin 1994) or nonverbal learning disorder (Rourke 1989), but the specific problems in shifting focus of attention that he describes may reflect impairments of perseverative obsessional thinking characteristic of some persons with OCD who may or may not also meet the diagnostic criteria for ADD and/or other disorders.

Many individuals with OCD have multiple anxiety disorders, including generalized anxiety disorder and panic disorder with or without agoraphobia (Brown 1998). Inquiry about one disorder may not elicit response about another. If queries about family psychiatric history have yielded any indications of blood-related family members with significant anxiety problems, Tourette syndrome, or a developmental disorder (e.g., pervasive developmental disorder or Asperger's disorder), even more detailed inquiry about the patient's experience with anxiety or OCD problems may be warranted. For more detailed inquiry about anxiety disorders in children, the Multidimensional Anxiety Scale for Children (MASC; March 1998a) is useful; adults can be queried with the Anxiety Disorders Interview Schedule for DSM-IV (ADIS-IV; DiNardo et al. 1994).

Often the clinician's query about excessive worries or related problems can open the door for a hesitant patient to discuss anxiety symptoms that may include those of OCD and/or other anxiety disorders. If the clinician is receptive and reassuring, even more detailed descriptions of OCD symptoms and related problems may be forthcoming from the patient. Clinicians need to keep in mind that whereas some patients with ADD often speak freely, if not excessively, about details of their life problems, patients with ADD and concurrent anxiety symptoms and/or OCD are likely to be much more cautious, especially early in the clinical relationship, regarding how much of their problems they disclose. These patients are often very quick to feel embarrassed or ashamed and may unwarrantedly assume that the clinician is feeling judgmental.

Sometimes it may be helpful in this inquiry for the clinician to give some specific examples of the wide variety of obsessions and compulsions. Brief vignettes can be offered—for example, a child who cannot get to sleep unless he performs a nightly ritual of raising and lowering each of his window shades in a ritualized sequence after which his closet door must be tightly closed; or a woman who is unable to park her car in her garage because the space is completely filled with old newspapers or magazines that she cannot bring herself to discard because she fears she may need to refer to old articles in them; or a student who feels a need to have all his music CDs arranged in alphabetical order and feels very uncomfortable when each is not in its appointed place. Offering such examples in a manner that makes clear that many people who are not "crazy" have such difficulties may help to reduce the patient's hesitations and facilitate symptom disclosure.

When evaluating children, clinicians should keep in mind that parents are not always aware of the anxiety symptoms of their children. Although parents are often better reporters of symptoms of disruptive behaviors in their sons and daughters than are the children themselves, it has been shown that, often, self-report from children may provide more adequate assessment of anxiety symptoms (Faraone et al. 1995). Given these findings, clinicians should ask both parents and their children about anxiety symptoms, and specifically about OCD symptoms, when screening for the range of disorders that may be comorbid with an ADD.

ASSESSMENT MEASURES FOR OCD SYMPTOMS

When initial screening indicates that OCD symptoms may be present, more systematic assessment of OCD and related symptoms is clearly indicated. Instruments for assessment of OCD have been reviewed by Goodman and Price (1990) and Taylor (1998). For assessment of children who may have OCD, the children's form of the Yale-Brown Obsessive Compulsive Scale (CY-BOCS), by Goodman and Price (1992), is currently considered the instrument of choice (March and Leonard 1996; Scahill et al. 1997). For assessment of adults who may have OCD, several measures are available—for example, the Maudsley Obsessive Compulsive Inventory (Rachman and Hodgson 1980) and the Yale-Brown Obsessive Compulsive Scale (Goodman et al. 1989a, 1989b). Of these, the Yale-Brown Obsessive Compulsive Scale is generally preferable because of its psychometrics and ease of use (Taylor 1998).

Some clinicians and researchers argue that a more broad-range symptom or personality assessment instrument is useful for assessment of OCD. Such measures include the Structured Clinical Interview for DSM-IV (First et al. 1996) and the Anxiety Disorders Interview Schedule for DSM-IV (DiNardo et al. 1994). Cloninger (1996) has argued for the use of more wide-range personality assessment measures, such as his Tridimensional Personality Questionnaire (Cloninger et al. 1994) or the NEO-Personality Inventory (Costa and McCrae 1991), in assessing patients who may have disorders on the impulsivity-compulsivity spectrum. Each of these more comprehensive measures can contribute information for assessment of OCD and other symptoms or personality traits that may be useful in guiding treatment of adults with OCD comorbid with ADD. However, these measures tend to be quite time-consuming, and clinicians who are pressed for time are likely to find the Yale-Brown Obsessive Compulsive Scale or the Children's Yale-Brown Obsessive Compulsive Scale more specific and cost-efficient for assessing OCD symptoms, both in making an initial assessment and in monitoring the effectiveness of treatments for OCD. Further suggestions for assessment and monitoring are available in the reviews by March and Leonard (1998) and Taylor (1998).

TREATMENT OF OCD SYMPTOMS AND COMBINED OCD AND ADDS

Medication Treatment for OCD Symptoms

Pigott and Seay (1998) reviewed the multiple studies which demonstrate that medications in the selective serotonin reuptake inhibitor (SSRI) group—for example, fluoxetine, sertraline, fluvoxamine—provide effective treatment for OCD symptoms in 55%–65% of adult patients with OCD while the patients are taking this medication. Similar findings of medication effectiveness for children and adolescents with OCD, though based on a more limited database, have been reported in the OCD practice parameters published by the American Academy of Child and Adolescent Psychiatry (AACAP) (King et al. 1998). It seems quite clear that medications in the SSRI group provide considerable relief of OCD symptoms for a majority, but not all, of the children, adolescents, and adults treated with these medications.

Pato et al. (1998) noted that some patients with OCD respond well to one medication in this group but do not respond to another. This highlights the usefulness of trying another agent(s) of the same class when the initial medication is not effective. Greist et al. (1995) found that 19% of patients who had not responded to clomipramine or fluoxetine did respond to fluvoxamine. It should be noted that medication response of OCD symptoms to an SSRI is not always prompt; sometimes trials for as long as 10–12 weeks are needed to determine whether an SSRI is effective for OCD symptoms (King et al. 1998).

When adequate trials of SSRI are not effective for treatment of significantly impairing OCD symptoms, other medications may be effective in an augmentation strategy. Clonazepam has been reported to be effective for augmentation of an SSRI (Leonard et al. 1994; Pigott et al. 1992). McDougle et al. (1994) reported haloperidol and risperidone to be more effective than placebo in augmenting fluvoxamine to alleviate OCD symptoms in adults with or without comorbid chronic tics or schizotypal personality disorder. These more complicated augmentation strategies may be particularly important for patients with pervasive developmental disorders or other complicated multiple comorbidities.

Follow-up studies indicate that sustaining the symptom remission accomplished by medication treatment of OCD usually requires continuation of the anti-OCD medication. Pigott and Seay (1998) reported on several studies which indicate that the majority of patients successfully treated for OCD with medication relapse rapidly when that medication is discontinued and/or replaced by placebo. Yet clinical experience indicates that many patients with OCD report that their symptoms tend to wax and wane such that continuous treatment with medication is not necessary for all patients with these symptoms. Sometimes OCD symptoms remit sufficiently on their own such that continuing medication is no longer necessary.

Interestingly, the rate of OCD patients' response to placebo is quite low. Whereas 30%–40% of patients with depression and 40%–50% of patients with panic disorder respond to placebo, few patients with OCD (8%–20%) respond to treatment with placebo (Pigott and Seay 1998). This suggests that the factors that sustain OCD symptoms may be more fully neurochemical than in some cases of depression and panic disorder and that medication is likely to play a central role in effective treatment of many cases of OCD.

Medication Treatment for Combined OCD and ADDs

Unfortunately, the class of medications demonstrated to be the most effective for treatment of OCD, the SSRIs, has not been found effective for treatment of the primary cognitive symptoms of ADD. Barrickman et al. (1991), reporting on a study of treatment of children with ADD symptoms with fluoxetine, found that fluoxetine was effective in alleviating some behavioral and affective symptoms associated with ADDs but that it did not effect any significant changes in focused attention. This is not surprising given the presumed centrality of dopamine in ADD, as discussed in the first chapter of this volume. Since there is currently no evidence that SSRIs are effective for treatment of the primary symptoms of ADD, this class of medications is not used to treat ADD symptoms, although such medications are often used in conjunction with stimulants to treat associated symptoms and comorbid disorders (cf. Chapters 3 and 9, this volume).

Just as SSRI medications useful for treatment of OCD are not effective for ADDs, so the stimulant medications used most frequently to treat ADDs are not effective in the treatment of OCD. One study suggested that D-amphetamine may have some benefit in alleviating some OCD symptoms in some patients, but this has not been replicated; other studies suggest that stimulants, particularly methylphenidate, may transiently induce overfocused, perseverative, or compulsive behavior (Borcherding et al. 1990; Solanto and Wender 1989). Practice guidelines for treatment of OCD published by the AACAP (King et al. 1998, p. 32S) note that stimulants have been used in children with OCD and concomitant ADHD without apparently exacerbating their OCD symptoms.

Given the demonstrated specific effectiveness of SSRI medications for the treatment of OCD symptoms and the demonstrated effectiveness of stimulant medications for the treatment of ADD symptoms, clinicians may wish to consider concurrent treatment with both a stimulant medication and an SSRI for individuals with both an ADD and OCD. Thus far, there are no controlled studies of this combination of medications and no studies specifically focused on the combined symptoms of an ADD and OCD. However, an open study of the combined use of stimulant medication and fluoxetine in children ages 9–17 years with both an ADD and comorbid depressive or anxiety symptoms has been reported by Gammon and Brown (1993). The authors found this combination of medications to be effective and well tolerated in 30 of 32 children in their sample.

Although the sample in Gammon and Brown's study was not specific to patients with the combination of ADD and OCD, the findings from this study, combined with anecdotal clinical experiences with this combination of medications for children, adolescents, and adults having both ADDs and OCD, suggest that further research on this combination of medications for persons with OCD with a concurrent ADD would be useful. Such research could be helpful for guiding clinical treatment of comorbid ADDs and OCD; it could also be helpful in illuminating the possible interaction of serotonin and dopamine in shaping certain aspects of brain function and behavior.

Behavioral Treatments for OCD Symptoms

Medication is not the only useful treatment for OCD. A variety of cognitive-behavioral interventions have also been demonstrated to be effective for OCD symptoms in children, adolescents, and adults. These interventions have been reviewed by Steketee (1993), Foa et al. (1998), March and Mulle (1998), and Stanley and Averill (1998).

The cognitive-behavioral treatments for OCD usually involve providing the patient and family accurate factual information about the nature, causes, and course of OCD, as well as highly individualized assessment of the specifics of the individual's obsessions and compulsions. This assessment is generally followed by systematic implementation of hierarchically presented exposures and response prevention strategies designed to challenge the irrational beliefs and behaviors. Usually 13–20 weekly sessions with the patient and some sessions with the patient's family are required for effective cognitive-behavioral treatment of OCD symptoms; sometimes longer duration or greater frequency is required.

Decisions as to whether treatment for OCD symptoms should be begun with medication alone, cognitive behavioral treatment alone, or the two modalities in combination need to be made in terms of each specific case. Guidelines for making these treatment decisions, based on a consensus from a panel of experts, have been published by March et al. (1997). These guidelines are summarized by March and Leonard (1998). The AACAP treatment guidelines for children with OCD (King et al. 1998) suggest that in relatively uncomplicated cases the initial treatment intervention might begin with cognitive-behavioral therapy or antiobsessional medication, either alone or in combination. These guidelines do suggest, however, that in cases complicated by comorbid depression, anxiety, or disruptive behavior, an SSRI should be included as one element of the initial treatment plan.

More Complicated Cases

Some of the more complicated cases of combined OCD and ADD involve many overlapping diagnoses, no one of which sufficiently describes the person's condition. Sometimes individuals with an ADD and OCD also meet the diagnostic criteria for Tourette syndrome (see Chapter 11, this volume). Others may have an ADD, OCD, and one or more mood disorders, anxiety disorders, substance abuse disorders, or personality disorders. Still others may demonstrate significant impairments in making and maintaining social relationships along with their having an ADD and OCD; this is often the case with individuals who qualify for the diagnosis of Asperger's disorder, pervasive developmental disorder, or other disorders on the autistic spectrum. For these very complicated cases in which the individual has an ADD, OCD, and many other complex concurrent disorders, the process of treatment usually involves a much more complicated process of ongoing assessment and cautious trials of various combinations of treatments tailored for the particular individual in the specifics of his or her current environment. Sometimes the treatments discussed in the foregoing subsections may be quite useful in these complex cases; in other cases, totally different treatment approaches are required.

REFERENCES

American Psychiatric Association: Diagnostic and Statistical Manual of Mental Disorders, 4th Edition. Washington, DC, American Psychiatric Association, 1994

Baer L, Minichiello WE: Behavior therapy for obsessive-compulsive disorder, in Obsessive-Compulsive Disorders: Theory and Management, 2nd Edition. Edited by Jenicke MA, Baer L, Minichiello WE. Chicago, IL, Year Book Medical, 1990, pp 203–232

Barrickman L, Noyes R, Kuperman S, et al: Treatment of ADHD with fluoxetine: a preliminary trial. J Am Acad Child Adolesc Psychiatry 30:762–767, 1991

Baxter LR, Schwartz JM, Guze BH, et al: Neuroimaging in obsessive-compulsive disorder: seeking the mediating neuroanatomy, in Obsessive-Compulsive Disorders: Theory and Management, 2nd Edition. Edited by Jenicke MA, Baer L, Minichiello WE. Chicago, IL, Year Book Medical, 1990, pp 167–188

Biederman J, Faraone SV, Keenan K, et al: Familial association between attention deficit disorder and anxiety disorders. Am J Psychiatry 148:251–256, 1991

Biederman J, Rosenbaum JA, Bolduc-Murphy EA, et al: A three-year follow-up of children with and without behavioral inhibition. J Am Acad Child Adolesc Psychiatry 32:814–821, 1993

Billett EA, Richter MA, Kennedy JL: Genetics of obsessive-compulsive disorder, in Obsessive-Compulsive Disorder: Theory, Research and Treatment. Edited by Swinson RP, Antony MM, Rachman S, et al. New York, Guilford, 1998, pp 181–206

Bland R, Newman S, Orn H: Lifetime prevalence of psychiatric disorders in Edmonton. Acta Psychiatr Scand Suppl 338:24–32, 1988

Bolton D, Luckie M, Steinberg D: Long-term course of obsessive-compulsive disorder treated in adolescence. J Am Acad Child Adolesc Psychiatry 34:1441–1450, 1995

Borcherding BG, Keysor CS, Rapoport JL, et al: Motor/vocal tics and compulsive behaviors on stimulant drugs: is there a common vulnerability? Psychiatry Res 33:83–94, 1990

Brody AL, Saxena S: Brain-imaging in obsessive-compulsive disorder: evidence for the involvement of frontal-subcortical circuitry in the mediation of symptomatology. CNS Spectrums 1:27–41, 1996

Brown TA: Relationship between obsessive-compulsive disorder and other anxiety-based disorders, in Obsessive-Compulsive Disorder: Theory, Research and Treatment. Edited by Swinson RP, Antony MM, Rachman S, et al. New York, Guilford, 1998, pp 207–226

Cloninger CR: Assessment of the impulsive-compulsive spectrum of behavior by the seven-factor model of temperament and character, in Impulsivity and Compulsivity. Edited by Oldham JM, Hollander E, Skodol AE. Washington, DC, American Psychiatric Press, 1996, pp 59–95

Cloninger CR, Przybeck TR, Svrakic DM, et al: The Temperament and Character Inventory (TCI): A Guide to Its Development and Use. St Louis, MO, Center for Psychobiology of Personality, Washington University, 1994

Costa PT Jr, McCrae R: Trait psychology comes of age. Nebr Symp Motiv 39:169–204, 1991

Cottraux J, Gerard D: Neuroimaging and neuroanatomical issues in obsessive-compulsive disorder: toward an integrative model—perceived impulsivity, in Obsessive-Compulsive Disorder: Theory, Research and Treatment. Edited by Swinson RP, Antony MM, Rachman S, et al. New York, Guilford, 1998, pp 154–180

Curry JF, Murphy LB: Comorbidity of anxiety disorders, in Anxiety Disorders in Children and Adolescents. Edited by March JS. New York, Guilford, 1995, pp 301–317

DiNardo P, Brown TA, Barlow DH: Anxiety Interview Schedule for DSM-IV. San Antonio, TX, Psychological Corporation, 1994

Faraone SV, Biederman J, Millberger S: How reliable are maternal reports of their children's psychopathology? One-year recall of psychiatric diagnoses of ADHD children. J Am Acad Child Adolesc Psychiatry 34:1001–10008, 1995

First MB, Spitzer RL, Gibbon M, et al: Structured Clinical Interview for DSM-IV Axis I Disorders—Patient Edition (SCID-I/P), Version 2.0. New York, New York Psychiatric Institute, Biometrics Research Unit, 1996

Foa EB, Franklin ME, Kozak MJ: Psychosocial treatments for obsessive-compulsive disorder: literature review, in Obsessive-Compulsive Disorder: Theory, Research and Treatment. Edited by Swinson RP, Antony MM, Rachman S, et al. New York, Guilford, 1998, pp 258–276

Freud S: The disposition to obsessional neurosis. A contribution to the problem of choice of neurosis (1913), in Standard Edition of the Complete Psychological Works of Sigmund Freud, Vol 12. Translated and edited by Strachey J. London, Hogarth, 1958, pp 317–326

Gammon GD, Brown TE: Fluoxetine and methylphenidate in combination for treatment of attention deficit disorder and comorbid depressive disorder. J Child Adolesc Psychopharmacol 3:1–10, 1993

Geller D, Beiderman J, Reed E, et al: Similarities in response to fluoxetine in the treatment of children and adolescents with obsessive-compulsive disorder. J Am Acad Child Adolesc Psychiatry 34:36–44, 1995

Geller DA, Biederman J, Griffin S, et al: Comorbidity of juvenile obsessive-compulsive disorder with disruptive behavior disorders. J Am Acad Child Adolesc Psychiatry 35:1637–1646, 1996

Geller D, Biederman J, Jones J, et al: Is juvenile obsessive-compulsive disorder a developmental subtype of the disorder? A review of the pediatric literature. J Am Acad Child Adolesc Psychiatry 37:420–427, 1998

Goldsmith T, Shapira NA, Phillips KA, et al: Conceptual foundations of obsessive-compulsive disorder in obsessive-compulsive disorder: theory, research and treatment. Edited by Swinson RP, Antony MM, Rachman S, et al. New York, Guilford, 1998, pp 397–425

Goodman WK, Price LW: Rating scales for obsessive-compulsive disorder, in Obsessive-Compulsive Disorders: Theory and Management, 2nd Edition. Edited by Jenicke MA, Baer L, Minichiello WE. Chicago, IL, Year Book Medical, 1990, pp 154–166

Goodman WK, Price LH: Assessment of severity and change on obsessive-compulsive disorder. Psychiatr Clin North Am 15:861–869, 1992

Goodman WK, Price LH, Rasmussen SA, et al: The Yale-Brown Obsessive Compulsive Scale, I: development, use, and reliability. Arch Gen Psychiatry 46:1006–1011, 1989a

Goodman WK, Price LH, Rasmussen SA, et al: The Yale-Brown Obsessive Compulsive Scale, II: validity. Arch Gen Psychiatry 46:1012–1016, 1989b

Goodwin DW, Guze S, Robins E: Follow-up studies in obsessional neurosis. Arch Gen Psychiatry 20:182–187, 1969

Greist JH, Jefferson JW, Kobak KA, et al: Efficacy and tolerability of serotonin transport inhibitors in obsessive-compulsive disorder. Arch Gen Psychiatry 52:53–60, 1995.

Hanna GL: Demographic and clinical features of obsessive-compulsive disorder in children and adolescents. J Am Acad Child Adolesc Psychiatry 34:19–27, 1995

Hollander E: Introduction, in Obsessive-Compulsive–Related Disorders. Edited by Hollander E. Washington, DC, American Psychiatric Press, 1993, pp 1–16

Hollander E, Cohen LJ: Psychobiology and psychopharmacology of compulsive spectrum disorders, in Impulsivity and Compulsivity. Edited by Oldham JM, Hollander E, Skodol AE. Washington, DC, American Psychiatric Press, 1996, pp 143–166

Insel TR, Winslow JT: Neurobiology of obsessive-compulsive disorder, in Obsessive-Compulsive Disorders: Theory and Management, 2nd Edition. Edited by Jenicke MA, Baer L, Minichiello WE. Chicago, IL, Year Book Medical, 1990, pp 118–131

Kagan J: Galen's Prophecy: Temperament in Human Nature. New York, Basic Books, 1994

King RA, Leonard H, March J: Practice parameters for the assessment and treatment of children and adolescents with obsessive-compulsive disorder. J Am Acad Child Adolesc Psychiatry 37(10, suppl):27S–45S, 1998

King RA, Leckman JF, Scahill L, et al: Obsessive-compulsive disorder, anxiety, and depression, in Tourette's Syndrome—Tics, Obsessions–Compulsions: Developmental Psychopathology and Clinical Care. Edited by Leckman JF, Cohen DJ. New York, Wiley, 1999, pp 43–62

Kinsbourne M: Overfocusing: an apparent subtype of attention deficit/hyperactivity disorder (1991), in Understanding, Diagnosing, and Treating AD/HD in Children and Adolescents: An Integrative Approach. Edited by Incorvaia JA, Mark-Goldstein BS, Tessmer D. Northvale, NJ, Jason Aronson, 1999, pp 131–152

Leckman JF, Grice DE, Boardman J, et al: Symptoms of obsessive-compulsive disorder. Am J Psychiatry 154:911–917, 1997

Leonard HL, Swedo S, Lenane M, et al: A 2- to 7-year follow-up study of 54 obsessive-compulsive children and adolescents. Arch Gen Psychiatry 50:429–439, 1993

Leonard HL, Topol D, Bukstein O, et al: Clonazepam as an augmenting agent in the treatment of childhood-onset obsessive-compulsive disorder. J Am Acad Child Adolesc Psychiatry 33:792–794, 1994

March JS: Multidimensional Anxiety Scale for Children (MASC). Toronto, Multi-Health Systems, 1998a

March JS: Obsessive-compulsive disorder, in Textbook of Pediatric Neuropsychiatry. Edited by Coffey CE, Brumback RA. Washington, DC, American Psychiatric Press, 1998b, pp 547–562

March JS, Leonard HL: Obsessive-compulsive disorder: a review of the past ten years. J Am Acad Child Adolesc Psychiatry 35:1265–1273, 1996

March JS, Leonard HL: Obsessive-compulsive disorder in children and adolescents, in Obsessive-Compulsive Disorder: Theory, Research and Treatment. Edited by Swinson RP, Antony MM, Rachman S, et al. New York, Guilford, 1998, pp 367–394

March JS, Mulle K: OCD in Children and Adolescents: A Cognitive-Behavioral Treatment Manual. New York, Guilford, 1998

March JS, Frances A, et al: Expert consensus guidelines: treatment of obsessive-compulsive disorder. J Clin Psychiatry 58 (no 4, suppl):1–72, 1997

McDougle CJ, Goodman WK, Leckman JF, et al: Haloperidol addition in fluvoxamine-refractory obsessive-compulsive disorder: a double-blind, placebo-controlled study in patients with and without tics. Arch Gen Psychiatry 51:302–309, 1994

Pato MT, Pato CN, Gunn SA: Biological treatments for obsessive-compulsive disorder: clinical applications, in Obsessive-Compulsive Disorder: Theory, Research and Treatment. Edited by Swinson RP, Antony MM, Rachman S, et al. New York, Guilford, 1998, pp 327–348

Pigott TA, Seay S: Biological treatments for obsessive-compulsive disorder: literature review, in Obsessive-Compulsive Disorder: Theory, Research and Treatment. Edited by Swinson RP, Antony MM, Rachman S, et al. New York, Guilford, 1998, pp 298–326

Pigott T, L'Heureux F, et al: A controlled trial of adjuvant clonazepam in clomipramine and fluoxetine treated patients with OCD. Presentation at the 145th annual meeting of the American Psychiatric Association, Washington, DC, May 2–7, 1992

Purcell R, Maruff P, Kyrios M, et al: Cognitive deficits in obsessive-compulsive disorder on tests of frontal-striatal function. Biol Psychiatry 43:348–357, 1998

Rachman S, Hodgson RJ: Obsessions and Compulsions. Englewood Cliffs, NJ, Prentice-Hall, 1980

Rapoport JL (ed): Obsessive-Compulsive Disorder in Children and Adolescents. Washington, DC, American Psychiatric Press, 1989

Rasmussen SA, Eisen JL: Epidemiology and clinical features of obsessive-compulsive disorder, in Obsessive-Compulsive Disorders: Theory and Management, 2nd Edition. Edited by Jenicke MA, Baer L, Minichiello WE. Chicago, IL, Year Book Medical, 1990, pp 10–27

Riddle M, Scahill L, King R, et al: Obsessive-compulsive disorder in children and adolescents: phenomenology and family history. J Am Acad Child Adolesc Psychiatry 29:776–772, 1990

Robins L, Helzer J, Weissman M, et al: Lifetime prevalence of specific psychiatric disorders in three sites. Arch Gen Psychiatry 41:958–967, 1984

Rosenberg DR, Keshavan MS: Toward a neurodevelopmental model of obsessive-compulsive disorder. Biol Psychiatry 43:623–640, 1998

Scahill L, Riddle MA, McSwiggin-Hardin M, et al: Children's Yale-Brown Obsessive Compulsive Scale: reliability and validity. J Am Acad Child Adolesc Psychiatry 36:844–852, 1997

Schmidtke K, Schorb A, Winkelmann G, et al: Cognitive frontal lobe dysfunction in obsessive-compulsive disorder. Biol Psychiatry 43:666–673, 1998

Solanto MV, Wender EH: Does methylphenidate constrict cognitive functioning? J Am Acad Child Adolesc Psychiatry 28:897–902, 1989

Stanley MA, Averill PM: Psychosocial treatments for obsessive-compulsive disorder: clinical applications, in Obsessive-Compulsive Disorder: Theory, Research and Treatment. Edited by Swinson RP, Antony MM, Rachman S, et al. New York, Guilford, 1998, pp 277–297

Steketee GS: Treatment of Obsessive-Compulsive Disorder. New York, Guilford, 1993

Swedo S, Rapoport JL, Leonard H, et al: Obsessive-compulsive disorder in children and adolescents. Arch Gen Psychiatry 46:335–341, 1989

Taylor S: Assessment of obsessive-compulsive disorder, in Obsessive-Compulsive Disorder: Theory, Research and Treatment. Edited by Swinson RP, Antony MM, Rachman S, et al. New York, Guilford, 1998, pp 229–257

Toro J, Cervera M, Osejo E, et al: Obsessive-compulsive disorder in childhood and adolescence: a clinical study. J Child Psychol Psychiatry 33:1025–1037, 1992

Weiss M, Hechtman LT, Weiss G: ADHD in Adulthood. Baltimore, MD, Johns Hopkins University Press, 1999

7 Attention-Deficit Disorders With Learning Disorders in Children and Adolescents

Rosemary Tannock, Ph.D.
Thomas E. Brown, Ph.D.

Many children experience a variety of problems at school, including failure to complete assignments, low marks, poor retention of learned material, difficulties in mastering specific academic skills, problems in planning and organization, failure to abide by rules, and interpersonal difficulties. Poor school performance may result from a variety of factors that may occur alone or in combination. These factors include severe environmental deprivation (e.g., poor nutrition, social disadvantage, abuse), low intellectual ability, developmental delay, sensory impairments (e.g., poor vision or hearing), emotional or behavioral disorders (e.g., anxiety, depression, attention-deficit disorders, conduct disorder), and specific learning disorders (also called specific developmental disorders).

The focus of this chapter is on attention-deficit/hyperactivity disorder (ADHD) and learning disorders, which are major problems of childhood that frequently co-occur and persist into adolescence and adulthood. Conservative estimates suggest that between 3% and 5% of children have ADHD and that

---

Preparation of this chapter was supported in part by a Scientist Award from the Medical Research Council of Canada and a grant from the National Institutes of Health (RO1 HD31714) to R. Tannock.

approximately one in four of these children has specific learning disabilities. Conversely, among the 5%–10% of children who have learning disorder, about one in three also has ADHD.

The terms *attention-deficit/hyperactivity disorder,* or ADHD, and *learning disability* are used generically throughout the chapter. That is, learning disorder includes all types of learning disability, such as reading disorder (dyslexia or developmental reading disorder), mathematical disabilities, disorder of written expression, developmental coordination disorder, specific language impairments, and central auditory processing disorder. ADHD is used to refer to DSM-IV (American Psychiatric Association 1994) subtypes of ADHD (predominantly inattentive type, predominantly hyperactive-impulsive type, combined type), the DSM-III-R (American Psychiatric Association 1987) category of attention-deficit hyperactivity disorder, the DSM-III (American Psychiatric Association 1980) categories of attention deficit disorder with hyperactivity and attention deficit disorder without hyperactivity, the DSM-II (American Psychiatric Association 1968) category of hyperkinetic reaction of childhood, and the categories of childhood hyperactivity or minimal brain dysfunction in the older literature.

Despite the prevalence of both ADHD and learning disorders, there is still widespread confusion over the differentiation of these two clinical entities. Are they merely alternative names for the same set of problems? Are the learning problems associated with ADHD secondary to the psychiatric aspects of the condition (inattention, impulsiveness, hyperactivity), a result of cognitive deficits associated with learning disorders, or due to other problems, such as psychosocial disadvantage, demoralization, and resultant decline in motivation, alone or in any combination? The answers to these questions have important implications for clinical practice and education, as well as for nosology and legal policy.

The confusion over how to differentiate ADHD and learning disorders may be ascribed to a number of factors, including the overlap of academic and attention problems associated with both conditions, the inconsistencies in definitions, the heterogeneity of definitional criteria for both conditions, and the frequent clinical presentation of both disorders within the same child. Also, much of this confusion results from the inevitable delay in the dissemination of recent advances in the conceptualization, definition, and classification of learning disorders and ADHD (B. A. Shaywitz et al. 1994).

In this chapter we first provide an update on the current conceptualizations of ADHD and learning disorders—disorders that may frequently co-occur in the same individual but that can clearly be distinguished from each other. In the remainder of the chapter we examine the impact of concurrent learning disorders on the clinical presentation, correlates, course, assessment, and clinical management of ADHD. Greatest emphasis is given to dyslexia, or reading disorder, because it is the most commonly observed learning disorder and more is known about its underlying mechanisms than about the mechanisms of any other type. In this chapter, we discuss learning disorders primarily with reference to children and adolescents; for a detailed discussion of learning disorders in adults, see Chapter 8, by Denckla, in this volume.

DISTINCTIONS BETWEEN ADDS AND LEARNING DISORDERS

Conceptual Distinctions

ADHD. Although traditionally considered to be primarily a disruptive behavior disorder, ADHD has been reconceptualized, on the basis of recent empirical evidence, as primarily a complex of cognitive impairments (Barkley 1997; Brown 1995, 1996; Douglas 1988; Pennington and Ozonoff 1996). The fundamental cognitive deficit of ADHD is unknown, and further research is needed to clarify the exact nature of the cognitive impairments in ADHD (Tannock 1998). (Core or primary deficits are universal [occur in all individuals with a specific disorder], specific [occur only in disorder A], and persistent [evident across the life span] [Pennington 1991].) Current proposals include those associated with self-regulation (Douglas 1988), response delay or response inhibition (Barkley 1997; Schachar et al. 1993; Sonuga-Barke et al. 1992), and executive control (Pennington 1991; Schachar and Logan 1990). At present, however, the psychiatric diagnostic system (i.e., DSM-III-R, DSM-IV) provides for a diagnosis of ADHD only on the basis of *behavioral* manifestations of inattention, impulsiveness, and hyperactivity within the individual (American Psychiatric Association 1987, 1994). These behavioral symptoms, which can occur in various combinations across school, home, and social settings, are first evident in early childhood (i.e., prior to age 7 years); they are persistent and unexpected (i.e., they cannot be explained by developmental or mental level or by other disorders, such as psychosis or affective disorders); and they cause significant impairment in social, academic, and occupational functioning (American Psychiatric Association 1994). DSM-IV distinguishes three subtypes: one defined exclusively by inattention (i.e., predominantly inattentive), a second defined by hyperactivity-impulsiveness (i.e., predominantly hyperactive-impulsive), and a third (i.e., combined type) defined by the presence of both inattention and hyperactivity-impulsiveness. It may be that the predominantly inattentive and predominantly hyperactive-impulsive subtypes can be mapped onto earlier concepts of cognitive and behavioral subtypes, respectively (August and Garfinkel 1989; Halperin et al. 1990; Healy et al. 1993). For recent reviews and discussion of the conceptualization of ADHD, see those by Brown (Chapter 1, this volume), Barkley (1997), Sergeant (1995), and B. A. Shaywitz et al. (1994).

Learning disorders. The category of learning disorder is applied to children who exhibit an unexpected failure to develop specific skills or abilities by the appropriate age despite an apparent normal capacity for learning. This term does not apply to children who have learning problems that are primarily the result of sensory impairments, neurological disease, severe emotional problems, environmental disadvantage/deprivation (including inadequate educational opportunities), or low intellectual ability. Consequently, not all children who perform poorly in school or exhibit difficulties learning can be considered to have a learning disorder.

In the United States, the term *learning disabilities* refers to a federal law disability category that is used to determine eligibility for special education services that must be provided by all public schools. Public Law 94-142, the Education for All Handicapped Children Act (1975), indicates that a designation of "specific learning disability" should be applied only to those children with a severe discrepancy between their potential for learning (as assessed by intelligence tests) and their actual academic achievement and who do not meet the specified exclusionary criteria:

> The term specific learning disability means *a disorder in one or more of the basic psychological processes involved in understanding or in using language, spoken or written,* which may manifest itself in an imperfect ability to listen, think, speak, read, write, spell, or do mathematical calculations. Such term includes such conditions as perceptual disabilities, brain injury, minimal brain dysfunction, dyslexia, and developmental aphasia. Such term does not include a learning problem that is primarily the result of visual, hearing, or motor disabilities, of mental retardation, of emotional disturbance, or of environmental, cultural, or economic disadvantage. (Individuals With Disabilities Education Act, June 4, 1997, §602.26a; emphasis added)

Note that this legal/educational definition of learning disabilities imputes cognitive or central nervous system deficits. This concept is best illustrated by dyslexia, or reading disorder, in which the core deficit, involving a specific component of the language system (i.e., phonological processing), is manifested by difficulties in single-word decoding (e.g., Brady and Shankweiler 1991; Goswami and Bryant 1990). However, evidence that poor readers who do not meet the discrepancy criteria also exhibit the core deficit in phonological processing challenges the requirement for evidence of a severe discrepancy between a child's intelligence and his or her actual reading achievement (Fletcher et al. 1994, 1998; S. E. Shaywitz et al. 1992; Stanovich and Siegel 1994).

In contrast, the medical/psychiatric definition considers that underlying abnormalities in cognitive processing are a possible, but not invariable, feature of learning disorders (American Psychiatric Association 1987, 1994). (What had been termed "academic skills disorders" and "language and speech disorders" in DSM-III-R are now referred to as "learning disorders" and "communication disorders," respectively, in DSM-IV. Also, it should be noted that learning disorders and communication disorders are now listed on Axis I [i.e., clinical disorders], along with ADHD, rather than on Axis II as in DSM-III-R.) Rather, the medical/psychiatric definition of learning disorders requires evidence that the disturbance in the specific skill produces *significant* impairment in academic achievement or in activities of daily living that require that skill and that the disturbance is not due primarily to other specified disorders (e.g., physical or neurological disorders, pervasive developmental disorders, mental retardation) or inadequate educational opportunities. (The term *disabilities* typically emphasizes the handicap/education aspect, whereas *disorder* implies a specific pathology/etiology. Ironically, the reverse appears to be the case for educational vs. medical definitions of learning disabilities.) This definition also requires evidence of a significant discrepancy between the individual's observed and potential level of achievement.

Finally, it should be noted that the medical/psychiatric category of learning disorders (based on the classification in DSM-IV) might appear to be more restricted than the legal/educational one because it includes only disorders of reading, mathematics, and written expression. However, disorders of language are listed under a separate category, communication disorders, which includes expressive language disorder, mixed receptive-expressive language disorder, phonological disorder, stuttering, and communication disorder not otherwise specified. Moreover, DSM-IV also identifies a motor skills disorder (developmental coordination disorder) that is not included in the legal/educational category of learning disorders even though the resultant motor difficulties interfere with school performance (e.g., poor handwriting, poor performance in sports). These disorders, which are usually first diagnosed in childhood or adolescence, are coded on Axis I in DSM-IV (a change from DSM-III-R, in which these disorders were coded on Axis II).

Empirical Distinctions

Substantial evidence from epidemiological, cognitive, neurobiological, and genetic linkage studies suggests that ADHD and learning disorders, particularly reading disabilities, are not alternative names for the same set of problems. ADHD and learning disorders exist independently of each other in the majority of cases, as demonstrated by epidemiological and clinical studies (for reviews, see DuPaul and Stoner 1994; Semrud-Clikeman et al. 1992). For example, when stringent criteria are used to define learning disorder, the overlap between ADHD and learning disorders is less than 20% (Frick et al. 1991; Semrud-Clikeman et al. 1992).

The two conditions are generally distinct in terms of their neuropsychological dysfunction and neurobiological basis. For example, there is growing evidence suggesting that deficits in central executive control functions, particularly in the ability to inhibit or delay a response, characterize ADHD but not reading disorder (e.g., Oosterlaan et al. 1998; Pennington and Ozonoff 1996; Schachar and Logan 1990). Nor are these deficits attributable to comorbid reading disorder or another learning disorder (Nigg et al. 1998; Seidman et al. 1997). Moreover, quantitative magnetic resonance imaging studies of ADHD indicate structural anomalies in the brain circuits associated with executive functions. Specifically, the reported anomalies include a smaller right prefrontal cortex, caudate (with loss of or reversal of the normal asymmetry), globus pallidus, and corpus callosum (for review, see Tannock 1998). A smaller splenial area of the corpus callosum may be specific to ADHD: it has not been observed in normally functioning control subjects or individuals with reading disorder or autism (Hynd et al. 1991c; J. P. Larsen et al. 1992; Filipek et al. 1992; Semrud-Clikeman et al. 1994). This anatomic variation in the corpus callosum is particularly interesting, given the role of this large-fiber tract in high-level functions, including the dynamic allocation of attention in response to task demands (Hoptman and Davidson 1994; Kennedy et al. 1991).

In contrast, neuropsychological studies indicate that phonological processing deficits are characteristic of reading disorder (for reviews, see Adams 1990; Goswami and Bryant 1990; Pennington 1991; Wagner and Torgesen 1987) but not ADHD (Dykman and Ackerman 1991; Pennington et al. 1993; B. A. Shaywitz and Shaywitz 1994; Siegel and Ryan 1988). Neuroimaging studies indicate a lack of the expected asymmetry (left > right) in the planum temporale and temporal lobe anomalies in children with language and learning disorders (Galaburda et al. 1985; Hynd et al. 1990, 1991b), although the findings are inconsistent (Filipek 1995). Also, one study reported that the reversed frontal area asymmetry (i.e., left > right) observed in children with reading disorder was related to poor reading of nonwords—the most reliable indicator of phonological processing deficits (Semrud-Clikeman et al. 1991).

Further evidence of the distinctions between ADHD and reading disorder is provided by twin studies and family genetic studies that consistently find evidence for a genetic etiology in ADHD and some forms of learning disorders (particularly reading disorder and spelling disorders). Moreover, these studies indicate that the ADHD and reading disorder are likely to be genetically independent, although the possibility of a small etiological subtype of combined ADHD and reading disorder has not been ruled out (Biederman et al. 1986, 1992; Faraone et al. 1993; Gilger et al. 1992; Gillis et al. 1992; Goodman and Stevenson 1989). Furthermore, preliminary findings from molecular genetic studies implicated genes within the dopaminergic system in the etiology of ADHD (e.g., LaHoste et al. 1996) and linked phonological deficits and word identification deficits with chromosomes 6 and 15, respectively (see, e.g., Grigorenko et al. 1997).

On the other hand, ADHD and reading disorder may share some common characteristics. For example, recent evidence suggests that deficits in speed of information processing, naming speed, motor skills, and time perception may be associated with both disorders (Barkley 1997; Barkley et al. 1997; Carte et al. 1996; Martinussen et al. 1998; Nicolson and Fawcett 1994; Nicolson et al. 1995; Nigg et al. 1998). Moreover, both disorders have been linked with subtle neuroanatomic anomalies in the cerebellum, a structure that is thought to play a major role in representing temporal information and the precise timing of motor responses and is part of a distributed neural network for motor control (Akshoomoff and Courchesne 1992; Berquin et al. 1998; Castellanos et al. 1996; Ivry 1997; Ivry and Keele 1989; Levinson 1990).

In summary, ADHD and learning disorders (particularly reading disorder) represent two distinct clinical entities that may co-occur in the same individual but can be distinguished from each other. Currently, ADHD is defined solely in terms of behavioral manifestations. Deficits in psychological processes are not incorporated into the diagnostic criteria, although ADHD is widely believed to have a cognitive or neuropsychological basis. By contrast, learning disorder is defined in terms of measured deficits in one or more basic psychological processes. Behavioral symptoms should play no part in the diagnosis of a learning disorder.

COMORBIDITY OF ADDS AND LEARNING DISORDERS

In this section, we consider how various types of learning disorders that co-occur with ADHD might alter the meaning of ADHD in terms of its clinical presentation, correlates, and treatment response. Numerous classification schemes exist for categorizing learning disorders, including schemes based on the modality of the disturbance (e.g., auditory vs. visual, verbal vs. nonverbal) and the skill or domain affected (e.g., reading, expressive language, mathematics calculation). We have opted to follow the DSM-IV classification system (American Psychiatric Association 1994), which uses a domain-based approach. This approach is useful from a clinical perspective because children present with problems in "reading," "arithmetic," or "speech," rather than with "auditory/verbal" or "right-hemisphere nonverbal" problems. On the other hand, such an approach provides little guidance in understanding the underlying psychological deficits. Accordingly, after discussing the epidemiology of these comorbidities, we present an overview of the current understanding of psychological processes that are implicated in each type of learning disorder before reviewing the impact of each disorder on the meaning of ADHD in terms of correlates and treatment response.

For simplicity, the various learning disorders that co-occur with ADHD are described separately. It is essential to recognize, however, that it is possible that many of these disorders have a common etiology. Thus, individuals may exhibit a severe disorder in one domain (e.g., spelling), moderate impairment in another (e.g., reading), and isolated difficulties in yet another domain (e.g., mathematics). Alternatively, some disorders may have different etiologies, so a child may exhibit two distinct disorders or may have severe impairment in one domain (mathematics) but may show high levels of competency in another (e.g., reading).

Epidemiology

About 20%–25% of children with ADHD are likely to present with specific learning disorders, with these estimates based on both epidemiological and clinical studies that use rigorous criteria to define ADHD and learning disorders (e.g., Semrud-Clikeman et al. 1992). Conversely, studies of nonreferred children with learning disorders indicate that about 17% of these children meet the criteria for a diagnosis of ADHD (S. E. Shaywitz et al. 1992).

The observed association between ADHD and learning disorders occurs at rates higher than would be expected by chance alone, given the base rates of each disorder in the community. Thus, the comorbidity of ADHD with one or more learning disorders is not simply a result of detection artifacts. For example, estimates of the prevalence of learning disorders based on epidemiological studies range from 2% to 10%, depending on the specific disorder, the definitions applied, and the method of ascertainment (e.g., Lewis et al. 1994; S. E. Shaywitz et al. 1990). Prevalence figures for ADHD range from 6% to 10% (Anderson et al. 1987; Bird et al. 1988; Offord et al. 1987). The association of ADHD and learning disorders expected by chance alone would range from 0.5% to 1% (product of the probability levels for each disorder alone), rates that are substantially lower than the observed association of 10%–25%. This high rate of overlap between ADHD and learning disorder, particularly among children referred to clinics, indicates the need for clinicians to routinely assess the psychoeducational functioning of children with ADHD. It also indicates, conversely, the need to assess for ADHD in children with learning disorders.

General Clinical Description

It is commonly assumed that learning disorders are manifested by frequent reversals of letters or numbers. Although this may hold true for some individuals with learning disorders, it does not for many others. Given the considerable diversity in this population, learning disorders may be manifested in many ways, some of which are readily observable in a clinic. For example, some children with comorbid ADHD and learning disorders appear "spacey" and fidgety rather than "driven" and overactive. They exhibit great difficulty following the conversation, particularly when there are more than two people involved and the conversation passes rapidly from one to another, with frequent use of puns, idioms, and metaphors. When talking, children with both ADHD and learning disorder use many nonspecific terms (e.g., "It did that . . .," "The thing he put there"), have difficulty finding the right word (e.g., "Um . . . the uh . . . the thing what you bang them with . . . uh . . . a hammer), mispronounce words (e.g., "aminals" instead of "animals"), and fail to use specific temporal or causal markers (e.g., words like first, next, finally, because). As a result, it is often very difficult to understand what the child is trying to say, and it is perhaps not surprising that many children with learning disorders tend to give up quickly and stop the conversation (e.g., "Oh forget it," "It doesn't matter," "I don't know").

In striking contrast to children with ADHD who do not have learning disorders, those with comorbid learning disorders frequently look puzzled and at a loss as to how to proceed when given instructions. Their response is often characterized by inaction and hesitation rather than by acting before thinking. They seem not to "get it," and upon inquiry they are often unable to repeat the instructions just given to them, may provide only part of the instructions, or may have completely misunderstood. Many are, surprisingly, unaware of basic routine information (days, months, the current date, numbers). For example, youngsters with comorbid ADHD and learning disorders, like children with learning disorders only, may be unable to list the alphabet or the months of the year in correct sequence or may have to start from the beginning of the sequence each time to know, for example, which letter follows "n" or which month comes after August. Some children with comorbid ADHD and learning disorders exhibit marked slowness with copying from a book or from the blackboard (e.g., they misalign numbers or decimal points, omit words, or copy incorrectly); their handwriting is messy, illegible, and poorly spaced, with many words misspelled. Most will exhibit great reluctance when asked to express their ideas in writing and produce only one or two sentences, with little elaboration of ideas but numerous mistakes in capitalization, punctuation, or grammar. Thus, the performance of children with comorbid ADHD and learning disorder tends to be slow and inaccurate rather than fast and inaccurate.

Motor problems and interpersonal and social difficulties are common among children with comorbid ADHD and learning disorders, and it is often these subtle personal/social features, observable when the youngsters enter the waiting room or office, that mark them as "different," well before more formal inquiry. For example, school-age youngsters may frequently collide with furniture in the office or clinic and knock over objects. They may be unable to rebutton clothing or close zippers after trips to the bathroom, and they may use crayons and pencils in an awkward manner. Adolescents may dress in a manner that is "odd" and sets them apart from their peers (e.g., wear shirts tucked in, pants pulled up high, and jacket hood up—a style that would be out of keeping with the current fashion). Many youngsters with comorbid ADHD and learning disorders fail to make eye contact during conversation and do not respond to conventional nonverbal social cues for opening or closing conversation (e.g., body stance, gesture, facial expression, looking at watch or at another person). Jokes, puns, or other forms of humor may pass without any response.

Although the general clinical presentation in ADHD with and without learning disorder varies, there is no consistent evidence of systematic differences in ADHD symptoms per se between the two groups (e.g., Pennington et al. 1993; Robins 1992). Thus, clinicians should not expect the ADHD profile to assist them in determining whether ADHD is primary or secondary.

Specific Comorbidities With Learning Disorders

ADHD With Reading Disorder

Reading disorder. Frequently called "dyslexia" or "specific reading disability," the category of reading disorder is applied to children who fail to learn to read despite intact sensory and intellectual abilities. Reading skills are complex, with several component dimensions contributing to word identification, reading fluency, and text comprehension. The most reliable indicator of reading disorder is failure to develop rapid, context-free word identification skills (Lovett 1992; Perfetti 1985; Stanovich 1986, 1994). Typically, the cause of this word identification failure is an underlying deficit in specific language-based skills, called *phonological processing* (for reviews, see Adams 1990; Brady and Shankweiler 1991; Vandervelden and Siegel 1996; Wagner et al. 1994; Wolf 1991). More recent models also implicate deficits in rapid automatized naming in the failure to develop efficient word identification skills (Bowers 1995; Meyer et al. 1998; Wolf 1991).

Phonological processing involves auditory skills that permit the recognition, differentiation, and manipulations of single speech sounds in words (termed *phonemes*), which in turn afford the ability to process oral and written language (Adams 1990; Wagner and Torgesen 1987; Wagner et al. 1994). It is a multidimensional construct that may include several latent abilities: 1) retrieval of phonological codes or pronunciations associated with letters, word segments, and whole words from a long-term store; 2) phonological analysis and synthesis, which refers to the ability to segment whole words into constituent units (e.g., phonemes) and to blend isolated phonemes to form whole words, respectively; and 3) phonological coding of information in working memory for short-term storage during ongoing processing (for in-depth reviews, see Adams 1990; Wagner and Torgesen 1987; Wagner et al. 1994; Wolf 1991). Deficits in these abilities makes the learning of letter-sound (grapheme-to-phoneme) correspondences very difficult because the child has no basis for segmenting orthographic (spelling) patterns corresponding to the sound units and either extracting rules for their synthesis or using them to decode by analogy (Lovett 1992).

Rapid naming, which demands the fast oral production of names of visual stimuli (letters, digits, colors, objects), is thought to be distinct from phonological processing and influences the development of word identification skills and, possibly, reading comprehension (Bowers 1995; Meyer et al. 1998; Wolf 1991). Deficiencies in naming speed may reflect inadequacies in a precise timing mechanism necessary to the development of orthographic codes and to their integration with phonological codes (Bowers and Wolf 1993). Children with deficits in both phonological awareness and visual naming speed (double-deficit) have been found to have more impairment and to be less responsive to treatment than individuals with phonological deficits only (Wolf 1991).

The effects of phonological processing deficits will have an impact throughout the language system and will likely affect other phonologically based linguistic processes, such as spelling, writing, word naming and retrieval, verbal memory, speech perception and production, and listening (B. A. Shaywitz et al. 1994). Typically, although not invariably, reading disorder is accompanied by deficits in speech and language development. Children (and adults) with reading disorder frequently present with a history of producing short and syntactically simple sentences, inaccurate pronunciation, and deficiencies in receptive vocabulary and object naming (see, e.g., Scarborough 1990). Also, they frequently experience an even greater difficulty with spelling, which remains a lifelong handicap even when the reading disability has improved (DeFries et al. 1991; Stevenson et al. 1993). Many also exhibit deficits in arithmetic fact retrieval, and this suggests a common underlying cognitive/neuropsychological deficit (for review, see Geary 1993). Moreover, longitudinal studies indicate not only that reading disorder has a chronic course but also that the individual differences in phonological processing abilities are remarkably stable (Bruck 1992; Byrne et al. 1992; Wagner et al. 1994).

These language-based reading problems are heritable and have been linked to chromosomes 6 and 15, although the mode of transmission is unclear (Cardon et al. 1994; DeFries and Gillis 1991; DeFries et al. 1987; Grigorenko et al. 1997; Pennington 1995; Pennington et al. 1991; Smith et al. 1990, 1994). Intriguingly, two distinct reading-related phenotypes—phonological coding and single-word reading—were found to be linked to two different chromosomal regions, although the findings have not yet been replicated (Grigorenko et al. 1997). However, in contrast to widespread beliefs, dyslexia does not appear to be a discrete entity (i.e., a specific syndrome), nor does it necessarily affect primarily boys (Flynn and Rahbar 1994; S. E. Shaywitz et al. 1990, 1992). For example, recent studies indicate that dyslexia most likely represents the lower tail of a normal distribution of reading abilities (Shaywitz et al. 1992). In other words, reading disorder is not a categorical (all-or-none) entity, but occurs, as does hypertension, in degrees along a continuum. Accordingly, there is no reason to expect qualitative differences (other than can be explained by IQ) between poor readers with and without a discrepancy between ability and achievement. This supposition has been confirmed empirically: both low-achieving poor readers and low-achieving readers who meet an ability-discrepancy criterion share the fundamental deficit in phonological processing (Fletcher et al. 1994, 1998; S. E. Shaywitz et al. 1992; Stanovich and Siegel 1994).

The belief that reading disorder primarily affects boys has been challenged by findings from an epidemiological study in which reading disorder was found to affect boys and girls equally (S. E. Shaywitz et al. 1990). The investigators in this study proposed that previous reports of differential gender ratios reflect a bias in sample selection: namely, a reliance on school-identified, as opposed to research-identified, samples. The overrepresentation of boys in school-identified samples may reflect teachers' mistaken tendencies to label boys as having reading disorder on the basis of behavioral problems (which are more common in boys) regardless of their reading ability. On the other hand, a subsequent epidemiological study of British schoolchildren (Lewis et al. 1994) suggested an alternative account of gender differences in reading disorder. The investigators in the British study reported an equal number of males and females among children with both reading and arithmetic disabilities but a preponderance of males among a group with reading disabilities only. (The co-occurrence of reading and arithmetic disabilities was not reported in the earlier study [S. E. Shaywitz et al. 1990].)

Overlap of reading disorder with ADHD. Epidemiological and clinical studies suggest a comorbidity rate of 15%–30% when relatively stringent criteria are used for defining the disorders (e.g., S. E. Shaywitz et al. 1992; Semrud-Clikeman et al. 1992). There is no consistent evidence to date that the presence of comorbid reading disorder systematically alters the behavioral profile of ADHD (e.g., Halperin et al. 1984; Pennington et al. 1993), although reading disorder may be more commonly associated with attention deficit disorder without hyperactivity (e.g., Barkley et al. 1990a; Hynd et al. 1991a). (The diagnostic category of attention deficit disorder without hyperactivity, included in DSM-III (American Psychiatric Association 1980), is currently believed to correspond to the predominantly inattentive subtype of ADHD in DSM-IV (American Psychiatric Association 1994). However, it is important to keep in mind that the DSM-III criteria required evidence of impulsivity, whereas the DSM-IV criteria do not.) Similarly, several studies based on DSM-IV criteria reported that academic problems and learning disabilities (particularly in arithmetic) are more common among children with the predominantly inattentive and combined subtypes of ADHD, suggesting that these problems are related to inattention rather than hyperactivity/impulsivity (Baumgaertel et al. 1995; Faraone et al. 1998; Gaub and Carlson 1997; Lahey et al. 1994; Marshall et al. 1997).

There is growing evidence that comorbid reading disorder adds to both the cognitive processing problems and the social problems associated with ADHD, although the nature of the impact of reading disorder in this context is not entirely clear. For example, most cognitive studies of ADHD, reading disorder, and comorbid ADHD and reading disorder (or subsets of this design) indicate that children with comorbid ADHD and reading disorder exhibit the deficits associated with reading disorder (i.e., deficits in phonological processing, naming speed, verbal memory deficits) and those associated with ADHD (i.e., deficits in sustained attention, response inhibition, and other executive functions) (e.g., Douglas and Benezra 1990; Felton and Wood 1989; Korkman and Pesonen 1994; Martinussen et al. 1998; Nigg et al. 1998; Narhi and Ahonen 1995).

On the other hand, some studies suggest that the comorbid group may exhibit some unique impairments that are not observed in the "pure" groups. For example, Korkman and Pesonen (1994) found that the group with comorbid ADHD and learning disorders had more pervasive attention problems and more visuomotor problems than the children with ADHD or learning disorders only. Likewise, Flicek's (1992) study of social behavior problems associated with learning disorders and ADHD revealed that only boys with comorbid ADHD and learning disorders were rejected by peers and associated with starting fights. The problems of the group of boys with comorbid ADHD and learning disorders in terms of popularity, leadership, and cooperation represented the contribution of learning disorders, and their high ratings for oppositional-defiant and disruptive behavior represented the contribution of ADHD (Flicek 1992). These findings are consistent with the hypothesis that comorbid ADHD and reading disorder represents an etiological subtype. According to this hypothesis, a third factor causes both disorders in an etiological subtype, but the two disorders are otherwise etiologically distinct (for discussion, see Pennington et al. 1993).

In contrast, a few studies indicate that the group with comorbid disorders exhibit the cognitive deficits of reading disorder but not of ADHD. For example, Pennington et al. (1993) conducted a study of two contrasting cognitive domains (phonological processing and executive functions) in four groups of children (those with reading disorder, ADHD, and comorbid ADHD and reading disorder and control subjects). The ADHD group was shown to have a significant impairment in executive function (compared with the control subjects and the group with reading disorder) but no impairment in phonological processing, whereas the group with reading disorder showed an impairment in phonological processing (compared with the control subjects and the group with ADHD) but not in executive function. This double dissociation between the group with ADHD only and the group with reading disorder only implies that ADHD and reading disorder represent two distinct clinical syndromes with separate underlying cognitive processes. The second major set of findings was that the group with comorbid ADHD and reading disorder resembled the group with reading disorder only on both cognitive domains (i.e., they exhibited an impairment in phonological processing but not in executive functions) and differed significantly from the group with ADHD only on both domains. These findings suggest that at least for some children with comorbid ADHD and reading disorder, the reading disorder may be the primary problem, leading to the behavioral symptoms of ADHD.

This pattern of findings has been interpreted as supportive of a "phenocopy hypothesis," which postulates that one disorder (in this case, reading disorder) leads to secondary symptoms but not the full syndrome of the second disorder (i.e., ADHD) (Pennington et al. 1993). Additional support for this phenocopy hypothesis is provided by a study of motor decision/response organization that used a response compatibility/incompatibility paradigm in a four-group design (Hall et al. 1997). Although both the ADHD and comorbid ADHD and reading disorder groups did not differ in accuracy of performance on the compatibility/incompatibility conditions (and both were less accurate than the reading disorder only group and the control group), they differed in speed of performance. The subjects in the ADHD group were slower in generating an incompatible response, a finding suggestive of impairments in motor-decision processes, whereas those in the group with comorbid ADHD and reading disorder were slower in generating a compatible response, a finding suggestive of difficulties in the basis timing of responses. However, other studies have failed to support the phenocopy hypothesis (e.g., Narhi and Ahonen 1995; Purvis 1999; Reader et al. 1994; Weyandt and Willis 1994).

To summarize, recent investigations of the causal basis of the development of the comorbidity between ADHD and reading disorder are consistent with two hypotheses: 1) reading disorder may lead to a phenocopy of ADHD (i.e., ADHD is secondary to reading disorder), and 2) comorbid ADHD and reading disorder is an etiological subtype. Underlying mechanisms for the comorbidity between ADHD and reading disorder have important implications for the treatment of this comorbid condition, particularly since the treatment approaches for ADHD and reading disorder are very different.

ADHD With Mathematics Disorder

Mathematics disorder. Learning disorders in the area of mathematics are relatively common: prevalence estimates range from 4% to 6% of children in elementary school and junior high school (Badian 1983; Baker and Cantwell 1985; Garnett and Fleischner 1987; Kosc 1974; Lewis et al. 1994; Share et al. 1988). Yet, despite their prevalence and overlap with reading disorder and disabilities (Ackerman and Dykman 1995; Badian 1983; Lewis et al. 1994; Richman 1983; Siegel and Ryan 1988), relatively little is known about mathematical learning disorders. Moreover, in contrast to research on children's reading, very little is known about the relations between early mathematical abilities (e.g., counting, understanding mathematical relations) and later success in mathematics (for insightful reviews, see Bryant 1995; Sokol et al. 1994).

Three types of cognitive deficits that might underlie mathematics disorder have been proposed: procedural aspects of computation, automatic retrieval of number facts from semantic memory, and visuospatial skills (for review, see Geary 1993). Also, problems with basic math concepts (number sense) and cognitive variables are likely to contribute to mathematics disorder (Geary 1993; McCall 1999).

Computational problems are manifested by the use of developmentally immature arithmetical procedures (e.g., counting on fingers), a high frequency of procedural errors, and low accuracy (Geary and Brown 1991). These difficulties tend to disappear by the end of second grade and may reflect a developmental delay in the acquisition of the underlying concepts (Geary et al. 1992).

Number fact problems are manifested by difficulties in acquiring and maintaining basic math facts at a level of automaticity that is adequate for the acquisition and use of higher math skills (Geary 1990; McCall 1999). Number facts, which are the most basic set of data in arithmetic, may be conceptualized as similar to a basic sight vocabulary in reading. They reflect isolated bits of information that can be used to complete a whole problem and are more useful if they can be recalled rapidly to allow greater attention to be given to higher-level processing. Accuracy and fluency in basic number facts are fundamental to proficiency in mathematics (Fleischner and Manheimer 1997). Children with this type of deficit retrieve fewer facts from memory, and when retrieval does occur, their retrieval speeds are slower and unsystematic and they exhibit a high error rate. These fact-retrieval deficits typically persist throughout the elementary school years and frequently co-occur with certain forms of language and reading verbal deficits, such as poor phonological awareness (Siegel and Linder 1984; Siegel and Ryan 1989). Recent epidemiological work suggests that approximately 2% of 9- to 10-year-old children exhibit both arithmetic and reading disabilities, with equal representation of boys and girls (Lewis et al. 1994). The overlap of mathematics disorder with reading disorder suggests a common underlying neuropsychological deficit in language-related processes, perhaps involving the posterior regions of the left hemisphere (Geary 1993).

Visuospatial deficits involve problems in the spatial representation and interpretation of numerical information, such as the misalignment of numbers in multicolumn arithmetic problems and the misinterpretation of place value (Rourke and Finlayson 1978; Share et al. 1988). Approximately 1% of school-age children, with an equal number of boys and girls, exhibit this type of deficit (Lewis et al. 1994). In contrast to the deficit associated with the semantic memory subtype, this deficit does not seem to be associated with phonetically based reading deficits. Rather, it is associated with visuospatial difficulties (Pennington 1991; Rourke and Finlayson 1978; Siegel and Linder 1984) and may be associated with right-hemisphere dysfunction, particularly in the posterior regions (Dahmen et al. 1982).

Basic math concepts, or number sense, include understanding of symbols, counting, decomposing and recombining numbers (e.g., 67 = 6 tens + 7 ones = 5 tens + 17 ones), place value, properties associated with each operation (e.g., commutative property of addition [a + b = b + a]), and estimation (Greeno 1991). Children with mathematics disorder exhibit a shakier foundation in basic math concepts (McCall 1999; Russell and Ginsberg 1984). Since these basic concepts tend to build on each other, children with mathematics disorder fall behind their peers at the earliest stage of number sense and then must struggle to catch up and/or continue to build on a shaky foundation.

Finally, it is possible that some children make arithmetical errors because of more general cognitive deficits rather than a specific mathematical deficit (Badian 1983). Associated deficits include those in working memory, short-term memory, long-term memory, processing speed, attentional allocation, and sequencing skills, as well as those in visuospatial skills mentioned previously (Geary 1993; Swanson 1993). These general deficits are not considered a deficit of a specific component skill in mathematics per se (Geary 1993).

Overlap of mathematics disorder with ADHD. Children with ADHD are particularly vulnerable to math difficulties as well as specific mathematical disabilities (Zentall et al. 1994). The overlap between ADHD and mathematics disorder is substantial, with estimates ranging from 10% to 60% (Barkley 1990; Frick et al. 1991; Semrud-Clikeman et al. 1992). It should be noted, however, that the estimates available were all derived from referred samples rather than epidemiological samples and may therefore be subject to inflation from biases of ascertainment (Berkson 1946). Also, the widely variable overlap depends in part on the stringency of the methods used to assess mathematics disorder (Barkley 1990; Semrud-Clikeman et al. 1992).

Comorbid mathematics disorder occurs more frequently in children with DSM-III attention deficit disorder without hyperactivity and those with DSM-IV predominantly inattentive and combined subtypes of ADHD, suggesting that mathematics disorder is more closely related to inattention than to hyperactivity/impulsivity (e.g., Hynd et al. 1991a; Faraone et al. 1998; Marshall et al. 1997).

The few investigations into the precise nature of the arithmetic problems associated with ADHD have identified two types of math difficulties: semantic memory and procedural disabilities. For example, ADHD children (with and without learning disorder) exhibit slower fact retrieval times compared with control children (Ackerman et al. 1986a, 1986b; Zentall 1990) and continue to use immature counting strategies through sixth grade (Ackerman et al. 1986a; Benedetto and Tannock 1999). In contrast, children with normally developing mathematical skills typically switch from a physical or mental counting strategy to a memory retrieval strategy by the fourth grade (Ashcraft and Fierman 1982). For example, children with ADHD were found to use finger-counting strategies more frequently than their peers, who were matched for both age and math achievement (Benedetto and Tannock 1999). These findings suggest that memory-retrieval problems may underlie both reading disorder (retrieval of phonological codes) and mathematics disorder (retrieval of basic math facts) in children with ADHD and account for the high rates of overlap of both types of learning disorder with ADHD.

In the elementary school–age years, children with ADHD also exhibit procedural deficits, particularly in subtraction that involves regrouping (Benedetto and Tannock 1999; S. Hoosen-Shakeel A. Ishak, A. Ickowicz, et al., submitted). However, one of the most salient problems is in productivity: children with ADHD complete fewer computation problems and make more errors than their normally functioning peers. Thus, it is not uncommon for their Academic Efficiency Scores to be one-third lower than those of their peers, even in the absence of comorbid mathematics disorder or general learning disorder (Benedetto and Tannock 1999; DuPaul and Rapport 1993; DuPaul et al. 1991). The Academic Efficiency Score reflects the number of problems completed correctly expressed as a proportion of the total number of problems to be completed (DuPaul et al. 1991).

Math vulnerability in ADHD may be attributable to a failure in automatization, which in turn results from a deficit in memory and in processing speed

(Ackerman et al. 1986a). Slow speed of retrieval impairs the acquisition and maintenance of number facts, and this impairment results in slow and inaccurate computation and subsequent impairment in the acquisition and use of more advanced mathematical procedures (Ackerman et al. 1986; Geary 1993). Alternatively, or in addition, the children's poor automaticity may be attributable to their tendency to avoid repetitive drills and limited attention skills (Marshall et al. 1997).

ADHD With Disorder of Written Expression

Disorder of written expression. Broadly defined in DSM-IV as "writing skills . . . that fall substantially below those expected given the individual's chronological age, measured intelligence, and age-appropriate education" (American Psychiatric Association 1994, p. 51), disorder of written expression is characterized by significant impairment in writing grammatically correct sentences and organized paragraphs.

Often the most striking evidence of disorder of written expression appears when an individual is articulate in expressing thoughts orally in conversation and yet manifests severe difficulties in expressing those same thoughts in written form. Such a student might work very slowly and laboriously to compose a few sentences or paragraphs, often complaining of an inability to think of any words to write; yet moments later in conversation, the same student may be able orally to address the same questions or topic articulately with much elaboration. Some individuals are severely constricted and chronically impaired in their ability to give written expression to thoughts and feelings that they can express quite fluently in oral speech.

Kellogg (1994) described the process of writing as including 1) collecting and retrieving relevant information; 2) planning and organizing specific ideas to communicate; 3) translating ideas into written words, sentences, and paragraphs of text; and 4) reviewing text to edit and integrate the product for communication to the reader. Presumably, disorder of written expression may derive from serious impairments in any or all of these component processes. Currently, little is known about the cognitive components, prevalence, long-term prognosis, or remediation of disorder of written expression; this is an area in which further research is urgently needed.

It is important that disorder of written expression not be confused with dysgraphia, which refers simply to extremely poor handwriting. According to DSM-IV, disorder of written expression may be accompanied by multiple spelling errors and excessively poor (i.e., illegible) handwriting. Yet DSM-IV notes that this diagnosis is not to be given if there are only spelling errors or poor handwriting in the absence of another problem in written expression. Spelling problems alone might indicate a reading disorder; extremely poor handwriting might be classified as a developmental coordination disorder (if the problem is attributable to motor incoordination).

Dysgraphia has been described by Deuel (1992, 1995) as having three distinguishable types, depending on the basis of the underlying problem: dyslexic dysgraphia, dysgraphia due to motor clumsiness, and dysgraphia due to problems in spatial discernment. *Dyslexic dysgraphia* is typically associated with language impairments and reading disorder and is characterized by poor written spelling (as poor as oral spelling), low productivity, and labored motoric output during spontaneous writing but not during drawing or copying of written text, both of which are relatively unimpaired. Shorter and simpler words are often written more neatly and evenly than long or unfamiliar words. By contrast, in individuals with *dysgraphia due to motor clumsiness,* copying of written text shows poor legibility and drawing is likely to be compromised, but reading and oral and written spelling are preserved. Also, this subtype may be distinguished from the other two types of dysgraphia by associated problems in fine-motor speed (finger tapping). The third type, *dysgraphia due to abnormal spatial perception,* is characterized by severe problems in drawing as well as poor legibility of copied written text. On the other hand, reading, oral and written spelling, and fine-motor speed (finger tapping) are all relatively preserved. Note that all three subtypes are associated with poor legibility of spontaneously written text; problems are evident in the spacing of writing on the total page; the spacing of sentences, words, and letters; the slant of the written text; and the formation of letters.

Overlap of disorder of written expression with ADHD. Since disorder of written expression is not yet widely recognized and differentiated, it is difficult to assess its overlap with ADHD. Those few studies that are relevant tend to lump impairments in written expression together with dysgraphia and poor spelling. Many children with ADHD exhibit poor written spelling and handwriting that is untidy, uneven, and often illegible (see, e.g., Barkley 1990). However, few systematic studies of this comorbidity have been conducted, so it is unclear whether the problems are correlates of comorbid reading disorder rather than of ADHD per se.

In an investigation of reading and written language abilities in a large clinical sample of two subgroups of children with attention-deficit disorders (83 children with hyperactivity, 32 without hyperactivity), Elbert (1993) found that both groups displayed significant underachievement in reading, written spelling, written sentence construction, and writing fluency. Also, both groups exhibited poorer performance on written spelling/language measures relative to performance on reading measures, but the difference was more prominent in the subgroup with attention-deficit disorder without hyperactivity. However, the high rate of comorbidity with reading disorder suggests that the written spelling/language problems may be attributable primarily to the reading disorder and that they also may reflect dyslexic dysgraphia (Deuel 1995).

ADHD With Developmental Coordination Disorder (Motor Skills Disorder)

Developmental coordination disorder. The essential features of developmental coordination disorder are "clumsiness" and "poor motor coordination" that interfere with academic achievement or routine daily activities (e.g., tying shoelaces, doing up buttons or zippers, playing ball, handwriting) and are not attributable to a general medical condition (e.g., cerebral palsy, muscular dystrophy) or pervasive developmental disorder. However, recent evidence derived from process-oriented approaches suggests that this is not a singular syndrome (Cermak 1985; Denckla and Roeltgen 1992; Dewey and Kaplan 1994). For example, Dewey and Kaplan (1994) distinguished three subtypes of developmental motor deficits among children who have been labeled "clumsy": deficits in motor sequencing, deficits in motor execution (reflected by deficits in balance, coordination, and gestural performance), and deficits in all motor skill areas. Moreover, differences in performance among individuals in these subtypes on measures of academic, language, visuoperceptual, and visuomotor skills provide support for the external validity of the subtypes. Specifically, deficits in motor sequencing may be associated with problems in language comprehension (Dewey and Kaplan 1994).

Overlap of developmental coordination disorder with ADHD. Many children with ADHD have concomitant visuomotor problems (Nigg et al. 1998; Taylor et al. 1991), and many of those with clumsiness also have attention disorders and behavior problems (Losse et al. 1991; Szatmari and Taylor 1984). Moreover, more anomalies of motor development (in terms of speed, rhythmicity, and precision) are exhibited by children with ADHD with comorbid reading disorder than by children with reading disorder only, and this suggests that the motor deficits are more closely linked with ADHD than with reading disorder (Denckla et al. 1985).

A pattern of deficits in attention, motor control, and perception (DAMP) is common in middle childhood. Results of an epidemiological study indicate that 1.2% of 7-year olds had severe DAMP and another 3%–6% had mild-to-moderate DAMP (Gillberg et al. 1982). Follow-up studies of population-based groups of children with attention-deficit disorders, motor/perceptual deficits, the combination of attention-deficit disorders and motor/perceptual deficits, and a comparison group of normally developing children indicate that the longer-term outcome and prognosis are much worse for the group with motor/perceptual deficits and the group with both attention-deficit disorders and motor/perceptual deficits than for the group with attention-deficit disorders and the comparison group (e.g., Hellgren et al. 1993, 1994). Specifically, at age 16 years (i.e., 10 years after diagnosis), speech/language difficulties, clumsiness, accidents leading to fractures, and depressive disorders were all more common in the group with both attention-deficit disorders and motor/perceptual deficits than in the group with attention-deficit disorders and the comparison group. Also, complex reaction times were significantly longer in the group with both attention-deficit disorders and motor/perceptual deficits than in the other clinical and comparison groups (Hellgren et al. 1993, 1994). In general, the outcome for the group with motor/ perceptual deficits only was considerably worse than that for the group with attention-deficit disorders only.

These findings suggest that the poorer health and psychiatric outcome in the group with both attention-deficit disorders and motor/perceptual deficits may be attributable more to factors related to the motor-perceptual problems than to factors specifically associated with attention deficits per se. But, Hellgren and colleagues (1993, 1994) cautioned that the conclusions are tentative given the limited numbers in the group with attention-deficit disorders and the group with motor/perceptual deficits. Nonetheless, it is tempting to speculate that the higher rate of driving-related accidents and injuries found for adolescents with ADHD relative to non-ADHD peers (Barkley et al. 1993; Pless et al. 1995) may be attributable to a subgroup with persisting motor-perceptual deficits rather than attention deficits per se. For more information about developmental coordination disorder and its overlap with attention-deficit disorders, see Chapter 12, by Gillberg and Kadesjö, in this volume.

ADHD With Communication Disorders

Communication disorders. A diagnosis of a communication disorder (also known as a speech/language impairment) is made when there is a failure of normal development of speech and/or language that cannot be explained in terms of mental or physical handicap, hearing loss, emotional disorder, or environmental deprivation (Bishop 1992). Communication disorders may be manifested by a wide range of signs that can occur alone or in different combinations. Traditionally, two broad categories have been distinguished: speech disorders (i.e., problems in the motor production of the sounds of one's language) and language disorders (i.e., problems in the comprehension and/or production of the arbitrary system of symbols and rules used to convey meaning).

Speech disorders include problems in *articulation* (frequent and recurring mispronunciations of one or more speech sounds), *fluency* (frequent pauses, hesitations, restarts that interrupt normal rhythm of speech), *voice quality* (abnormal pitch, loudness, nasality, or hoarseness), and *rate of speech* (too slow or too rapid so that speech is rendered unintelligible).

Language disorders include problems in comprehending the meaning of words or sentence structures (*receptive* language disorder) and problems in retrieving words, pronouncing multisyllabic words, formulating sentences and ordering the words grammatically to convey a meaningful message, organizing ideas, and communicating ideas across various contexts (*expressive* language disorders). Mixed receptive and expressive language disorders are present in many cases. Also, there is a growing awareness of language-related problems that may not necessarily reflect deficits in the basic subsystems of language (i.e., phonology, syntax, semantics) but rather involve problems in the appropriate use of language within social, situational, and communicative contexts. These problems are known as *pragmatic disorders.* Pragmatic skills include both verbal and nonverbal communication, as well as the ability to adjust language for various audiences and for specific contexts (e.g., addressing the school principal vs. chatting to a peer).

DSM-IV uses a different classification of communication disorders:

- Phonological disorder, which was formerly called developmental articulation disorder in DSM-III-R, but now includes problems in production (articulation) and in linguistic categorization (phonological processing) of the sounds of one's language
- Expressive language disorder
- Mixed receptive-expressive language disorder, in recognition of the fact that receptive language problems rarely occur in isolation without accompanying expressive problems
- Stuttering, a disturbance in the normal fluency and time patterning of speech
- Communication disorder not otherwise specified, which subsumes voice disorders

Overlap of communication disorders with ADHD. A specific link between ADHD and speech and language impairments is suggested by several epidemiological and clinical studies of children with psychiatric disorders and children with language impairments (for reviews, see Baker and Cantwell 1992; Cantwell and Baker 1991; Prizant et al. 1990; Tannock and Schachar 1996). Estimates of the overlap varies from a low of 8% to a high of 90%, depending on the precise definitions of speech and language impairments, the nature of the communication problems, the source and type of sample, and the type of methods used to diagnose ADHD. The association between ADHD and speech and language impairments is greater than would be expected by chance alone, suggesting that the comorbidity is not an artifact of ascertainment bias. Of particular concern is that many children referred solely for disruptive behavior disorders have moderate to severe speech and language impairments that have not been recognized previously and are identified only on systematic assessment (N. Cohen et al. 1993; Oram et al. 1999; Tannock et al. 1995a; Warr-Leeper et al. 1994).

Given the high rates of language impairments in ADHD, surprisingly little is known about the precise nature of these impairments and how they might affect the children's everyday function. This is because few studies have examined language abilities in ADHD per se, and no study to date has examined a wide spectrum of language abilities in children with rigorously diagnosed disorders. Moreover, few of the existing studies have taken into account other comorbid disorders (e.g., learning disabilities, anxiety, conduct disorders) when describing language abilities in ADHD.

The limited available evidence suggests that speech disorders are less strongly related to ADHD than are language problems. When speech disorders are present, they typically coexist with language problems (e.g., Beitchman et al. 1989; Cantwell and Baker 1991). The onset of language (as assessed by the appearance of first words and short sentences) may be delayed in ADHD, although findings are inconsistent (Gross-Tsur et al. 1991; Hartsough and Lambert 1985; Ornoy et al. 1993; Szatmari et al. 1989). Also, problems in both receptive and expressive language abilities have been reported in children with ADHD, with expressive language being particularly impaired (Baker and Cantwell 1992; Beitchman et al. 1987; Oram et al. 1999). Children with ADHD are likely to exhibit word retrieval problems when asked to name pictures or to describe events that require highly specific vocabulary (Tannock et al. 1993, 1995a). These problems are manifested by the use of nonspecific words (e.g., stuff, that thing, they) and circumlocutions (e.g., "the thing you hit with"). Also, children with ADHD may have problems formulating precise sentences and more complex sentences (Oram et al. 1999). However, recent studies suggest that receptive and expressive impairments in the basic language systems (phonology, semantics, syntax) may be more closely linked with developmental reading disorder than with ADHD per se (Purvis and Tannock 1997; Tannock et al. 1994; Wood and Felton 1994). Longitudinal studies suggest that hyperactive preschool-age children with comorbid language impairments are at high risk for the development of comorbid learning disabilities, particularly reading disorders, which persist through adolescence (McGee et al. 1991; Ornoy et al. 1993).

In contrast, pragmatic deficits occur even in those with adequate phonological, morphological, syntactic, and semantic abilities (Humphries et al. 1994; Ludlow et al. 1978; Purvis and Tannock 1997). Moreover, although pragmatic dysfunction is also evident in children with learning disabilities (Lapadat 1991), it appears to be more strongly associated with ADHD. For example, Humphries et al. (1994) found that 60% of boys with attention problems exhibited pragmatic deficits, compared with 15% of boys with learning disabilities and 7% of normally developing children.

Pragmatic deficits evident in children with ADHD include the following:

1. Excessive verbal output during spontaneous conversations and task transitions and in play settings (Barkley et al. 1983; Zentall 1988)
2. Decreased verbal output and more dysfluencies when confronted with tasks that require planning and organization of verbal responses, as in storytelling or when giving directions (Hamlett et al. 1987; Tannock et al. 1993; Zentall 1988)
3. Difficulties in maintaining and changing topics appropriately and in negotiating smooth turn taking during conversation (Humphries et al. 1994; Zentall et al. 1983)
4. Problems in being specific, accurate, and concise in the selection and use of words to convey information in an unambiguous manner (Tannock et al. 1993)
5. Difficulties in adjusting language to the listener and to specific contexts (Landau and Milich 1988; Whalen et al. 1979; Zentall 1988)

ADHD With Central Auditory Processing Disorder

Central auditory processing disorder. The subtype of learning disorder referred to as central auditory processing disorder (CAPD) is not distinguished in DSM-IV: it is included here because of a relatively recent increase in interest in the overlap of this disorder with ADHD (see, e.g., Riccio et al. 1994).

Broadly defined by the American Speech-Language-Hearing Association (1992) as a deficit in processing audible signals that cannot be attributed to impaired peripheral hearing sensitivity or intellectual impairment, CAPD is manifested by severe problems in processing information presented in the auditory modality; visual information is processed normally. Children with CAPD are described as poor listeners, with short attention span to auditory information. They have problems following directions, particularly in settings that are noisy or have poor acoustics, and may misorder words and phrases. A history of severe or recurrent otitis media is common among these children. CAPD may also involve distractibility and inattentiveness as well as possible difficulties in memory, reading, spelling, and written language (American Speech-Language-Hearing Association 1992).

Testing for CAPD tends to be conducted by specially trained audiologists in sound-treated testing booths and with specialized equipment that affords precise control of the auditory stimuli. Measures used to evaluate CAPD may include dichotic tests (e.g., Staggered Spondaic Word Test; Katz 1962), tests of filtered speech (e.g., Low Pass Filtered Speech Test; Willeford 1977), and tests of pattern recognition (e.g., Pitch Pattern Sequence Test; Pinheiro 1977). Impaired performance on one or more of these audiometric measures can be considered evidence of CAPD (Katz and Wilde 1985).

Overlap of CAPD with ADHD. There is consistent evidence that children with ADHD have impairment on measures of central auditory function (Cook et al. 1993; Gascon et al. 1986; Keith and Engineer 1991; Keith et al. 1989; Ludlow et al. 1983; Pearson et al. 1991; Riccio et al. 1994). Moreover, preliminary studies suggest that the rate of comorbidity between ADHD and CAPD ranges from 45% to 75% (Cook et al. 1993; Keith et al. 1989; Riccio et al. 1994).

The high level of comorbidity between ADHD and CAPD may reflect the difficulties in making a differential diagnosis, given that attention is included in the conceptualization of both CAPD and ADHD (Riccio et al. 1994). Alternatively, the high frequency of language-based learning disabilities found in children with CAPD and ADHD and in those with CAPD only (Riccio et al. 1994) suggests that central auditory processing deficits may be an underlying factor in the co-occurrence of language-based learning disabilities and ADHD (Keith and Engineer 1991). Thus, for some children the behavioral symptoms of ADHD (inattentiveness, impulsiveness, hyperactivity) may be secondary to specific auditory/linguistic problems rather than the result of an ADHD syndrome per se (August and Garfinkel 1990; Baker and Cantwell 1987; Riccio et al. 1994; Weinberg and Emslie 1991).

SCREENING AND ASSESSMENT FOR COMORBIDITY OF ADHD AND LEARNING DISORDERS

Referrals and Comorbidities

Assessment of possible comorbidity between ADHD and learning disorders may begin with a referral because of recognized learning problems when the possibility of ADHD is to be considered. Or it may begin with an established diagnosis of ADHD when the possibility of a concurrent learning disorder is being raised. Or a referral may be made simply because the individual is having significant difficulties functioning in school, home, or community but no determination of relevant diagnostic categories has yet been made.

Whatever the reason for referral, the evaluating clinician will want to hold in mind the possibility that the individual being assessed may have multiple comorbidities. For example, it is quite possible for a person fully to meet the diagnostic criteria for ADHD, reading disorder, expressive language disorder, generalized anxiety disorder, cannabis dependence, conduct disorder, and major depressive disorder all at the same time. One diagnosis does not rule out another. Adequate assessment should consider the full range of diagnoses that are potentially relevant in conceptualizing the current strengths and functional impairments of the person being assessed. For more information about the assessment process, see Chapter 15, by Quinlan, in this volume.

Nonacademic Impairments

In considering that one or more learning disorders may be comorbid with ADHD in a given individual, it is important to look not only at the person's academic functioning but also at the broader range of his or her functioning in social relationships, family, and the wider community. Learning disorders are often noticed first in the school setting, where they clearly have an impact on activities such as reading school textbooks, doing math homework, writing assigned essays, and understanding teachers' instructions. As important, but perhaps less well recognized, is that they may also result in impairment in a wide range of everyday activities in nonacademic settings; careful assessment often reveals such impairment. Silver (1989) has described many ways in which learning disabilities are "life disabilities" that tend to produce secondary emotional, social, and family problems in multiple domains at each stage of psychosocial development.

Learning disorders may result in, for example, impairments in the ability to 1) understand and carry on conversation with peers or family members, 2) order a meal in a restaurant, 3) sequence a series of errands, 4) negotiate conflicts with parents or peers, 5) recall and follow directions to a friend's house, and 6) participate effectively in playground games or athletic competition.

For some, the impairments from learning disorders are rather circumscribed, affecting just some academic tasks and only very limited aspects of their social and family functioning; these individuals may be exceptionally competent in other domains. For others, the frustrations and embarrassments caused in school by their learning disorder impairments extend pervasively into almost every aspect of their daily functioning. To fully assess the possible importance of impairments due to comorbid learning disorders and ADHD for an affected individual, the clinician should sensitively inquire not only about school functioning but also about the impact of the impairments on other aspects of the individual's daily functioning.

Stages of Assessment for Comorbidity Between Learning Disorders and ADHD

Assessment of possible comorbidity between ADHD and learning disorders involves several stages: 1) an initial screening, which should be included in any assessment for attention-deficit disorder and/or learning disorder; 2) indicators of the need for further evaluation; 3) a more systematic screening when indicators of this comorbid combination are present: and 4) a comprehensive evaluation when indicated by the initial screening.

Routine Initial Screening

The following are suggested guidelines for the initial screening for ADHD and learning disorders:

1. Recognize the high rate and clinical significance of learning disorders in patients with ADHD, particularly in clinical samples of children. Also, recognize the persistence of these learning disorders, which are likely to be present in adults with ADHD (see Chapter 8, this volume).
2. Recognize that teachers and parents of children with ADHD may focus on the more salient disruptive behavior symptoms, attributing academic problems to inattentiveness or oppositional behavior, and thus may overlook the possibility of concurrent specific learning disorders.
3. Recognize that the phonological processing deficits that underlie reading

disorder will likely have an impact throughout the language system. Consideration of current abilities in receptive and expressive language and in mathematics is an essential part of the assessment of reading disorder. Conversely, children with ADHD with current or past speech and language impairments are at the highest risk for learning disorders, particularly reading disorder, and should be monitored accordingly.

4. Recognize that many factors such as anxiety, depression, low self-esteem, poor reading skills, and problems in executive control and attention allocation can lead to underachievement in mathematics (Ashcraft and Faust 1994; Badian 1983; Muth 1984). However, real deficits exist that affect mathematical learning and performance. Mathematical abilities, along with reading ability, should routinely be assessed in children with ADHD. (For a thoughtful commentary on clinical assessment of mathematical abilities, see Jordan 1995.)
5. Recognize that children with poor written expression may have problems with poor handwriting (dysgraphia) and/or impaired ability to convert thought and oral speech into written text. Either problem can put children at a major disadvantage for a large part of the school day because virtually every academic subject requires substantial written expression to take notes or to communicate understanding of subject matter content on quizzes or tests (Deuel 1995; McHale and Cermak 1992). Disorder of written expression could be the primary etiology of low productivity in the classroom and failure to complete homework assignments. Routine screening of written expression in children with ADHD is indicated.
6. Recognize that CAPD has yet to be validated as a diagnostic entity that is distinct from language-based learning disabilities and ADHD. Thus, routine evaluation for CAPD per se is not warranted at this time. On the other hand, it is important to be aware that many children with ADHD are likely to exhibit auditory processing problems and other language-based learning difficulties. It is also important to recognize that some of these children's behavioral and learning difficulties may be attributable to their difficulties in processing the language of instruction in the classroom and the language of social interaction in the playground and at home.
7. Routinely assess abilities in and screen for deficits in reading, mathematics, oral communication, written expression, and motor coordination in children with ADHD. (At this time there is insufficient evidence to warrant routine assessment of central auditory processing abilities and screening for CAPD.) Specific recommendations for screening instruments are listed later in this section.

8. Recall that a diagnosis of ADHD is based solely on behavioral manifestations of inattention and/or hyperactivity/impulsiveness that have an onset prior to age 7 years and cause significant impairment in social, academic, and occupational functioning. Evidence is derived from a detailed developmental and medical history and profile of presenting problems obtained from parents, teachers, and self-report through clinical interviews and rating scales. In contrast, learning disorder is defined in terms of measured deficits in one or more basic psychological processes, as estimated by the child's performance on standardized tests with established norms; behavioral symptoms play no part in the diagnosis of learning disorder.

   a. Probe the child's developmental and family history during the clinical interview with parents for correlates and risk factors associated with learning disorders (e.g., familial history of reading disorder; delayed developmental milestones, particularly in language or fine-motor domain; current educational difficulties in terms of difficulty following directions, problems in reading and spelling; and poor social interaction skills).
   b. Obtain teacher ratings of academic performance in specific domains (e.g., reading, mathematics, spelling, penmanship, written expression). (Suggested scales are listed at the end of this section.)
   c. Note overt signs of comprehension and communication problems in the child during the assessment, including frequent dysfluencies and nonspecific words ("the thing," "the . . . uh . . . what's it called?"), requests for repetitions (e.g., "Huh?," "What?"), and frequent topic shifts during conversation.
   d. Probe more specifically for symptoms of learning disorder by asking the child to write his or her name and the date, to provide routine sequenced information (e.g., "What month comes after June?"), and to draw a picture and write a brief paragraph about it. The Symbol Language and Communication Battery (Weinberg and Harper 1995) may be a useful tool for clinical practice.
   e. Screen for concurrent anxiety, depression, and low self-esteem, each of which could contribute to or partially account for the learning difficulties.

Indications for Further Evaluation

Some children and adolescents referred for assessment of possible ADHD have already been identified by their school as having a specific learning disorder and may be receiving special education services to address problems related to their learning disorder. For these children, the evaluating clinician will want to include in the assessment a review of the reports of educational and psychological evaluations already completed by the school. The assessment should also include up-to-date information from teachers about how the student is functioning both in the mainstream school program and in the special education services, if any, that are being provided. Evaluation in these instances is addressed to determine the presence and severity of ADHD symptoms that may be impairing academic functioning and possibly exacerbating the impairments of the already identified learning disorder problems and interfering with the ability of the student to make good use of the special education services being provided.

Yet many students who have both ADHD and one or more problems related to learning disorders are referred with a presumption of their having only ADHD. When a student has both ADHD and learning disorder problems, it is often the ADHD problems that are most readily apparent; this is particularly likely if the ADHD is the combined type and includes hyperactive-impulsive behaviors that are disruptive in the classroom. For these children it is often assumed that if the ADHD symptoms can be alleviated, both classroom behavior and academic achievement will improve. If, in fact, the student also has one or more impairments related to learning disorders, it is likely that more than the usual ADHD interventions may be required. Some clinicians respond to such situations by simply treating the ADHD symptoms and then reevaluating for possible learning disorders after the ADHD treatments have been adjusted and stabilized. Others arrange systematic assessment for both ADHD and learning disorders in the initial evaluation.

Given the high rate of comorbidity of ADHD and learning disorders, we recommend that any child being evaluated for ADHD should be screened for the possibility of a comorbid learning disorder if there is any suggestion in the academic or clinical history of a possible learning disorder. Such screening might be done by a review of appropriate testing already done by the school. If such testing has not been done, the clinician might arrange for the student to receive such a screening at school or in an independent clinical setting.

Brief screening for reading disorder and mathematics disorder can be done with the Wide Range Achievement Test–3 (Wilkinson 1993) or with the screener of the Wechsler Individual Achievement Test (WIAT; Psychological Corporation 1992) or the Mini-Battery of Achievement (MBA; Woodcock et al. 1994). Both of these instruments are normed for use with children and adolescents; only the MBA is normed for use through adulthood. Both the WIAT and the MBA include a measure of reading comprehension and not just a measure of ability to call the words. Unfortunately, none of the screeners currently available provide an effective way to screen for disorder of written expression; screening for this learning disorder problem may be done by careful history and examination of informal writing samples.

More Systematic Screening for Learning Disorders

When preliminary screening suggests the possibility of a learning disorder concurrent with ADHD, more extensive assessment for the learning disorder should be arranged. For general clinical practice, the following markers are suggested as potentially important indicators of a clinically meaningful discrepancy, *any one of which* warrants further testing to confirm a possible diagnosis of specific learning disabilities:

1. *Report of student's chronic difficulty or teacher or parent suspicion.* Student report of long-standing difficulty with a particular type of learning (e.g., reading, mathematics, written expression, speech/language) or report that an individual's parent or recent or current teachers have suspected the possibility of a specific learning disorder.
2. *Report of family history.* An individual's having had difficulty with a particular type of learning (e.g., reading, mathematics, written expression, speech/language) that parallels similar impairments in blood-related members of that person's family who have been identified as having a specific learning disability.
3. *Screener score significantly below Full Scale IQ.* Score on the reading, arithmetic, or writing subtest of the MBA or WIAT that is at least 20 standard score points below the Full Scale IQ (Education for All Handicapped Children Act 1977; Frick et al. 1991; Semrud-Clikeman et al. 1992).
4. *Screener score in the low average range or below.* Standard scores on the reading, mathematics, or writing subtest of the MBA or WIAT that are 90 or less (at or below the 25th percentile) (Fletcher et al. 1998).

Evaluation and Diagnosis of Learning Disorders

When the aforementioned indicators or other elements of screening indicate need for full assessment for a possible learning disorder, the evaluating clinician should arrange for full assessment of the relevant domains by an appropriately qualified professional. Depending on the available resources and complexity of the case, evaluation for a learning disorder might be done by school staff (e.g., school psychologist and educational evaluator) or by a neuropsychologist or certified private educational evaluator.

Evaluation for a possible learning disorder should include, at a minimum, a full IQ test (e.g., Wechsler Intelligence Scale for Children, 3rd Edition [WISC-III; Wechsler 1991] or Woodcock-Johnson Test of Cognitive Abilities [Woodcock and Mather 1989]) and a full achievement test battery (e.g., WIAT or Woodcock-Johnson Tests of Achievement—Revised [Woodcock and Johnson 1989]). Other standardized measures useful for a comprehensive assessment of learning disorders include the Developmental Test of Visual Motor Integration (Beery 1997) to assess visuoperceptual and motor skills, and the Wide Range Assessment of Memory and Learning (Sheslow and Adams 1990) or Children's Memory Scale (M. Cohen 1996) to assess visual and verbal memory functions.

Additional useful information may be obtained by teacher rating scales that include an evaluation of academic skills and fine-motor coordination. These scales include the Multigrade Inventory for Teachers (Agronin et al. 1992); Child Behavior Checklist, Teacher Report Form (Achenbach 1991, 1993); and Academic Performance Rating Scale (DuPaul et al. 1991). Also, the Checklist of Written Expression Skills (Poteet 1980) may be used to obtain teacher ratings of handwriting and written spelling/language.

Many additional standardized tests are available for assessing specific academic skills. Examples provided below are used to illustrate the range of measures and do not indicate an endorsement of any specific test. Standardized tests for assessing word identification skills that are strong predictors of reading ability include the Goldman-Fristoe-Woodcock Sound-Symbol Tests (Goldman et al. 1974), Word Attack and Word Identification subtests of the Woodcock Reading Mastery Tests—Revised (Woodcock 1987), and the Broad Reading Cluster of the Woodcock-Johnson Tests of Achievement—Revised (Woodcock and Johnson 1989). Children with at least low average intelligence who score below the 25th percentile on two or more of these tests would be considered to have a specific reading disability.

Standardized assessment of mathematical abilities include KeyMath—Revised (Connolly 1991); Test of Early Mathematical Abilities (Ginsberg and Baroody 1990), ideally used with standardized probes developed by Ginsberg (1990); Arithmetic subtest of the Wide Range Achievement Test–III (Wilkinson 1993); and Broad Mathematics Cluster of the Woodcock-Johnson Tests of Achievement—Revised (Woodcock and Johnson 1989).

Age- and grade-normed tests for handwriting, written composition, and spelling include Repeated Patterns Test (Waber and Bernstein 1994), Test of Written Language (Hammill and Larsen 1988), Test of Written Spelling (S. C. Larsen and Hammill 1994), Test of Written Expression (McGee et al. 1995), Written Expression Cluster of the Woodcock-Johnson Tests of Achievement—Revised (Woodcock and Johnson 1989), and Oral and Written Language Scales (Carrow-Woolfolk 1996).

Measurement of the Discrepancy Between Ability and Achievement

The benchmark criterion, according to both the educational/legal and the medical/psychiatric definitions, is an *unexpected* disability in one or more academic domains that is not predicted by general intellectual competence or socioeducational opportunities. In practical terms, this criterion has been translated into a statistical assessment of the difference between a child's objectively measured ability in a given domain (e.g., reading, arithmetic, receptive language) and his or her general intelligence (as assessed by an individually administered intelligence test). Indeed, in the United States, evidence of IQ-based discrepancies is often required to determine eligibility for provision of special education services. Typically, little effort is spent in ascertaining whether the child is at a sociocultural disadvantage or exhibits deficits in "specific psychological processes," or whether adequate educational instruction has been provided. The last issue has particular relevance for assessing learning disabilities in children with ADHD. Children with ADHD may miss a substantial amount of instruction for several reasons: 1) they tend to spend a great deal of time out of the classroom (e.g., in the principal's office) as a result of their disruptive behavior, and 2) their attention difficulties may render them "unavailable" for instruction even when they are in the classroom.

The IQ-based discrepancy approach to diagnosis appears straightforward, but since neither the magnitude of the discrepancy nor the methods for measuring ability and intelligence were specified in the professional and legal guidelines, misunderstandings and confusion have arisen. Which achievement tests should we use? Should we test reading comprehension as well as basic reading (i.e., reading isolated words)? Do we require the child to simply recognize or produce the correct spelling (or the correct answer to a computational problem in arithmetic)? Should we define a "significant discrepancy" as a 15-point or a 22-point difference between standard scores on an intelligence test and an achievement test? Should we include children who are 1 year behind their peers in arithmetic or in reading, or should we require them to be 2 years behind? These questions may appear to be pedantic pondering, but the way in which we define learning disabilities has important implications for who is eligible to receive special educational services. Too broad a definition may include many children who do not need these services and will place an impossible fiscal strain on school systems at a time that is marked by massive federal deficits and budget cutbacks. On the other hand, a definition that is too restrictive runs the risk of denying services to those children who really need them.

Clinicians in the United States should also be aware that, in contrast to learning disabilities, ADHD itself is not specified by the federal law (PL 94-142) as falling within the range of disorders eligible for provision of special educational services. However, a policy clarification memorandum from the U.S. Department of Education (Davila et al. 1991) indicates that children with ADHD may qualify for special education services in several ways. First, a child with ADHD may qualify for PL 94-142 assistance if he or she meets the eligibility criteria for one of the existing disability categories (e.g., learning disabilities) defined in the Individuals With Disabilities Education Act (IDEA) of 1990 (i.e., the reauthorization of the Education for All Handicapped Children Act, PL 94-142), which became Public Law 105-17 on June 4, 1997. Second, the memorandum indicates that children with ADHD should be classified as eligible for special education services under the category of other health impairment when the disorder results in limited alertness, which adversely affects educational performance. The potential for inclusion of ADHD under other health impairment is now stated *explicitly* in the 1999 amendment to the *Code of Federal Regulations*:

> Other health impairment means having limited strength, vitality or alertness, including a heightened alertness to environmental stimuli, that results in limited alertness with respect to the educational environment, that (i) is due to chronic or acute health problems such as asthma, *attention deficit hyperactivity disorder,* diabetes, epilepsy, a heart condition, hemophilia, lead poisoning, leukemia, nephritis, rheumatic fever, and sickle cell anemia; and (ii) adversely affects a child's educational performance. (34 CFR 300.7[c][9], July 1, 1999; emphasis added)

None of the available definitions of learning disabilities are operationally precise because they do not specify the magnitude of the discrepancy between academic achievement and intellectual ability (nor do they provide guidance on how to verify the deficit in psychological processes or the dysfunction of the central nervous system). The number of children classified as "learning disabled" will vary according to the definition used (e.g., Barkley 1990; Semrud-Clikeman et al. 1992). Thus, the definition has important implications for determining who is eligible to receive special educational services.

Several approaches have been used in determining learning disabilities in the United States and in research studies (for an insightful discussion of this issue, see Fletcher et al. 1998). In one approach, standard scores on intelligence tests (e.g., WISC-III) are compared with those on achievement tests for reading and arithmetic (e.g., Woodcock-Johnson Psychoeducational Battery—Revised, WIAT). The magnitude of the required discrepancy is specified in units of standard deviation (SD) (e.g., 1-, 1.5-, or 2-SD gap) or in number of standard score points (e.g., gap of 10, 15, or 22 standard score points) (Education for All Handicapped Children Act 1977; Frick et al. 1991). (Standard scores are scores whose distribution has a mean of 100 and a SD of 15.) One problem with an approach with a criterion based on a discrepancy between IQ and achievement is that it overestimates the prevalence of learning disorder in children with IQs in the superior range (e.g., 120–140) and underestimates the prevalence in those with lower IQs (e.g., 80–90). For example, the discrepancy criterion would be met in the case of a child with an IQ of 130 and a reading score of 100, yet investigation is likely to reveal adequate performance in school and, more important, no evidence of deficits in phonological abilities that are characteristic of reading disabilities. Another problem with this approach is that the standardized intelligence tests must be administered by someone who has been specifically trained to administer them and to score and interpret the results (e.g., a registered clinical psychologist). The tests are somewhat costly to administer, and therefore such testing is not offered routinely by school systems unless there is a good reason to suspect a marked discrepancy between a child's intelligence and academic achievement. This means that medical practitioners and other clinicians may need the assistance of a psychologist or psychoeducational specialist for the use and interpretation of the standardized tests of ability and achievement. Similarly, the assistance of a speech/language pathologist may be required for the standardized assessment of speech and language abilities.

A second approach to determining whether a child has a learning disability involves the use of a regression formula, which adjusts the comparison of IQ and achievement for the correlation of the two measures (Fletcher et al. 1998). This adjustment is required to prevent overidentification of children with higher IQs and underidentification of children with lower IQs as being learning disabled because of regression to the mean (Reynolds 1984). This approach requires access to tables of reliability quotients when one is assessing psychometric data and is therefore cumbersome for general clinical practice, although it may be the preferred approach for psychologists and researchers.

A third approach is to base the definition solely on low achievement (Siegel 1988, 1992). One advantage of this approach is that it simplifies the definition of learning disabilities and avoids the psychometric and statistical problems associated with the discrepancy approach. This approach also has potential problems, such as the criterion for severity and the identification of learning disorders in children with IQs at the upper and lower ends of the IQ range (Fletcher et al. 1998).

A recent approach proposes an evaluation of domain-specific achievement skills and of abilities correlated with these skills (Fletcher et al. 1998; Morris et al. 1998; Torgesen and Wagner 1998). This approach is best illustrated by its application to the assessment of reading disorder, which includes an evaluation of reading, phonological processing, naming speed, verbal short-term memory, and other language skills (see, e.g., Torgesen and Wagner 1998). This approach is likely to identify a very different group of children for services than are currently being served in the public schools as "reading disabled" who were identified by an IQ-achievement discrepancy approach. The implications of this approach for services are substantial. It would require an expansion of resources for providing special instructional programs, because children whose reading is impaired but not discrepant from their IQ scores would no longer be excluded from the category of reading disorder (and thus from services). On the other hand, the instructional needs of children with a similar profile of weaknesses (e.g., in the phonological processing domain) would be very similar. Moreover, the instruction could start prior to or simultaneously with the start of formal reading instruction (Torgesen and Wagner 1998).

Integration of Assessment Results Into Planning and Monitoring

Whatever the method used to assess discrepancy and to arrive at a diagnosis that either recognizes or rules out comorbid ADHD and learning disorders, it is critically important that the results of the diagnostic assessment be integrated and presented in understandable terms to the student and family as well as to the educators and clinicians involved (Kaufman 1994; Prifitera and Saklofske 1998). Careful systematic assessment of strengths and weaknesses of the individual student is the basis on which planning for both educational and clinical interventions should be done. Yet the value of such an assessment cannot be derived unless findings are shared and understood by all those involved so that plans for appropriate and effective interventions can be developed in a collaborative atmosphere in the school setting and at home. This planning for interventions should also include development of ongoing mechanisms for monitoring the effectiveness of all interventions for each individual with comorbid ADHD and learning disorder.

IMPLICATIONS OF COMORBIDITY OF ADHD AND LEARNING DISORDERS FOR TREATMENT

Development of Treatment Plans

Once ADHD has been diagnosed in comorbidity with one or more learning disorder, a plan for treatment interventions should be developed. Usually the school, in collaboration with the student, parents, and clinicians, will develop an *individualized educational plan,* or IEP, for a student identified with either a specific learning disability or ADHD, or both. DuPaul and Power, in Chapter 19 of this volume, discuss how clinicians can collaborate with educators in developing and monitoring the individualized plan for intervention.

Usually school plans developed for children with learning disorders with or without comorbid ADHD focus solely on in-school educational interventions and do not include suggestions for medication or other interventions implemented outside of school. Often school teams are reluctant to suggest such interventions lest the school thereby be called on to finance the suggested interventions. Parents and clinicians may need to take initiative to raise the issue and assess the appropriateness of such out-of-school interventions.

Medications in the Treatment of Comorbid ADHD and Learning Disorders

Among the possible interventions for ADHD comorbid with a learning disorder, medication is the most widely used. Psychostimulant medication, particularly methylphenidate, is the most common treatment for ADHD in North America, with approximately 750,000 children (i.e., more than 2% of the school-age population) being treated with these drugs annually (Safer and Krager 1988). Moreover, it is often the sole treatment received (Wolraich et al. 1990), despite strong recommendations for multimodal treatment (e.g., S. E. Shaywitz and Shaywitz 1991). Treatment with psychostimulants typically produces immediate improvements in the behavioral symptoms of ADHD as well as in some aspects of cognitive, academic, and social function. These short-term benefits have been documented in an extensive number of well-controlled trials (for reviews, see Gadow 1986; Jacobvitz et al. 1990; Rapport and Kelly 1991; Schachar et al. 1996).

In contrast, the effects of psychotropic medication on the psychological processes underlying learning disorders comorbid with ADHD are not well understood. Also, the longer-term benefits of stimulant treatment on the core and associated problems of ADHD are less clear (for reviews, see Jacobvitz et al. 1990; Schachar and Tannock 1993). These limitations in our knowledge are of concern given the high rates of comorbidity with learning disorders and the average duration of stimulant treatment, which is estimated at 2–7 years, depending on the age of the child (Barkley et al. 1990b; Safer and Krager 1988). In the next subsection, we review empirical evidence for the effects of stimulants on the various types of learning disorders that coexist with ADHD.

Effects of Stimulants on Learning Disorders Comorbid With ADHD

Reading Disorder/Mathematics Disorder

Numerous well-controlled medication trials have demonstrated that stimulants produce beneficial short-term effects on academic productivity (for reviews, see Carlson and Bunner 1993; Elia et al. 1993; Pelham 1993; Swanson et al. 1991). For example, children with ADHD who are treated with stimulant medication attempt and correctly answer more reading comprehension questions and complete more arithmetic problems than at baseline or on placebo (see, e.g., Balthazor et al. 1991; Elia et al. 1993; Forness et al. 1992; Pelham et al. 1985). The magnitude of these beneficial effects on academic productivity is substantial: 25%–40% improvement over baseline or placebo. The positive findings of stimulants on academic productivity have been replicated across studies, laboratories, settings, and tasks (including experimental or laboratory analog tasks, classroom and study hall assignments, quiz and test scores, and teacher lectures) (see, e.g., Douglas et al. 1986; DuPaul and Rapport 1993; Elia et al. 1993; Pelham et al. 1991; Rapport et al. 1986). They hold for girls with ADHD as well as boys (Pelham et al. 1989) and for adolescents with ADHD (S. W. Evans and Pelham 1991; Pelham et al. 1991) as well as school-age children. Also, the beneficial effects apply to long-acting preparations and other stimulants such as pemoline and dextroamphetamine (Elia et al. 1993; Pelham et al. 1990). Moreover, improvements in academic productivity appear to be sustained with extended stimulant treatment (Forness et al. 1992; Richardson et al. 1988). Furthermore, the positive effects of stimulants on one aspect of reading performance—number of comprehension questions attempted and completed correctly—have been reported to be comparable in ADHD children with and without comorbid reading disorder, although the comorbid samples were too small for a firm conclusion to be drawn (Elia et al. 1993; Forness et al. 1992). It is important to note that although the *statistical* significance of stimulant effects on academic productivity has been demonstrated reliably, the *clinical* significance of these effects in terms of normalizing performance is less impressive (see, e.g., DuPaul and Rapport 1993). Approximately 25% of children with ADHD fail to show normalized levels of academic productivity.

In contrast to the beneficial effects on academic productivity, there is no evidence that stimulants have any impact on the specific cognitive processes underlying reading disorder (e.g., phonological processing) or mathematics disorder (e.g., memory retrieval). That is, stimulant medication may enhance verbal retrieval mechanisms involved in word recognition (Ballinger et al. 1984; R. W. Evans et al. 1986; Peeke et al. 1984; Richardson et al. 1988), but it does not produce direct effects on phonological processing per se (Balthazor et al. 1991; Richardson et al. 1988). Similarly, although findings from some studies suggest that stimulants may speed the children's computation (addition) as well as their ability to move from problem to problem (Carlson et al. 1991) and reduce the reliance of finger-counting strategies (Benedetto and Tannock 1999; S. Hoosen-Shakeel A. Ishak, A. Ickowicz, et al., submitted), it is not yet clear whether stimulants have a direct impact on computational procedures, number-fact retrieval, or other psychological processes underlying the different types of mathematics disorder. These findings suggest that the beneficial effects of stimulants on academic productivity in reading and arithmetic may be mediated by the behavioral response to stimulants or by nonspecific enhancement of information processing, rather than by specific effects on phonological processing and other processes (Balthazor et al. 1991; Richardson et al. 1988).

The apparently generalized beneficial impact of stimulants on information processing for a variety of cognitive functions raises interesting questions for further research on both ADHD and learning disorders. Although it seems clear that stimulants cannot directly modify many of the impairments associated with learning disorders, there is reason to consider that the generalized effects of stimulants on cognitive information processing may help to facilitate improvement in some aspects of functions impaired in learning disorders. One specific component of information processing that may be relevant is working memory.

Working memory is a term used by Baddeley (1993) to describe a system of short-term memory that allows several pieces of information to be held simultaneously in mind for interactive processing. This working memory function has been described as playing a critical role in learning and execution of a wide variety of cognitive information-processing tasks, including learning to read and reading comprehension (Baddeley 1986, 1993; Gathercole and Baddeley 1993); mathematics fact retrieval, procedural recall, computation, and problem solving (Geary 1994); writing composition (Kellogg 1994); and learning a foreign language (Baddeley 1993).

As was discussed in the introductory chapter of this book, Barkley (1997) and Brown (1995, 1996) proposed that impairment of working memory be considered an aspect of ADHD; it may be that working memory impairments also play a significant role in learning disorders. Relative impairment of working memory has been demonstrated in children with impaired reading comprehension (Baddeley 1993; Gathercole and Baddeley 1993) and in children with procedural and/or fact-retrieval deficits of mathematics disorder (Geary 1994). If the effects of stimulant medication in generally enhancing information processing within the brain include enhancement of working memory function, this treatment may significantly contribute to alleviation of some aspects of learning disorders comorbid with ADHD. Preliminary evidence indicates that stimulant medication does enhance working memory in children with ADHD, provided that the children do not exhibit comorbid anxiety disorders (Tannock et al. 1995b). Further study of the role of working memory in ADHD and learning disorders, as well as research on the effects of stimulants on working memory, is needed to determine the role of medication in treatment of these overlapping disorders.

The deficient phonological processing abilities of children with reading disorder (in the absence of ADHD) have been shown to be amenable to remedial educational treatment (Lovett et al. 1990, 1994; Olson and Wise 1992). For example, an intensive and focused remediation program that provides 35 hours of training in phonological analysis and blending skills at the levels of both oral and printed language is effective in improving both speech- and print-based phonological processing deficits in children with reading disorder (Lovett et al. 1994). It is not known whether children with ADHD and comorbid reading disorder could obtain similar benefits from this intervention approach alone. Perhaps the use of stimulant medication to reduce the ADHD symptoms and to enhance the impaired information processing might enable children with comorbid ADHD and reading disorder to tolerate and benefit from an intense phonologically oriented instruction, although this proposition is challenged by the negative findings from previous studies in which a combined treatment approach was used (Gittelman et al. 1983; Richardson et al. 1988). However, this issue is currently under investigation in Tannock's laboratory, in a randomized controlled trial of Lovett's remediation programs with and without adjunctive stimulant medication for children with ADHD and comorbid reading disorder (Medical Research Council of Canada Grant MT13366).

To date, there is insufficient evidence to conclude that stimulant medication is an appropriate treatment for mathematics disorder per se: yet, as with reading disorder, it is possible that stimulant medication may help the individual with mathematics disorder to benefit from special educational interventions more than would be possible without such medication treatment. However, medication cannot reasonably be expected to remedy underlying deficits in mathematics skills; these will likely require specific educational intervention.

Research has demonstrated that effective intervention for mathematics disorder requires more than just repetitive instruction. Retrieval does not substantially improve for many children with mathematics disorder, even with extensive drilling (e.g., Howell et al. 1987). Further research is urgently needed to identify effective interventions for the various subtypes of mathematics disorder and to assess whether stimulants might help to render affected individuals more accessible to remedial educational interventions, perhaps by facilitating improved functioning of working memory.

Disorder of Written Expression/Dysgraphia

Stimulants have consistently been shown to have a pronounced beneficial effect on handwriting or penmanship in children with ADHD; published samples of handwriting show the magnitude of this effect (e.g., Schain and Reynard 1975; Taylor 1979). The findings also appear to hold for children with extremely poor handwriting (Lerer et al. 1977). Children's writing is neater and more legible when they are receiving stimulant treatment; handwriting deteriorates rapidly when treatment is stopped.

In contrast to the beneficial aspects on motor skills, the effects of stimulants on other aspects of written expression (e.g., spelling, sentence structure and grammar, and the organization of ideas) have not yet been adequately tested. For example, modest improvements have been reported for children's performance on regular and nonsense word spelling tasks (e.g., Stephens et al. 1984), but findings are not always consistent (e.g., Douglas et al. 1986; Pelham et al. 1985). Although there have been anecdotal clinical reports of stimulant-induced improvements in flow of written expression (see Chapter 1, this volume), there are not, at present, sufficient controlled research data to allow one to draw definite conclusions about the possible role of medications in treatment of disorder of written expression.

Developmental Coordination Disorder

Other aspects of fine and gross motor coordination and performance on perceptual motor tasks may also be enhanced by stimulant treatment. Stimulants have been found to improve motor steadiness (Knights and Hinton 1969) and to facilitate the acquisition of gross motor skills, such as balance (Wade 1976). However, it is unclear whether the findings apply to ADHD children with comorbid developmental coordination disorder per se.

Communication Disorders/Central Auditory Processing Disorder

The effects of stimulant medication on everyday use of language are virtually unexplored, and the few existing psychopharmacological studies have yielded contradictory findings (Tannock 1998). For example, Ludlow et al. (1978) found that stimulants improved but did not normalize disruptive talk and that only the less hyperactive children exhibited benefits from stimulant treatment on task-related talk. There is no evidence that stimulants improve dysfluency, enhance communicative effectiveness, or increase the amount of appropriate task-related talk (Hamlett et al. 1987; Ludlow et al. 1978; Whalen et al. 1979). Moreover, findings from some studies suggest that the effects of methylphenidate on children's everyday use of language may not all be beneficial. For example, methylphenidate has been found to increase talkativeness in children with ADHD (e.g., Barkley 1990; Creager and Van Riper 1967; see also reviews by Barkley 1977; Gadow 1986).

Since children with ADHD are often excessively and inappropriately talkative, these data suggest an adverse effect of stimulants on some children's use of language. Yet some individuals with ADHD tend to be excessively constricted in their spontaneous speech; for those more inhibited speakers, stimulant medication may help to facilitate a more adaptive flow of expressive speech. Moreover, there is some suggestion that stimulants may enhance the quality of expressive speech. Findings from a recent (uncontrolled) study by Berk and Potts (1991) suggest that stimulants may promote children's use of a more mature and internalized form of self-regulatory speech that is strongly associated with focused attention and motor quiescence. Further research to determine the effects of stimulant medication on the everyday use of language by children with ADHD is urgently required (a randomized controlled trial is currently under way in Tannock's laboratory).

Stimulant treatment prescribed for ADHD may improve some aspects of the communication disorder (e.g., pragmatic dysfunction), but it is unlikely to have any impact on deficits in the basic language systems (i.e., phonology, syntax, semantics). Deficits in the basic language systems require specific adjunctive interventions in consultation with speech/language pathologists.

The few studies to address the impact of stimulants on CAPD provide consistent evidence that psychostimulant medication, particularly methylphenidate, improves performance on measures of auditory vigilance and auditory processing in children with ADHD (Cook et al. 1993; Gascon et al. 1986; Keith and Engineer 1991). Moreover, stimulant medication also improves the behavioral symptoms of ADHD in children who meet the diagnostic criteria for both ADHD and CAPD (Cook et al. 1993). The sensitivity of both ADHD and CAPD measures to stimulant therapy suggests a close relationship between these two disorders.

In-School Interventions for Comorbid ADHD and Learning Disorders

Even when medication treatment for ADHD comorbid with learning disorders is maximally effective, medication alone cannot generally provide sufficient remediation. Educational interventions within school are usually needed to adjust curriculum requirements or classroom modifications (e.g., extended time for tests), to provide alternative and/or remedial modes of instruction, to provide assistance in study skills, organization, and planning of assignments, and so forth. Such in-school modifications and interventions are developed for individual students by teams of educators in collaboration with the student and parents according to federal and state regulations. The role of clinicians in collaborating with educators, students, and parents to develop and monitor these in-school interventions is discussed by Du Paul and Power in Chapter 19 of this volume.

Outside-of-School Interventions for Comorbid ADHD and Learning Disorders

In-school interventions for students with combined ADHD and learning disorders usually need to be supplemented by out-of-school interventions that are generally arranged by the parents and students rather than by the school. The most common of these is stimulant medication, but other interventions may be at least equally important. Additional outside-of-school interventions for consideration include computer training and usage, books-on-tape, supplementary videos, parent guidance, and counseling for the student. At present, there is little research available from which to assess the effectiveness of these outside-of-school interventions, but clinical reports indicate that such interventions may play an especially important role for students with comorbid ADHD and learning disorder.

Computer Training and Usage

Although most schools in North America now offer training for their students in computer keyboarding skills and software applications, such instruction is often not provided until late elementary or junior high school. For students with comorbid ADHD and learning disorders, particularly those with disorder of written expression, there may be benefit in developing keyboarding and word-processing proficiency by the middle elementary years. For these students the computer can become not simply a way to play interesting interactive games but a powerful adjunct for cognitive skill development, content research and review, and written expression.

To gain the potential benefits of the computer, students with comorbid ADHD and learning disorders need to develop early in their schooling sufficient proficiency in keyboarding and enough familiarity with relevant software so that these functions can become automatized; usually this requires that the child have earlier and more intensive keyboarding instruction and access to computer time than most elementary school classrooms provide.

Some parents are able to provide such instruction by making available a computer and appropriate instructional software at home; others may arrange for extra computer time at the school or with a neighbor or friend. Since the early stages of developing keyboarding profiency are rather boring, some parents find that they need to provide gamelike typing instruction software, possibly with added extrinsic incentives for reaching certain levels of proficiency or for putting in effort at brief daily practice periods.

Once word-processing skills have been developed and automatized so the student can efficiently compose and edit text for writing notes and homework assignments on the screen, the computer may serve to compensate for some of the impairments of working memory that often accompany ADHD, particularly with comorbid disorder of written expression. When the student can see many lines of his or her writing on the computer screen and can readily edit and revise without needing to recopy, the task of writing and revision can be less onerous and may become less intimidating.

Computers can also facilitate content learning and review with interactive instruction and assist in research for term projects with CD-ROM or on-line reference resources. These computer resources can be helpful for any student; they can be especially valuable for many students with comorbid ADHD and learning disorder.

Books on Tape and Supplementary Videos

For many students with combined ADHD and learning disorders, particularly those with language impairments or reading disorder, long reading assignments commonly given for homework in high school, junior high school, and sometimes earlier can be particularly difficult. When the assigned reading is a classic play or popular novel, it may be possible for parents to help the student to borrow or rent a videotape that can provide a visual preview of the story or play; viewing the tape prior to the reading may help the student to gain an overview of the story line and characters, which can make it considerably easier to read and understand the assignment. In using such previews, students should be reminded that video adaptations of novels and plays are invariably different in some ways from the written form and should be used not as a substitute for but rather as a supplement to reading the assigned text.

Another way to assist students with comorbid ADHD and learning disorders to cope with very slow or impaired reading of long assignments is to provide audio versions of reading assignments. These may be locally prepared tapes of textbooks or other assigned readings; or the national service of books-on-tape, available for individuals with documented reading disorder or other learning disorder, may be used. With proper documentation of need, these materials may be ordered from the Recording for the Blind and Dyslexic, 20 Roszel Road, Princeton, New Jersey 08540 (Phone: 1-800-803-7201; http://www.rfbd.org).

Counseling and Support for Students and Parents

Often academic and social problems of students with comorbid ADHD and learning disorders produce chronic stresses in the students and/or in their interactions with their parents. Especially during adolescence, self-esteem problems may exacerbate as students with combined ADHD and learning disorders repeatedly encounter reminders of many things they "just don't get" and of how much harder they have to work to complete academic tasks that are much easier for most of their peers. These issues tend to become especially problematic in later years of high school, when students face the inevitable questions about what sort of postsecondary education and/or work they will undertake. For any of these issues, it may be helpful for the student to talk individually on a scheduled or as-needed basis with a mentor or counselor who can empathically understand the nature and frustrations of the combined ADHD and learning disorder, offer accurate information about available resources, and help the student effectively to confront important stresses and decisions in light of a clear understanding of the comorbid ADHD and learning disorder.

Sometimes counseling support is needed not just for the individual problems of the student but for problematic interaction patterns of the student and family. Parents of children with impairments from ADHD and comorbid learning disorders may be very helpful in providing support and advocacy for their children. Yet parents can readily get caught up in stressful chronic conflicts with their sons and daughters over homework and study habits, especially during adolescence, when homework demands increase and expectations for autonomy from parents escalate. Sometimes such conflicts can result in a student's refusing to do assignments, to take needed medication, or to attend their classes and comply with school rules. All the usual conflicts common in any parent-child interactions may be found in family relationships of students with comorbid ADHD and learning disorders, but these conflicts may be intensified by the stresses of the impairments that not only affect competence and motivation for academic tasks but also may impair communication skills that are needed to negotiate and resolve such problems in the family.

Counselors or psychotherapists familiar with ADHD, learning disorders, family dynamics, and the stresses to which adolescents and their parents are exposed may be very helpful in offering support and guidance to parents and their children, either separately or in conjoint sessions, to help them to gain understanding, to adjust expectations, and to develop more adequate and developmentally appropriate ways to cope with these ongoing dilemmas.

Additionally, some adolescents and parents may find help in reading materials that explain learning disorders and attention-deficit disorders without excessive technical language. For parents, these include *The Misunderstood Child: A Guide for Parents of Children With Learning Disabilities,* 2nd Edition (Silver 1992), *How to Reach and Teach ADD/ADHD Children* (Rief 1993), *Educational Care: A System for Helping Children With Learning Problems* (Levine 1994), and *When You Worry About the Child You Love: Emotional and Learning Problems in Children* (Hallowell 1996). Adolescents might benefit from *Keeping a Head in School: A Student's Book About Learning Abilities and Learning Disorders* (Levine 1990).

REFERENCES

Achenbach TM: Manual for the Child Behavior Checklist/4-18 and 1991 Profile. Burlington, VT, Department of Psychiatry, University of Vermont, 1991

Achenbach TM: Empirically Based Taxonomy: How to Use Syndromes and Profile Types Derived From the CBCL/4-18, TRF, and YSR. Burlington, VT, Department of Psychiatry, University of Vermont, 1993

Ackerman PT, Dykman RA: Reading-disabled students with and without comorbid arithmetic disability. Developmental Neuropsychology 11:351–371, 1995

Ackerman PT, Anhalt JM, Dykman RA: Arithmetic automatization failure in children with attention and reading disorders: associations and sequelae. J Learn Disabil 19:222–232, 1986a

Ackerman PT, Anhalt JM, Holcomb PJ, et al: Presumable innate and acquired automatic processes in children with attention and/or reading disorders. J Child Psychol Psychiatry 27:513–529, 1986b

Adams MJ: Beginning to Read: Thinking and Learning About Print. Cambridge, MA, MIT Press, 1990

Agronin ME, Holahan JM, Shaywitz BA, et al: The Multi-Grade Inventory for Teachers (MIT): scale development, reliability, and validity of an instrument to assess children with attentional deficits and learning disbilities, in Attention Deficit Disorder Comes of Age. Edited by Shaywitz SE, Shaywitz BA. Austin, TX, Pro-Ed, 1992, pp 89–116

Akshoomoff NA, Courchesne E: A new role for the cerebellum in cognitive operations. Behav Neurosci 106:731–738, 1992

American Psychiatric Association: Diagnostic and Statistical Manual of Mental Disorders, 2nd Edition. Washington, DC, American Psychiatric Association, 1968

American Psychiatric Association: Diagnostic and Statistical Manual of Mental Disorders, 3rd Edition. Washington, DC, American Psychiatric Association, 1980

American Psychiatric Association: Diagnostic and Statistical Manual of Mental Disorders, 3rd Edition, Revised. Washington, DC, American Psychiatric Association, 1987

American Psychiatric Association: Diagnostic and Statistical Manual of Mental Disorders, 4th Edition. Washington, DC, American Psychiatric Association, 1994

American Speech, Language, Hearing Association: Report of the Ad Hoc Committee on Central Auditory Processing Disorders. Washington, DC, American Speech, Language, Hearing Association, 1992

Anderson JC, Williams S, McGee R, et al: DSM-III-R disorders in preadolescent children: prevalence in a large sample from the general population. Arch Gen Psychiatry 44:69–76, 1987

Ashcraft MH, Faust MW: Mathematics anxiety and mental arithmetic: an exploratory investigation. Cogn Emotion 8:97–125, 1994

Ashcraft MH, Fierman BA: Mental addition in third, fourth, and sixth graders. J Exp Child Psychol 33:216–234, 1982

August GJ, Garfinkel BD: Behavioral and cognitive subtypes of ADHD. J Am Acad Child Adolesc Psychiatry 28:739–748, 1989

August GJ, Garfinkel BD: Comorbidity of ADHD and reading disability among clinic referred children. J Abnorm Child Psychol 18:29–45, 1990

Baddeley AD: Working Memory. Oxford, UK, Oxford University Press, 1986

Baddeley AD: Your Memory: A User's Guide. London, Multimedia Books, 1993

Badian NA: Dyscalculia and nonverbal disorders of learning, in Progress in Learning Disabilities, Vol 5. Edited by Myklebust HR. New York, Grune & Stratton, 1983, pp 235–264

Baker L, Cantwell DP: Developmental arithmetic disorder, in Comprehensive Textbook of Psychiatry/IV, 4th Edition. Edited by Kaplan HI, Sadock BJ. Baltimore, MD, Williams & Wilkins, 1985, pp 1697–1700

Baker L, Cantwell DP: Comparison of well, emotionally disordered, and behaviorally disordered children with linguistic problems. J Am Acad Child Adolesc Psychiatry 26:193–196, 1987

Baker L, Cantwell DP: Attention deficit disorder and speech/language disorders. Comprehensive Mental Health Care 2:3–16, 1992

Ballinger CT, Varley CK, Nolen PA: Effects of methylphenidate on reading in children with attention deficit disorder. Am J Psychiatry 141:1590–1593, 1984

Balthazor MJ, Wagner RK, Pelham WE: The specificity of effects of stimulant medication on classroom learning-related measures of cognitive processing for attention deficit disorder children. J Abnorm Child Psychol 19:35–52, 1991

Barkley RA: A review of stimulant drug research with hyperactive children. J Child Psychol Psychiatry 18:137–165, 1977

Barkley RA (ed): Attention Deficit Hyperactivity Disorder: A Handbook for Diagnosis and Treatment. New York, Guilford, 1990

Barkley RA: Behavioral inhibition, sustained attention, and executive functions: constructing a unifying theory of ADHD. Psychol Bull 121:65–94, 1997

Barkley RA, Cunningham C, Karlsson J: The speech of hyperactive children with their mothers: comparisons with normal children and stimulant effects. J Learn Disabil 16:105–110, 1983

Barkley RA, DuPaul GJ, McMuray MB: A comprehensive evaluation of attention deficit disorder with and without hyperactivity as defined by research criteria. J Consult Clin Psychol 58:775–789, 1990a

Barkley RA, Fischer M, Edelbrock CS, et al: The adolescent outcome of hyperactive children diagnosed by research criteria, I: an 8-year prospective follow-up study. J Am Acad Child Adolesc Psychiatry 29:546–557, 1990b

Barkley RA, Guevremont DC, Anastopoulos AD, et al: Driving-related risks and outcomes of attention deficit hyperactivity disorder in adolescents and young adults: a 3- to 5-year follow-up survey. Pediatrics 92:212–218, 1993

Barkley RA, Koplowicz S, Anderson T, et al: Sense of time in children with ADHD: effects of duration, distraction, and stimulant medication. Journal of the International Neuropsychological Society 3:359–369, 1997

Baumgaertel A, Wolraich M, Dietrich M: Comparison of diagnostic criteria for attention deficit disorders in a German elementary school sample. J Am Acad Child Adolesc Psychiatry 34:629–638, 1995

Beery KE: The Visual-Motor Integration Test, 4th Edition: Administration, Scoring, and Teaching Manual. Austin, TX, Pro-Ed, 1997

Beitchman J, Tuckett M, Batth S: Language delay and hyperactivity in preschoolers: evidence for a distinct group of hyperactives. Can J Psychiatry 32:683–687, 1987

Beitchman JH, Hood J, Rochon J, et al: Empirical classification of speech/language impairment in children, II: behavioral characteristics. J Am Acad Child Adolesc Psychiatry 28:118–123, 1989

Benedetto-Nash E, Tannock R: Math computation performance and error patterns of children with attention deficit hyperactivity disorder. Journal of Attention Disorders 3:121–134, 1999

Berk L, Potts M: Development and functional significance of private speech among attention-deficit hyperactivity disordered and normal boys. J Abnorm Child Psychol 19:357–377, 1991.

Berkson J: Limitations of the application of fourfold table analysis to hospital data. Biometrics 2:47–53, 1946

Berquin PC, Giedd JN, Jacobsen LK, et al: Cerebellum in attention-deficit hyperactivity disorder: a morphometric MRI study. Neurology 50:1087–1093, 1998

Biederman J, Munir K, Knee D, et al: A family study of patients with attention deficit disorder and normal controls. J Psychiatr Res 20:263–274, 1986

Biederman J, Faraone SV, Keenan K, et al: Further evidence for family genetic risk factors in attention deficit hyperactivity disorder: patterns of comorbidity in probands and relatives in psychiatrically and pediatrically referred samples. Arch Gen Psychiatry 49:728–738, 1992

Bird H, Canino G, Rubio-Stipec M, et al: Estimates of the presence of childhood maladjustment in a community survey in Puerto Rico. Arch Gen Psychiatry 45: 1120–1126, 1988

Bishop DVM: The underlying nature of specific language impairment. J Child Psychol Psychiatry 33:3–66, 1992

Bowers PG: Tracing symbol naming speed's unique contribution to reading disabilities over time. Reading and Writing: An Interdisciplinary Journal 7:189–216, 1995

Bowers PG, Wolf M: Theoretical links among naming speed, precise timing mechanisms and orthographic skills in dyslexia. Reading and Writing: An Interdisciplinary Journal 5:69–85, 1993

Brady SA, Shankweiler DP (eds): Phonological Processes in Literacy: A Tribute to Isabelle Y. Liberman. Hillsdale, NJ, Erlbaum, 1991

Brown TE: Differential diagnosis of ADD vs. ADHD in adults, in Comprehensive Guide to Attention Deficit Disorder in Adults. Edited by Nadeau KG. New York, Brunner/Mazel, 1995, pp 93–108

Brown TE: Manual for Brown Attention Deficit Disorder Scales. San Antonio, TX, Psychological Corporation, 1996

Bruck M: Persistence of dyslexics' phonological awareness deficits. Dev Psychol 28:874–886, 1992

Bryant P: Children and arithmetic. J Child Psychol Psychiatry 36:3–32, 1995

Byrne B, Freebody P, Gates A: Longitudinal data on the relations of word-reading strategies to comprehension, reading time, and phonemic awareness. Reading Research Quarterly 27:141–151, 1992

Cantwell DP, Baker L: Psychiatric and Developmental Disorders in Children With Communication Disorder. Washington, DC, American Psychiatric Press, 1991

Cardon LR, DeFries JC, Filker DW, et al: Quantitative trait locus for reading disability on chromosome 6. Science 266:276–279, 1994

Carlson CL, Bunner MR: Effects of methylphenidate on the academic performance of children with attention-deficit hyperactivity disorder and learning disabilities. School Psychology Review 22:184–198, 1993

Carlson CL, Pelham WE, Swanson JM, et al: A divided attention analysis of the effects of methylphenidate on the arithmetic performance of children with attention deficit hyperactivity disorder. J Child Psychol Psychiatry 32:463–471, 1991

Carrow-Woolfolk E: Oral and Written Language Scales. Circle Pines, MN, American Guidance Services, 1996

Carte ET, Nigg JT, Hinshaw SP: Neuropsychological functioning, motor speed, and language processing in boys with and without ADHD. J Abnorm Child Psychol 24:481–498, 1996

Castellanos FX, Giedd JN, Marsh WL, et al: Quantitative brain magnetic resonance imaging in attention-deficit hyperactivity disorder. Arch Gen Psychiatry 53: 607–616, 1996

Cermak SA: Developmental dyspraxia, in Neuropsychological Studies of Apraxia and Related Disorders. Edited by Roy EA. Amsterdam, North Holland, 1985, pp 225–248

Cohen M: Manual for Children's Memory Scale: An Assessment of Memory and Learning. San Antonio, TX, Psychological Corporation, 1996

Cohen N, Davine M, Horodezky N, et al: Unsuspected language impairment in psychiatrically disturbed children: prevalence and language and behavioral characteristics. J Am Acad Child Adolesc Psychiatry 32:595–603, 1993

Connolly AJ: Key Math Revised: A Diagnostic Inventory of Essential Mathematics. Circle Pines, MN, American Guidance Service, 1991

Cook JR, Mausbach T, Burd L, et al: A preliminary study of the relationship between central auditory processing disorder and attention deficit disorder. J Psychiatry Neurosci 18:130–137, 1993

Creager P, Van Riper C: The effect of methylphenidate on the verbal productivity of children with cerebral dysfunction. Journal of Speech and Hearing Research 10: 623–628, 1967.

Dahmen W, Hartje W, Bussing A, et al: Disorders of calculation in aphasic patients—spatial and verbal components. Neuropsychologia 20:145–153, 1982

Davila RR, Williams ML, MacDonald JT: Clarification of policy to address the needs of children with attention deficit disorders within general and/or special education. Unpublished letter to Chief State School Officers, U.S. Department of Education, September 16, 1991

DeFries JC, Gillis JJ: Etiology of reading deficits in learning disabilities: quantitative genetic analysis, in Neuropsychological Foundations of Learning Disabilities: A Handbook of Issues, Methods, and Practice. Edited by Obrzut JE, Hynd GW. Orlando, FL, Academic Press, 1991, pp 29–47

DeFries JC, Fulker DW, LaBuda MC: Evidence for a genetic aetiology in reading disability of twins. Nature 329:537–539, 1987

DeFries JC, Stevenson J, Gillis JJ, et al: Genetic etiology of spelling deficits in the Colorado and London twin studies of reading disability. Reading and Writing: An Interdisciplinary Journal 3:271–283, 1991

Denckla MB, Roeltgen DP: Disorders of motor function and control, in Handbook of Developmental Neuropsychology, Vol 6: Child Neuropsychology. Edited by Rapin I, Segalowitz SJ (Boller F, Grafman J, Series Editors). Amsterdam, Elsevier, 1992, pp 455–476

Denckla MB, Rudel RG, Chapman C, et al: Motor proficiency in dyslexic children with and without attentional disorders. Arch Neurol 42:228–231, 1985

Deuel RK: Motor skill disorder, in Developmental Disorders: Diagnostic Criteria and Clinical Assessment. Edited by Hooper SR, Hynd GW, Mattison RE. Hillsdale, NJ, Erlbaum, 1992, pp 239–281

Deuel RK: Developmental dysgraphia and motor skills disorders. J Child Neurol 10(suppl):S6–S8, 1995

Dewey D, Kaplan BJ: Subtyping of developmental motor deficits. Developmental Neuropsychology 10:265–284, 1994

Douglas VI: Cognitive deficits in children with attention deficit disorder with hyperactivity, in Attention Deficit Disorder: Critique, Cognition, and Intervention. Edited by Bloomingdale L, Sergeant J. New York, Pergamon, 1988, pp 65–82

Douglas VI, Benezra E: Supraspan verbal memory in attention deficit disorder with hyperactivity, normal and reading-disabled boys. J Abnorm Child Psychol 18: 617–638, 1990

Douglas VI, Barr RG, O'Neill ME, et al: Short term effects of methylphenidate on the cognitive, learning and academic performance of children with attention deficit disorder in the laboratory and classroom. J Child Psychol Psychiatry 27:191–211, 1986

DuPaul GJ, Rapport MD: Does methylphenidate normalize the classroom performance of children with attention deficit disorder? J Am Acad Child Adolesc Psychiatry 32:190–198, 1993

DuPaul GJ, Stoner G: ADHD in the Schools: Assessment and Intervention Strategies. New York, Guilford, 1994

DuPaul GJ, Rapport MD, Perriello LM: Teacher ratings of academic skills: the development of the Academic Performance Rating Scale. School Psychology Review 20:284–300, 1991

Dykman RA, Ackerman PT: Attention deficit disorder and specific reading disability: separate but often overlapping disorders. J Learn Disabil 24:96–103, 1991

Education for All Handicapped Children Act (PL 94-142). Federal Register 42: 42496-7, 1977

Elbert JC: Occurrence and pattern of impaired reading and written language in children with attention deficit disorders. Annals of Dyslexia 43:26–43, 1993

Elia J, Welsh PA, Gullotta CS, et al: Classroom academic performance: improvement with both methylphenidate and dextroamphetamine in ADHD boys. J Child Psychol Psychiatry 34:785–804, 1993

Evans RW, Gualtieri CT, Amara I: Methylphenidate and memory: dissociated effects in hyperactive children. Psychopharmacology (Berl) 90:211–216, 1986

Evans SW, Pelham WE: Psychostimulant effects on academic and behavioral measures for ADHD junior high school students in a lecture format classroom. J Abnorm Child Psychol 19:537–552, 1991

Faraone SV, Biederman J, Lehman BK, et al: Evidence for the independent familial transmission of attention deficit hyperactivity disorder and learning disabilities: results from a family genetic study. Am J Psychiatry 150:891–895, 1993

Faraone SV, Biederman J, Weber W, et al: Psychiatric, neuropsychological, and psychosocial features of DSM-IV subtypes of attention-deficit/hyperactivity disorder: results from a clinically referred sample. J Am Acad Child Adolesc Psychiatry 37:185–193, 1998

Felton RH, Wood FB: Cognitive deficits in reading disability and attention deficit disorder. J Learn Disabil 22:3–13, 1989

Filipek PA: Neurobiological correlates of developmental dyslexia: how do dyslexics' brains differ from those of normal readers? J Child Neurol 10 (suppl 1): S62–S69, 1995

Filipek PA, Richelme C, Kennedy DM, et al: Morphometric analysis of the brain in developmental language disorders and autism (abstract). Ann Neurol 32:475, 1992

Fleischner JE, Manheimer MA: Math interventions for students with learning disabilities: myths and realities. School Psychology Review 26:397–413, 1997

Fletcher JM, Shaywitz SE, Shankweiler DP, et al: Cognitive profiles of reading disability: comparisons of discrepancy and low achievement definitions. Journal of Educational Psychology 86:6–23, 1994

Fletcher JM, Francis DJ, Shaywitz SE, et al: Intelligent testing with the discrepancy model for children with learning disabilities. Learning Disabilities: Research and Practice 13:186–203, 1998

Flicek M: Social status of boys with both academic problems and attention-deficit hyperactivity disorder. J Abnorm Child Psychol 20:353–366, 1992

Flynn JM, Rahbar MH: Prevalence of reading failure in boys compared with girls. Psychology in the Schools 31:66–70, 1994

Forness SR, Swanson JM, Cantwell DP, et al: Stimulant medication and reading performance: follow-up on sustained dose in ADHD boys with and without conduct disorders. J Learn Disabil 25:115–123, 1992

Frick PJ, Kamphaus RW, Lahey BB, et al: Academic underachievement and the disruptive behavior disorders. J Consult Clin Psychol 59:289–294, 1991

Gadow KD: Hyperactivity, in Children on Medication, Vol 1: Hyperactivity, Learning Disabilities, and Mental Retardation. Edited by Gadow KD. Boston, MA, Little, Brown, 1986, pp 31–95

Galaburda AM, Livingstone M: Evidence for a magnocellular deficit in developmental dyslexia. Ann N Y Acad Sci 682:70–82, 1985

Garnett K, Fleischner JE: Mathematical disabilities. Pediatr Ann 16:159–176, 1987

Gascon GG, Johnson R, Burd L: Central auditory processing and attention deficit disorders. J Child Neurol 1:27–33, 1986

Gathercole SE, Baddeley AD: Working Memory and Language. Hillsdale, NJ, Erlbaum, 1993

Gaub M, Carlson CL: Behavioral characteristics of DSM-IV ADHD subtypes in a school-based population. J Abnorm Child Psychol 25:103–111, 1997

Geary DC: A componential analysis of an early learning deficit in mathematics. J Exp Child Psychol 49:363–383, 1990

Geary DC: Mathematical disabilities: cognitive, neuropsychological, and genetic components. Psychol Bull 114:345–362, 1993

Geary DC: Children's Mathematical Development: Research and Practical Applications. Washington, DC, American Psychological Association, 1994

Geary DC, Brown SC: Cognitive addition: strategy choice and speed-of-processing differences in gifted, normal, and mathematically disabled children. Dev Psychol 27:398–406, 1991

Geary DC, Bow-Thomas CC, Yao Y: Counting knowledge and skill in cognitive addition: a comparison of normal and mathematically disabled children. J Exp Child Psychol 54:372–391, 1992

Gilger JW, Pennington BF, DeFries C: A twin study of the etiology of comorbidity: attention deficit hyperactivity disorder and dyslexia. J Am Acad Child Adolesc Psychiatry 31:343–348, 1992

Gillberg C, Rasmussen P, Carlstrom G, et al: Perceptual, motor and attentional deficits in six-year-old children. Epidemiological aspects. J Child Psychol Psychiatry 23:131–144, 1982

Gillis JJ, Gilger JW, Pennington BF, et al: Attention deficit hyperactivity disorder in reading disabled twins: evidence for a genetic etiology. J Abnorm Child Psychol 20:303–315, 1992

Ginsberg HP: The Test of Early Mathematics Ability: Assessment Probes and Instructional Activities. Austin, TX, Pro-Ed, 1990

Ginsberg HP, Baroody AJ: The Test of Early Mathematics Ability, 2nd Edition. Austin, TX, Pro-Ed, 1990

Gittelman R, Klein DF, Feingold I: Children with reading disorders, II: effects of methylphenidate in combination with reading remediation. J Child Psychol Psychiatry 24:193–212, 1983

Goldman R, Fristoe M, Woodcock R: Goldman-Fristoe-Woodcock Sound-Symbol Tests. Circle Pines, MN, American Guidance Service, 1974

Goodman R, Stevenson J: A twin study of hyperactivity, II: the etiological role of genes, family relationships and perinatal adversity. J Child Psychol Psychiatry 5:691–709, 1989

Goswami U, Bryant P: Phonological Skills and Learning to Read. Hillsdale, NJ, Erlbaum, 1990

Greeno JG: Number sense as situated in knowing in a conceptual domain. Journal of Research in Mathematics 22:170–218, 1991

Grigorenko EL, Wood FB, Meyer MS, et al: Susceptibility loci for distinct components of developmental dyslexia on chromosomes 6 and 15. Am J Hum Genet 60:27–39, 1997

Gross-Tsur V, Shalev RS, Amir N: Attention deficit disorder: association with familial-genetic factors. Pediatr Neurol 7:258–261, 1991

Hall SJ, Halperin JM, Schwartz ST, et al: Behavioral and executive functions in children with attention-deficit hyperactivity disorder and reading disability. Journal of Attention Disorders 1:235–247, 1997

Hallowell E: When You Worry About the Child You Love: Emotional and Learning Problems in Children. New York, Simon & Schuster, 1996

Halperin JM, Gittelman R, Klein DF, et al: Reading disabled hyperactive children: a distinct subgroup of attention deficit disorder with hyperactivity? J Abnorm Child Psychol 12:1–14, 1984

Halperin JM, Newcorn JH, Sharma V, et al: Inattentive and noninattentive ADHD children: do they constitute a unitary group? J Abnorm Child Psychol 18:437–449, 1990

Hamlett KW, Pellegrini DS, Connors CK: An investigation of executive processes in the problem solving of attention deficit disorder–hyperactive children. J Pediatr Psychol 12:227–240, 1987

Hammill DD, Larsen SC: Test of Written Language, 2nd Edition. Austin, TX, Pro-Ed, 1988

Hartsough CS, Lambert NM: Medical factors in hyperactive and normal children: prenatal, developmental, and health history findings. Am J Orthopsychiatry 55:190–201, 1985

Healy JM, Newcorn JH, Halperin JM, et al: The factor structure of ADHD items in DSM-III-R: internal consistency and external validation. J Abnorm Child Psychol 21:441–453, 1993

Hellgren L, Gillberg C, Gillberg IC, et al: Children with deficits in attention, motor control and perception (DAMP) almost grown up: general health at 16 years. Dev Med Child Neurol 35:881–892, 1993

Hellgren L, Gillberg IC, Bagenholm A, et al: Children with deficits in attention, motor control and perception (DAMP) almost grown up: psychiatric and personality disorders at age 16 years. J Child Psychol Psychiatry 35:1255–1271, 1994

Hoptman MJ, Davidson RJ: How and why do the two cerebral hemispheres interact? Psychol Bull 116:195–219, 1994

Howell R, Sidorenko E, Jurica J: The effects of computer use on the acquisition of multiplication facts by a student with learning disabilities. J Learn Disabil 20: 336–341, 1987

Humphries T, Koltun H, Malone M, et al: Teacher-identified oral language difficulties among boys with attention problems. J Dev Behav Pediatr 15:92–98, 1994

Hynd GW, Semrud-Clikeman M, Lorys AR, et al: Brain morphology in developmental dyslexia and attention deficit disorder/hyperactivity. Arch Neurol 47:919–926, 1990

Hynd GW, Lorys AR, Semrud-Clikeman M, et al: Attention deficit disorder without hyperactivity: a distinct behavioral and neurocognitive syndrome. J Child Neurol 6(suppl):S37–S43, 1991a

Hynd GW, Marshall RM, Semrud-Clikeman M: Developmental dyslexia, neurolinguistic theory and deviations in brain morphology. Reading and Writing: An Interdisciplinary Journal 3:345–362, 1991b

Hynd GW, Semrud-Clikeman M, Lorys AR, et al: Corpus callosum morphology in attention deficit-hyperactivity disorder: morphometric analysis of MRI. J Learn Disabil 24:141–146, 1991c

Ivry R: Cerebellar timing systems. Int Rev Neurobiol 41:555–573, 1997

Ivry RB, Keele SW: Timing functions of the cerebellum. J Cogn Neurosci 1:136–152, 1989

Jacobvitz D, Sroufe LA, Stewart M, et al: Treatment of attentional and hyperactivity problems in children with sympathomimetic drugs: a comprehensive review. J Am Acad Child Adolesc Psychiatry 29:677–688, 1990

Jordan NC: Clinical assessment of early mathematics disabilities: adding up the research findings. Learning Disabilities Research and Practice 10:59–69, 1995

Katz J: The use of staggered spondaic words for assessing the integrity of the central auditory nervous system. Journal of Auditory Research 2:327–337, 1962

Katz J, Wilde L: Auditory perceptual disorders in children, in Handbook of Clinical Audiology, 3rd Edition. Edited by Katz J. Baltimore, MD, Williams & Wilkins, 1985, pp 664–688

Kaufman AS: Intelligent Testing With the WISC-III. New York, Wiley, 1994

Keith RW, Engineer P: Effects of methylphenidate on the auditory processing abilities of children with attention deficit-hyperactivity disorder. J Learn Disabil 24: 630–636, 1991

Keith RW, Rudy J, Donahue PA, et al: Comparison of SCAN results with other auditory and language measures in a clinical population. Ear Hear 10:383–386, 1989

Kellogg RT: Psychology of Writing. New York, Oxford University Press, 1994

Kennedy H, Meisserel C, Dehay C: Callosal pathways and their compliancy to general rules governing the organization of corticocortical connectivity, in Neuroanatomy of the Visual Pathways and Their Development. Edited by Dreher B, Robinson SR. Boca Raton, FL, CRC, 1991, pp 324–359

Knights RM, Hinton GG: The effects of methylphenidate (Ritalin) on the motor skills and behavior of children with learning problems. J Nerv Ment Dis 148:643–653, 1969

Korkman M, Pesonen AE: A comparison of neuropsychological test profiles of children with attention deficit-hyperactivity disorder and/or learning disability. J Learn Disabil 27:383–392, 1994

Kosc L: Developmental dyscalculia. J Learn Disabil 7:46–58, 1974

Lahey BB, Applegate B, McBurnett K, et al: DSM-IV field trials for attention-deficit/hyperactivity disorder in children and adolescents. Am J Psychiatry 151:1673–1685, 1994

LaHoste GJ, Swanson JM, Wigal SB, et al: Dopamine D4 receptor gene polymorphism is associated with attention deficit hyperactivity disorder. Mol Psychiatry 1:121–124, 1996

Landau S, Milich R: Social communication patterns of attention-deficit-disordered boys. J Abnorm Child Psychol 16:69–81, 1988

Lapadat JC: Pragmatic language skills of students with language and/or learning disabilities: a quantitative synthesis. J Learn Disabil 24:147–158, 1991

Larsen JP, Hoien T, Odegaard H: Magnetic resonance imaging of the corpus callosum in developmental dyslexia. Cogn Neuropsychol 9:123–134, 1992

Larsen SC, Hammill DD: Test of Written Spelling, 3rd Edition. Austin, TX, Pro-Ed, 1994

Lerer RJ, Lerer MP, Artner J: The effects of methylphenidate on the handwriting of children with minimal brain dysfunction. J Pediatrics 91:127–132, 1977

Levine MD: Keeping a Head in School: A Student's Book About Learning Abilities and Learning Disorders. Cambridge, MA, Educator's Publishing Service, 1990

Levine MD: Educational Care: A System for Helping Children With Learning Problems. Cambridge, MA, Educator's Publishing Service, 1994

Levinson HN: The diagnostic value of cerebellar vestibular tests in detecting learning disabilities, dyslexia, and attention deficit disorder. Percept Motor Skills 71:67–82, 1990

Lewis C, Hitch GJ, Walker P: The prevalence of specific arithmetic difficulties and specific reading difficulties in 9- to 10-year-old boys and girls. J Child Psychol Psychiatry 35:183–292, 1994

Losse A, Henderson SE, Elliman D, et al: Clumsiness in children—do they grow out of it? A 10-year follow-up study. Dev Med Child Neurol 33:55–68, 1991

Lovett MW: Developmental dyslexia, in Handbook of Neuropsychology, Vol 7: Child Neuropsychology. Edited by Segalowitz SJ, Rapin I (Boller F, Grafman J, Series Editors). Amsterdam, Elsevier, 1992, pp 163–185

Lovett MW, Warren-Chaplin PM, Ransby MJ, et al: Training the word recognition skills of dyslexic children: treatment and transfer effects. Journal of Educational Psychology 82:769–780, 1990

Lovett MW, Borden SL, DeLuca T, et al: Treating the core deficits of developmental dyslexia: evidence of transfer-of-learning following strategy- and phonologically based reading training programs. Dev Psychol 30:805–822, 1994

Ludlow C, Rapoport J, Basich C, et al: Differential effects of dextroamphetamine on language performance in hyperactive and normal boys, in Treatment of Hyperactive and Learning Disordered Children. Edited by Knights R, Bakker D. Baltimore, MD, University Park Press, 1978, pp 185–205

Ludlow CL, Cudahy EA, Bassich C, et al: Auditory processing skills of hyperactive, language impaired and reading disabled boys, in Central Auditory Processing Disorders: Problems of Speech, Language, and Learning. Edited by Lasky EZ, Katz J. Baltimore, MD, University Park Press, 1983, pp 163–184

Marshall RM, Hynd GW, Handwerk MJ, et al: Academic underachievement in ADHD subtypes. J Learn Disabil 30:635–642, 1997

Martinussen R, Frijters J, Tannock R: Naming speed and stimulant effects in attention-deficit/hyperactivity disorder. Poster presented at the annual meeting of the American Academy of Child and Adolescent Psychiatry, Anaheim, CA, October–November 1998

McCall CA: Math computation difficulties in grade 7 and 8 students. Unpublished doctoral dissertation, University of Toronto, Ontario, Canada, 1999

McGee R, Partridge F, Williams S, et al: A twelve-year follow-up of preschool hyperactive children. J Am Acad Child Adolesc Psychiatry 30:224–232, 1991

McGee R, Bryant BR, Larsen SC, et al: Test of Written Expression (TOWE). Austin, TX, Pro-Ed, 1995

McHale K, Cermak SA: Fine motor activities in elementary school: preliminary findings and provisional implications for children with fine motor problems. Am J Occup Ther 46:898–903, 1992

Meyer MS, Wood FB, Hart LA, et al: Selective predictive value of rapid automatized naming in poor readers. J Learn Disabil 31:106–117, 1998

Morris RD, Stuebing KK, Fletcher JM, et al: Subtypes of reading disability: variability around a phonological core. Journal of Education Psychology 90:347–373, 1998

Muth KD: Solving arithmetic word problems: role of reading and computational skills. Journal of Educational Psychology 76:205–210, 1984

Narhi V, Ahonen T: Reading disability with and without attention deficit hyperactivity disorder: do attentional problems make a difference? Dev Neuropsychol 11:337–350, 1995

Nicolson RI, Fawcett AJ: Reaction times and dyslexia. Q J Exp Psychol A 47:29–48, 1994

Nicolson RI, Fawcett AJ, Dean P: Time estimation deficits in developmental dyslexia: evidence of cerebellar involvement. Proc R Soc Lond B 259:43–47, 1995

Nigg JT, Hinshaw SP, Carte ET, et al: Neuropsychological correlates of childhood attention-deficit/hyperactivity disorder: explainable by comorbid disruptive behavior or reading problems? J Abnorm Psychol 107:468–480, 1998

Offord DR, Boyle MH, Szatmari P, et al: Ontario Health Study: six-month prevalence of disorder and rates of service utilization. Arch Gen Psychiatry 44:832–836, 1987

Olson RK, Wise BW: Reading on the computer with orthographic and speech feedback. Reading and Writing: An Interdisciplinary Journal 4:107–144, 1992

Oosterlaan J, Logan GD, Sergeant JA: Response inhibition in AD/HD, CD, comorbid AD/HD+CD, anxious, and control children: a meta-analysis of studies with the stop task. J Child Psychol Psychiatry 39:411–425, 1998

Oram J, Fine J, Okamoto C, et al: Assessing the language of children with attention deficit hyperactivity disorder: role of executive function. American Journal of Speech-Language Pathology 8:72–89, 1999

Ornoy A, Uriel L, Tennenbaum A: Inattention, hyperactivity and speech delay at 2–4 years of age as a predictor for ADD-ADHD syndrome. Isr J Psychiatry Relat Sci 30:155–163, 1993

Pearson DA, Lane DM, Swanson JM: Auditory attention switching in hyperactive children. J Abnorm Child Psychol 19:479–492, 1991

Peeke S, Halliday R, Callaway E, et al: Effects of two doses of methylphenidate on verbal information processing in hyperactive children. J Clin Psychopharmacol 4: 82–88, 1984

Pelham WE: Pharmacotherapy for children with attention-deficit hyperactivity disorder. School Psychology Review 22:199–227, 1993

Pelham WE, Bender ME, Caddell J, et al: Methylphenidate and children with attention deficit disorder: dose effects on classroom academic and social behavior. Arch Gen Psychiatry 42:948–952, 1985

Pelham WE, Walker JL, Sturges J, et al: The comparative effects of methylphenidate on ADD girls and boys. J Am Acad Child Adolesc Psychiatry 28:773–776, 1989

Pelham WE, Greenslade KE, Vodde-Hamilton MA, et al: Relative efficacy of long-acting CNS stimulants on children with attention deficit-hyperactivity disorder: a comparison of standard methylphenidate, sustained-release methylphenidate, sustained-release dextroamphetamine, and pemoline. Pediatrics 86:226–237, 1990

Pelham WE, Vodde-Hamilton M, Murphy DA, et al: The effects of methylphenidate on ADHD adolescents in recreational, peer group, and classroom settings. J Clin Child Psychol 20:293–300, 1991

Pennington BF: Diagnosing Learning Disorders: A Neuropsychological Framework. New York, Guilford, 1991

Pennington BF: Genetics of learning disabilities. J Child Neurol 1(suppl):S69–S77, 1995

Pennington BF, Ozonoff S: Executive functions and developmental psychopathology. J Child Psychol Psychiatry 37:51–87, 1996

Pennington BF, Gilger J, Pauls D, et al: Evidence for major gene transmission of developmental dyslexia. JAMA 266:1527–1534, 1991

Pennington BF, Groisser D, Welsh MC: Contrasting cognitive deficits in attention deficit hyperactivity disorder versus reading disability. Dev Psychol 29:511–552, 1993

Perfetti CA: Reading Ability. New York, Oxford University Press, 1985

Pinheiro M: Tests of central auditory function in children with learning disabilities, in Central Auditory Dysfunction. Edited by Keith RW. New York, Grune & Stratton, 1977, pp 223–256

Pless IB, Taylor HG, Arsenault L: The relationship between vigilance and traffic injuries involving children. Pediatrics 95:219–224, 1995

Poteet JA: Informal assessment of written expression. Learning Disability Quarterly 3:88–98, 1980

Prifitera A, Saklofske D: WISC-III Clinical Use and Interpretation. San Diego, CA, Academic Press, 1998

Prizant BM, Audet LR, Burke GM, et al: Communication disorders and emotional/behavioral disorders in children and adolescents. J Speech Hear Disord 55:179–192, 1990

Psychological Corporation: Wechsler Individual Achievement Test. San Antonio, TX, Psychological Corporation, 1992

Purvis KL: Contrasting cognitive abilities in children with attention deficit hyperactivity disorder and reading disability. Unpublished doctoral dissertation, University of Toronto, Ontario, Canada, 1999

Purvis KL, Tannock R: Language abilities in children with attention deficit hyperactivity disorder, reading disabilities, and normal controls. J Abnorm Child Psychol 25:133–144, 1997

Rapport MD, Kelly KL: Psychostimulant effects on learning and cognitive function: findings and implications for children with attention-deficit hyperactivity disorder. Clin Psychol Rev 11:61–92, 1991

Rapport MD, DuPaul GJ, Stoner G, et al: Comparing classroom and clinic measures of attention deficit disorder: differential, idiosyncratic, and dose-response effects of methylphenidate. J Consult Clin Psychol 54:334–341, 1986

Reader MJ, Harris EL, Schuerholz LJ, et al: Attention deficit hyperactivity disorder and executive dysfunction. Developmental Neuropsychology 10:493–512, 1994

Reynolds CR: Critical measurement issues in learning disabilities. Journal of Special Education 18:451–456, 1986

Riccio CA, Hynd GW, Cohen MJ, et al: Comorbidity of central auditory processing disorder and attention-deficit hyperactivity disorder. J Am Acad Child Adolesc Psychiatry 33:849–857, 1994

Richardson E, Kupietz SS, Winsberg BG, et al: Effects of methylphenidate dosage in hyperactive reading-disabled children, II: reading achievement. J Am Acad Child Adolesc Psychiatry 27:78–87, 1988

Richman LC: Language-learning disability: issues, research, and future directions, in Advances in Developmental and Behavioral Pediatrics, Vol 4. Edited by Wolraich M, Routh DK. Greenwich, CT, JAI Press, 1983, pp 87–107

Rief SF: How to Reach and Teach ADD/ADHD Children. West Nyack, NY, Center for Applied Research in Education, 1993

Robins PM: A comparison of behavioral and attentional functioning in children diagnosed as hyperactive or learning disabled. J Abnorm Child Psychol 20:65–82, 1992

Rourke BP, Finlayson MAJ: Neuropsychological significance of variations in patterns of academic performance: verbal and visual-spatial abilities. J Abnorm Child Psychol 6:121–133, 1978

Russell RL, Ginsberg HP: Cognitive analysis of children's mathematics difficulties. Cognition and Instruction 1:217–244, 1984

Safer DJ, Krager JM: A survey of medication treatment for hyperactive/inattentive students. JAMA 260:2256–2258, 1988

Scarborough HS: Very early language deficits in dyslexic children. Child Dev 61:1728–1743, 1990

Schachar R, Logan G: Impulsivity and inhibitory control in normal development and childhood psychopathology. Dev Psychol 26:710–720, 1990

Schachar R, Tannock R: Childhood hyperactivity and psychostimulants: a review of extended treatment studies. J Child Adolesc Psychopharmacol 3:81–97, 1993

Schachar R, Tannock R, Logan G: Inhibitory control, impulsiveness, and attention deficit hyperactivity disorder. Clin Psychol Rev 13:721–739, 1993

Schachar R, Tannock R, Cunningham C: Treatment of childhood hyperactivity, in Hyperactive Disorders. Edited by Sandberg S. Cambridge, UK, Cambridge University Press, 1996, pp 433–476

Schain RJ, Reynard CL: Observations on effects of central stimulant drug (methylphenidate) in children with hyperactive behavior. Pediatrics 55:709–716, 1975

Seidman LJ, Biederman J, Faraone SV, et al: Towards defining a neuropsychology of attention deficit-hyperactivity disorder: performance of children and adolescents from a large clinically referred sample. J Consult Clin Psychol 65:150–160, 1997

Semrud-Clikeman M, Hynd GW, Novey ES, et al: Dyslexia and brain morphology: relationships between neuroanatomical variation and neurolinguistic tasks. Learning and Individual Differences 3:225–242, 1991

Semrud-Clikeman M, Biederman J, Sprich-Buckminster S, et al: Comorbidity between ADDH and learning disability: a review and report in a clinically referred sample. J Am Acad Child Adolesc Psychiatry 31:439–448, 1992

Semrud-Clikeman M, Filipek PA, Biederman J, et al: Attention-deficit hyperactivity disorder: magnetic resonance imaging morphometric analysis of the corpus callosum. J Am Acad Child Adolesc Psychiatry 33:875–881, 1994

Sergeant JA: A theory of attention: an information processing perspective, in Attention, Memory, and Executive Function. Edited by Lyon GR, Krasnegor NA. Baltimore, MD, Paul H Brookes, 1995, pp 57–69

Share DL, Moffitt TE, Silva PA: Factors associated with arithmetic-and-reading disability and specific arithmetic disability. J Learn Disabil 21:313–320, 1988

Shaywitz BA, Shaywitz SE: Learning disabilities and attention disorders, in Pediatric Neurology, 2nd Edition. Edited by Swaiman KF. St Louis, MO, CV Mosby, 1994, pp 1119–1151

Shaywitz BA, Fletcher JM, Shaywitz SE: A conceptual framework for learning disabilities and attention-deficit/hyperactivity disorder. Canadian Journal of Special Education Summer 1994

Shaywitz SE, Shaywitz BA: Attention deficit disorder: diagnosis and role of Ritalin in management, in Ritalin: Theory and Patient Management. Edited by Greenhill L, Osman B. New York, Mary Ann Liebert, 1991, pp 209–231

Shaywitz SE, Shaywitz BA, Fletcher JM, et al: Prevalence of reading disability in boys and girls: results of the Connecticut Longitudinal Study. JAMA 264:998–1002, 1990

Shaywitz SE, Escobar MD, Shaywitz BA, et al: Evidence that dyslexia may represent the lower tail of a normal distribution of reading ability. N Engl J Med 326:145–150, 1992

Sheslow D, Adams W: Wide Range Assessment of Memory and Learning. Wilmington, DE, Jastak Associates, 1990

Siegel LS: Evidence that IQ scores are irrelevant to the definition and analysis of reading disability. Canadian Journal of Psychology 42:202–215, 1988

Siegel LS: Dyslexic vs. poor readers: is there a difference? J Learn Disabil 25:618–629, 1992

Siegel LS, Linder BA: Short-term memory processes in children with reading and arithmetic disabilities. Dev Psychol 20:200–207, 1984

Siegel LS, Ryan EB: Reading disability as a language disorder. Remedial and Special Education 5:28–33, 1988

Siegel LS, Ryan EB: The development of working memory in normally achieving and subtypes of learning disabled children. Child Dev 60:973–980, 1989

Silver LB: Psychological and family problems associated with learning disabilities: assessment and intervention. J Am Acad Child Adolesc Psychiatry 28:319–325, 1989

Silver LB: The Misunderstood Child: A Guide for Parents of Children With Learning Disabilities, 2nd Edition. New York, McGraw-Hill, 1992

Smith SD, Pennington BF, Kimberling WJ, et al: Familial dyslexia: use of genetic linkage data to define subtypes. J Am Acad Child Adolesc Psychiatry 29:204–213, 1990

Smith SD, Pennington B, Fulker DW, et al: Evidence for a gene influencing reading disability on chromosome 6p in two populations (abstract). Am J Hum Genet 55:A203, 1994

Sokol SM, Macaruso P, Gollan TH: Developmental dyscalculia and cognitive neuropsychology. Developmental Neuropsychology 10:413–441, 1994

Sonuga-Barke EJS, Taylor E, Sembi S, et al: Hyperactivity as delay aversion, I: the effect of delay on choice. J Child Psychol Psychiatry 33:387–398, 1992

Stanovich KE: Explaining the variance in reading ability in terms of psychological processes: what have we learned? Annals of Dyslexia 15:67–96, 1986

Stanovich KE: Explaining the differences between the dyslexic and the garden-variety poor reader: the phonological-core variable-difference model. J Learn Disabil 21:590–604, 1988

Stanovich KE: Annotation: does dyslexia exist? J Child Psychol Psychiatry 35:579–595, 1994

Stanovich KE, Siegel LS: Phenotypic performance profile of children with reading disabilities: a regression-based test of the phonological-core variable-difference model. Journal of Educational Psychology 86:24–53, 1994

Stephens RS, Pelham WE, Skinner R: The state-dependent and main effects of methylphenidate and pemoline on paired-associates learning and spelling in hyperactive children. J Consult Clin Psychol 52:104–113, 1984

Stevenson J, Pennington BF, Gilger JW, et al: Hyperactivity and spelling disability: testing for shared genetic aetiology. J Child Psychol Psychiatry 34:1137–1152, 1993

Swanson HL: Working memory in learning disability subgroups. J Learn Disabil 20:3–7, 1993

Swanson JM, Cantwell D, Lerner M, et al: Effects of stimulant medication on learning in children with ADHD. J Learn Disabil 24:219–230, 1991

Szatmari P, Taylor DC: Overflow movements and behaviour problems: scoring and using a modification of Fog's test. Dev Med Child Neurol 26:297–310, 1984

Szatmari P, Offord DR, Boyle MH: Ontario Child Health Study: prevalence of attention deficit disorder with hyperactivity. J Child Psychol Psychiatry 30:219–230, 1989

Tannock R: Attention deficit hyperactivity disorder: advances in cognitive, neurobiological, and genetic research. J Child Psychol Psychiatry 39:65–99, 1998

Tannock R, Schachar R: Executive dysfunction as an underlying mechanism of behavior and language problems in attention deficit hyperactivity disorder, in Language, Learning and Behaviour Disorders: Developmental, Biological, and Clinical Perspectives. Edited by Beitchman JH, Cohen N, Konstantareas MM, et al. Cambridge, UK, Cambridge University Press, 1996, pp 128–155

Tannock R, Purvis K, Schachar R: Narrative abilities in children with attention deficit hyperactivity disorder and normal peers. J Abnorm Child Psychol 21:103–117, 1993

Tannock R, Corkum P, Schachar R, et al: Phonological processing in children with attention deficit hyperactivity disorder. Poster presentation at the Annual Child Psychiatry Day, The Hospital for Sick Children, Toronto, Ontario, Canada, February 1994

Tannock R, Ickowicz A, Oram J, et al: Language impairment and audiological status in ADHD: preliminary results. Poster presentation at the Annual Child Psychiatry Day, The Hospital for Sick Children, Toronto, Ontario, Canada, February 1995a

Tannock R, Ickowicz A, Schachar R: Differential effects of methylphenidate on working memory in ADHD children with and without comorbid anxiety. J Am Acad Child Adolesc Psychiatry 34:886–896, 1995b

Taylor E: The use of drugs in hyperkinetic states: clinical issues. Neuropsychopharmacology 18:951–958, 1979

Taylor E, Sandberg S, Thorley G, et al: The Epidemiology of Childhood Hyperactivity (Maudsley Monographs No 33). London, Institute of Psychiatry, 1991

Torgesen JK, Wagner RK: Alternative diagnostic approaches for specific developmental reading disabilities. Learning Disabilities: Research and Practice 13:220–232, 1998

Vandervelden MC, Siegel LS: Phonological recoding deficits and dyslexia: a developmental perspective, in Language, Learning, and Behavior Disorders: Developmental, Biological, and Clinical Perspectives. Edited by Beitchman JH, Cohen NJ, Konstantareas MM, et al. New York, Cambridge University Press, 1996, pp 224–246

Waber DP, Bernstein JH: Repetitive graphomotor output in learning-disabled and nonlearning-disabled children: the Repeated Patterns Test. Developmental Neuropsychology 10:51–65, 1994

Wade MG: Effects of methylphenidate on motor skill acquisition of hyperactive children. J Learn Disabil 9:443–447, 1976

Wagner RK, Torgesen JK: The nature of phonological processing and its causal role in the acquisition of reading skills. Psychol Bull 101:192–212, 1987

Wagner RK, Torgesen JK, Rashotte CA: Development of reading-related phonological processing abilities: new evidence of bidirectional causality from a latent variable longitudinal study. Dev Psychol 30:73–87, 1994

Warr-Leeper G, Wright NA, Mack A: Language disabilities of antisocial boys in residential treatment. Behavioral Disorders 19:159–169, 1994

Wechsler D: Manual for the Wechsler Intelligence Scale for Children—Third Edition (WISC-III). San Antonio, TX, Psychological Corporation, 1991

Weinberg WA, Emslie GJ: Attention-deficit hyperactivity disorder: the differential diagnosis. J Child Neurol 6(suppl):S23–S37, 1991

Weinberg WA, Harper CR, Brumback RA: Use of the Symbol Language and Communication Battery in the physician's office for assessment of higher brain functions. J Child Neurol 1(suppl):S23–S31, 1995

Weyandt LL, Willis WG: Executive functions in school-aged children: potential efficacy of tasks in discriminating clinical groups. Developmental Neuropsychology 10:27–38, 1994

Whalen CK, Henker B, Collins BE, et al: Peer interaction in a structured communication task: comparisons of normal and hyperactive boys and of methylphenidate (Ritalin) and placebo effects. Child Dev 50:388–401, 1979

Wilkinson GS: Wide Range Achievement Test–3. Wilmington, DE, Jastak Associates, 1993

Willeford J: Assessing central auditory behavior in children: a test battery approach, in Central Auditory Dysfunction. Edited by Keith R. New York, Grune & Stratton, 1977, pp 43–72

Wolf M: Naming speed and reading: the contribution of the cognitive neurosciences. Reading Research Quarterly 26:123–141, 1991

Wolraich ML, Lindgren S, Stromquist A, et al: Stimulant medication use by primary care physicians in the treatment of attention deficit hyperactivity disorder. Pediatrics 86:95–101, 1990

Wood FB, Felton RH: Separate linguistic and attentional factors in the development of reading. Topics in Language Disorders 14:42–57, 1994

Woodcock RW: Woodcock Reading Mastery Tests—Revised. Circle Pines, MN, American Guidance Service, 1987

Woodcock RW, Johnson MB: Woodcock-Johnson Psycho-Educational Battery—Revised. Allen, TX, DLM Teaching Resources, 1989

Woodcock RW, Mather N: Woodcock-Johnson Tests of Cognitive Ability: Manual. Allen, TX, DLM Teaching Resources, 1989

Woodcock RW, McGrue K, Werder J: Mini-Battery of Achievement. Chicago, IL, Riverside Publishing, 1994

Zentall SS: Production deficiencies in elicited language but not in the spontaneous verbalizations of hyperactive children. J Abnorm Child Psychol 16:657–673, 1988

Zentall SS: Fact-retrieval automatization and math problem solving by learning disabled, attention-disordered, and normal adolescents. Journal of Educational Psychology 82:856–865, 1990

Zentall SS, Gohs DE, Culatta B: Language and activity of hyperactive and comparison children during listening tasks. Exceptional Children 50:255–266, 1983

Zentall SS, Smith YN, Yung-Bin BL, et al: Mathematical outcome of attention-deficit hyperactivity disorder. J Learn Disabil 27:510–519, 1994

8 Learning Disabilities and Attention-Deficit/Hyperactivity Disorder in Adults: Overlap With Executive Dysfunction

Martha Bridge Denckla, M.D.

This chapter offers an exposition of current knowledge regarding the neurological basis of learning disabilities in adults. *Learning disabilities,* as defined here, are "difficulties in the acquisition *and use of*" any one of a number of skills, including academic reading, spelling, writing, and mathematics (Interagency Committee on Learning Disabilities 1987; emphasis added). The specification "and use of" a skill is particularly relevant to adults with learning disabilities.

Put another way, a learning disability is a circumscribed mental disability; persons with learning disabilities have impairment in a minority (rather than a majority, as is the case for persons with mental retardation) of cognitive modules encompassed by the mental status domain. For the behavioral neurologist, adults with learning disabilities more closely resemble patients with a focal insult to some part of the brain that subserves cognition than patients

---

This chapter is a revised version of an earlier article: Denckla MB: "The Child With Developmental Disabilities Grown Up: Adult Residua of Childhood Disorders." *Neurologic Clinics* 11:105–125, 1993. Used with permission of W. B. Saunders.

Preparation of this manuscript was supported, in part, by P50 HD25806. Grateful acknowledgment is made to Pamula D. Yerby for her help in the preparation of this manuscript.

with dementia. Unlike the adult with a focal insult and a well-localizable cognitive deficit, however, the adult with developmental learning disabilities presents not with a dramatic, high-contrast syndrome, but rather with subtle and often well-hidden deficits.

Some adults with well-documented childhood-onset learning disabilities may seek follow-up evaluation to determine the degree to which they have compensated for their disabilities and the degree to which they show residual difficulties. Other adults with learning disabilities are being referred for evaluation for the first time. These adults may self-refer because of what they have read or heard about learning disabilities or because other professionals, usually educators, psychologists, or psychiatrists, may suspect learning disabilities in them. Questions of whether adults have dyslexia or attention-deficit/hyperactivity disorder (ADHD) most commonly impel those whose learning disabilities have not been previously diagnosed to seek a behavioral-neurological evaluation. Still others are referred preponderantly by psychologists or psychiatrists who have been alerted to seek neurological factors in adults with a wide variety of psychosocial complaints or maladjustments. The adults in this group are not referred for specific academic underachievement as often as those in other age groups.

Adults with ADHD frequently seek a diagnosis because the disorder has been diagnosed in one of their children. These adults, after hearing or reading about the described characteristics of the child, may recognize themselves in the profile (Barkley 1991). Because ADHD is commonly associated with school failure, or at least academic underachievement, and its relationship with learning disabilities is intimately interwoven, it is virtually impossible to predict from the referral question whether the condition resembling ADHD (in a child or in an adult) will be just that, whether it will evolve into another unexpected cognitive deficit (what educators call a "processing deficit"), or whether it will turn out to be the surface presentation of a mixture of modular deficits. Conversely, dyslexia, as a starting point for referral, may turn out to be underachievement stemming from cognitive characteristics indistinguishable from those connected with the history-based diagnosis of ADHD. This situation is not unlike that familiar to behavioral neurologists who see adults with acquired deficits; a chief complaint, such as poor memory, may turn out to be indicative of aphasia, executive dysfunction, or memory deficit.

As with ADHD, adults may believe they have dyslexia because it has been diagnosed in one of their children. Or they may have inferred the possibility from a comment, provoked by the spelling or grammar in a term paper, from a college professor who has taught students with dyslexia. Or, perhaps, they may have been cued to the possibility by a comment from a mental health professional who picked up the possibility of dyslexia from the patient's school history or language characteristics (expressive or receptive) in therapy sessions.

As noted earlier, some adults with learning disabilities (still the smallest group of adults referred for evaluation of learning disabilities) are most often referred by mental health professionals. The diagnosis of these individuals' learning disabilities is difficult and largely inferential. These individuals are young, exhibit social ineptness and emotional disturbances, and usually are diagnosed with nonverbal learning disabilities or right-hemisphere dysfunction (Semrud-Clikeman and Hynd 1990).

Given that a broad range of intelligence, as well as disabilities, is represented by grouping learning disabilities together, it is not surprising that adult college students with learning disabilities (who are more likely to be women) have less severe deficits than adults with learning disabilities in vocational training (Minskoff et al. 1989; Zvi and Axelrod 1992). On the question of whether there are specific or consistent (from childhood) subtypes of learning disabilities, the literature is not concordant. Most adults with learning disabilities underachieve in both reading and arithmetic, with only a few individuals having a significant discrepancy in achievement between the two. Those who do show this discrepancy exhibit the predicted underlying cognitive profile: better linguistic ability predicts better reading skill, whereas better visuospatial ability predicts better arithmetic skill (McCue et al. 1986).

Studies that address the issue of learning disabilities that persist into adulthood indicate that a minority of adults maintain a profile similar to the one with which they presented 15 years earlier (Spreen and Haaf 1986). Children with linguistic impairments tend to exhibit global low achievement later in life, and this raises the possibility that linguistic factors often preclude compensation in the realm of academic achievement. In children with learning disabilities and visuospatial impairments, the deficits appear to persist into adulthood, with more selective underachievement in arithmetic/mathematics.

Neurological signs correlate with the severity of learning disabilities but not with any specific subtype; therefore, analysis based on psychoeducational discrepancy patterns does not give much support to the concept of stable, discrete subtypes of learning disabilities in adults (Spreen and Haaf 1986). Rather, the impact over time of underlying cognitive processing deficits may be more revealing; the circumscribed mental disabilities (linguistic and visuospatial) may have longitudinal life histories that interact with other factors to determine which academic skill is deficient.

The sections that follow address dyslexia, ADHD, and nonverbal learning disabilities of the right hemisphere. First, dyslexia is examined in its adult incarnation, because this disorder has received the most intense focus in the research literature. In the section on ADHD, the impact of the executive function factor is examined as one important codeterminant of adult outcome. The concluding section describes cognitive impairments of adults with nonverbal learning disorders as these shape social-emotional functioning.

DYSLEXIA IN ADULTS

The term *dyslexia* antedates the vocabulary of learning disabilities and is linked conceptually to neurological syndromes of alexia. Before specific measurements of aptitude and achievement and calculations of discrepancies between them were introduced, the clinical diagnosis was largely one of exclusion (e.g., "unexpected reading failure"), embellished by personal and family history of difficulties with speech, language, reading, spelling, and foreign language acquisition. These embellishments were built up from the converging clinical experiences being reported in the lay press.

Later, clinical data inspired a generation of research that documented multifaceted language-related deficits in dyslexia—deficits in naming, repetition, syntax, and verbal working memory—all of which may emanate from deficient phonological representation, a circumscribed language weakness (Vellutino and Denckla 1991). It is striking that such convergence of clinical findings was reached, especially since researchers used very different population samples and widely different criteria for dyslexia.

Research on adults with dyslexia indicates that dyslexia is likely to be not only a specific language disability (language affected, nonlanguage spared) but also a disorder that affects specific aspects of language. This suggests that generic language development may be unimpeachable and that there may be impairment in the orthographic-phonological interface—the portion of language in which written language must be built on oral. There is still room for heterogeneity in the mechanism whereby this interface may fail to develop smoothly, but such heterogeneity may be still more microscopic than it is when subtyped under language disorders. Conversely, because the orthographic-phonological interface is so focal and detailed in cognition, totally nonlinguistic endowments—attention and executive function—may be crucial for its operative integrity.

The Genetics of Dyslexia

The study of adults has, for obvious reasons, been necessary for pinpointing the genetics of dyslexia. Familial occurrence has been known since early this century but within the past decade evidence has moved from familial data to data supporting genetic heterogeneity in the transmission of dyslexia. Recent research points to a partially dominant major gene or genes (Pennington 1990). Chromosome 15 and chromosome 6 have received attention. The former is significantly linked with markers in apparently dominantly transmitting families; the latter is more linked with Geschwind's theory that immune system–related human leukocyte antigen (HLA) regions may be linked. Behaviorally, spelling and phonological coding are demonstrably more heritable than reading per se or orthographic coding. There is much convergence among researchers on the validity of neuropsychological analyses of what most significantly predicts unexpected reading difficulty and what is heritable (i.e., the phonological coding deficit). It is estimated that 30% of the cognitive phenotype in poor reading is heritable and, again, that the phonological coding domain is primarily responsible (Pennington 1990).

Varieties of Dyslexia

Clinically, the research literature is valid. The heterogeneity among adults who had or who still have dyslexia comes from either the depth (historical evidence) or breadth (evidence from current assessment) of language disorder as well as from evidence of inadequate attention and executive function. Not all language disorders are equal in their impact on reading; paradoxically, some adults with the most profoundly impairing language disorders (receptive), which affect comprehension in daily life and certainly in academic pursuits, may read quite adequately, in the sense of decoding the printed word. As reading material increases in linguistic complexity, these adults fail to comprehend what they read; however, their comprehension does not improve when listening to the same material.

In contrast, adults with dyslexia who have no history or current evidence of receptive or expressive-semantic spoken language disorder may comprehend text far better than they can read text aloud. Such adults, who are often described as "very verbal" and who characteristically are slow readers, describe themselves as capable of learning through lectures or discussions. Although the phonological inefficiencies of adults with "pure" dyslexia may result in imprecise pronunciation, hesitant word retrieval, and even some difficulty with rote memorization, the language deficit is subtle outside academic, book-oriented pursuits.

On the other hand, dyslexia-plus, which spreads beyond the verbal or linguistic domain, is a difficult issue to avoid even in adults. The term *dys-*

lexia-plus was introduced by Denckla and Hughes to refer to the overlap between dyslexia and attention deficits (not necessarily full-blown ADHD but impairment along the attention–executive function dimension of cognition) (Denckla 1978). The dyslexia-plus issue, a persistent source of confusion in the literature concerning childhood cases, does not disappear in the adult population. Dyslexia-plus has not yet been systematically investigated as a contributor to compensation-resistant adult dyslexia, but such investigation is under way. The model for dyslexia-plus as a persistent adult state is that mild to moderate phonological deficits require good to excellent attention–executive function resources as mediating variables in compensation. Reports of "cures" for adult dyslexia with stimulant medication are likely to reflect amelioration of the attention factor in compensation in dyslexia-plus cases.

Diagnostic Issues

When adult patients with no history or documentation of dyslexia (or even dysreading difficulties) present for the first time and ask whether they have dyslexia, how might the clinician approach diagnosis? The most reasonable way to proceed is to investigate personal and family history and, on assessment, neuropsychological (cognitive) deficits reported in the literature. Contrary to what may appear to be common sense, reading tests per se will not help clinicians make the diagnosis, because an adult without prior documentation of dyslexia is unlikely to show the clear discrepancy between aptitude and achievement enshrined in the more straightforward literature on childhood dyslexia.

Adults whose dyslexia is subtle may demonstrate to clinicians a belief in what may be called, somewhat ironically or facetiously, "the right to be dyslexic," implying that current overload is causing decompensation. Clinicians must seek, first, a suggestive (rarely well-documented) history of family members who allegedly underachieve in reading, spelling, or foreign-language study. Spelling is one of the most useful residual areas of adult deficit in the detection of subtle dyslexia (M. Rutter, personal communication, 1991); therefore, getting written samples from family members may be the most telling. Personal history of delayed or peculiarly imprecise speech (the latter difficult to get from any but the most sophisticated families) and recollections of struggle with reading acquisition (e.g., "I didn't read until the fourth grade") and especially spelling may be helpful.

The most usual marker for a diagnosis of dyslexia is the individual's personal recognition of slow, effortful reading even after he or she appeared to have accomplished reading acquisition. Finding out that a patient needs to look up simple words repeatedly and has difficulty mastering a foreign language is helpful to clinicians. Sometimes teachers, family members, or other professionals add observations about the patient's "illiterate appearing" written expression or difficulty following syntactically complex sequential directions. Such difficulties are usually of recent onset and related to heavy reading requirements or timed multiple-choice tests such as SATs, LSATs, or even medical or law board examinations.

On assessment, the adult with subtle dyslexia usually does well on tests related to spatial cognition, including perception, reproduction, construction, and memory of heavily configurational visual presentations. In contrast, these adults show deficiencies in confrontation naming, sentence repetition, phonologically based word fluency (e.g., naming all the words that rhyme with eel in 1 minute), and memorization that involves phonological word mixing. More variable is a relative deficiency in unraveling complex syntax, yet a substantial number of adults with subtle dyslexia show long latencies when interpreting the syntax correctly and relatively low scores on tests with passive constructions, embedded clauses, and multiple conditional clauses. (This syntactic subdomain of linguistic competence has not yet received the research scrutiny it merits.)

Errors made by an adult with dyslexia are similar to errors made by adults with "deep" dyslexia. The term *deep dyslexia* is used in the literature to describe adults who read "deeply" beneath the phonology to semantic fields, rather than responding to the speech sound level (e.g., "cake" is substituted for "cookies" and "dog" for "puppy"). On tests of memorization (e.g., California Verbal Learning Test), for example, "jacket" may be recalled as "coat." On tests of confrontation naming, similar substitutions may be mingled with phonological distortions and, most common, circumlocution in the form of descriptions of the depicted item's function. Semantic word fluency (e.g., demonstrated by naming a category of items for 1 minute) may be far superior to controlled word association ("F-A-S" lists) and rhyming. Repetition, especially of nonsense words or meaningless sentences, will bring out the phonological processing deficit. Narrative speech (as patients give their history) may also provide telling examples of phonological imprecision. (For example, one intelligent college graduate, attempting the expression "I am loathe to admit," said, "I am woe to admit.") Written samples done in the clinician's office under time pressure may bring out spelling, grammar, and word-usage deficiencies no longer seen in written work.

Taking into account all these subtle deficiencies together with historical clues, the clinician arrives at a diagnostic formulation that characterizes the patient as showing the underlying neurobiological weaknesses that add up to "the right to be dyslexic" under stress. The recommendations are usually for nonstandard (e.g., extended time) test administration and rearranging course load to accommodate slower reading. Career counseling and cognitive therapy focusing on personal goals often emanate from discussion with the adult with newly diagnosed dyslexia.

ADHD IN ADULTS

Strictly speaking, it is not permissible to make a de novo diagnosis of ADHD in adults; only ADHD documented in childhood is permissible (Barkley 1991; Kane et al. 1990). As is the case with dyslexia, adults seek diagnosis based most often on articles they read in the lay press, information they obtained from radio or television shows, or the diagnosis of ADHD in their own child (on the basis of which it is easier to make a neurobiological case for ADHD historically). However, on direct assessment, most of these adults may prove to have subtle impairment. Without a childhood history convincingly characteristic of ADHD, the differential diagnosis in the adult patient is difficult because of the frequency in which a variety of psychiatric disorders are associated with impaired attention and because of the genuine comorbidity of ADHD with affective disorders, alcoholism, and conduct disorder.

Even in the hands of experts, however, it is difficult to rely solely on the patient's memory or description of current events. Many adults attended school before their teachers' comments about their behavior were reported in terms that can translate into current ADHD constructs; therefore, school records frequently are not useful. Parents, siblings, friends, and spouses are useful for interviewing and filling out rating scales. Barkley (1991) compared the scores of adults with the norms for 16-year-olds on the Child Behavior Checklist and 17-year-olds on the Conner Parent Rating Scale—Revised. Direct assessment of attention and closely related neuropsychological characteristics is not sufficient for making a differential diagnosis, because many psychiatric disorders that either coexist with or are the sole correct alternative to ADHD will result in the same set of impairments (Denckla 1991b; Kane et al. 1990). For example, head injury (very common as a complication of ADHD) is often the source of frontal lobe deficits. Therefore, although useful for understanding learning disabilities and planning the patient's treatment, assessment cannot rescue the clinician from the diagnostic dilemma of whether or not the adult has the disorder known as ADHD (Barkley 1991; Kane et al. 1990).

Some critics question whether a syndrome as common as ADHD should be considered a disorder. This is an example of a more pervasive problem that plagues the study of all developmental disorders without retardation: Are these disorders per se or, in each instance, the extreme end of a continuous distribution? The issue of categorical versus dimensional understanding of dyslexia, ADHD, or any learning disability is beyond the scope of this chapter. I believe, however, that if an extreme position on a distribution causes an individual to experience distress, by analogy to mental retardation, it is equivalent to a disorder.

Neuroanatomic research has just begun to elucidate the neurobiology of adult ADHD. Functional neuroimaging, using positron emission tomography technology, of adults with ADHD who were selected because they are parents of well-studied children with ADHD has demonstrated an overall 8% reduction in metabolism during an attention task compared with the metabolism of control subjects. The hypometabolism was most striking in the right frontal region (Zametkin et al. 1990). Because of the difficulty inherent in diagnosing ADHD in adults, this remains the only published study on in vivo localization of attention deficit in this population.

What can be gleaned from the electrophysiological literature on adult ADHD often must be "backed into" by means of post hoc analyses within groups of adults with dyslexia. Thus, failure to mobilize frontal attention systems (as indicated by frequency band shifts or reduced amplitude of P300, a late-component evoked potential) has been reported in dyslexia-plus subgroups in populations of adults with dyslexia (Duncan et al. 1994; Rumsey et al. 1989). Along the dimension implied by dyslexia-plus (i.e., attention impairment, even if subjects are not overtly in the category ADHD), electrophysiological studies of adults implicate anterior brain regions classically associated not only with attention but also with effortful processing.

The neurobiological status of adult ADHD is supported by genetic approaches (Barkley 1991; see also Chapter 2, this volume). The cross-generational symptomatic similarity has already been noted (with the child-to-parent chain of clinical referral as a frequent starting point), and studies now indicate that 20%–32% of siblings and parents of persons with childhood ADHD also share ADHD characteristics. Twin studies support a genetic component; identical twins were concordant for hyperactivity and inattention much more frequently than fraternal twins (Barkley 1991; see also Chapter 2, this volume). The heritability for ADHD has been estimated as 30%–50%, with environmental factors accounting for 10% of the variance in ADHD traits. Only a small minority of ADHD appears to be accounted for by disease or injury to the nervous system independent of genetic predisposing factors (Kane et al. 1990).

The most reliable source of our understanding of ADHD remains the literature on follow-up of individuals in the known childhood-onset group as they moved into adolescence and adulthood. The bulk of this research has been summarized by Weiss and Hechtman (1986) and Hechtman (see Chapter 14, this volume). ADHD symptoms persisted in 50%–65% of those followed into young adulthood (30 years or younger). Twenty-five percent to 45% expressed some antisocial behavior, with the lower figure (25%) referring to those who qualified for a diagnosis of antisocial personality disorder. In the 12% who abused substances, alcohol was the most likely substance to be abused; this proportion of the sample overlapped with the 25% with antisocial conduct by 50% (Weiss and Hechtman 1986). Substance abuse in early adulthood tended to lessen with time; therefore, by their mid-20s, members of the ADHD groups and control groups did not differ.

The relevance of ADHD to learning disabilities is supported by evidence of underachievement in the follow-up groups. The magnitude of academic failures among siblings in adulthood differed even more significantly from that among children with ADHD (Gittelman et al. 1985; Weiss and Hechtman 1986). Only 5% of children with ADHD earned a college degree. Employment, less skilled than if education had been pursued successfully, appeared to be more satisfactory among young adults with ADHD as long as they were supervised. Employers tended to rate adults with ADHD as less able to work independently, less persistent in task completion, and less likely to get along well with supervisors. Adults with ADHD changed jobs (both by quitting and by being laid off) more frequently than control subjects; they also changed residence more frequently than control subjects (Weiss and Hechtman 1986). Therefore, their adult instability with respect to jobs and homes constituted adult hyperactivity, drawn on the larger canvas, as it were, of an adult time and place matrix. Physical height and weight, regardless of childhood treatment with stimulant medication, was not found to be significantly different from that of other adults (Gittelman et al. 1985; Weiss and Hechtman 1986).

If childhood aggressivity is factored out of the follow-up studies, antisocial and emotionally unstable outcomes drop out of the profile of adults with ADHD. Predictors of the highest educational level completed turned out to be a combination of childhood intelligence, parental socioeconomic status, parental child-rearing style, emotional climate of the home, and severity of the child's ADHD symptoms. No single element of a child's ADHD characteristics predicted good adult outcome (i.e., the 35%–50% who will have "normal" functioning); however, a high level of intelligence and the absence of aggressivity (within the individual) combined with favorable family environment (around the individual) to predict benign adult status (Gittelman et al.

1985; Weiss and Hechtman 1986). The entire group remains at greater risk for academic problems and ultimate underachievement, educationally and hence vocationally, than for any other kind of outcome (Kane et al. 1990; Weiss and Hechtman 1986).

Probably the most important cognitive characteristics affecting outcome in people with ADHD are those I have discussed elsewhere as "executive dysfunction" (Denckla 1991b, 1991c, 1994, 1996a, 1996b; Denckla and Reader 1992). These impairments, over and above intelligence measures and emotional stability indicators, best explain why adults with ADHD may be regarded as having learning disabilities. Executive dysfunction is the zone of overlap between ADHD and learning disabilities. Adults are expected to have full executive functional capacity, regardless of intelligence; the use of these critical capacities is limited by ADHD.

Briefly, executive dysfunction refers to a neuropsychological weakness, hypothesized to originate from dysfunction of the frontal lobes or of its interconnected regions, which results in impairments in a variety of abilities that can have both academic and interpersonal consequences. These problems involve the cognitive competencies of selective and sustained attention, inhibition of verbal and nonverbal responses, strategic memorization, organization, self-monitoring, planning and sequencing of complex behaviors, and management of time and space. The onset is often first noted in childhood or adolescence and appears to have a chronic course, although it is unknown whether some "outgrow" executive dysfunction (Denckla 1991b, 1991c, 1994, 1996a, 1996b; Denckla and Reader 1992).

These problems are endemic but not restricted to populations "officially" identified as having learning disabilities or ADHD or populations at risk for either of these disorders, including those with Tourette syndrome. In fact, the relationship between executive dysfunction and certain types of developmental disabilities appears to overlap. That is, executive dysfunction appears to be common in those who are diagnosed with ADHD, although there are children and adults who have executive dysfunction without ADHD. Executive dysfunction unaccompanied by ADHD appears to be particularly common in bright children with learning problems (with or without an identifiable learning disability) and in adolescents and adults who underachieve. The implications for psychosocial adjustment are important.

The term *executive dysfunction* refers to dysfunction in the system within the brain that engages in cognition control and future-oriented processes. Impairment of this system can wreak havoc on the affected individual. Consider the professional whose job includes both administrative and clinical responsibilities. A typical workday might include numerous appointments, telephone calls in various stages of being processed, incidental consultations or chats, and, of course, emergency situations. In addition, the same individual might be juggling domestic and personal responsibilities that require performing countless home-based tasks, including organizing meals, coordinating schedules of various family members, picking up children at various locations, monitoring the whereabouts of adolescents, trying to regulate finances, and finding time for family and friends. The relatively successful person uses schedules, organizes his or her time, sets priorities, concentrates on completing tasks, and minimizes inefficiency in his or her use of time. In other words, the individual depends on what is called "executive functioning."

The adult with executive dysfunction might be very intelligent but nonetheless inefficient—a person who seems to go through his or her day in a very nonproductive manner. Such a person might be unsure about what is due from subordinates or what is owed to superiors; he or she might play "telephone tag" all day and never return all phone calls. He or she might be very distractible and, during a meeting, shift from one activity to another, allowing outside interruptions (e.g., extraneous phone calls and unexpected visitors) or going off on a tangent (e.g., reacting to thoughts immediately). Although the person might be a charming individual and a brilliant colleague, his or her inefficiency may infuriate others. A demanding job might take substantially longer or be performed in an inferior manner, both qualitatively and quantitatively. At home, such a person forgets to pay taxes and bills, renew registrations and licenses, or show up at social functions. The individual with executive dysfunction often refers to the problem as always being "a day late and a dollar short."

Executive dysfunction is easier to diagnose than ADHD in adults because adult-normed neuropsychological tests and measures (Denckla 1991b; Denckla and Reader 1992) are available. Deviance can be documented in all but a handful of brilliant persons who can pass any short-term test. The diagnosis of executive dysfunction is usually made after completion of a battery of neuropsychological tests, which includes tests that tap the executive dysfunction construct. Conceptually relevant neuropsychological measures, or, more specifically, selected scores from several neuropsychological measures, are used to help characterize the patient. The measures/scores most frequently include 1) the Wisconsin Card Sorting Test (Heaton et al. 1991) (number of perseverations, set breaks, and categories); 2) a 20-minute continuous performance test (Greenberg et al. 1999) (errors of omission and commission, average reaction time, variability in reaction time, and comparison of all scores on the first and second half of administration); 3) the Rey-Osterreith Complex Figure (Bernstein and Waber 1996) (organization score derived from the copy and two delayed recalls); and 4) word fluency (Benton et al. 1978) (perseverations and rule breaks). For adults, the interference score from the Stroop Color-Word Test (Golden 1978) and the process-related scores (clustering, intrusions, and perseverations) from the California Verbal Learning Test (Delis et al. 1994) are used.

These various scores can be organized or clustered in several ways, such as by dividing them into higher executive function abilities (interference control, organization, and strategy utilization) or into more basic neuropsychological abilities, including focusing, shifting, sustaining, or dividing attention. The actual diagnosis is contingent on the quantitative scores, the qualitative nature of performance, and a brief neurological examination. The neurological examination is useful inasmuch as the results are neighborhood signs of control and inhibition, because the motor system is physically located in proximity to the frontal lobes and its interconnected regions, including the basal ganglia. Persistent immature patterns, such as extraneous associated overflow, contribute to characterizing adults as disinhibited or disorganized in basic ways, not susceptible to much psychodynamic interpretation (Denckla 1991b; Denckla and Reader 1992).

Many adults who present themselves for diagnosis of learning disabilities, even with the question of whether they may have dyslexia, turn out to have executive dysfunction on evaluation and history taking, even though they do not fulfill the Wender or Barkley criteria for ADHD (Kane et al. 1990; Spreen and Haaf 1986; P. Wender, personal communication, 1989). Frequently, the academic focus of the chief complaint masks a more general dishevelment in the patient's life. Executive dysfunction history must be elicited if it is not volunteered. Executive dysfunction revealed by assessment will inspire the clinician to probe for the relevant history; again, ADHD-related questionnaires and rating scales may not suffice.

These adults with executive dysfunction are academic underachievers who may have acquired all academic skills but fail to use them effectively. If some linguistic or spatial weaknesses are also present in the cognitive makeup of these individuals, the combined effect makes its impact on academic areas most affected by the weak domain of cognition, for which the individual with executive dysfunction fails to compensate. In other words, the dismissive cliché "everyone is a little bit learning disabled" may contain a grain of truth, because it is the combination of a relative cognitive weakness and executive dysfunction, rather than the relative cognitive weakness alone, that determines the academic shortfall of many adult patients seen in clinics. If the executive dysfunction is severe enough, underachievement may occur in the absence of any relative cognitive weakness.

In summary, adults whose learning disabilities combine linguistic dysfunction and executive dysfunction are by far the most common. In adults, pure linguistic deficits underlie dyslexia accompanied by academically poor language-related skills. Pure executive deficits underlie dyslexia with demonstrated global underachievement in which basic skills (e.g., reading, spelling, calculating, and writing) are usually spared. This underachievement gets progressively worse as these adults are required to perform more independent, integrated, and long-term assignments (in school or on the job).

NONVERBAL LEARNING DISABILITIES IN ADULTS

Nonverbal learning disabilities (NVLDs), sometimes referred to (with perhaps a premature inferential leap) as learning disabilities of the right hemisphere, are a complex group of disorders that occur less commonly than either dyslexia or ADHD (Tranel et al. 1987; Weintraub and Mesulam 1983). NVLDs overlap with ADHD or the construct of executive dysfunction because the anterior portion of the right hemisphere is suspected to be extremely important in subserving attention, orientation, and preparedness to underlie self-regulation and executive function. Much of what is written about NVLDs (whether overtly tied to the right hemisphere or not) involves executive dysfunctional descriptors (Rourke 1989; Rourke et al. 1986, 1989). Terms and phrases such as "spacy," "being in a fog," and "disorganized in a disoriented way" abound in the literature on NVLDs (see Semrud-Clikeman and Hynd 1990 for detailed review of the past 20 years of research contributions on this topic).

There is as yet no literature on the neuropathology, neuroimaging, neurophysiology, or neurogenetics of NVLDs. Adults with NVLDs are initially defined by what they do not have (i.e., dyslexia)—with their symptoms overlapping with ADHD, although not specifically announced to show this overlap—and are characterized neuropsychologically (Denckla 1991a; Tranel et al. 1987). From this perspective, Weintraub and Mesulam (1983) described a group of young adults who presented with social-emotional complaints but who were found to have left-sided motoric deficits and cognitive deficit profiles implicating right hemisphere involvement. Another neuropsychologist, Rourke, started, as special educators had, with index symptoms and signs of relatively isolated poor mathematical skills and expanded the characterization of the person from the academic to the socioemotional level (Rourke et al. 1989).

In Rourke's well-articulated model (Rourke 1989), primary tactile and visual perceptual deficits (hence the term "nonverbal") are the basis of the problems of adults with NVLDs. Also identified by Rourke as primary were deficits in complex psychomotor coordination, often more marked on the left side (as may be the sensory-perceptual deficits), and in impaired orientation to novelty. The deficits that adults with NVLDs show in their deployment of selective and sustained attention to tactile and visual input are called "secondary level" deficits. At a tertiary level, Rourke located tactile and visual memory deficits; impaired concept formation, generation of strategies, and problem solving; and impaired ability to flexibly explore novel or complex situations. Further, although these disabilities are described as nonverbal, Rourke found deficits in the right hemisphere–dependent types of verbal functions (prosody, pragmatics, and higher-order verbal representations) in this group.

The academic and socioemotional impairments in adults with NVLDs are, in Rourke's view, outgrowths of these hierarchically characterized neuropsychological deficits; motor aspects of speech and handwriting are the only deficits said to improve with age (Rourke et al. 1986). On the opposite end of the natural history of NVLDs, Rourke saw serious psychiatric risk of depression and suicide in adults followed by his clinic; he reported that adults with NVLDs experienced both vocational and social failure even when they were academically successful (Rourke et al. 1989). Thus, adults with NVLDs are not necessarily academic underachievers (except in subjects involving mathematics), but rather they tend to generate in themselves and others expectations for vocational and social achievement they cannot fulfill. Their most vulnerable moments occur when they complete education and attempt independent adult living, often failing (because of ineptitude in social skills) even in jobs less demanding than those for which their education would appear to qualify them (Rourke et al. 1986). It is the socioemotional component of the NVLD syndrome, rather than the mathematical learning disability, that leads to vocational and social failure, depression, and risk of suicide (Rourke et al. 1989; Voeller 1991).

People with NVLDs who do well academically but not socially are referred for evaluation for the first time as adults; however, the following items are lacking from the research-based characterization: 1) follow-up from childhood of those with index disability in arithmetic (later mathematics), and 2) operationalization of deficits at the primary, secondary, and tertiary levels of Rourke's model in neuropsychological status reports at crucial points in development. Until such follow-up is undertaken, it is not possible to determine how many of those first seen for specific arithmetic disorder will have such serious neuropsychiatric disabilities as adults. Another problem is that

Rourke's model is so behaviorally and anatomically inclusive (it is easy to discern executive function components) that those whom it describes seem to have nothing in their cognitive repertoire except a kind of linguistic savant status. Indeed, Rourke's concept does not confine NVLDs to the right hemisphere but includes white matter lesions widely dispersed through the brain as an underlying factor in the NVLDs (as in cases of head injury) (Rourke 1989).

A systematic epidemiological search for involvement of right-hemisphere systems might allow us to identify different subtypes of NVLDs (Denckla 1991a). If right anterior were found to be separated from right posterior and right-posterior perceptual functions were further subdivided, one might look for 1) a variety of executive dysfunction characterized by a particularly high level of disorientation, 2) a spatial disability (see Denckla 1991a), and 3) a social skills disability (see Voeller 1991). Without knowing at the outset whether the brain substrate would in fact turn out to be the right hemisphere, such neuropsychological fractionation would have the heuristic advantage of differentiating those at risk for serious psychiatric sequelae.

Only individuals with complicated or severe cases of NVLDs are likely to come to clinical attention; therefore, dire consequences implied by specific arithmetic disorder may be overestimated. If a person's specific arithmetic disorder is based on spatial disability, he or she may present to a clinic only if the disorder coexists with executive dysfunction that precludes elaboration of compensatory strategies (Denckla 1991a). Individuals with spatial disability and early signs of mathematical ineptitude who nevertheless possess sufficient executive function to compensate for them may never arrive at a clinic for treatment of learning disabilities. Their spatial disability may impair them in ways that do not trigger referral for evaluation because the impairments are likely to be nonacademic and, hence, dismissed as "lack of talent." Those who exhibit social ineptness are most likely to be ignored until emotional distress is evident and they are sent to mental health facilities (Rourke et al. 1986, 1989; Voeller 1991; Weintraub and Mesulam 1983).

Behavioral neurologists and neuropsychologists, therefore, are biased toward seeing only adults with NVLDs whose referral is determined primarily by having the most inclusive set of cognitive impairments. The greatest difficulty in making the differential diagnosis of NVLDs is simultaneously distinguishing depressive overlay (Brumback and Weinberg 1990) and separating learning disabilities from autistic spectrum disorders, in which social skills are markedly deficient (Voeller 1991). At present, the diagnostician must rely heavily on history (i.e., the past and developmental trajectory of the individual) in clearing away the depressive and autistic overlaps to discern the NVLD.

Adults with NVLDs who unequivocally have neither depression nor autistic-like behaviors still demonstrate core cognitive impairments. Such adults have been noted, by both educators and neuropsychologists, to manifest not only visuospatial difficulties but also deficient visualization, visual imagery, and configurational processing even when no external perception is involved. Having an overly local and partly oriented cognitive style, such adults manifest "forest for trees disease"—that is, they miss the "big picture" and get stuck on detail. Despite good verbal skills, they write poorly because they do not summarize or relate pieces of information. Asked for the main idea, the overarching concept, or the hierarchy (rather than the sequence) of priorities inherent in academic or vocational material, the adult with NVLD will be baffled (Denckla 1991a).

It is important to recognize these cognitive characteristics that invade verbally mediated adult pursuits, because, otherwise, the results of neuropsychological tests may be dismissed as relevant only to visuospatial activities such as art or carpentry, which the adult and his or her referring source may never have intended as vocational choices. Tests that are performed for neuropsychological assessment, such as copying designs, completing puzzles, and matching patterns, are perceived as remote from the postsecondary school or job requirements of adults with NVLDs. The tests may be more easily aligned with the experiences of these adults' getting lost, having difficulty with fitting furniture into rooms, or being unable to remember where possessions have been stored. In this sense, the adult with NVLDs is better able than the child with NVLDs (who does little or no independent travel or domestic organization) to correlate direct visuospatial assessment in the clinic with realistic activities.

The behavioral neurologist or neuropsychologist has to work hard to explain the workings, inside the "mind's eye" of the brain, of processes that hold thoughts, images, words, or external objects together simultaneously, visualize, rotate into various mental perspectives, and integrate elements of cognition in a way that is far from obvious and certainly not literally tactile or visual. In fact, as Rourke et al. (1986, 1989) pointed out, it is most difficult to understand and gain insight into the disabilities of adults with NVLDs.

Nevertheless, remedial academic approaches to help adults with NVLDs have been undertaken. Anecdotal evidence demonstrates that approaches involving verbal mediation have been modestly successful in helping adults with NVLDs compensate for deficient academic skills (comprehension of and writing about complex verbal material). Success usually depends on establishing a balance between verbal mediation and more global "grasp." Step-by-step formulas for actively encoding larger headings and classificatory schemata have been employed by some special education tutors, who reported improvement in the academic work of adults with NVLDs (Foss 1991). It is not known whether such strategies are being used flexibly and outside the field of special education tutoring or whether they can be generalized beyond the college setting.

Adults with NVLDs also need social cognitive training (Foss 1991; Rourke et al. 1986; Voeller 1991). Often imperceptive of the messages conveyed by the facial expressions, postures, and vocal tones of others, adults with NVLDs may antagonize and alienate superiors and peers (in school or at work). Social skills training is an underdeveloped special education undertaking at any age, but it is particularly so for adults. Tests of social cognition are not developed outside research laboratories. Mental health professionals, rather than special educators, even on college campuses, are likely to be charged with the treatment of social skills deficits, but the appropriate group setting in which this could be best accomplished is often lacking. Some one-to-one social skills training, mainly applicable to simulated teacher-student and employer-employee interactions, can be carried out in cognitive therapy by a mental health professional. No data are available on the effectiveness of this social skills training, especially because anecdotal case reports, the only available findings on such tests, do not precisely characterize the extent or severity of the patient's neuropsychological deficits, even when the lack of social-cognitive measures is taken into account.

Little progress has been made since 1983 in the clinical field of socio-emotional learning disabilities; therefore, "guilt by association" remains the method for diagnosis: neighborhood signs of left-sided motor deficit and nonlinguistic neuropsychological impairment, encompassing poor visuospatial and visuoconstructive skills. The degree to which executive dysfunction exists in adults who exhibit social ineptness is not known, much less whether in NVLDs executive dysfunction has a peculiarly disoriented presence because persons with these disorders are spatially and socially "out of it." The clinician, therefore, is limited to recognition of the existence of a type of learning disability, an NVLD, that is characterized better by what is spared—well-developed linguistic elements, rote verbal memory, basic reading (i.e., decoding), and spelling skills—than by what is deficient.

Subtypes within NVLDs have not yet been described, but the convergence of the ADHD literature on right frontostriatal dysfunction and NVLD elements (flexibility and organization) that seem to emphasize the cognitive overlap zone of executive dysfunction makes it likely that the vocabulary and perspectives from different fields may be obscuring underlying identities (i.e., neuropsychologists may not talk about ADHD; educators will not note left-sided signs). Characterizing each adult with an NVLD in nontheoretical, assessment-bound terms will certainly be more useful in developing the individual's treatment plan and also may prove to be a better contributor to the analysis of NVLDs in future research.

Instruments designed for determining whether ADHD is present should be given to patients with NVLDs; arithmetic or mathematical ineptitude on the academic testing side and social ineptitude on the psychosocial history side should be pursued if visuospatial deficit is documented. In addition, the examiner should be alert to the subtle impact of global and local and holistic and piecemeal cognitive imbalances on ostensible verbal thinking (classification, main idea summation, and appreciation of metaphor and humor). Finally, if endogenous rather than reactive depression is present, it is imperative to refrain from firm conclusions about NVLDs until the depression is treated, because many right-hemisphere neuropsychological profiles are, in part or in the main, expressions of a complex relationship between depressive mood and cognition, with neurotransmitters as the common mediator (Brumback and Weinberg 1990; Voeller 1991).

CONCLUSION

My clinic, which specializes in learning disabilities, receives referrals for adult assessments that parallel the three major reasons for referral in the pediatric and adolescent school-age population: to determine whether the patient has dyslexia, ADHD, or some kind of learning disability. The first, dyslexia, has the most secure neuroscientific background and in some ways the most straightforward conceptualization; yet it is still controversial in terms of the subtle and well-masked ways in which its manifestations may be seen. Aptly placed in the second and, hence, middle position, straddling dyslexia and learning disabilities, is that sprawling and emphatically heterogeneous collection of observations agglomerated under the rubric ADHD and affiliated with the pharmacotherapy of stimulants. Yet for all its sprawl, ADHD stands in relation to its cognitive overlap zone, executive dysfunction, as symptoms do to signs, and executive dysfunction, especially in adults, appears to be a cognitive-deficit cluster of special importance to the persistence of uncompensated or clinically significant learning disabilities.

The real question to be answered about adults with learning disabilities is, Why haven't they compensated for cognitive deficits, or if they have acquired basic academic skills, why haven't they been able to use these skills? Unless linguistic or spatial deficits are extremely severe, academic skills can usually be acquired by compensatory strategies and, once acquired, can be used. Ability to compensate (and to generalize the compensation) is crucial in determining outcome of adult learning disabilities. Less is understood about nonacademic skills, the social domain of which seems least optional (i.e., most pervasively important). Spatially based skills are the least difficult to avoid. With the exception of severe linguistic or spatial cognitive deficits, the most central neuropsychological issues in studies on learning disabilities in adults are executive dysfunction and social imperception and ineptitude. Much remains to be learned about assessing and treating these impairments, both of which may be important to adults who seek assessment for ADHD.

REFERENCES

Barkley RA: Attention deficit hyperactivity disorder. Psychiatric Annals 21:725–733, 1991

Benton AL, Hamsher D deS, Sivan AB: Multilingual Aphasia Examination, 3rd Edition—Manual of Instructions. Iowa City, IA, AJA Associates, 1978

Bernstein JH, Waber DP: Developmental Scoring System for the Rey-Osterreith Complex Figure—Professional Manual. Odessa, FL, Psychological Assessment Resources, 1996

Brumback RA, Weinberg WA: Pediatric behavioral neurology: an update on the neurologic aspects of depression, hyperactivity, and learning disabilities. Neurol Clin 8:677–703, 1990

Delis DC, Kramer JH, Kaplan E, et al: California Verbal Learning Test—Children's Version (CVLT-C). San Antonio, TX, Psychological Corporation, 1994

Denckla MB: Critique of EEG correlates of dyslexia, in Dyslexia: An Appraisal of Current Knowledge. Edited by Benton AL, Pearl D. New York, Oxford University Press, 1978, pp 243–249

Denckla MB: Academic and extracurricular aspects of nonverbal learning disabilities. Psychiatric Annals 21:717–724, 1991a

Denckla MB: Attention deficit hyperactivity disorder—residual type. J Child Neurol 6(suppl):S44–S48, 1991b

Denckla MB: Foreword, in Diagnosing Learning Disorders. Edited by Pennington BF. New York, Guilford, 1991c, pp vii–x

Denckla MB: Measurement of executive function, in Frames of Reference for the Assessment of Learning Disabilities. Edited by Lyon GR. Baltimore, MD, Paul H Brookes, 1994, pp 117–142

Denckla MB: Research on executive function in a neurodevelopmental context: application of clinical measures. Developmental Neuropsychology 12:5–15, 1996a

Denckla MB: A theory and model of executive function, in Attention, Memory and Executive Function. Edited by Lyon GR, Krasnegor NA. Baltimore, MD, Paul H Brookes, 1996b, pp 263–278

Denckla MB, Reader MJ: Educational and psychosocial interventions, in Handbook of Tourette Syndrome and Related Tic and Behavioral Disorders. Edited by Kurlan R. New York, Marcel Dekker, 1992, pp 431–451

Duncan CC, Rumsey JM, Wilkniss SM, et al: Developmental dyslexia and attention dysfunction in adults: brain potential indices of information processing. Psychophysiology 31:386–401, 1994

Foss JM: Nonverbal learning disabilities and remedial interventions. Annals of Dyslexia 41:128–140, 1991

Gittelman R, Mannuzza S, Shenker R, et al: Hyperactive boys almost grown up, I: psychiatric status. Arch Gen Psychiatry 42:937–947, 1985

Golden CJG: Stroop Color and Word Test (Cat. No. 30150M). A Manual for Clinical and Experimental Uses. Wood Dale, IL, Stoetling Publishing, 1978

Greenberg LM, Kindschi CL, Corman CL: Test of Variables of Attention—Clinical Guide. Los Alamitos, CA, Universal Attention Disorders, 1999

Heaton RD, Chelune GJ, Talley JL, et al: Wisconsin Card Sorting Test Manual—Revised and Expanded. Odessa, FL, Psychological Assessment Resources, 1991

Interagency Committee on Learning Disabilities: A Report to the U.S. Congress. Washington, DC, U.S. Government Printing Office, 1987

Kane R, Mikalac C, Benjamin S, et al: Assessment and treatment of adults with ADHD, in Attention Deficit Hyperactivity Disorder: A Handbook for Diagnosis and Treatment. Edited by Barkley RA. New York, Guilford, 1990, pp 613–654

McCue M, Goldstein G, Shelly C, et al: Cognitive profiles of some subtypes of learning disabled adults. Arch Clin Neuropsychol 1:13–23, 1986

Minskoff E, Hawks R, Steidle EF, et al: A homogeneous group of persons with learning disabilities: adults with severe learning disabilities in vocational rehabilitation. J Learn Disabil 22:521–528, 1989

Pennington BF: The genetics of dyslexia. J Child Psychol Psychiatry 31:193–201, 1990

Rourke BP: Nonverbal Learning Disabilities: The Syndrome and the Model. New York, Guilford, 1989

Rourke BP, Young GC, Strang JD, et al: Adult outcomes of central processing deficiencies in childhood, in Neuropsychological Assessment in Neuropsychiatric Disorders: Clinical Methods and Empirical Findings. Edited by Grand I, Adams KM. New York, Oxford University Press, 1986, pp 244–267

Rourke BP, Young GC, Leenaars AA: A childhood learning disability that predisposes those afflicted to adolescent and adult depression and suicide risk. J Learn Disabil 22:169–175, 1989

Rumsey JM, Coppola R, Denckla MB, et al: EEG spectra in severely dyslexic men: rest and word and design recognition. Electroencephalogr Clin Neurophysiol 73: 30–40, 1989

Semrud-Clikeman M, Hynd GW: Right hemispheric dysfunction in nonverbal learning disabilities: social, academic, and adaptive functioning in adults and children. Psychol Bull 107:196–209, 1990

Spreen O, Haaf RG: Empirically derived learning disability subtypes: a replication attempt and longitudinal patterns over 15 years. J Learn Disabil 19(3):170–180, 1986

Tranel D, Hall LE, Olson S, et al: Evidence for a right-hemisphere developmental learning disability. Dev Neuropsychol 3:113–127, 1987

Vellutino FR, Denckla MB: Cognitive and neuropsychological foundations of word identification in poor and normally developing readers, in Handbook of Reading Research, Vol II. Edited by Barr R, Kamil ML, Mosenthal P, et al. New York, Longman, 1991, pp 571–608

Voeller KKS: Social-emotional learning disabilities. Psychiatric Annals 21:735–741, 1991

Weintraub S, Mesulam M-M: Developmental learning disabilities of the right hemisphere: emotional, interpersonal, and cognitive components. Arch Neurol 40:463–468, 1983

Weiss G, Hechtman L: Hyperactive Children Grown Up. New York, Guilford, 1986

Zametkin AJ, Nordahl T, Gross M, et al: Cerebral glucose metabolism in adults with hyperactivity of childhood onset. N Engl J Med 323:1361–1366, 1990

Zvi JC, Axelrod LT: Learning disabled college students: an analysis of the factors emerging from initial assessment (abstract). J Clin Exp Neuropsychol 14:119, 1992

9 Attention-Deficit/Hyperactivity Disorder With Substance Use Disorders

Timothy E. Wilens, M.D.
Thomas J. Spencer, M.D.
Joseph Biederman, M.D.

The overlap between attention-deficit/hyperactivity disorder (ADHD) (the term as used here also refers to previous definitions of the disorder) and the addictive disorders has been the subject of increased interest (for reviews, see Kaminer 1992; Levin and Kleber 1995; Schubiner et al. 1995; Wilens et al. 1995, 1996). Both disorders are highly prevalent, severe neuropsychiatric conditions associated with high morbidity and disability. While ADHD affects 6%–9% of children and adolescents (Anderson et al. 1987; Bird et al. 1988; Safer and Krager 1988) and a sizable number of adults, the substance use disorders (including drug and alcohol abuse and dependence) affect 10%–30% of adults and a sizable number of juveniles (Kessler et al. 1994; Windle 1991).

Both disorders share several important characteristics. There appears to be similarity in the familiality of these two disorders. Although the etiology of ADHD remains unknown, family, adoption, and twin studies, as well as segregation analysis, have indicated that genetic risk factors may be operant in this disorder (Biederman et al. 1990, 1992; Faraone et al. 1992). Likewise, both familial/genetic and environmental risk factors appear to operate in the pathogenesis and maintenance of substance use disorders (Cadoret 1991; Cloninger et al. 1981; Kandel and Faust 1975; National Institute on Drug

Abuse 1991; Tsuang et al. 1996). High rates of comorbidity are also seen with each of these disorders. Adult and juvenile populations with substance use disorders have been shown to have elevated rates of psychopathology, including conduct and antisocial, mood, and anxiety disorders (Bukstein et al. 1989; DeMilio 1989; Groves et al. 1986; Kaminer 1991; Kashani et al. 1985; Ross et al. 1988; Rounsaville et al. 1991; Tarter and Edwards 1988), similar to the comorbidity reported with ADHD (Biederman et al. 1991, 1993). Conversely, adolescents and adults with psychiatric disorders appear to be at increased risk for substance use disorders (Christie et al. 1988; Kaminer 1991; Kashani et al. 1985; Mezzich et al. 1992). Hence, both substance use disorders and ADHD are major complex public health problems in themselves, and each confers additional risk for further psychopathology and morbidity.

The study of comorbidity between ADHD and substance use disorders is relevant to both research and clinical practice in developmental pediatrics, psychology, and psychiatry, with implications for diagnosis, prognosis, treatment, and health care delivery. The identification of specific risk factors of substance use disorders within ADHD may permit more targeted treatments for both disorders at earlier stages of their expression, potentially dampening the morbidity, disability, and poor long-term prognosis in adolescents and adults with this comorbidity. In the following sections, we present important associations between ADHD and substance use disorders.

ASSOCIATIONS BETWEEN ADHD AND SUBSTANCE USE DISORDERS

Comorbidity of ADHD and Substance Use Disorders

Substance use disorders occur at a higher rate in individuals with ADHD than in psychiatrically healthy adolescents; conversely, ADHD is more prevalent in individuals with substance use disorders. More recently, three studies incorporated structured psychiatric diagnostic interviews to assess ADHD and other disorders in substance abusing groups of adolescents. DeMilio and colleagues (see DeMilio 1989), applying DSM-III criteria, reported that one-quarter of 57 inpatient adolescents with substance use disorders had current ADHD as well as conduct and mood disorders. Similarly, in juvenile offenders there were significantly higher rates of ADHD in those with substance use disorders (23%) than in juveniles without substance use disorders (0%) (Milin et al. 1991). Additionally, higher rates of ADHD were reported in juveniles with drug abuse compared with those with alcohol abuse (Milin et al. 1991). In another study of psychiatric comorbidity in 52 inpatient adolescents with substance use disorders, 31% had ADHD, and no differences in the types of substances abused in the ADHD vs. non-ADHD groups of substance abusers were reported (Hovens et al. 1994). In these studies, higher rates of ADHD were reported in juveniles (i.e., those 18 years and younger) with drug use disorders than with alcohol use disorders, and mood disorders (depression and bipolar disorder) and disorders of juvenile delinquency (conduct disorder) were frequently observed in youths with ADHD and comorbid substance use disorders.

Findings from studies of adults with substance use disorders are similar to those from studies of adolescents in terms of comorbidity with ADHD (Table 9–1). For example, the rates of ADHD among adults with alcoholism ranged from 35% to 71% (Goodwin et al. 1975; Tarter et al. 1977; Wilens et al. 1995). From 15% to 25% of adults with addictions and alcoholic adults have current ADHD (Levin et al. 1997). Furthermore, adults with ADHD and comorbid substance use disorders have been reported to have substance use disorder of earlier onset and more severity than do adults with substance use disorders but no comorbid ADHD (Carroll and Rounsaville 1993; Levin et al. 1997; Wilens et al. 1997).

An overrepresentation of substance use disorders has also been consistently observed in studies of adults with ADHD. All eight investigations of adults with ADHD reported higher rates of substance use disorders in adults with ADHD than in the general population: alcohol abuse or dependence and drug abuse or dependence are present in 17%–45% and 9%–30% of adults with ADHD, respectively (Wilens et al. 1996). The risk of developing a substance use disorder over the life span among individuals with ADHD is nearly twice that among adults without ADHD (52% vs. 27%, respectively) (Biederman et al. 1995).

ADHD as Risk Factor for Substance Use Disorders

ADHD is a risk factor for substance use disorder; however, certain co-occurring behavioral disorders confer an even greater risk when co-occurring with ADHD. The association of ADHD and substance use disorder is particularly compelling from a developmental perspective, since ADHD manifests itself earlier than substance use disorder; therefore, substance use disorder as a risk factor for ADHD is unlikely.

Prospective studies of children with ADHD have provided evidence that

Table 9–1. Representative studies of ADHD in the context of substance use disorders

Study	*N*	SUD	Diagnostic criteria	Study group	ADHD rate (%)	Comment(s)
Goodwin et al. 1975	14[a]	Alcohol	Questionnaire	Adult male adoptees	71	Childhood ADHD diagnosis; criteria not well defined
Tarter et al. 1977	72	Alcohol	MMPI, Utah Criteria, questionnaire	Adult inpatients and outpatients	Elevated[b]	More severe and earlier-onset alcohol use with ADHD; diagnosis not well defined
Schuckit 1978	100	Multiple drugs	Semistructured questionnaire	Adults in residential treatment	17	Problematic assessments; high rate (53%) of ASPD; highly variable rate of ADHD based on criteria
Eyre et al. 1982	157	Opiates	Questionnaire, SADS	Adult outpatients	22	Retrospective; very high rate (91%) of CD
Wood et al. 1983	33	Alcohol	SADS, RDC, DSM-III criteria, Utah criteria	Adults in residential treatment	33	Small sample size; single interviewer; alcohol use not related to ADHD
R. D. Weiss et al. 1988	149	Opiates	DSM-III	Adult inpatients	5	Problematic assessments; low rates of ADHD
DeMilio 1989	57	Multiple	DSM-III-R, SCID	Adolescent psychiatric inpatients	21	Mixed population; no family data; high rates of CD (42%) and depression (35%)
Rounsaville et al. 1991, 1993	298	Cocaine	DSM-III-R SADS	Treatment-seeking adult outpatients	35	More severe and earlier-onset cocaine use with ADHD; high rates of CD (93%) and ASPD (47%)
Levin et al. 1996	294	Cocaine	DSM-IV SCID, SADS	Treatment-seeking adults	22[c]	Additional 15% with "late onset" ADHD-like symptoms

Note. All studies were cross sectional; longitudinal studies are not included in this table. ADHD = attention-deficit/hyperactivity disorder; ASPD = antisocial personality disorder; CD = Conduct Disorder; MMPI = Minnesota Multiphasic Personality Inventory; RDC = Research Diagnostic Criteria; SADS = Schedule for Affective Disorders and Schizophrenia; SCID = Structured Clinical Interview for DSM; SUD = substance use disorder. [a]Study included 119 control subjects. [b]Specific rate not reported. [c]Full or partial.

ADHD is a risk factor for substance use disorders (Table 9–2); however, the group with conduct disorder or bipolar disorder (characterized by severe moodiness, irritability, and mood swings) co-occurring with ADHD has the poorest outcome with respect to developing substance use disorders and major morbidity (Barkley et al. 1990; Biederman et al. 1997; Gittelman et al. 1985; Hechtman and Weiss 1986; Mendelson et al. 1971; Mannuzza et al. 1991, 1993; G. Weiss et al. 1985). For example, in 5- and 8-year follow-up studies, more alcohol use was found among adolescents with ADHD, most of whom had conduct disorder, than among control subjects without ADHD (Blouin et al. 1978; Satterfield et al. 1982). Moreover, our group found, as part of an ongoing prospective study of ADHD, differences in the risk for developing substance use disorders among adolescents with ADHD (mean age: 15 years) compared with control subjects without ADHD, with these differences accounted for by comorbid conduct or bipolar disorders (Biederman et al. 1997). Of interest, in the older siblings with ADHD, ADHD was found to be a risk factor for substance use disorders. These data support retrospectively derived data from studies of adults with ADHD indicating an earlier age at onset of substance use disorders in adults with ADHD compared with control subjects without ADHD (mean age: 19 vs. 22 years, $P < 0.01$) (Wilens et al. 1997) and findings among adults of substance use disorders of an earlier onset and more severe course associated with ADHD (Carroll and Rounsaville 1993).

Symptom clusters within ADHD that have been linked to later development of substance use disorders include aggression and impulsivity, with evidence of lessened risk of developing substance use disorders when these symptoms are reduced (Loney et al. 1981). The secondary problems caused by long-standing attention problems, resulting in underachievement and demoralization, also appear to mediate development of substance use disorders, albeit to a lesser degree.

High rates of ADHD-like symptoms are consistently reported in children who later develop substance use disorders. If ADHD is a risk factor for substance use disorders, then ADHD should be overrepresented in those children and adolescents who develop substance use disorders. Longitudinal research of children who later develop substance use disorders also indicates that ADHD may be an important antecedent in some individuals who develop substance use disorders. For instance, in the Chicago-based Woodlawn Study (Kellam et al. 1980), children who were rated as aggressive, impulsive, and inattentive as first-graders had higher rates of substance use 10 years later as adolescents. Although not clearly articulated in these studies, the patterns of behavior described are consistent with ADHD and other comorbidities commonly associated with ADHD.

Table 9–2. Longitudinal studies of substance use disorders in children with ADHD

Study	*N*	Instrument	Age at follow-up (study length)	Findings	Comment(s)
Mendelson et al. 1971	108	Questionnaires	12–16 years (2–5 years)	15% with excessive drinking	SUD correlated with continuation of aggression, impulsivity
Blouin et al. 1978	45 64 control subjects	Questionnaires, Conners rating scales, WRAT	14 years (5 years)	50% of adolescents with ADHD using alcohol more than once a month	Problematic assessments; comorbidity not assessed; problematic control
Hechtman and Weiss 1986	61 41 control subjects	SCID, SADS, GAS	21–23 years (15 years)	SUDs in ADHD: alcohol (16%), cocaine (5%), marijuana (6%); ASPD, 23%	SUDs largely found in subjects with ADHD and comorbid CD; males only assessed
Gittelman et al. 1985; Mannuzza et al. 1993	91 95 control subjects	DIS, SCID	23–30 years (13–19 years)	Drug dependence, 16%; alcohol dependence, 6%; ASPD, 18%	Low rate of ADHD persistence (8%); SUDs largely found in subjects with ADHD and comorbid CD
Barkley et al. 1990	123 66 control subjects	Conners rating scales, CBCL, SCID	12–20 years (8 years)	In ADHD: cigarettes (48%), alcohol (40%), marijuana (17%), stimulants (6%); SUD, 14%	High rate (44%) of CD in subjects with ADHD; SUDs largely found in subjects with ADHD and comorbid CD
Mannuzza et al. 1991	94 78 control subjects	DIS (parent and child versions), DSM-III-R criteria	16–21 years (8–14 years)	In ADHD: SUD, 30%	SUDs largely found in subjects with ADHD and comorbid CD; males only assessed
Biederman et al. 1997	128 120 control subjects	DSM-III-R (parent and child), Kiddie-SADS	16–21 years (4 years)	In ADHD and control subjects: 15% at mean age	Higher rates of SUD associated with comorbid CD; males only assessed

Note. ADHD = attention-deficit/hyperactivity disorder; ASPD = antisocial personality disorder; CBCL = Child Behavior Checklist; CD = Conduct Disorder; DIS = Diagnostic Interview Schedule; GAS = Global Assessment Scale; Kiddie-SADS = Child version of the Schedule for Affective Disorders and Schizophrenia; MMPI = Minnesota Multiphasic Personality Inventory; RDC = Research Diagnostic Criteria; SADS = Schedule for Affective Disorders and Schizophrenia; SCID = Structured Clinical Interview for DSM. SUD = substance use disorder; WRAT = Wide Range Achievement Test.

ADHD as Factor in Onset of Substance Use Disorders

ADHD is associated with an earlier onset of alcohol and drug use disorders and plays a role in particular pathways of their development and remission. Cigarette smoking in youths is often a gateway to more severe alcohol and drug use disorders (Kandel and Faust 1975). The literature suggests that juveniles with ADHD are at increased risk of cigarette smoking and substance use disorders during adolescence. In a sample of boys with ADHD, Milberger et al. (1997) demonstrated an increased risk for cigarette smoking (by age 15 years) that was heightened in those with comorbid bipolar disorder or conduct disorder.

ADHD influences the transition into and out of substance use disorders. ADHD was shown to be related to an acceleration in the transition from less severe alcohol or drug abuse to more severe dependence (1.2 years in individuals with ADHD vs. 3 years in control subjects; $P < 0.05$) (Wilens et al. 1998). Furthermore, ADHD heightens the risk of developing a drug use disorder, particularly in individuals with an established alcohol problem (Biederman et al. 1998). Although anxiety and depressive disorders comorbid with ADHD do not bestow additive risk for the development of substance use disorders, youths with ADHD and comorbid bipolar disorder or conduct disorder are at risk of developing substance use disorders very early in life (i.e., before 16 years of age). Adolescents and adults with ADHD prefer drugs to alcohol, with marijuana being the most commonly abused agent (Biederman et al. 1995). The aggregate literature indicates that youths with ADHD disproportionately become involved first with cigarettes, then alcohol, and finally drugs (Milberger et al. 1997).

ADHD also affects remission of substance use disorders. In a study of 130 referred adults with ADHD and 71 adults without ADHD, all of whom had a history of substance use disorders, the rate of remission and duration of substance use disorders differed significantly between the two groups (Wilens et al. 1998). The median time to remission of the substance use disorder was more than twice as long in individuals with ADHD as in control subjects (144 vs. 60 months, respectively), with the substance use disorder lasting over 3 years longer in the ADHD adults compared with their non-ADHD peers (Wilens et al. 1998). Hence, the aggregate data indicate that ADHD and associated conditions developmentally influence the onset of, transitions to, and recovery from SUD.

Familial and Genetic Factors in ADHD and Substance Use Disorders

Family studies are highly informative in examining the nature of the association between two co-occurring disorders. If, for instance, the relationship between ADHD and substance use disorders has a familial or genetic component, then family members of individuals (probands) with ADHD or a substance use disorder should be at elevated risk for the other disorder.

The higher prevalence of substance use disorders in the relatives of children with ADHD has been noted for many years. Elevated rates of alcoholism have been consistently found in the parents of youths with ADHD. Morrison and Stewart (1971) and Cantwell (1972), in independent studies, found elevated rates of alcoholism in the parents of youths with ADHD. The transmission of substance use disorders in families with ADHD remains under study, with family genetic studies showing a preferentially elevated risk of substance use disorders in relatives of ADHD children with conduct disorder, as well as independent transmission of ADHD and substance use disorders. Conversely, child and adolescent offspring of alcoholic persons have been reported, in controlled studies, to have abnormal cognitive and behavioral traits, including lower attention spans and higher impulsivity, aggressiveness, and hyperactivity, as well as elevated rates of ADHD, compared with control subjects (Aronson and Gilbert 1963; Fine et al. 1976; Steinhausen et al. 1984; Wilens 1994). For example, Earls et al. (1988) found elevated rates of ADHD in children of alcoholic persons compared with children of control subjects; the rates were more robust in families when both parents had substance use disorders.

Although the influence of prenatal substance exposure is confounded by many factors (Griffith et al. 1994; Richardson and Day 1994), several reports have documented increased risk of postnatal complications, including neuropsychiatric abnormalities, in the offspring of alcohol- and cocaine-dependent mothers (Abel and Sokol 1989; Finnegan 1976; Steinhausen et al. 1993; Volpe 1992). One study has shown that three-quarters of children diagnosed with fetal alcohol syndrome manifest ADHD in adolescence (Steinhausen et al. 1993). Data in youths exposed to cocaine are complex, suggesting that confounding variables such as poverty and poor prenatal care, and not cocaine exposure per se, may be the major factors leading to ADHD-like symptoms (Griffith et al. 1994; Wilens et al. 1996). In addition, since family genetic data are generally lacking, it is unknown to what extent reported outcomes are due to exposure to substances, the contribution of parental psychopathology, and a gene-environment interaction.

PUTATIVE MECHANISMS DRIVING SUBSTANCE USE DISORDERS IN INDIVIDUALS WITH ADHD

Although a robust relationship between ADHD and substance use disorders is supported in the literature, the nature of this association remains unclear. In studies of drug- and alcohol-dependent populations, the amelioration of psychiatric symptoms and deficits with substances of abuse has been forwarded as a plausible explanation for substance use disorders (Khantzian 1997). This self-medication hypothesis is compelling in ADHD, considering that the disorder is chronic and often associated with demoralization and failure (Biederman et al. 1993; Mannuzza et al. 1993; G. Weiss 1992), factors frequently associated with substance use disorders in adolescents and young adults (Kandel and Logan 1984; Yamaguchi and Kandel 1984). Moreover, the accompanying poor judgment, aggression, and impulsivity in these youths may be particularly conducive to development of substance use disorder, considering that adolescence is a time of high risk for the development of substance use disorders (Tarter and Edwards 1988).

Despite a paucity of systematically derived data (Bukstein et al. 1989; Kaminer 1992), a subgroup of ADHD individuals appear to be self-medicating. Data exist supporting a developmental progression from ADHD to conduct disorder, with resulting demoralization, failure, substance use, and eventually substance use disorder (Gittelman et al. 1985). Other evidence includes a disproportionate use of the class of drugs over alcohol in ADHD adolescents and adults compared with their non-ADHD peers (Biederman et al. 1995, 1997). Along these lines, one small study involving inpatient substance-abusing adolescents found that adolescents with ADHD continued substance use in order to alter their mood; in contrast, the adolescents without ADHD reported continuing drug use for the euphorogenic properties (Horner and Scheibe 1997).

The potential importance of self-medication needs to be tempered against more systematic data showing the strongest relationship between ADHD and substance use disorders being mediated by the presence of conduct, bipolar, and antisocial disorders—both in the individual and in the family (Biederman et al. 1990; Cantwell 1972; Earls et al. 1988; Stewart et al. 1980). Furthermore, substance use disorders in youths with ADHD may be accounted for largely by family history of substance use disorders (Milberger et al. 1998). The robust findings of a family genetic nature, coupled with recent findings of the association of postsynaptic dopamine D_4 receptor polymorphisms with ADHD (LaHoste et al. 1996), suggest that a polygenic mechanism may be operant. It may also be that ADHD and early-onset substance use disorders represent variable expressivity of a shared risk factor (Comings et al. 1991; Ebstein et al. 1996). Clearly, more work needs to be done in examining the contribution of psychiatric symptoms and deficits to explain the relationship of ADHD with substance use disorders.

CLINICAL IMPLICATIONS OF COMORBIDITY OF ADHD AND SUBSTANCE USE DISORDERS

The comorbidity of ADHD and substance use disorders is of high clinical and public health concern. Clinically, the symptoms of one disorder may exacerbate those of the other. For instance, impulsivity may impair a patient's quality of life while adversely affecting substance moderation or abstinence and treatment retention (Tarter and Edwards 1988). Comorbidity of substance use disorders and ADHD has been associated with chronicity, treatment difficulties, and poorer outcomes of substance use disorders (Carroll and Rounsaville 1993; Levin et al. 1996; Schubiner et al. 1997; Tarter et al. 1977). The identification and treatment of ADHD-related symptoms may improve treatment of the substance use disorder and reduce associated morbidity (Khantzian 1983; Levin et al. 1998a, 1998b; Wender et al. 1981). From the public health perspective, the identification of subtypes of individuals with ADHD and comorbid substance use disorders may be helpful for prevention, early intervention, and treatment for those affected as well as for children at high risk of developing these disorders (Mrazek and Haggerty 1994; Tarter and Edwards 1988; Wilens and Biederman 1993).

Diagnosis and Treatment Guidelines

Evaluation and treatment of comorbid ADHD and substance use disorders should be part of a plan in which consideration is given to all aspects of the adolescent or adult's life. Any intervention in this group should follow a careful evaluation of the patient, including psychiatric, addiction, social, cognitive, educational, and family evaluations (Table 9–3). A thorough history of substance use should be obtained, including past and current usage and treatments. Careful attention should be paid to the differential diagnosis or diagnoses, including medical and neurological conditions whose symptoms may overlap those of ADHD (hyperthyroidism) or be a result of the substance use disorder (e.g., withdrawal, intoxication, or overactivity). Current environmen-

Table 9–3. Evaluation of substance abuse for patients with ADHD

Assessment	Components
Psychiatric evaluation	Personal interview Semistructured interviews Cognitive screen (i.e., for learning disorders)[a]
Addiction history	Interview Questionnaires Urine toxicology screen[a]
Sources of information	Interview with multiple sources: patient with mate or parents Information from other caregivers
Psychosocial	Query about current stressors and available supports
Family concerns	Family history of psychiatric disorders or learning problems (underachievement)
Differential diagnosis issues	Addiction-related issues (i.e., intoxication, withdrawal) Medical concerns (i.e., endocrinopathies) Neurological issues (i.e., seizures, infections) Psychiatric comorbidity (i.e., mood, anxiety, antisocial disorders)
Discussion of treatment strategies	Review of expectations for treatment Need for multimodal treatment Psychotherapy (group and/or individual) for addiction treatment, maladaptive behavioral patterns, intrapsychic distress, and interpersonal difficulties Pharmacotherapy for ADHD and psychiatric comorbidity

[a]As indicated by clinical presentation.

tal factors contributing to the clinical presentation, such as family discord, need to be explored.

Although no specific guidelines exist for evaluating the patient with an active substance use disorder(s), in our experience at least 1 month of abstinence is useful in accurately and reliably assessing for ADHD symptoms. Semistructured psychiatric interviews are invaluable aids for the systematic diagnostic assessments of this group. In individuals with ADHD and substance use disorders, special attention has to be given to the presence of other psychiatric and learning disorders. As with ADHD symptoms, a history of psychiatric symptoms not referable to the substance use disorder (i.e., bipolarity) needs to be reviewed with the adolescent or adult and their family. This evaluation provides a basis for a multimodal treatment plan tailored for the patient.

The treatment needs of individuals with ADHD and comorbid substance use disorders should be considered simultaneously; however, the substance use disorder needs to be addressed first (Riggs 1998). If the substance use disorder is active, immediate attention should be paid to control of the addiction. Depending on the severity and duration of the substance use disorder, adolescents or adults may require inpatient treatment. Self-help groups offer a helpful treatment modality for many persons with substance use disorders. In parallel with addiction treatment, patients with ADHD and comorbid substance use disorders require intervention(s) for the ADHD (and, if applicable, for comorbid psychiatric disorders). Education of the individual, family members, and other caregivers is a useful initial step in improving recognition of the ADHD (Riggs 1998).

The family and individual's expectations need to be explored, and realistic goals of treatment need to be clearly delineated. ADHD patients with psychological distress should be directed to appropriate psychotherapeutic intervention with clinicians knowledgeable in ADHD and the addictive disorders. It appears that effective psychotherapy for patients with this comorbidity combines structured and goal-directed sessions, active therapist involvement, and knowledge of substance use disorders and ADHD (see Chapter 18, this volume, for discussion of cognitive therapy approaches). Often, substance use disorders and ADHD therapeutic interventions are completed in tandem with interventions from other addiction modalities (i.e., Alcoholics and Narcotics Anonymous, Rational Recovery), including pharmacotherapy.

Medication serves an important role in reducing the symptoms of ADHD and other concurrent psychiatric disorders (Table 9–4). Effective agents for

Table 9–4. Pharmacotherapy considerations in the treatment of comorbid ADHD and substance use disorders

Class	Medication
Atypical antidepressants	Bupropion
Tricyclic antidepressants	Desipramine, nortriptyline, and others
Stimulants	Pemoline, methylphenidate, amphetamines
Antihypertensives	Clonidine, guanfacine, propranolol, and others
MAOIs (antidepressants)	Tranylcypromine, pargyline

Note. MAOIs = monoamine oxidase inhibitors.
Source. Adapted from Riggs 1998; Spencer et al. 1996.

ADHD include the stimulants, antidepressants, and antihypertensives (Spencer et al. 1996). Findings from short-term open trials suggest that stimulants (pemoline and methylphenidate) and antidepressants (bupropion) administered to adolescents and adults with ADHD and comorbid substance use disorders assist in ameliorating the ADHD symptoms while reducing, and not exacerbating, substance misuse or cravings (Levin et al. 1998b; Riggs et al. 1996). For example, Levin and associates showed that in cocaine-addicted adults with ADHD, methylphenidate administration reduced cocaine craving (Levin et al. 1998b); in another study, these authors found that bupropion reduced ADHD and substance misuse concurrently (Levin et al. 1998a). Similar results were found in an open trial with pemoline in substance-abusing adolescents with ADHD who exhibited delinquent behavior (Riggs et al. 1996).

Study of the critical influence of long-term ADHD treatment on later development of substance use disorders remains hampered by methodological issues such as the inability to disentangle positive or deleterious effects of treatment from the severity of the underlying condition. Although concerns of the abuse liability and potential kindling of specific types of abuse (i.e., cocaine) secondary to stimulant treatment of children with ADHD have been raised (Drug Enforcement Administration 1995), the preponderance of clinical data (Hechtman 1985) and consensus in the field do not appear to support such a contention. For example, two nonrandomized investigations evaluated substance use disorder outcome in adolescents and young adults with ADHD who had been naturalistically treated with stimulants 5 years previously as youths (Loney et al. 1981). The individuals with ADHD who were untreated and those who had poorer responses to psychostimulants later engaged in more illegal substance use than those who had been successfully treated (Loney et al. 1981).

Biederman and colleagues (1999) recently reported that medicated youths with ADHD were at lower risk for subsequent substance use disorder than were their unmedicated ADHD peers. In this 4-year follow-up study of ADHD in which medicated ADHD (n = 117), unmedicated ADHD (n = 45), and unmedicated non-ADHD control youths (n = 344) were evaluated in midadolescence, baseline ADHD pharmacotherapy was strongly associated with lower rates of substance use disorders, including alcohol, cocaine, stimulant, and other illicit drugs, in midadolescence compared with unmedicated ADHD youths. Of note, no significant baseline differences between the medicated and unmedicated ADHD groups on independent predictors of substance use disorder (e.g., conduct disorder, family history of substance use disorder) were evident. Moreover, rates of substance use disorders were similar between the medicated ADHD and non-ADHD control groups.

Clearly, more prospectively derived studies are necessary to evaluate the protective or deleterious effects and mechanisms of the influence of ADHD, as well as its associated comorbidity and treatment, on later substance use, misuse, abuse, and dependence.

For adolescents and adults with ADHD and comorbid substance use disorders, an emerging consensus suggests that the antidepressants (bupropion, tricyclics, venlafaxine) and longer-acting stimulants with lower abuse liability (e.g., pemoline) are the medications of choice (Riggs 1998). When choosing antidepressants, one should be mindful of potential drug interactions with substances of abuse. Preclinical and human studies suggest variable profiles of stimulants, with methylphenidate having less abuse liability than amphetamine or methamphetamine (Table 9–2) (Drug Enforcement Administration 1995). Despite a lack of evidence of stimulant treatment leading to stimulant use disorders or other substance use disorders (Hechtman 1985), an increase in oral and intranasal abuse of methylphenidate, generally by youths without ADHD, has been reported in adolescents (Drug Enforcement Administration 1995). Families and patients should be educated about the concern of diversion of stimulants from individuals being treated for ADHD to others for whom the medications are not prescribed. In individuals with ADHD and comorbid substance use disorders, frequent monitoring of pharmacotherapy should be undertaken and should include evaluation of compliance with treatment, use of random urine toxicology screens, and coordination of care with other caregivers.

Clinical Case

The following case is typical of cases in which patients present with ADHD and comorbid substance use disorder:

> C.M. is a 31-year-old female presenting for treatment for ADHD. The patient reports lifelong ADHD symptoms, including inattentiveness and distractibility, marked impulsivity, and hyperactivity as a child. The patient also notes a history of alcohol abuse from ages 19 to 21 years and marijuana dependence from ages 18 to 28 years, and she is active in Rational Recovery. On further questioning, C.M. reports long-standing poor self-esteem and intermittent depressive episodes since age 14. The patient reports being reared in the presence of family discord. The family psychiatric history is notable for her father's alcohol dependence and one of her brother's "long-standing school difficulties" and drug de-

pendency. C.M. has an 8-year-old son with ADHD who is being treated with behavioral modification and methylphenidate C.M. reported chronic academic underachievement, and she wishes to attempt college courses again. Cognitive testing revealed a Full Scale IQ of 115, and no learning disorders were identified.

C.M. was enrolled in cognitive therapy and simultaneously was started on desipramine up to a total daily dose of 150 mg. Although C.M. noted improvement in her depressive and anxiety symptoms, her ADHD symptoms were only partially ameliorated. Subsequently, methylphenidate, 10 mg twice daily, was added to the desipramine, with good control of the ADHD symptoms.

CONCLUSION

There is a robust literature supporting a relationship between ADHD and substance use disorders. Noncomorbid ADHD appears to confer an intermediate risk factor for development of substance use disorders, although conduct disorder and bipolar disorder appear to heighten the risk for early onset of substance use disorders in youths. Family data indicate that youths of parents with substance use disorders, antisocial disorder, and ADHD are at particular risk for development of substance use disorders. Both genetic and self-medication influences appear to be related to the development and continuation of substance use disorders in persons with ADHD. Children, adolescents, and adults with ADHD and comorbid substance use disorders require multimodal intervention incorporating addiction and mental health treatment. Pharmacotherapy for individuals with ADHD and comorbid substance use disorders needs to take into consideration abuse liability, potential drug interactions, and compliance concerns.

Although existing literature has provided important information on the relationship between ADHD and substance use disorders, it points to a number of areas in need of further study. The effect of stimulant and nonstimulant pharmacotherapy in promoting or reducing subsequent substance use disorders needs to be assessed. Given the prevalence and major morbidity and impairment caused by the comorbidity of ADHD and substance use disorders, prevention and treatment strategies for patients with this comorbidity need to be further developed and evaluated.

REFERENCES

Abel EL, Sokol RJ: Alcohol consumption during pregnancy: the dangers of moderate drinking, in Alcoholism: Biomedical and Genetic Aspects. Edited by Goedde HW, Agarwal DP. Boston, MA, Pergamon, 1989

Anderson JC, Williams S, McGee R, et al: DSM-III disorders in preadolescent children. Arch Gen Psychiatry 44:69–76, 1987

Aronson H, Gilbert A: Preadolescent sons of male alcoholics. Arch Gen Psychiatry 8:235–241, 1963

Barkley RA, Fischer M, Edelbrock CS, et al: The adolescent outcome of hyperactive children diagnosed by research criteria, I: an 8-year prospective followup study. J Am Acad Child Adolesc Psychiatry 29:546–557, 1990

Biederman J, Faraone SV, Keenan K, et al: Family genetic and psychosocial risk factors in DSM-III attention deficit disorder. J Am Acad Child Adolesc Psychiatry 29: 526–533, 1990

Biederman J, Newcorn J, Sprich S: Comorbidity of attention deficit hyperactivity disorder with conduct, depressive, anxiety, and other disorders. Am J Psychiatry 148: 564–577, 1991

Biederman J, Faraone SV, Keenan K, et al: Further evidence for family genetic risk factors in attention deficit disorder: patterns of comorbidity in probands and relatives in psychiatrically and pediatrically referred samples. Arch Gen Psychiatry 49:728–738, 1992

Biederman J, Faraone SV, Spencer T, et al: Patterns of psychiatric comorbidity, cognition, and psychosocial functioning in adults with attention deficit hyperactivity disorder. Am J Psychiatry 150:1792–1798, 1993

Biederman J, Wilens TE, Mick E, et al: Psychoactive substance use disorders in adults with attention deficit hyperactivity disorder (ADHD): effects of ADHD and psychiatric comorbidity. Am J Psychiatry 152:1652–1658, 1995

Biederman J, Wilens T, Mick E, et al: Is ADHD a risk for psychoactive substance use disorder? Findings from a four-year follow-up study. J Am Acad Child Adolesc Psychiatry 36:21–29, 1997

Biederman J, Wilens T, Mick E, et al: Does attention-deficit hyperactivity disorder impact the developmental course of drug and alcohol abuse and dependence. Biol Psychiatry 44:269–273, 1998

Biederman J, Wilens TE, Mick E, et al: Protective effects of ADHD pharmacotherapy on subsequent substance abuse: a longitudinal study. Pediatrics 104(2):e20, 1999

Bird HR, Canino G, Rubio-Stipec M, et al: Estimates of the prevalence of childhood maladjustment in a community survey in Puerto Rico. Arch Gen Psychiatry 45: 1120–1126, 1988

Blouin A, Bornstein R, Trites R: Teenage alcohol use among hyperactive children: a five-year follow-up study. J Pediatr Psychol 3:188–194, 1978

Bukstein OG, Brent DA, Kaminer Y: Comorbidity of substance abuse and other psychiatric disorders in adolescents. Am J Psychiatry 146:1131–1141, 1989

Cadoret RJ: Genetic and environmental factors in initiation of drug use and the transition to abuse, in Vulnerability to Drug Abuse. Edited by Glantz M, Pickens R. Washington, DC, American Psychological Press, 1991, pp 99–114

Cantwell D: Psychiatric illness in the families of hyperactive children. Arch Gen Psychiatry 27:414–417, 1972

Carroll KM, Rounsaville BJ: History and significance of childhood attention deficit disorder in treatment-seeking cocaine abusers. Compr Psychiatry 34:75–82, 1993

Christie KA, Burke JD, Regier DA, et al: Epidemiologic evidence for early onset of mental disorders and higher risk of drug abuse in young adults. Am J Psychiatry 145:971–975, 1988

Cloninger CR, Bohman M, Sigvardsson S: Inheritance of alcohol abuse: cross-fostering analysis of adopted men. Arch Gen Psychiatry 38:861–868, 1981

Comings D, Comings B, Muhleman D, et al: The dopamine D2 receptor locus as a modifying gene in neuropsychiatric disorders. JAMA 266:1793–1800, 1991

DeMilio L: Psychiatric syndromes in adolescent substance abusers. Am J Psychiatry 146:1212–1214, 1989

Drug Enforcement Administration: Methylphenidate Review Document No. 20537. Washington, DC, Office of Diversion Control, Drug and Chemical Evaluation Section, Drug Enforcement Administration, 1995

Earls F, Reich W, Jung KG, et al: Psychopathology in children of alcoholic and antisocial parents. Alcoholism Clin Exp Res 12:481–487, 1988

Ebstein R, Novick O, Umansky R, et al: Dopamine D4 receptor exon III polymorphism associated with the human personality trait of novelty seeking. Nat Genet 12:78–80, 1996

Eyre SL, Rounsaville BJ, Kleber HD: History of childhood hyperactivity in a clinic population of opiate addicts. J Nerv Ment Disord 170:522–529, 1982

Faraone SV, Biederman J, Chen WJ, et al: Segregation analysis of attention deficit hyperactivity disorder. Psychiatr Genet 2:257–275, 1992

Fine EW, Yudin LW, Holmes J, et al: Behavioral disorders in children with parental alcoholism. Ann N Y Acad Sci 273:507–517, 1976

Finnegan LP: Clinical effects of pharmacologic agents on pregnancy, the fetus and the neonate. Ann N Y Acad Sci 281:74–89, 1976

Gittelman R, Mannuzza S, Shenker R, et al: Hyperactive boys almost grown up, I: psychiatric status. Arch Gen Psychiatry 42:937–947, 1985

Goodwin DW, Schulsinger F, Hermansen L, et al: Alcoholism and the hyperactive child syndrome. J Nerv Ment Disord 160:349–535, 1975

Griffith DR, Azuma SD, Chasnoff IJ: Three-year outcome of children exposed prenatally to drugs. J Am Acad Child Adolesc Psychiatry 33:20–27, 1994

Groves JB, Batey SR, Wright HH: Psychoactive-drug use among adolescents with psychiatric disorders. American Journal of Hospital Pharmacy 43:1714–1718, 1986

Hechtman L: Adolescent outcome of hyperactive children treated with stimulants in childhood: a review. Psychopharmacol Bull 21:178–191, 1985

Hechtman L, Weiss G: Controlled prospective fifteen year follow-up of hyperactives as adults: non-medical drug and alcohol use and anti-social behaviour. Can J Psychiatry 31:557–567, 1986

Horner B, Scheibe K: Prevalance and implications of ADHD among adolescents in treatment for substance abuse. J Am Acad Child Adolesc Psychiatry 36:30–36, 1997

Hovens JG, Cantwell DP, Kiriakos R: Psychiatric comorbidity in hospitalized adolescent substance abusers. J Am Acad Child Adolesc Psychiatry 33:476–483, 1994

Kaminer Y: The magnitude of concurrent psychiatric disorders in hospitalized substance abusing adolescents. Child Psychiatry Hum Dev 22:89–95, 1991

Kaminer Y: Clinical implications of the relationship between attention-deficit hyperactivity disorder and psychoactive substance use disorders. Am J Addict 1:257–264, 1992

Kandel D, Faust R: Sequence and stages in patterns of adolescent drug use. Arch Gen Psychiatry 32:923–932, 1975

Kandel DB, Logan JA: Patterns of drug use from adolescence to young adulthood, I: periods of risk for initiation, continued use, and discontinuation. Am J Public Health 74:660–666, 1984

Kashani JH, Keller MB, Solomon N, et al: Double depression in adolescent substance abusers. J Affect Disord 8:153–157, 1985

Kellam SG, Ensminger ME, Simon MB: Mental health in first grade and teenage drug, alcohol, and cigarette use. Drug Alcohol Depend 5:273–304, 1980

Kessler RC, McGonagle KA, Zhao S, et al: Lifetime and 12-month prevalence of DSM-III-R psychiatric disorders in the United States. Arch Gen Psychiatry 51: 8–19, 1994

Khantzian EJ: An extreme case of cocaine dependence and marked improvement with methylphenidate treatment. Am J Psychiatry 140:784–785, 1983

Khantzian EJ: The self-medication hypothesis of substance use disorders: a reconsideration and recent applications. Harv Rev Psychiatry 4:231–244, 1997

LaHoste GJ, Swanson JM, Wigal SB, et al: Dopamine D4 receptor gene polymorphism is associated with attention deficit hyperactivity disorder. Mol Psychiatry 1:121–124, 1996

Levin FR, Kleber HD: Attention-deficit hyperactivity disorder and substance abuse: relationships and implications for treatment. Harv Rev Psychiatry 2:246–258, 1995

Levin F, Evans SM, Lugo L, et al: ADHD in cocaine abusers: psychiatric comorbidity and pattern of drug use. College of Problems of Drug Dependence, 1996 Annual Meeting, San Juan, Puerto Rico, 1996, p 56

Levin F, Evans SM, Rosenthal M, et al: Psychiatric comorbidity in cocaine abusers in outpatient settings or a therapeutic community. College of Problems on Drug Dependence, 1997 Annual Meeting, Nashville, TN, 1997, p 91

Levin F, Evans S, McDowell D, et al: Bupropion treatment for adult ADHD and cocaine abuse. College of Problems on Drug Dependence, 1998 Annual Meeting, Scottsdale, AZ, 1998a, p 79

Levin FR, Evans SM, McDowell DM, et al: Methylphenidate treatment for cocaine abusers with adult attention-deficit/hyperactivity disorder: a pilot study. J Clin Psychiatry 59:300–305, 1998b

Loney J, Klahn M, Kosier T, et al: Hyperactive boys and their brothers at 21: predictors of aggressive and antisocial outcomes. Paper presented at the Society for Life History Research, Monterey, CA, 1981

Mannuzza S, Klein RG, Bonagura N, et al: Hyperactive boys almost grown up, V: replication of psychiatric status. Arch Gen Psychiatry 48:77–83, 1991

Mannuzza S, Klein RG, Bessler A, et al: Adult outcome of hyperactive boys: educational achievement, occupational rank, and psychiatric status. Arch Gen Psychiatry 50:565–576, 1993

Mendelson W, Johnson N, Stewart M: Hyperactive children as teenagers: a followup study. J Nerv Ment Dis 153:273–279, 1971

Mezzich AC, Tarter RE, Hsieh Y, et al: Substance abuse severity in female adolescents: association between age at menarche and chronological age. Am J Addict 1:217–221, 1992

Milberger S, Biederman J, Faraone S, et al: ADHD is associated with early initiation of cigarette smoking in children and adolescents. J Am Acad Child Adolesc Psychiatry 36:37–43, 1997

Milberger S, Faraone S, Biederman J, et al: Familial risk analysis of the association between ADHD and PSUD, in College of Problems on Drug Dependence. Scottsdale, AZ, College of Problems on Drug Dependence, 1998, p 97

Milin R, Halikas JA, Meller JE, et al: Psychopathology among substance abusing juvenile offenders. J Am Acad Child Adolesc Psychiatry 30:569–574, 1991

Morrison JR, Stewart MA: A family study of the hyperactive child syndrome. Biol Psychiatry 3:189–195, 1971

Mrazek PJ, Haggerty RJ: Reducing Risks for Mental Disorders: Institute of Medicine. Washington, DC, National Academy Press, 1994

National Institute on Drug Abuse: Monitoring the Future, 1990: National High School Senior Drug Abuse Survey. Rockville, MD, National Institute on Drug Abuse, U.S. Department of Health and Human Services, 1991

Richardson GA, Day NL: Detrimental effects of prenatal cocaine exposure: illusion or reality? J Am Acad Child Adolesc Psychiatry 33:28–34, 1994

Riggs P: Clinical approach to treatment of ADHD in adolescents with substance use disorders and conduct disorder. J Am Acad Child Adolesc Psychiatry 37:331–332, 1998

Riggs PD, Thompson LL, Mikulich SK, et al: An open trial of pemoline in drug dependent delinquents with attention deficit hyperactivity disorder. J Am Acad Child Adolesc Psychiatry 35:1018–1024, 1996

Ross HE, Glaser FB, Germanson T: The prevalence of psychiatric disorders in patients with alcohol and other drug problems. Arch Gen Psychiatry 45:1023–1031, 1988

Rounsaville BJ, Anton SF, Carroll K, et al: Psychiatric diagnoses of treatment-seeking cocaine abusers. Arch Gen Psychiatry 48:43–51, 1991

Safer DJ, Krager JM: A survey of medication treatment for hyperactive/inattentive students. JAMA 260:2256–2258, 1988

Satterfield JH, Hoppe CM, Schell AM: A prospective study of delinquency in 110 adolescent boys with attention deficit disorder and 88 normal adolescent boys. Am J Psychiatry 139:795–798, 1982

Schubiner H, Tzelepis A, Isaacson JH, et al: The dual diagnosis of attention-deficit/hyperactivity disorder and substance abuse: case reports and literature review. J Clin Psychiatry 56:146–150, 1995

Schubiner H, Tzelepis A, Schoener E, et al: Prevalence of ADHD among substance abusers. College of Problems on Drug Dependence, 1997 Annual Meeting, Nashville, TN, 1997, p 135

Schuckit MA, Petrich J, Chiles J: Hyperactivity: diagnostic confusion. J Nerv Ment Disord 166:79–87, 1978

Spencer T, Biederman J, Wilens T, et al: Pharmacotherapy of attention deficit disorder across the life cycle. J Am Acad Child Adolesc Psychiatry 35:409–432, 1996

Steinhausen H, Gobel D, Nestler V: Psychopathology in the offspring of alcoholic parents. J Am Acad Child Adolesc Psychiatry 23:465–471, 1984

Steinhausen HC, Willms J, Spohr HL: Long-term psychopathological and cognitive outcome of children with fetal alcohol syndrome. J Am Acad Child Adolesc Psychiatry 32:990–994, 1993

Stewart MA, DeBlois CS, Cummings C: Psychiatric disorder in the parents of hyperactive boys and those with conduct disorder. J Child Psychol Psychiatry 21:283–292, 1980

Tarter RE, Edwards K: Psychological factors associated with the risk for alcoholism. Alcoholism Clin Exp Res 12:471–480, 1988

Tarter RE, McBride H, Buonpane N, et al: Differentiation of alcoholics. Arch Gen Psychiatry 34:761–768, 1977

Tsuang MT, Lyons MJ, Eisen SA, et al: Genetic influences on DSM-III-R drug abuse and dependence: a study of 3,372 twin pairs. Am J Med Genet 67:473–477, 1996

Volpe JJ: Effect of cocaine use on the fetus. N Engl J Med 327:399–406, 1992

Weiss G: Attention-Deficit Hyperactivity Disorder. Philadelphia, PA, WB Saunders, 1992

Weiss G, Hechtman L, Milroy T, et al: Psychiatric status of hyperactives as adults: A controlled prospective 15-year followup of 63 hyperactive children. J Am Acad Child Adolesc Psychiatry 24:211–220, 1985

Weiss RD, Mirin SM, Griffin ML, et al: Psychopathology in cocaine abusers. J Nerv Ment Disord 176:719–725, 1988

Wender PH, Reimherr FW, Wood DR: Attention deficit disorder ('minimal brain dysfunction') in adults: a replication study of diagnosis and drug treatment. Arch Gen Psychiatry 38:449–456, 1981

Wilens TE: The children and adolescent offspring of alcoholic parents. Curr Opin Psychiatry 7:319–323, 1994

Wilens T, Biederman J: Psychopathology in preadolescent children at high risk for substance abuse: a review of the literature. Harv Rev Psychiatry 1:207–218, 1993

Wilens T, Spencer T, Biederman J: Are attention-deficit hyperactivity disorder and the psychoactive substance use disorders really related? Harv Rev Psychiatry 3:260–262, 1995

Wilens TE, Biederman J, Spencer T: Attention deficit hyperactivity disorder and the psychoactive substance use disorders, in Pediatric Substance Use Disorders. Edited by Jaffee S. Philadelphia, PA, WB Saunders, 1996, pp 73–91

Wilens TE, Biederman J, Mick E, et al: Attention deficit hyperactivity disorder (ADHD) is associated with early onset substance use disorders. J Nerv Ment Dis 185:475–482, 1997

Wilens T, Biederman J, Mick E: Does ADHD affect the course of substance abuse? Findings from a sample of adults with and without ADHD. Am J Addict 7:156–163, 1998

Windle M: Alcohol use and abuse. Alcohol Health Res World 15:5–10, 1991

Wood D, Wender PH, Reimherr FW: The prevalence of attention deficit disorder, residual type, or minimal brain dysfunction in a population of male alcoholic patients. Am J Psychiatry 140:95–98, 1983

Yamaguchi K, Kandel DB: Patterns of drug use from adolescence to young adulthood, III: predictors of progression. Am J Public Health 74:673–681, 1984

10 Attention-Deficit Disorders With Sleep/Arousal Disturbances

Thomas E. Brown, Ph.D.
Edward J. Modestino, A.L.B., M.L.A.

Sleep/arousal disturbances include difficulties in falling asleep, in awakening, and in maintaining adequate alertness for daily activities. Many individuals with attention-deficit disorders (ADDs) report chronic difficulties with one or more of these sleep/arousal disturbances, often from early childhood. The high frequency of sleep/arousal disturbances reported by persons with ADDs is not surprising given the close linkage between brain systems involved in regulation of sleep/arousal and those involved in the regulation of attention and affect. Dahl (1996) identified the prefrontal cortex as playing a critical role in regulation of arousal, sleep, affect, and attention. From this point of view, developmental impairment in one of these domains is very likely to be linked to impaired functioning in another.

Dahl (1996) described sleep and arousal as the polar extremes of a single continuum in which sleep is "a categorical diminution of awareness and responsiveness to the environment" in contrast to "a state of high responsiveness (vigilance) . . . a high arousal state [that] precludes the ability to sleep" (p. 4). He noted the substantial developmental changes in sleep/arousal patterns that occur from infancy when sleep is the primary activity of the child through preschool years and after, when sleep and wakefulness are more evenly balanced.

Many individuals with ADDs report that they are not able to develop or maintain developmentally adequate balance between sleep and wakefulness. Not only do they report chronic difficulties in falling asleep and/or awakening, many also report chronic difficulties in attaining and maintaining a sufficient level of alertness and arousal so that they can be activated and energized sufficiently for work and many other daily activities. Frequently, complaints of excessive procrastination and difficulties in task completion often reflect not only problems in organization, prioritizing, and sequencing but also serious difficulties in mustering and maintaining the necessary levels of activation and arousal required to feel "motivated" for getting started and sustaining effort to complete tasks in a reasonable time. As discussed in the first chapter of this book, an adequate model of attention must incorporate elements of arousal, activation, and effort.

At present, there is a dearth of adequate research data on comorbidity of sleep/arousal disturbances and ADDs. As Corkum et al. (1998, 1999) noted, it has not yet been established whether the sleep and arousal disturbances frequently reported by ADD patients and their families are due to the essential pathophysiology of ADDs or are aspects of comorbid disorders (e.g., of mood or anxiety). Most discussions of ADDs do not incorporate disturbance of sleep or arousal in their conceptualization of the disorder. Yet, further research may yield evidence to support and explain the frequent clinical reports from patients with ADDs that they have chronic difficulties in achieving and sustaining alertness and/or in transitioning from sleep to wakefulness or vice versa.

Whatever the mechanisms, many clinicians working with children, adolescents, and adults with ADDs have found that these sleep disturbances appear with striking frequency among these patients and, when present, warrant clinical attention, because inadequate sleep or alertness can significantly exacerbate the impairments of ADD symptoms (Dahl 1995; Dahl et al. 1991). In this chapter we describe these three sleep disturbances commonly associated with ADD, address how these might be related to currently emerging understandings of ADDs, and, in concluding, discuss the treatment interventions that may be useful for persons whose ADDs are accompanied by comorbid sleep and/or arousal disturbances.

It should be noted that this chapter does not discuss all types of sleep disturbances. Some types—for example, difficulties in staying asleep, nightmares, sleep apneas, sleepwalking, and excessive movement during sleep—are mentioned only briefly or are not discussed in this chapter because there is currently no substantial evidence of their being more common or problematic in persons with ADDs than in other persons. (For a review of the wider range of sleep disorders, see Anders and Eiben 1997 and Ferber and Kryger 1995.)

EARLIER CONCERNS ABOUT ADDS AND SLEEP PROBLEMS

Much of the sparse literature on ADDs and sleep has focused on two issues tangential to the concerns of this chapter: insomnia secondary to treatment of an ADD with stimulant medications, and excessive movement of the person with an ADD during sleep. Insomnia can be a side effect of the stimulant medications commonly used to treat ADD symptoms. Usually the insomnia results from the individual's receiving a dose of stimulant too late in the day; since individuals vary widely in their sensitivity to stimulants and in the rate at which these medicines are excreted, there is considerable variability from one person to another in how stimulant administration should be timed to avoid causing insomnia. Yet, recent studies and anecdotal clinical reports suggest that some persons with ADD find it easier, not more difficult, to sleep if they are given a small dose of stimulant late in the day. The impact of stimulant medication on sleep is discussed more fully in a subsequent section of this chapter.

The other commonly discussed aspect of overlap between sleep problems and ADD is excessive movement during sleep by persons with ADD. DSM-III (American Psychiatric Association 1980) listed "moves about excessively during sleep" as a symptom of the hyperactive type of ADD, but this was dropped from subsequent editions of the manual for lack of evidence. Picchietti and Walters (1996) discussed the comorbidity of restless legs syndrome with ADHD, but the comorbidity appears to be a relatively infrequent problem. In this chapter we focus on chronic difficulties in falling asleep, waking up, and maintaining alertness that appear to affect many with an ADD diagnosis.

DIFFICULTIES IN SLEEP COMMONLY REPORTED IN ADDS

Difficulties in Falling Asleep

Parents of children with ADDs often report that from infancy their son or daughter has had great difficulty in getting to sleep. Often they complain that their young child is unable or unwilling to take a nap, even when obviously exhausted. Some describe battles every evening with a child who is overtired and unable to settle into sleep until absolute exhaustion has set in, long past the point when other family members are longing for respite from the persistent antics and demands of the child's overactive behavior. Many clinicians have documented these frequent complaints of parents about difficulties of their young children with ADDs who have these chronic and severe problems in settling into sleep (Brown and Gammon 1992; Carskadon et al. 1993; Corkum et al. 1998; Greenhill et al. 1983; Morrison et al. 1992; Porrino et al. 1983).

Reluctance or inability to settle into sleep at a designated time may be due to many different factors (see Broughton 1994). For some children it may be simply lack of an adequate routine for gradually tapering down the level of activity and stimulation near the end of the day. Yet some other children are often unable to get to sleep at an appropriate time even when parents have worked hard to establish appropriate routines. Bedtimes may be beset nightly with a child's persistent refusal to stop ongoing play or watching television. Some children persist in innumerable "curtain calls," asking or demanding "one more story" or "one more glass of water" or "just a little more time" to stay up with the grownups. Others cry or tantrum protractedly if a parent will not lie in bed with them until they are fully asleep.

Such demandingness at bedtime may reflect a child's chronically oppositional behavior pattern or chronic anxiety about frightening dreams and imaginings or realities within or outside the family that may appear terrifying to the child. Or the chronic difficulty in falling asleep may be due to chronic impairments in the physiological mechanisms regulating sleep and wakefulness. It often is not easy to disentangle factors contributing to a child's chronic difficulty in getting to sleep.

Chronic disturbances in sleep are characteristic not only of children with ADD; many adolescents and adults with ADD report similar disturbances. These older individuals, too, may have inadequate wind-down routines to prepare for sleep, may have excessive obsessional worries, or may experience evening family conflicts. Yet there appears to be a significant number of individuals with ADD who report a lifelong pattern of consistently becoming more alert in the evening, feeling more energized and more ready to engage in work or social activities after dark than in the daytime.

These "night owls" often describe a pattern of not being able to fall asleep until very late at night; as preschoolers they may not have been able to settle and fall into sleep until 10 or 11 P.M. on many nights. As adolescents or adults they may chronically feel too restless and may be unable to shut down their activity or thought processes enough to sleep until 2 or 3 A.M. or later. Others report that they stay up because they get involved in enjoyable activities and just do not feel tired while reading or writing, surfing the Internet, or socializing, until long past the time they need to be asleep in order to get sufficient rest for the next day.

At present, it is not clear how these chronic problems in getting to sleep are related to the pathophysiology of ADD. Dahl emphasized that there is a strong relationship between the control of sleep and the regulation of mood and behavior in waking states. He also noted, however, that "[o]ur current knowledge of these complex relationships between sleep, development and psychiatric well-being is at an embryonic state" (Dahl 1995, p. 151). These issues are discussed later in this chapter.

Difficulties in Awakening

Not surprisingly, persons who chronically stay up very late, either because they choose to or because they are simply unable to get to sleep earlier, often report chronic difficulty in morning awakening. Although individuals vary widely in the amount of sleep they need, everyone has some minimum of sleep and an established rhythm of sleep and awakening that they need to maintain in order to function effectively. The difficulties in adjusting these circadian rhythms to the realities of biological and social needs, especially during adolescence, are discussed by Ferber (1995, p. 93).

Some "night owls" are fortunate enough that they can arrange their schedule for work, classes, or other obligations in a way that usually allows going to bed late and getting up late so they can meet at least their minimal, if not their optimal, sleep requirements. Many are not so fortunate, however; they often find themselves unable to avoid trying to function on insufficient sleep, which is likely to exacerbate their ADD symptoms and further impair their functioning.

Yet difficulties in morning awakening are not limited to persons who stay up excessively late because of insomnia or staying involved too late in work or pleasurable activities. Some individuals with ADD report that they have chronic difficulty in awakening, even when they have had adequate sleep the night before. They note that they tend to sleep very soundly and are often unresponsive to the loudest of alarm clocks or strenuous efforts of others to awaken them. This resistance to awakening often persists even when they have felt strong need and intentions to get up on time for a particular activity or event.

Chronic difficulty in awakening can cause persistent stress in a household where one or more members of a family are daily burdened with the protracted task of urging, pleading, or trying to force a sleepy, resistant person out of bed and into morning routines to prepare for school or work. In addition to family stresses, severe and persistent problems of this sort may have substantial consequences for the affected individual in school or work. Many high schools withhold academic credit for courses in which a student has been late to class too many times. College students may fail courses when their chronic difficulty in getting up for morning lectures or examinations is too persistent. Employees may lose their jobs if they repeatedly fail to get to work on time.

Despite determination to avoid such consequences, some persons with ADDs have chronic difficulties in getting themselves awake and out to school or work on time. Many affected persons do not live with someone who is able and willing to provide reliable daily wakeup service. Even those who live in the same household are often not willing daily to confront a soundly sleeping person who, at least at the time of the needed awakening, may be very resistant to being wakened or quite persistent in resuming sleep or refusing to get out of bed, even when apparent wakefulness has been achieved. One family reported often having to struggle, with repeated calls, pokings, and proddings, for almost an hour to wake their adolescent son and to get him on his feet, undressed, and into the shower, only to find him shortly afterward soundly asleep as he sat on the floor of his shower with water pouring over him.

Chronic difficulties in awakening also occur in persons without ADD, but such difficulties, in varying degrees of severity, are quite common among persons with ADD. Causes of such chronic difficulties in awakening may be quite complex: comorbid mood problems, physiological abnormalities in the sleeper, motivational conflicts, interpersonal or family dynamics, and secondary gains may all play a part.

Difficulties in Maintaining Alertness

The third type of sleep disturbance often reported by persons with ADD, especially those with the predominantly inattentive type, is difficulty in staying alert when not engaged in stimulating mental action or lively physical activity. Many persons with an ADD diagnosis note that even when they are adequately rested, they often have much difficulty in staying alert if they have to sit still or do a routinized or unstimulating task. These individuals, some of whom appear to be have "borderline narcolepsy," report that even after a very adequate night's sleep, they tend quickly to become very drowsy when they sit still to attend a meeting, listen to a lecture, read a book, or, for some, drive a car (Brown 1993, 1995, 1996). At such times these persons often find that they have to keep wiggling around, changing activities, or giving themselves frequent breaks in order to avert falling asleep. Some college students report repeatedly falling asleep in lectures, even when well rested and wanting to take good notes so they could be prepared for an imminent exam. Some working adults report repeated yawning and having to persistently fight sleep during important business meetings, even when they are aware of being in clear view of their colleagues and supervisors.

Often these individuals note a sudden improvement in their level of alertness as soon as they get up and start moving or if something exciting occurs to liven up an otherwise boring activity. They emphasize that their drowsiness seems not to be a pervasive sense of fatigue such as occurs when they have had insufficient sleep. Instead, it appears to be an inability to maintain a sufficient level of alertness or arousal unless engaged in significant physical movement or in mental activity that they find consistently stimulating.

The most extreme form of this difficulty in maintaining alertness is narcolepsy. Yoss (1970), Navelet and Anders (1976), Duane (1991), and Dahl et al. (1994) have each studied persons with diagnoses of ADDs and narcolepsy. Some of their cases suggest that children or adolescents with narcolepsy may have their condition misdiagnosed as an ADD. Others of their case reports are more consistent with the possibility that both narcolepsy and an ADD were present.

Another approach to conceptualizing ADDs with chronic problems in maintaining alertness has been suggested by Weinberg and Brumback (1990) and Weinberg and Harper (1993), who proposed the term *primary disorder of vigilance* to replace the diagnosis of ADD for describing a syndrome involving inattentiveness, boredom, restlessness, and sleepiness. They presented case studies to illustrate how individuals with this syndrome tend to be hyperactive in order to ward off drowsiness; the observation was made that these persons tend to fall asleep several times daily if not adequately stimulated. Weinberg and Harper (1993) claimed that persons with primary disorder of vigilance do not have the type of sleep attacks characteristic of narcolepsy, but they did not report use of the blood test commonly used in differential diagnosis of narcolepsy (Carlander et al. 1993; Moscovitch et al. 1991). They reported that primary disorder of vigilance responds well to treatment with the stimulants commonly used to treat ADDs. Thus far, Weinberg et al.'s case reports have called attention to the overlap of some cases of ADD with excessive daytime somnolence and other aspects of impaired vigilance, but these investigators have not yet established a case for their alternative diagnostic category.

Data regarding the chronic problems of persons with ADDs in maintaining alertness can be found in the manual for the Brown Attention Deficit Disorder Scales (Brown 1996) for adolescents and adults. These self-report scales, developed from interviews with individuals who met the DSM diagnostic criteria for attention-deficit disorders, query about chronic problems in maintaining alertness, energy, and effort for work tasks and about chronic problems with sustaining attention and concentration, in addition to other clusters of ADD symptoms. Clusters of items related to chronic difficulties in maintaining alertness and effort for work and of items related to problems in sustaining attention and concentration were found to correlate quite well (0.80 and 0.85, respectively), with total scores for ADD symptoms in adolescents and in adults with diagnosed ADDs. These data suggest that chronic problems with maintaining alertness and sustaining attention may be an important aspect of ADD symptoms for many who meet the established diagnostic criteria for an ADD.

The notion that ADDs intrinsically involve dysfunction in regulation of arousal or an impaired ability to sustain alertness is not new. Virginia Douglas (1988, p. 66) included "regulation of arousal and alertness to meet task demands" among the aspects of self-regulation she considered impaired in ADD. Yet the emphasis on symptoms of hyperactivity and the relative neglect of cognitive impairments of ADDs in recent years have contributed to the lack of attention paid to this important area of impairment.

It is not clear from existing research what the similarities and differences between ADDs and narcolepsy and other problems of excessive daytime sleepiness might be. Copeland and Copps (1995, pp. 287–288) have noted similarities between the chronic underarousal characteristic of narcolepsy and that of some persons with ADDs. They have observed that persons diagnosed with narcolepsy often complain of memory problems similar to those associated with ADDs; they have also speculated that the neurochemistry of narcolepsy may parallel that of ADDs. Further research is needed to clarify the exact nature of these linkages.

ADDITIONAL SLEEP ABNORMALITIES NOTED IN STUDIES OF ADDS

Thus far, polysomnographic studies of ADDs within sleep laboratories have not produced much consistent empirical data to support the complaints of individuals with ADDs about their sleep disturbances. Corkum et al. (1998) have discussed some factors that may contribute to this lack of confirmatory data from laboratory studies.

Some abnormal findings have been documented in comparisons of ADD patients and control subjects. These include an increased latency to REM onset (Busby et al. 1981) in contrast to a decreased latency to REM onset (Khan 1982) and a decrease in overall REM activity (Greenhill et al. 1983). Other polysomnographic abnormalities include an increase in delta wave sleep (Ramos-Platon et al. 1990) and sleep spindles (Kiesow and Surwillo 1987). Irregular sleep behaviors include excessive movement, frequent awakenings, and general restless sleep (Busby et al. 1981; Porrino et al. 1983; Ramos-Platon et al. 1990; Simmonds and Parraga 1984). Simmonds and Parraga (1984) also showed an increase in head banging and snoring among those with ADDs, compared with control subjects.

The mechanisms and meanings of these findings are not yet clear, but this research has thus far been limited by small sample sizes, an almost exclusive focus on young children (predominantly boys who were hyperactive), and lack of data for sustained trials of sleep in naturalistic settings. Just as individuals with ADDs often do not manifest some of their behavioral impairments in the novel situation of a clinician's office, it is likely that some of the sleep problems of persons with ADDs may not be observable in one or two nights of sleep within a sleep laboratory. More research with a wider age sampling and more sustained measures in more natural settings is needed to increase understanding of the problems that lead so many persons with ADDs to report chronic impairments in their regulation of sleep and alertness.

DIFFERENTIAL DIAGNOSIS OF ADDS AND SLEEP AROUSAL DISORDERS

It has been suggested by some researchers that primary sleep disorders may sometimes be misdiagnosed as ADDs. They observe that daytime behaviors of those with a wide variety of sleep disorders (e.g., sleep apnea, narcolepsy, periodic leg movements of sleep, sleep schedule disorders, insufficient sleep) can mimic the symptoms of ADDs by manifesting short attention span, hyperactivity, and impulsivity (Ferber and Kryger 1995; Sheldon 1996). This view is consistent with those of Navelet et al. (1976), Dahl et al. (1994), and Kotagal and Swink (1996).

Narcolepsy is not the only sleep disorder that may be missed in favor of an ADD diagnosis. Other clinicians have noted that restless legs syndrome and periodic limb movement syndrome are disorders that may be misdiagnosed as ADD (Hickey et al. 1992; Picchietti and Walters 1994; Walters et al. 1994, 1996). Hickey et al. (1992) reported three case studies of children with restless legs syndrome who were misdiagnosed with ADD. Picchietti and Walters (1994) reported that 34% of a group of children with ADHD had sufficient symptoms of periodic limb movement syndrome to qualify for that diagnosis. Brooks (1993) reported that sleep apnea can often be misdiagnosed as an ADD because many children with sleep apnea are often hyperactive. Likewise, Ferber and Kryger (1995) claimed that sleep apnea can cause impaired daytime alertness and hyperactivity that may lead to an ADD diagnosis.

It remains to be determined whether the overlap of these patients with ADDs and concurrent sleep disorders is due to misdiagnosis or to a genuine comorbidity of ADD with these various disorders of sleep, or to a common pathophysiology of the mechanisms for self-regulation of sleep and waking-time behaviors. Systematic studies are needed to address these questions.

ASSESSMENT AND EVALUATION OF SLEEP AROUSAL DISORDERS

At the clinical level, careful assessment of each individual with complaints of ADD symptoms or sleep disorder symptoms is needed to determine whether the primary diagnosis is ADD, a sleep disorder, or both. For assessment of sleep disorders in children and adolescents, Ferber (1995, 1996) presented an excellent protocol; Sheldon et al. (1992) included in their book a useful appendix that serves as a guide for differential diagnosis. Methods for assessment of ADDs are described in Chapter 15 of this volume.

The beginning point of effective intervention for sleep disturbances associated with ADD is a thorough assessment of the nature and history of the patient's difficulties with sleep and arousal. Every assessment for possible ADD should include inquiry about sleep routines—for example, usual time for going to bed, time required to fall asleep after getting into bed, frequency and duration of awakening during sleep, degree of difficulty in awakening and getting up as needed, and so forth. This inquiry should also address the frequency and circumstances of daytime drowsiness. The assessing clinician should also inquire about the frequency and duration of naps taken during the day; it is not uncommon for some adolescents or adults to take a lengthy nap in late afternoon or early evening, thereby making it difficult for them to get to sleep at an appropriate time in the evening.

In taking the history of sleep patterns, it is most important to get an accurate picture of current patterns and their variability. Yet when patients report current difficulties in any aspect of sleep, it is also important to get more details about the history and persistence of that difficulty. For example, if it is reported that a child has slept reasonably well until a pattern of difficulty falling asleep began several months ago, it is important to inquire about other changes in the child's life that may have occurred about the same time—for example, sickness of a family member, parental divorce, a burglary in the neighborhood, viewing a frightening film or news story, moving into a different bedroom, and starting a new medication.

In an evaluation it is also important to inquire about how the patient's sleep and/or awakening problems are usually responded to by the family. Is there frequent frustration and conflict within the family about the sleep difficulties? Are parents often battling with each other about how best to manage the problem? Are parents often losing time they need for their own sleep or their private life because of daily struggles with a child who cannot or will not go to bed at a reasonable time? Does the entire household start each day with harsh yelling and rushing to get a somnolent adolescent out of bed in time to catch the school bus? Is a parent often late to work because he or she drives a tardy child to school? Usually a few simple questions and careful listening to the emotional undercurrents of family members' responses will give clear indications of how much stress is associated with the chronic sleep problems of a particular family member. This information may give some clues about the complexities of individual motives, family dynamics, and environmental constraints that may sustain the problem and/or help to alleviate it.

TREATMENT INTERVENTIONS FOR SLEEP DISTURBANCES WITH ADDS

Chronic Difficulties in Falling Asleep

Sleep hygiene. If the assessment indicates a significant chronic problem with falling asleep (e.g., sleep latency of more than 30 minutes on most nights), the first step to be suggested is a review of bedtime routines, often called *sleep hygiene,* to determine that appropriate behavioral measures are being taken. Persons with difficulty in falling asleep may be helped by maintaining a consistent bedtime and regularly following a routine that allows them gradually to reduce their level of activity and move toward relaxation. For children this may include having a snack, taking a warm bath and then brushing teeth, getting into pajamas, having a story read by or with a parent, having quiet conversation while a parent gives a back rub, engaging in relaxing imagery, and so forth. For adolescents or adults it might mean activities such as watching television, reading enjoyable magazines or books, and listening to music.

The main strategy here is to try to condition the individual to a consistent sequence of activities to wind down from excitement and gradually to relax in preparation for sleep. It is sometimes surprising to see how some children are encouraged in very active play or to be engaged in exciting television shows or video games just prior to bedtime and then are expected simply to lie down and go to sleep without any intervening quieting activities to facilitate the transition to sleep.

Other aspects of sleep hygiene relate to setting. It is usually helpful if the bedroom is quiet, but some find that music or quiet television is experienced as more calming. Comfortable temperature, ventilation, and sleepwear are also desirable. Climate control/temperature regulation via air conditioners, heating, humidifiers, and dehumidifiers may also help to make for a more conducive sleep environment. Sound screens may muffle bothersome sounds, and night masks may screen out excessive light.

If sleep hygiene measures alone are not sufficient to cope with chronic problems in getting to sleep, other interventions may be needed. One method used by some parents of young children with ADDs to cope with their child's chronic difficulty in getting to sleep is *co-sleeping* (i.e., the parent lies down with the child until the child is asleep or may sleep with the child for the entire night). One variant of this occurs when the child falls asleep in his or her own bed and then awakens sometime during the night and comes to the parent's bed and sleeps for the rest of the night with the parent.

Often parents of children with ADDs who report co-sleeping with their child to clinicians are embarrassed and apologetic, saying things like, "I know this is not the way it is supposed to be, but we have tried everything else and this is the only way we can all get a decent night's sleep." Clinicians should reassure such parents that they are not alone; many parents find themselves in a similar situation with their young children with ADD. This can then lead to discussion about how well this strategy is working and whether it should be continued or modified to meet the needs of this particular child and family.

Lozoff (1995) has reminded us that the practice of co-sleeping is very common in many cultures and that in the United States until the last century most families were co-sleeping. She notes that few non-Western cultures expect young children to fall asleep alone or to sleep through the night by themselves. Studies in the United States indicate that over 50% of families with young children report at least some degree of co-sleeping, although there have been significant socioeconomic and ethnic differences in reported patterns.

For regular (more than two or three times per week) all-night co-sleeping, the highest incidence is reported for lower-socioeconomic-level families in which separate beds and bedrooms are less likely to be available. Across socioeconomic levels, black families report 50%, Hispanic families 21%, and white families 10% of regular co-sleeping (Lozoff 1995, p. 70). Yet it is not known whether these reported differences reflect actual differences in co-sleeping practices or simply different levels of withholding information because of social expectations.

Regardless of the actual incidence, there is not yet clear evidence that parents' co-sleeping with their young children, particularly children who have chronic and severe difficulty getting to sleep, is intrinsically helpful or not. Some studies suggest that children who regularly co-sleep with parents have more sleep problems; other studies do not support this finding (Lozoff 1995, p. 71). None of these studies thus far has adequately addressed the question of whether the co-sleeping may be a response of parents to their young child's chronic difficulties in falling asleep.

When parents of children with ADDs have been co-sleeping with their child, eventually there comes a point when it is clearly to the advantage of the parents and/or child to have the child sleep alone. To work toward that goal parents may encourage the child to sleep with a pet dog or cat or to use a favorite blanket, doll, teddy bear, or other object to assist the transition. Some children are helped by having a night-light or ready access to a flashlight at bedside. Some children respond to incentive plans in which rewards are given for each night they are able to "be brave" or "more grown up" by sleeping all night in their own bed. If a school-age child has extraordinary difficulty in making the transition to sleeping alone, a clinical evaluation might be useful to consider whether biochemical factors and/or emotional/family factors may be disrupting the child's capacity to learn to sleep adequately without the comfort of sleeping with a parent.

Medications. If adequate sleep hygiene is not sufficient to alleviate chronic problems in getting to sleep, and if there is no evidence of contributory emotional or family factors that can be directly addressed, the clinician may want to consider a trial of medication. However, before adding a new medication to address sleep problems, the clinician must be certain that the patient is not taking some medication that may be contributing to chronic difficulty in falling asleep.

Stimulants used to treat ADDs may contribute to difficulties in falling asleep in two different ways. Sometimes an individual with an ADD who is responding well to stimulant medication taken during the day may have insomnia resulting from taking a dose too close to bedtime. For most persons taking stimulants, an interval of at least 4–6 hours from ingestion of the last dose of the day will allow sufficient washout of the medication for sleep onset. Yet there are some who are able to get to sleep easily within just a few hours of taking a dose, and others who need an interval of 6–8 hours or more from time of ingestion of their last dose before they are able to fall asleep.

Sleep of a person with an ADD may also be delayed because of insufficient stimulant medication later in the day. Many clinicians still encourage patients to avoid taking a dose of stimulant in mid- or late afternoon because they fear medication-induced insomnia. Often this plan backfires because of rebound agitation or irritability occurring in late afternoon or early evening after the last dose of stimulant has worn off. Kent et al. (1995) reported that administration of a late-afternoon dose of methylphenidate tended to help alleviate ADD symptoms without adversely affecting sleep. Tirosh et al. (1993) reported that methylphenidate given late in the afternoon tends actually to improve sleep for many patients with ADDs. Clinicians whose patients taking stimulants for ADDs are having chronic difficulty in falling asleep should consider both of two possibilities: the patient may need less stimulant coverage in late afternoon, or he or she may need an additional smaller dose in late afternoon or early evening.

When sleep hygiene measures are ineffective for a person with an ADD and stimulant medication does not appear to be causing the insomnia, and when chronic difficulty in falling asleep is causing serious problems, there are some other options for intervention that have been reported to be effective. Brown and Gammon (1992) reported a sequence of interventions for such patients. Those with sleep latency in excess of 30 minutes who did not respond to sleep hygiene measures were given a trial of Benadryl (diphenhydramine hydrochloride), in liquid or tablets, about 1 hour prior to sleep time. For some this was sufficient support for getting to sleep. For a few patients the antihistamine had a paradoxical effect of inducing agitation; in these cases it was immediately discontinued and the second step was taken.

The second level of intervention used by Brown and Gammon with a group of children with ADD and chronic difficulty in falling asleep, all of whom had responded well to methylphenidate during the daytime and did not benefit from Benadryl, was administration of a small dose of clonidine (one-half of a 0.1-mg tab) given about 90 minutes before bedtime. Of 18 children (ages 6–17 years), only one had the medication discontinued because of side effects (headaches). After 5 days the dose of clonidine was increased to 0.1 mg if sleep latency was not reduced to less than 45 minutes. Seven children remained on the 0.05-mg dose, and 10 increased to the full 0.1-mg dose. There was no correlation between the size of the dose needed and age or body weight. After 3 weeks the mean sleep latency for the group had decreased from the baseline of 1.9 hours to 0.5 hour.

More substantial samples of children and adolescents with ADDs treated with clonidine for sleep disturbance have been reported by Wilens et al. (1994) and Prince et al. (1996). In a systematic chart review of 62 cases in which clonidine was used to treat chronic difficulty in falling asleep, 85% of the patients reported significant improvement maintained over a mean of 3 years. In this sample no association was found between response and age group, gender, comorbidity, or concurrent pharmacotherapy; those whose insomnia existed prior to stimulant use and those whose insomnia was caused or exacerbated by stimulants responded equally well to clonidine given to help sleep (Prince et al. 1996).

Recently, there has been some controversy about the combined use of stimulant medications with clonidine, after a few case reports of sudden death in children who had been treated with this combination of medications. The Food and Drug Administration investigated and did not find sufficient evidence of a causal relationship to issue any warning. For thoughtful discussions of this controversy and its implications for clinical practice, see Popper 1995, Cantwell et al. 1997, and Wilens et al. 1999.

Other medications that have been reported to be useful for treatment of chronic difficulties in getting to sleep are tricyclic antidepressants and trazodone. Tricyclic antidepressants (e.g., desipramine, nortriptyline) have been demonstrated to be effective for treatment of ADDs (for review, see Spencer 1996; Chapter 16, this volume), although there is some question about whether they ameliorate the cognitive symptoms as effectively as they do the behavioral symptoms of ADDs. These medications, often administered in a single dose at bedtime, are frequently helpful in alleviating chronic difficulties in getting to sleep.

Many clinicians are reluctant to use tricyclics with prepubescent children, however, because of a highly toxic potential of these agents if taken in overdose, and because of the small number of case reports of sudden death associated with use of seemingly appropriate dosing of desipramine in 9- and 10-year-old children (for review, see Popper 1995). Since the sudden death incidents have not involved any adolescents or adults, use of this class of medications with fully pubescent patients or with adults is more common and has been found to be effective in treating ADD symptoms and depressive symptoms, including chronic difficulty in falling asleep.

An alternative medication with demonstrated effectiveness for addressing insomnia in adults is trazodone. Nierenberg et al. (1994) demonstrated that trazodone, a sedating triazolopyridine antidepressant, is superior to placebo for persistent primary insomnia and for insomnia induced or exacerbated by antidepressants. Although their report did not assess patients with ADDs, uncontrolled anecdotal reports indicate that similar results have been found with adults with severe chronic difficulty in falling asleep and concurrent ADD.

Difficulties in Awakening

When individuals with ADDs chronically have severe difficulties in awakening, the first intervention is to be certain that they are getting adequate sleep. If an individual is chronically having difficulty in falling asleep at a reasonable time, or is having very disrupted sleep, and is therefore getting insufficient sleep, it is not surprising when that person also has chronic difficulty in awakening. The first task is to assess factors that may be contributing to the difficulty in falling asleep or disruption of sleep and to take appropriate remedial actions. This may include assessment for sleep apnea, narcolepsy, or other specific sleep disorders.

If patients are having great difficulty in awakening despite apparently adequate sleep, it may be useful to talk with them to ascertain whether they may have a mood disorder or whether there may be some reason why they have intense conflict between their wish to awaken for school, work, or whatever and their wish to avoid getting to that activity. Such inquiry is especially important if the difficulty in awakening is of relatively recent onset rather than a lifelong problem.

If the problem in awakening, with or without daytime hypersomnia, is associated with other depressive symptoms, the possibility of an underlying mood disorder should be considered. The assessment and treatment of depression comorbid with ADDs are discussed extensively by Spencer et al. elsewhere in this volume (see Chapter 3).

Sometimes difficulty in getting out of bed is simple avoidance that needs to be addressed in terms of both the specific factors sustaining the wish to avoid the activity and any secondary gains that may be involved. For example, by not getting up in time to catch the school bus, a student may avoid an intensely disliked class or a frightening social situation and/or may be able to spend more time at home with a parent, playing video games, and so forth.

When the difficulty in awakening does not appear to be associated with simple avoidance or with comorbid depression, especially if this has been a lifelong pattern of someone with an ADD, it may be useful to consider an early-morning dose of stimulant prior to getting up for the day. Brown and Gammon (1992) reported on a small sample of children and adolescents with ADDs whose chronic difficulty in awakening responded to their being awakened about 30–45 minutes prior to the time they actually needed to get up. At that time the parent administered a dose of stimulant to the child while he or she was still in bed. After taking the medication and a drink of juice or water, the child was encouraged to go back to sleep and was then reawakened 30–45 minutes later to get up and out of bed after the stimulant had time to take effect.

For college students or other adults who may not have someone living with them who is able or willing to awaken them for this early-morning dose, the same approach has been used with a self-administration strategy. The patient is encouraged to obtain two alarm clocks, setting one on a bedside table to sound 45 minutes prior to the actual wake-up time desired and the other on the opposite side of the room set to go off at the time the patient actually wants to get out of bed.

When the first clock goes off, the patient awakens and self-administers the premeasured dose of stimulant that has been set out with a glass of water on the bedside table. The patient then goes back to sleep and, hopefully, is able to respond to the second alarm clock by getting out of bed and walking over to turn it off. The reason for the second clock is that patients with this problem are often unsuccessful in accurately resetting the bedside alarm clock before they go back to sleep.

Difficulties in Maintaining Alertness

For patients with ADDs who report significant chronic problems in maintaining alertness, the first task is to take a careful history to assess for depression and/or sleep disorders (e.g., obstructive sleep apnea or narcolepsy), any of which may be masked by ADD symptoms. Obstructive sleep apnea, most common in overweight males, is characterized by chronic loud snoring interspersed with frequent episodes of silence during which the sleeper briefly stops breathing. The resulting disruption of sleep can cause severe daytime drowsiness, failure of concentration, and many other symptoms (Parkes 1985). Narcolepsy is characterized by chronic and severe daytime sleepiness; sudden loss of muscle tone; vivid, dreamlike images during the transition into sleep; and unusual persistence of sleep muscle paralysis after awakening. Yet not all persons with narcolepsy present with all these characteristics.

Dahl et al. (1994) cautioned that many persons with narcolepsy are not diagnosed correctly until adulthood. In one study of narcoleptic adults, 59% reported that their narcoleptic symptoms began before age 15 years, but only 4% had received the correct diagnosis by that age (Yoss and Daly 1960). If any patient with an ADD reports severe problems in maintaining daytime alertness, a full sleep assessment should be done to rule out narcolepsy, chronic obstructive sleep apnea, and other sleep disorders. If there is reason to suspect a significant sleep disorder, referral to a specialist for a laboratory sleep study may be indicated.

Some ADD patients report chronic difficulties in maintaining alertness. Some of these patients may, in fact, qualify for a diagnosis of narcolepsy or obstructive sleep apnea by sleep laboratory criteria. Many, however, have significant problems in maintaining alertness that do not meet the full sleep laboratory criteria for narcolepsy or any other major sleep disorder, yet they may experience significant problems at work or school or in social and family relationships because of chronic difficulties in maintaining adequate arousal. It appears that some persons with ADDs have "borderline narcolepsy," being alert enough when they are up and moving around or otherwise engaged in lively physical or mental activity. Yet these individuals quickly become drowsy when they have to sit still and be quiet. They readily fall asleep when trying to read or when sitting in meetings or classrooms in which they are not very active. These individuals appear to have chronic difficulty in maintaining alertness that is not truly a comorbid disorder but rather a manifestation of the sleep/arousal problems that appear to be one important diagnostic feature for many who qualify for an ADD diagnosis. As Segalowitz et al. (1994) noted, the relationship between sleep, arousal, and attention is not simple. Much remains to be learned about the relationship between sleep, arousal, and allocation of arousal in persons with normal functioning and in those with ADDs with or without comorbid sleep disorders.

Some patients with ADDs and a history of chronic difficulty in maintaining alertness report that they are much better able to maintain appropriate alertness when their ADD is treated with stimulants. Often patients for whom maintaining alertness is an especially problematic symptom need more extensive coverage with stimulant medications than do other patients with a different ADD symptom profile. For example, they may need more closely spaced doses of stimulant to combat rapid excretion with rebound fatigue, and/or they may need stimulant coverage for more hours of the day than do many others with ADDs.

Unlike some ADD patients who need stimulants only for times when they are working and are able to be without stimulants on nonworking days, patients with chronic difficulties in maintaining alertness may need coverage of stimulant medications every day, especially for times when they are driving or socializing. In short, their use of stimulant medication more closely resembles the regimen generally used for treating patients with narcolepsy. For any patients whose symptoms are more complicated or who do not respond well to such treatment for an ADD, a full evaluation by a specialist in sleep disorders may be indicated.

CONCLUSION

As the foregoing pages suggest, problems in regulation of sleep and arousal appear to be an important aspect of the impairments associated with the broadly defined construct of attention-deficit disorder described in the opening chapter of this volume. Regulation of alertness would seem to be central to the exercise of executive functions in the brain. Fuller implications of these connections should emerge as more is learned from research on the neurochemistry of brain functions. Meanwhile, clinicians should be alert to the possibility that chronic difficulties in getting to sleep, in awakening, and in maintaining alertness, as well as other sleep-related disturbances, are likely to need careful attention in assessment and treatment of persons with ADDs.

REFERENCES

American Psychiatric Association: Diagnostic and Statistical Manual of Mental Disorders, 3rd Edition. Washington, DC, American Psychiatric Association, 1980

American Psychiatric Association: Diagnostic and Statistical Manual of Mental Disorders, 4th Edition. Washington, DC, American Psychiatric Association, 1994

Anders TF, Eiben LA: Pediatric sleep disorders: a review of the past 10 years. J Am Acad Child Adolesc Psychiatry 36:9–20, 1997

Brooks LJ: Diagnosis and pathophysiology of obstructive sleep apnea in children. Ear Nose Throat J 72:58–60, 1993

Broughton R: Important underemphasized aspects of sleep onset, in Sleep Onset: Normal and Abnormal Processes. Edited by Ogilvie RD, Harsh JR. Washington, DC, American Psychological Association, 1994, pp 19–35

Brown TE: Attention deficit disorders without hyperactivity. CHADDER 7(Spring/Summer):7–9, 1993

Brown TE: Differential diagnosis of ADD versus ADHD in adults, in A Comprehensive Guide to ADD in Adults: Research, Diagnosis and Treatment. Edited by Nadeau KG. New York, Brunner/Mazel, 1995, pp 93–108

Brown TE: Manual for Brown Attention Deficit Disorder Scales. San Antonio, TX, Psychological Corporation, 1996

Brown TE, Gammon GD: ADHD-associated difficulties falling asleep and awakening: clonidine and methylphenidate treatments. Poster presented at annual meeting of the American Academy of Child and Adolescent Psychiatry, Washington, DC, October 1992

Busby K, Firestone P, Pivik RT: Sleep patterns in hyperkinetic and normal children. Sleep 4:366–383, 1981

Cantwell DP, Swanson J, Conner DF: Case study: adverse response to clonidine. J Am Acad Child Adolesc Psychiatry 36:539–544, 1997

Carlander B, Eliaou JF, Billiard M: Autoimmune hypothesis in narcolepsy. Neurophysiol Clin 23:15–22, 1993

Carskadon MA, Pueschel SM, Millman RP: Sleep-disordered breathing and behavior in three risk groups: preliminary findings from parental reports. Childs Nerv Syst 9:452–457, 1993

Copeland ED, Copps SC: Medications for Attention Disorders (ADHD/ADD) and Related Medical Problems (Tourette's Syndrome, Sleep Apnea, Seizure Disorder): A Comprehensive Handbook. Plantation, FL, Specialty Press, 1995, pp 287–288

Corkum P, Tannock R, Moldofsky H: Sleep disturbances in children with attention-deficit/hyperactivity disorder. J Am Acad Child Adolesc Psychiatry 37:637–646, 1998

Corkum P, Moldofsky MD, Hogg-Johnson S: Sleep problems in children with attention-deficit/hyperactivity disorder: impact of subtype, comorbidity, and stimulant medication. J Am Acad Child Adolesc Psychiatry 10:1285–1293, 1999

Dahl RE: Sleep in behavioral and emotional disorders, in Principles and Practice of Sleep Medicine in the Child. Edited by Ferber R, Kryger M. Philadelphia, PA, WB Saunders, 1995, pp 147–153

Dahl RE: Regulation of sleep and arousal: development and psychopathology. Dev Psychopathol 8:3–27, 1996

Dahl RE, Pelham WB, Wierson MC: The role of sleep disturbance in attention deficit disorder symptomatology. J Pediatr Psychol 16:229–239, 1991

Dahl RE, Holttum J, Trubnik L: A clinical picture of child and adolescent narcolepsy. J Am Acad Child Adolesc Psychiatry 33:834–841, 1994

Douglas V: Cognitive deficits in children with attention deficit disorder with hyperactivity, in Attention Deficit Disorder: Criteria, Cognition, Intervention. Edited by Bloomingdale LM, Sergeant JA. New York, Pergamon, 1988, pp 65–81

Duane DD: Letter to the Editor. J Pediatr 118:489–490, 1991

Ferber R: Circadian rhythm sleep disorders in childhood, in Principles and Practice of Sleep Medicine. Edited by Ferber R, Kryger M. Philadelphia, PA, WB Saunders, 1995, pp 91–98

Ferber R: Clinical assessment of child and adolescent sleep disorders. Child Adolesc Psychiatr Clin N Am 5:569–579, 1996

Ferber R, Kryger M: Principles and Practice of Sleep Medicine in the Child. Philadelphia, PA, WB Saunders, 1995

Greenhill L, Puig-Antich J, Goetz R, et al: Sleep architecture and REM sleep measures in prepubertal children with attention deficit disorder with hyperactivity. Sleep 6:91–101, 1983

Hickey K, Walters A, Hening W: Hyperactivity and growing pains as a possible misdiagnosis in young-age onset restless leg syndrome. Sleep Res 21:209, 1992

Kent JD, Blader JC, Koplewicz HS, et al: Effects of late afternoon methylphenidate administration on behavior and sleep in attention-deficit hyperactivity disorder. Pediatrics 96:320–325, 1995

Khan AU: Sleep REM latency in hyperkinetic boys. Am J Psychiatry 139:1358–1360, 1982

Kiesow NA, Surwillo WW: Sleep spindles in the EEG's of hyperactive children. Psychol Rep 60:139–144, 1987

Kotagal S, Swink TD: Excessive daytime sleepiness in a 13-year-old. Semin Pediatr Neurol 3:170–172, 1996

Lozoff B: Culture and family: influences on childhood sleep practices and problems, in Principles and Practice of Sleep Medicine. Edited by Ferber R, Kryger M. Philadelphia, PA, WB Saunders, 1995, pp 69–73

Morrison DN, McGee R, Stanton WR: Sleep problems in adolescence. J Am Acad Child Adolesc Psychiatry 31:94–99, 1992

Moscovitch A, Partinent M, Guilleminault C: The positive diagnosis of narcolepsy and narcolepsy's borderland. Neurology 43:55–60, 1991

Navelet Y, Anders T, Guilleminault C: Narcolepsy in children, in Narcolepsy: Proceedings of the First International Symposium on Narcolepsy (Advances in Sleep Research, Vol 3). Edited by Guilleminault C, Dement WC, Passouant P. New York, Spectrum, 1976, pp 171–177

Nierenberg A, Adler L, Peselow E, et al: Trazodone for antidepressant-associated insomnia. Am J Psychiatry 151:1069–1072, 1994

Parkes JD: Sleep and Its Disorders. Philadelphia, PA, WB Saunders, 1985

Picchietti DL, Walters AS: Attention-deficit hyperactivity disorder and PLMD in childhood. Sleep Research 23:303, 1994

Picchietti DL, Walters AS: Restless legs syndrome and periodic limb movement disorder in children and adolescents: comorbidity with attention-deficit hyperactivity disorder. Child Adolesc Psychiatr Clin N Am 5(3):729–740, 1996

Popper CW: Combining methylphenidate and clonidine: pharmacologic questions and news reports of sudden death. J Child Adolesc Psychopharmacol 5:157–166, 1995

Porrino LJ, Rapoport JL, Behar D, et al: A naturalistic assessment of the motor activity of boys, I: comparison with normal controls. Arch Gen Psychiatry 40:681–687, 1983

Prince JB, Wilens TE, Biederman J, et al: Clonidine for sleep disturbances associated with attention-deficit hyperactivity disorder: a systematic chart review of 62 cases. J Am Acad Child Adolesc Psychiatrry 35:599–605, 1996

Ramos-Platon MJ, Vela-Bueno A, Espinar-Sierra J, et al: Hypnopolygraphic alterations in attention deficit disorder (ADD) children. Int J Neurosci 53(2–4):87–101, 1990

Sandeh A, Anders TF: Infant sleep problems: origins, assessment, intervention. International Mental Health Journal 14:17–34, 1993

Segalowitz SJ, Velikonja D, Storrie-Baker J: Attentional allocation and capacity in waking arousal, in Sleep Onset: Normal and Abnormal Processes. Edited by Ogilvie RD, Harsh JR. Washington, DC, American Psychological Association, 1994, pp 351–368

Sheldon SH, Spire JP, Levy HB: Pediatric Sleep Medicine. Philadelphia, PA, WB Saunders, 1992

Sheldon SH: Evaluating Sleep in Infants. Philadelphia, PA, Lippincott-Raven, 1996

Simmonds JF, Parraga H: Sleep behaviors and disorders in children and adolescents evaluated at psychiatric clinics. J Dev Behav Pediatr 5:6–10, 1984

Spencer T, Biederman J, Wilens T, et al: Pharmacotherapy of attention-deficit hyperactivity disorder across the life cycle. J Am Acad Child Adolesc Psychiatry 35:409–432, 1996

Tirosh E, Sadeh A, Munvez R, et al: Effects of methylphenidate on sleep in children with attention-deficit hyperactivity disorder: an activity monitor study. American Journal of Diseases of Children 147:1313–1315, 1993

Walters AS, Picchietti DL, Ehrenberg BL, et al: Case reports: restless leg syndrome in childhood and adolescence. Pediatr Neurol 11:241–245, 1994

Walters AS, Hickey K, Maltzman J, et al: A questionnaire study of 138 patients with restless leg syndrome: the 'Night-Walkers' Survey. Neurology 46:92–95, 1996

Weinberg WA, Brumback RA: Primary disorder of vigilance: a novel explanation of inattentiveness, boredom, restlessness, and sleepiness. J Pediatr 116:720–725, 1990

Weinberg WA, Harper CR: Vigilance and its disorders. Neurol Clin 11:59–78, 1993

Wilens TE, Biederman J, Spencer T: Clonidine for sleep disturbances associated with attention-deficit hyperactivity disorder. J Am Acad Child Adolesc Psychiatry 33:424–426, 1994

Wilens TE, Spencer TJ, Swanson JM, et al: Combining methylphenidate and clonidine: a clinically sound medication option. J Am Acad Child Adolesc Psychiatry 38:614–619, 1999 [discussion: J Am Acad Child Adolesc Psychiatry 38:619–622, 1999]

Yoss RE: The inheritance of diurnal sleepiness as measured by pupillography. Mayo Clin Proc 45:426–437, 1970

Yoss RE, Daly DD: Narcolepsy in children. Pediatrics 25:1025–1030, 1960

11 Attention-Deficit/ Hyperactivity Disorder With Tourette Syndrome

David E. Comings, M.D.

Because Tourette syndrome is characterized by visible rather than subjective symptoms, it is one of the easiest of the neurobehavioral diagnoses to make. Despite this, suppressibility of the symptoms is one of the characteristics of the disorder that often results in the diagnosis being missed. The DSM-IV diagnosis of Tourette syndrome is made on the basis of the development, prior to age 21 years, of motor and vocal tics that occur many times a day nearly every day, or intermittently, for a period of a year or more. The most common motor tics are eye blinking, facial grimacing, mouth opening, shoulder shrugging, crotch touching, and pulling at the clothing. The most common vocal tics are throat clearing, sniffing, snorting, barking, spitting, and making "huh" noises. However, the tics may be suppressed for minutes to hours. Since this suppression is especially likely to occur in the doctor's office, asking about chronic tics is an important part of the history taking. If the appropriate questions are not asked, or if the parents or the patient is not believed, the diagnosis frequently will be missed.

I first became interested in Tourette syndrome in 1980. As a human geneticist, I have a particular interest in hereditary neurological disorders. The distinctive nature of the motor and vocal tics made it easy to identify those members of the family who appeared to be carrying the Gilles de la Tourette, or Gts, genes. After seeing my first 100 patients, one of the single most striking features of Tourette syndrome was that the majority of affected children also had attention-deficit/hyperactivity disorder (ADHD). This was of particular interest to me because the mechanism of inheritance of ADHD was unknown, and many even doubted that it was a genetic, or even a biological, disorder. Since Tourette syndrome was clearly a genetic disorder, and since the prevalence of ADHD was 10 times greater in Tourette syndrome patients than in the general population, at least the subset of ADHD related to the Gts genes was genetic in origin.

Figure 11–1 shows a typical pedigree that illustrates several of the issues to be discussed in this chapter. If a 7-year-old boy (no. 1) came into the office presenting with symptoms that met the DSM criteria for ADHD and a family history was not taken, the diagnosis would simply be ADHD, and one might reasonably begin treating him with methylphenidate. However, if a family history showed that his 10-year-old brother (no. 2) with ADHD also had a history of rapid eye blinking, facial grimacing, shoulder shrugging, throat clearing, and sniffing since age 7 years, then one would be justified in suspecting that the ADHD was associated with Gts genes and that the patient's condition actually might represent an incipient case of Tourette syndrome. Having read the *Physicians' Desk Reference* warning that methylphenidate should not be given to patients with Tourette syndrome or a family history of Tourette syndrome, many clinicians might then decide not to prescribe methylphenidate. The family history also shows that the mother has chronic depression, her brother has ADHD and dyslexia, and her sister is 100 pounds overweight. Since the uncle (no. 3) also had a childhood history of ADHD, the criteria for ADHD, residual type, would be fulfilled for him. Finally, the father had exhibited eye blinking and facial grimacing for 5 years as a child and now has problems with alcohol and drug abuse. His brother is addicted to cocaine and his sister has been diagnosed as having a manic-depressive disorder and is taking lithium.

This pedigree illustrates many of the issues surrounding the question of the relationship between ADHD and Tourette syndrome and the comorbid disorders of both. Since my first realization that Tourette syndrome and ADHD were in many cases clinically and genetically related, evidence that the two disorders are very similar has continued to grow. In this chapter I discuss some of the evidence that has led me to believe that *Tourette syndrome is simply ADHD with tics.* The presentation of this evidence will simultaneously illustrate many of the issues that come up in the treatment of ADHD patients who have tics, develop tics, or have a family history of tics.

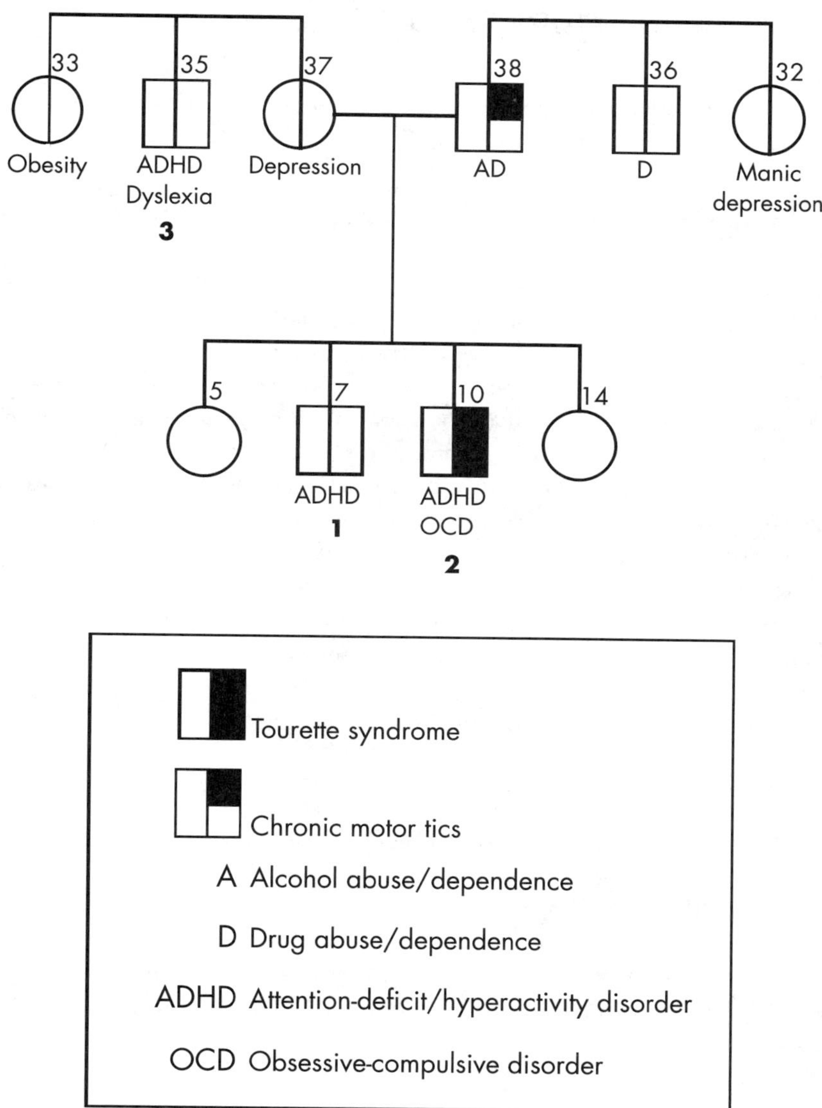

Figure 11–1. A typical pedigree for an ADHD proband with a family history of tics (see text for details).

EVIDENCE FOR A RELATIONSHIP BETWEEN ADHD AND TOURETTE SYNDROME

Many lines of evidence support a relationship between ADHD and Tourette syndrome, as described in the following subsections.

High Prevalence of ADHD in Tourette Syndrome

Virtually all studies agree that between 25% and 85% of Tourette syndrome probands have comorbid ADHD or attention-deficit disorder (ADD) (i.e., ADHD with or without hyperactivity) (D. E. Comings and Comings 1984, 1988; Shapiro et al. 1988). As the severity of the Tourette syndrome increases, the frequency of comorbid ADD also increases. Thus, in two of our series, involving 250 and 247 Tourette syndrome patients, respectively, ADD was present in 47% of mild cases, 58% of moderate cases, and 83% of severe cases of Tourette syndrome (D. E. Comings and Comings 1984, 1987a, 1988). Since the severity of Tourette syndrome, based on tics and other behaviors, is related to the number or degree of expression of the Gts genes, and since the prevalence of ADHD increases with severity, it is reasonable to conclude that the presence of ADHD also represents a greater number or greater degree of expression of the Gts genes. Simply put, the more severe the global rating of the Tourette syndrome, the more likely it is that ADHD is also present.

High Prevalence of Tics in Relatives of ADHD Probands

When a family history is carefully taken, including detailed questions about the presence of chronic motor tics, 20%–50% of ADHD probands are found to have a first-, second-, or third-degree relative with chronic motor or vocal tics. Figure 11–1 provides a typical pedigree for an ADHD proband with a family member with tics.

Presence of ADHD Prior to the Onset of Tics

The first symptom in the majority of Tourette syndrome patients is not the presence of tics but the appearance of ADHD. Although the precise age at onset of ADHD is more difficult to determine than that of tics, in general, onset of ADHD precedes the development of the tics by about 2.4–3.0 years (D. E. Comings and Comings 1984, 1987a, 1988). However, we also see many cases in which the onset of the ADHD closely coincides with the onset of the tics. The temporal, clinical, and genetic interrelatedness of Tourette syndrome and ADHD is illustrated in the following case:

> G.S. is a 10-year-old male. He was very active in the first year of life and was expelled from nursery school because he was too hyperactive and often left the building. At age 4 years, he developed motor tics consisting of facial grimacing and mouth opening and vocal tics consisting of throat clearing and barking. He picked at his fingers until they bled and had complex finger tics. At this same age he was diagnosed with ADHD but no treatment was recommended. He started kindergarten at age 5 but was immediately expelled because of hyperactive and disruptive behavior. Just before starting kindergarten, he was treated with methylphenidate 10 mg tid. This resulted in a considerable decrease in the motor hyperactivity and no increase or decrease in the motor or vocal tics. In first grade he was immediately placed in special education classes, but even in that setting the teacher was constantly calling his parents and complaining about his behavior. The addition of transdermal clonidine to the methylphenidate resulted in cessation of the tics and a decrease in the disruptive behaviors.

The pedigree for G.S., shown in Figure 11–2, illustrates the genetic interrelatedness of ADHD and Tourette syndrome in that both parents had a history of childhood ADHD. It is not difficult to envision a polygenic threshold model of inheritance in which a few Gts-ADHD genes that are present in sufficient number to produce ADHD in both parents come together in the child in even higher numbers and produce ADHD and Tourette syndrome.

The nearly simultaneous development of tics and ADHD is often striking. It can be particularly devastating for a child who performed superbly in grade school to develop both tics and ADHD in junior high school. We have observed this so many times that we feel that the DSM diagnostic criterion that ADHD must start before age 7 years is unduly restrictive. Although the tics may be mild enough to pose no problem, the comorbid ADHD can be devastating. Instead of the classwork being easy, as it once was, it now requires a major effort for such children to learn and keep up with their peers. Unless recognized, diagnosed, and treated, their condition may simply be explained away as teenage laziness and poor motivation.

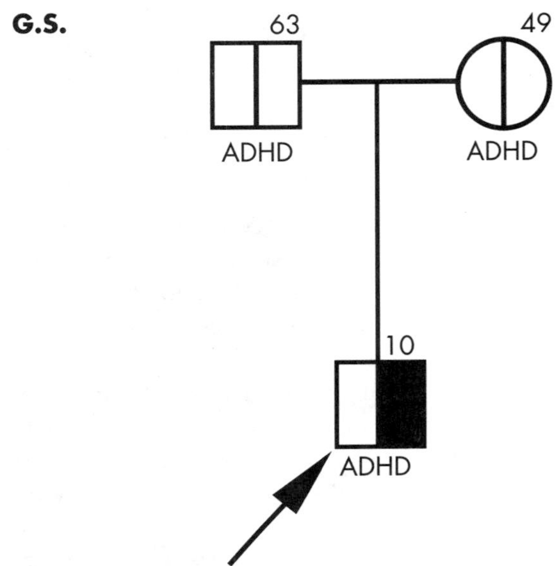

Figure 11–2. The pedigree of G.S., illustrating the presence of childhood attention-deficit/hyperactivity disorder (ADHD) in both parents of a proband with Tourette syndrome and ADHD. The pedigree is consistent with a polygenic threshold model of inheritance, in which genes are contributed by both parents and, after a certain genetic threshold is surpassed, can be expressed, resulting in Tourette syndrome and ADHD.

Similar Natural Histories of ADHD and Tourette Syndrome

The studies of Burd and co-workers provide an excellent demonstration of the fact that many children with Tourette syndrome outgrow the tics as they grow older. These studies indicated that within the same defined geographic area, the prevalence of Tourette syndrome was 10 times greater in children (Burd et al. 1986b) than in adults (Burd et al. 1986a). In my clinical practice, where individual cases are followed over the period from childhood to adolescence, in over 50% of the cases the tics subside sufficiently in the teenage years to such an extent that treatment for the tics is no longer required. Similar results were reported by Bruun (1988), Erenberg et al. (1987), and Shapiro et al. (1988). This trend is similar to that seen in ADHD, in which the symptoms tend to disappear over time in about half the subjects (Gittelman et al. 1985; Mannuzza et al. 1991). As discussed later in this chapter, although the tics and motor hyperactivity of both Tourette syndrome and ADHD may diminish with age, other problems, such as substance abuse, depression, and anxiety, may develop. The following case illustrates these intertwining patterns of comorbidities in the natural histories of ADHD and Tourette syndrome:

> R.P. is a 28-year-old male. In the first year of life, he slept poorly and was very active and "unruly." The hyperactivity was so severe that he was treated with methylphenidate at 3 years of age. The medication was not helpful and was discontinued. After attending kindergarten for only 1 month, R.P. was expelled because of aggressive behavior and poor attention span. In first grade, these problems persisted, and he was treated with methylphenidate intermittently over the next 2 years. The medication was finally discontinued because of the patient's lethargy. R.P. was expelled from fourth grade because of aggressive and disruptive behaviors, compounded by short attention span, and was placed in a special day class. He did much better in that setting because of the small class and specially trained teacher.
>
> At 10 years of age, in the fifth grade, R.P. developed tics involving mouth opening, head jerking, and facial grimacing. Throat-clearing tics began the following year. His parents were divorced, and in eighth grade R.P. was sent to live on a farm with his father. "They didn't worry about me getting lost because they could always tell where I was because of my noises."
>
> R.P. graduated from high school, despite barely passing all his classes, and joined the Navy. While there he began to have problems with alcohol abuse. After leaving the Navy, he worked as a porter in Las Vegas. During the subsequent 5 years, R.P. developed severe problems with drug dependence, using predominantly cocaine and methamphetamine. He was fired from most jobs because of losing his temper or other inappropriate behaviors.
>
> When seen in the clinic, R.P. had facial-grimacing and horizontal head-jerking tics of moderate severity. The diagnosis consisted of Tourette syndrome, ADHD—residual type, and psychoactive substance abuse. Treatment was initiated with clonidine transdermal patch TTS-1, beginning with 0.25 patch per week. At a dose of 1.5 patches per week, R.P.'s tics disappeared, and he felt calmer and less angry and irritable. He has continued off cocaine and methamphetamine.

The pedigree for R.P., shown in Figure 11–3, illustrates the family history of substance abuse and other behavioral problems on both the maternal and parental side of the family and the frequent absence of motor or vocal tics in

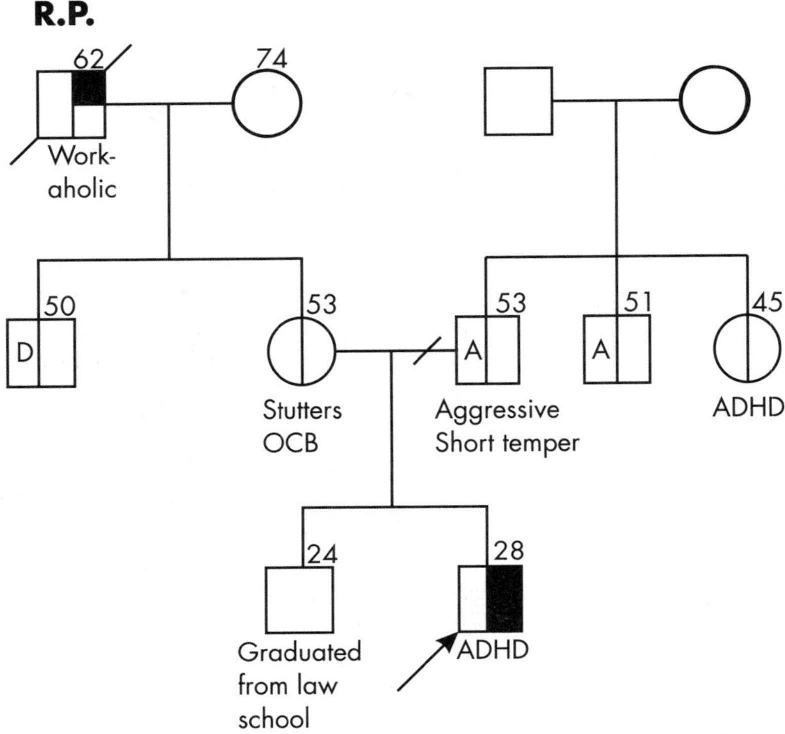

Figure 11–3. The pedigree of R.P., illustrating the frequent occurrence of substance abuse in the relatives of Tourette syndrome and attention-deficit/hyperactivity disorder (ADHD) probands. Note the absence of chronic tics in either parent of the Tourette syndrome proband. This occurs very often and supports the concept that the pattern of inheritance of Tourette syndrome is more complex than that described by an autosomal dominant model with reduced penetrance. A = alcohol abuse/dependence; D = drug abuse/dependence; OCB = obsessive-compulsive behavior.

the parents. These features are consistent with a complex, probably polygenic, mode of inheritance. This case history illustrates the frequent presence of comorbid substance abuse in both ADHD and Tourette syndrome.

Increased Prevalence of ADHD in Relatives of Tourette Syndrome Patients

An alternative hypothesis for the high frequency of ADDs in Tourette syndrome was proposed by Pauls et al. (1986). They suggested that the presence of ADD simply represented ascertainment bias. *Ascertainment bias* refers to the tendency for subjects who seek medical care to have more than one disorder. Thus, people with two or three problems, which are possibly independent of one another, are more likely to seek medical care for one of them than are those with a single disorder. Closely related to this is the tendency for more severely affected individuals to seek medical care before mildly affected individuals. The person in the family who seeks medical care is called the *proband,* and thus the term *proband ascertainment bias* has been applied to refer to this tendency.

The easiest way to rule out proband ascertainment bias is to examine relatives of the proband who also have tics. We refer to these individuals as *nonproband Tourette syndrome relatives.* The relatives without Tourette syndrome or chronic tics are referred to as *non–Tourette syndrome relatives.*

In their original article, Pauls et al. (1986) observed that if the Tourette syndrome probands had ADHD, 17.2% of the relatives had ADD or ADHD, whereas if the Tourette syndrome probands did not have ADHD, 2.2% of the relatives had ADD or ADHD. When the analysis was restricted to the relatives with tics, when the proband had ADHD, 25% (4 of 16) of the relatives had ADD or ADHD, whereas if the proband did not have ADHD, none (0 of 14) of the relatives had ADD or ADHD. From these findings, Pauls et al. concluded that Tourette syndrome and ADHD were segregating independently and were unrelated entities and that the presence of ADHD in Tourette syndrome was due to ascertainment bias. However, this study involved a small sample size, and thus there was a risk for type II errors. In contrast to this study, a prior study in which the authors participated found that the proband did not have ADHD, and yet 33% of the relatives with tics had ADHD (Kurlan et al. 1986).

To test the ascertainment bias hypothesis, we examined 24 of the families used in our linkage studies. In this sample, when the proband had ADD, 37% of the nonproband Tourette syndrome relatives had ADD. When the proband did not have ADD, 21% of the nonproband Tourette syndrome relatives had ADD. There was a highly significant difference in the frequency of ADD in the nonproband Tourette syndrome relatives (34%) versus the non–Tourette syndrome relatives (4.6%).

In a later study, we again examined this question (Knell and Comings 1993). As a way of avoiding ascertainment bias, 338 first-degree relatives of 131 Tourette syndrome probands were examined with a structured questionnaire. Of the relatives with Tourette syndrome, 61% had ADD and 36% had ADHD. Of the relatives with chronic tics, 41% had ADD and 26% had ADHD. A log-linear analysis showed a major significant association between tics and ADHD. If the proband had ADHD, 17.5% of the relatives had ADHD. This association was significantly greater than that in the control group ($P < 0.0001$).

If the proband did not have ADHD, 9.7% of the relatives had ADHD ($P < 0.05$). There was a significant difference between male and female probands in terms of rates of ADHD among relatives. For male probands with ADHD, 21.3% of the relatives had ADHD. If the male proband did not have ADHD, 20.0% of the relatives had ADHD. Both of these associations were significantly different from those in the group of control subjects. For female probands with ADHD (vs. control subjects), 14.0% of the relatives had ADHD ($P < 0.0001$); for female probands without ADHD, 0% of the relatives had ADHD (not significant). As discussed later in this chapter, in another independent study there was a significantly greater frequency of ADHD in the nonproband Tourette syndrome relatives than in the non–Tourette syndrome relatives. Pauls et al. (1993) also reexamined this question. On the basis of a study of 85 Tourette syndrome probands, the authors concluded that there is a genetic relationship between Tourette syndrome and some cases of ADHD.

Two further methods of eliminating ascertainment bias—epidemiological and prospective studies—are discussed below.

Increased Prevalence of ADHD in Epidemiologically Ascertained Tourette Syndrome Subjects

Epidemiological studies eliminate ascertainment bias because the cases are selected independently of whether or not the subjects have sought medical care. In the study by Caine et al. (1988), the combined prevalence of Tourette syndrome among males was 1 in 1,400. Of the males with Tourette syndrome, 27% had ADHD, 27% had sleep problems, 17% had conduct disorder, and 7% had obsessive-compulsive disorder. Further, 27% had repeated a grade, and 24% had learning disorders. These frequencies all were manyfold higher than those in the general population.

To determine the prevalence of Tourette syndrome in schoolchildren, we monitored 3,000 students in kindergarten through grade 7 (D. E. Comings et al. 1990b). The prevalence of Tourette syndrome in boys was 1 in 95. Ten of the boys ascertained in this study were subsequently seen in the clinic, and all were diagnosed with ADHD.

Increased Prevalence of ADHD in a Prospective Study of Relatives of Tourette Syndrome Patients

The only prospective study performed to date, that by Carter et al. (1994), involved children or siblings of Tourette syndrome probands who entered the study at an early age, before they developed tics. In a preliminary report, of the 21 subjects followed to 7–10 years of age, 42.8% developed tics and 23.8% had ADHD, 19% had obsessive-compulsive behaviors, 23.8% had anxiety disorders, and 23.8% had speech problems—rates that were all significantly higher than those in the general population.

Shared Spectrum of Comorbid Disorders in Tourette Syndrome and ADHD Patients and Their Relatives

Many chapters in this book illustrate the fact that ADHD is a spectrum disorder—that is, in addition to ADHD, the probands and their relatives show a high frequency of a range of other disorders, including conduct disorder, depression, anxiety, learning problems, and drug and alcohol dependence. The same spectrum of disorders is also present in Tourette syndrome probands and their relatives.

Comorbidity in Tourette Syndrome Probands

The comorbid disorders occurring in Tourette syndrome probands, reviewed elsewhere (D. E. Comings and Comings 1993), include ADHD, depression, mania, alcoholism, drug abuse, inappropriate sexual behaviors, migraine headaches, panic attacks, phobias, agoraphobia, generalized anxiety disorder, conduct disorder, eating disorders, learning disorders, obsessive-compulsive disorder, sleep disorders, somatoform disorders, and speech disorders.

The three studies that have used structured instruments to examine the presence of comordid disorders in Tourette syndrome are those of D. E. Comings and B. G. Comings (B. G. Comings and Comings 1987; D. E. Comings and Comings 1987a, 1987b, 1987c, 1987d, 1987e), Pauls et al. (1988; see also D. E. Comings and Comings 1993), and Singer and Rosenberg (1989). These studies demonstrated the increased frequency of ADHD, substance abuse, depression, anxiety, conduct problems, schizoid behavior, and speech problems in Tourette syndrome probands, but they did not answer the question of whether these problems were due to the Gts genes themselves or to ascertainment bias. To answer this question would require examining nonproband Tourette syndrome subjects.

Comorbidity in Nonproband Tourette Syndrome Subjects

In our clinic, every new patient—and, when available, both parents and siblings—are required to fill out a 31-page structured questionnaire based on the

Diagnostic Interview Schedule (Robins et al. 1981) and DSM-III-R (American Psychiatric Association 1987). The 720 variables cover 32 different DSM-III-R diagnoses, many demographic variables, and questions about tics (D. E. Comings 1990b). To date, more than 4,400 subjects with a range of diagnoses are represented in this computerized database. This database allows us to examine many questions concerning the spectrum of behavioral disorders present in probands and their relatives.

Examination of the presence or absence of comorbid behaviors in relatives of Tourette syndrome subjects who themselves have Tourette syndrome (i.e., nonproband Tourette syndrome relatives) allows us to avoid the problem of proband ascertainment bias, since the subjects are not probands. An ideal control group would be relatives who do not have Tourette syndrome, since they would be from the same families and thus provide a perfect match for socioeconomic, ethnic, and other, related variables.

The following groups would be expected to have progressively less genetic loading for Gts genes: 1) Tourette syndrome probands, 2) nonproband Tourette syndrome relatives, 3) non–Tourette syndrome relatives, and 4) control subjects. If the frequency of specific behaviors is significantly correlated with the degree loading for the Gts genes, it is probable that the behavior is, at least in part, associated with those genes. If there is a significantly higher frequency of that behavior in nonproband Tourette syndrome relatives compared with non–Tourette syndrome relatives, one can rule out effects of both ascertainment bias and the inappropriate choice of controls. This concept is illustrated in Figure 11–4.

We have used this approach to show that comorbid alcohol and drug abuse, problematic sexual behaviors, oppositional defiant disorder and conduct disorder (Figure 11–5), somatoform disorder, and depression (Figure 11–6) (D. E. Comings 1994a, 1994b, 1994c; 1995a, 1995b) are associated with Gts genes. Similar results were obtained with ADHD probands and their relatives.

Table 11–1 summarizes the results of these studies in relation to a range of comorbid disorders and behaviors. The frequency of the disorder or behavior in nonproband Tourette syndrome relatives vs. non–Tourette syndrome relatives (third column in the table) is the most important comparison because it allows us to rule out ascertainment bias and inappropriateness of the controls. For this comparison, the results were significant ($P < 0.001$) for all problems except those related to smoking, reading, eating, gambling, and somatization. However, some of the results were highly significant for a subset of the Tourette syndrome relatives (data not shown). For example, the P value for eating problems among those with obsessive-compulsive behaviors

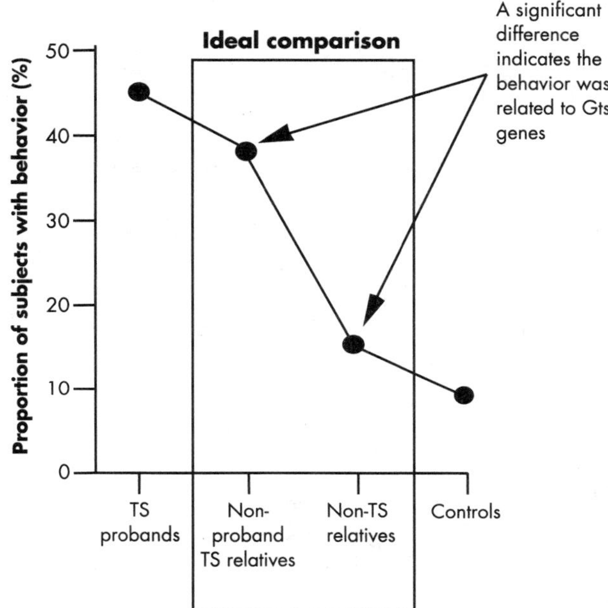

Figure 11–4. Model for examining association of behaviors with Gilles de la Tourette (Gts) genes to avoid proband ascertainment bias or inappropriate choice of controls. If a behavior, such as that illustrated here, shows a significant decrease in frequency going from Tourette syndrome (TS) probands to relatives with Tourette syndrome, to relatives without Tourette syndrome, to control subjects, that behavior is assumed to be associated with Gts genes. The ideal comparison is between relatives with Tourette syndrome (nonproband Tourette syndrome relatives) and relatives without Tourette syndrome (non–Tourette syndrome relatives). When the frequency of the behavior is significantly higher in nonproband Tourette syndrome relatives than in non–Tourette syndrome relatives, problems with proband ascertainment bias or inappropriate choice of controls can be ruled out.

was $<10^{-9}$, as was the *P* value for obsessive-compulsive behaviors. I refer to this as "association by association." In a similar vein, the association with smoking was highly significant among those with alcohol or drug abuse, that with reading problems was highly significant among subjects with learning disorders, and that with gambling was highly significant among subjects with obsessive-compulsive behaviors. Some examples of the results of these comparisons for oppositional defiant disorder and conduct disorder and for symptoms of depression are shown in Figures 11-5 and 11-6, respectively. The *P* values represent the comparisons between the nonproband Tourette syndrome relatives and the non–Tourette syndrome relatives. The results of these studies show that the comorbid behaviors in Tourette syndrome are very similar to the comorbid behaviors in ADHD, as discussed throughout out this book. The similarities in frequency of comorbid behaviors in these disorders are summarized in Table 11–2.

The results from these family studies are all consistent with the conclusion that Tourette syndrome and ADHD either are related to the same gene or genes or have a significant number of genes in common. Further evidence for the similar or shared genetic basis of these disorders comes from examining specific genes at the molecular level.

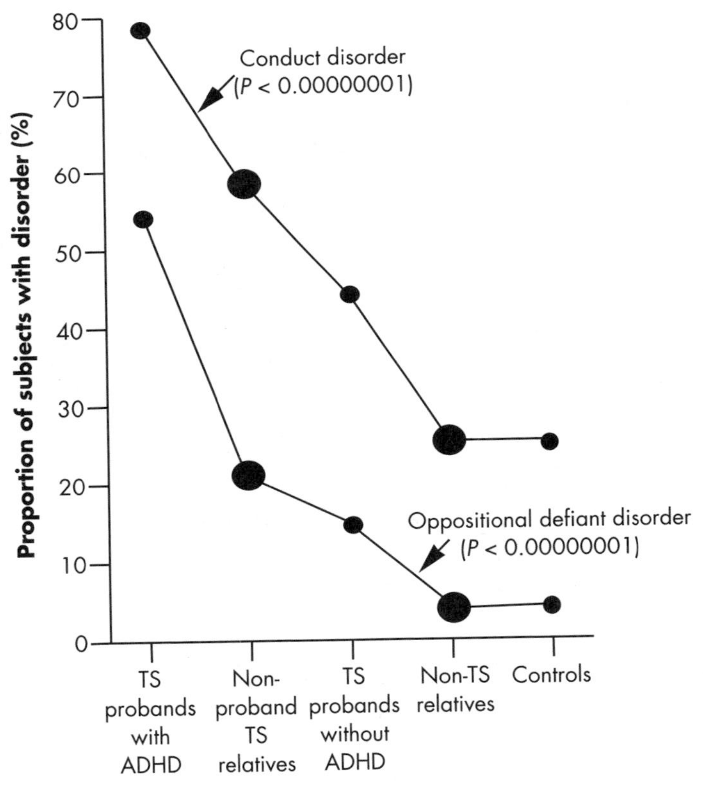

Figure 11–5. Association between conduct disorder and oppositional defiant disorder and genetic loading for the Gilles de la Tourette (Gts) genes. The larger dots represent the comparison of nonproband Tourette syndrome (TS) relatives with relatives without Tourette syndrome. *P* values refer to this comparison. ADHD = attention-deficit/hyperactivity disorder.

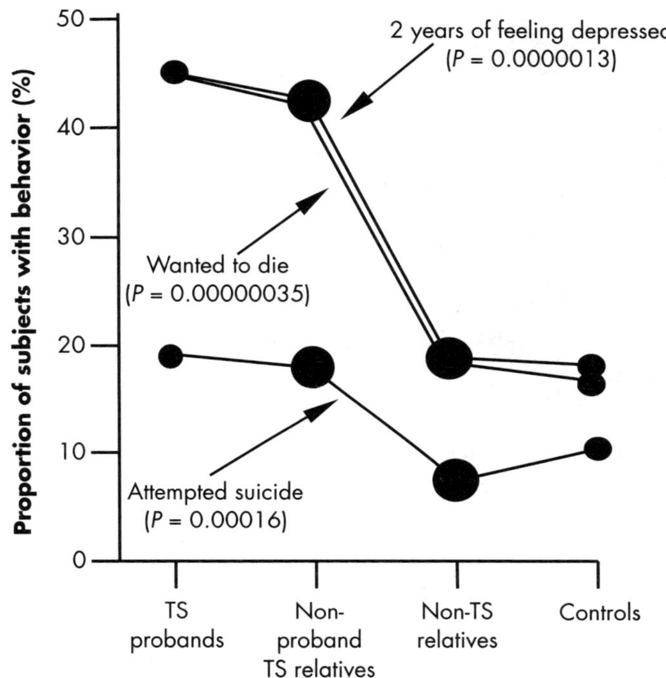

Figure 11–6. Association between depressive symptoms of "2 years of feeling depressed," "wanted to die," and "attempted suicide" and genetic loading for the Gilles de la Tourette (Gts) genes. The larger dots represent the comparison of nonproband Tourette syndrome (TS) relatives with relatives without Tourette syndrome. *P* values refer to this comparison.

Similarities in the Genes Involved in Tourette Syndrome and ADHD

One of the major hypotheses concerning the cause of ADHD is that of a defect in dopaminergic pathways. Lesions of the frontal lobe dopaminergic neurons in newborn rats resulted in a behavioral syndrome similar to ADHD (Shaywitz et al. 1976b). Like ADHD, the syndrome responded to the administration of dopaminergic agonists such as amphetamine (Shaywitz et al. 1976a). Defects in dopamine metabolism frequently have been proposed as the cause of Tourette syndrome (Chase et al. 1986; D. E. Comings 1987; Devinsky 1983).

Table 11–1. Prevalence (%) of comorbid disorders and behaviors in a clinic sample of Tourette syndrome (TS) probands and their relatives (with or without TS)

Comorbid disorder or condition	TS[a] (*n* = 361)	Relatives: +TS[b] (*n* = 113)	Relatives: –TS[c] (*n* = 380)	Controls (*n* = 68)
ADHD	61.5^{9}	50.9^{9}	7.4^{9}	7.4
Obsessive-compulsive behaviors	57.3^{9}	47.8^{9}	12.6^{9}	10.3
Alcohol abuse	15.0^{3}	23.0^{4}	9.2^{5}	1.5
Drug abuse	22.7^{4}	30.1^{6}	10.8^{7}	8.8
Smoking	16.3^{1}	20.4^{2}	12.6^{2}	11.8
Discipline problems	56.9^{7}	40.0^{9}	15.1^{8}	20.6
Learning disorders	37.7^{7}	16.8^{9}	4.5^{6}	5.9
Reading problems	34.3^{3}	23.9^{9}	14.5^{2}	14.7
Stuttering	28.2^{4}	19.6^{9}	5.3^{6}	7.7
Phobias	50.1^{2}	60.2^{8}	28.9^{9}	38.2
Panic attacks	55.7^{4}	59.1^{9}	30.1^{8}	31.3
Generalized anxiety	40.7^{4}	38.9^{9}	18.7^{6}	17.6
Eating problems	32.6^{1}	34.9^{2}	25.1^{2}	27.9
Gambling	20.2^{2}	18.6^{5}	9.5^{3}	10.3
Depression	43.9^{5}	39.3^{9}	18.8^{6}	17.6
Manic symptoms	51.5^{9}	47.8^{9}	10.8^{9}	4.4
Somatization	46.1^{3}	46.6^{7}	28.2^{3}	25.0
Sleep problems	38.8^{4}	38.9^{9}	11.8^{9}	17.6
Sexual problems	55.1^{5}	57.5^{9}	24.7^{9}	29.4
Schizoid behaviors	45.4^{7}	40.4^{9}	14.4^{5}	13.2

Note. ADHD = attention-deficit/hyperactivity disorder.

[a]Tourette syndrome probands. Superscripts represent negative logs of the *P* values for the chi-square comparisons of the frequency of the listed problem in the Tourette syndrome probands vs. control subjects.

[b]Nonproband Tourette syndrome relatives. Superscripts represent negative logs of the *P* values for chi-square analyses for a linear trend progressing from Tourette syndrome probands to nonproband Tourette syndrome relatives to non–Tourette syndrome relatives to control subjects.

[c]Non–Tourette syndrome relatives. Superscripts represent the negative logs of the *P* values of the chi-square comparisons of the frequency of the behavior in nonproband Tourette syndrome subjects and non–Tourette syndrome relatives.

Table 11–2. Frequency (%) of comorbid behaviors in Tourette syndrome and ADHD probands

Comorbid disorder or behavior	Tourette syndrome[a]	ADHD[b]
ADD	50–90	100
ADHD	25–80	100
Affective disorders	10–30	15–75
Alcoholism, drug abuse	30[c]	5–20
Anxiety disorder, panic attacks	30	25
Conduct disorder	30–50	30–50
Exhibitionism	2–20	5–20
ODD	30–50	35
Learning disabilities	20–50	10–90
Obsessive-compulsive behaviors	40–60	25–35
Schizoid behaviors	11–12	5–8
Self-abusive behaviors	20–30	15–30
Sleep disorders	20–45	30–40
Stuttering	25–45	20–25

Note. ADD = attention-deficit disorder; ADHD = attention-deficit/hyperactivity disorder; ODD = oppositional defiant disorder.
[a]See D. E. Comings and Comings 1993.
[b]See Biederman et al. 1991, 1992.
[c]Severe Tourette syndrome.

In 1990, Blum et al. (1990) reported a significant increase in the prevalence of the *Taq*I A1 allele of the dopamine D_2 receptor gene in patients with severe alcoholism compared with control subjects. Although subsequent studies have both confirmed and denied this relationship, a recent review indicates that the D_2 A1 allele is associated with severity in at least some forms of alcoholism (Noble 1993). The association of this allele with drug addiction has been more robust (D. E. Comings et al. 1994; Noble et al. 1993; Smith et al. 1992).

We wondered if the variability in these results might be attributed in part to the D_2 A1 allele's being more strongly associated with a behavioral trait or disorder that is present in some alcoholic persons but not in others. As shown in Table 11–3, we found a significant increase in the prevalence of the D_2 A1 allele in individuals with polysubstance abuse, Tourette syndrome, ADHD, conduct disorder, autism, and posttraumatic stress disorder (D. E. Comings et al. 1991). In the context of this chapter, it is interesting to note that the prevalence of the D_2 A1 allele was very similar in both Tourette syndrome and

Table 11–3. Prevalence of the *Taq*I A1 allele of the dopamine$_2$ (D_2) receptor gene (*DRD2*) in control subjects and in subjects with various impulsive/compulsive disorders

Diagnosis	n	Proportion with 1 allele (%)	χ^2	P
Control	378	24.6		
Alcoholism/drug abuse or dependence	104	42.3	12.57	0.0007
Tourette syndrome				
Moderate	108	39.8	9.64	0.002
Severe	39	59.0	20.80	0.0001
Total sample	147	44.9	20.65	0.0001
ADHD	104	46.2	18.30	0.0001
Autism	33	54.5	13.63	0.0005
Conduct disorder	7	85.7	11.94	0.0009
PTSD	35	45.7	7.35	0.007

Note. ADHD = attention-deficit/hyperactivity disorder; PTSD = posttraumatic stress disorder.
Source. Data from D. E. Comings et al. 1991.

ADHD subjects. This is the first gene shown to be involved in either Tourette syndrome or ADHD, and its prevalence was comparably elevated in both disorders.

We examined the role of two other dopamine genes in Tourette syndrome and ADHD: those for dopamine β-hydroxylase (*DBH*) and the dopamine transporter (*DAT1*). The dopamine β-hydroxylase enzyme is responsible for conversion of dopamine to norepinephrine, another neurotransmitter frequently implicated in ADHD (McCracken 1991; Mefford and Potter 1989). The dopamine transporter is responsible for transporting dopamine from the synapse back to the presynaptic neuron from which it was released. We were interested in the gene for the dopamine transporter because the dopamine transporter is the site of action of methylphenidate and dextroamphetamine sulfate, the two most widely used drugs for treatment of ADHD. We found that each of these genes also played a significant role in Tourette syndrome and ADHD and that genetic variants of all three genes—*DRD2, DBH,* and *DAT1*—were additive in their effect (D. E. Comings 1996; D. E. Comings et al. 1996b). These three genes play a role in many of the disorders that are comorbid with Tourette syndrome and ADHD. Thus, the severity scores for problems with ADHD, oppositional defiant behavior, conduct disorder, manic symptoms, tics, substance abuse, obsessive-compulsive behaviors, and other behaviors were highest for those individuals who inherited the relevant alleles of all three genes, lower for those who inherited two of three or one of three, and lowest for those who did not inherit any of the markers. Cook et al. (1995) also found an association between *DAT1* and ADHD. Using single-photon emission computed tomography scanning, Malison et al. (1995) reported an increase in the activity of the dopamine transporter, an indication of increased expression of *DAT1,* in the caudate region of Tourette syndrome subjects.

Specific markers of a fourth dopamine gene, the dopamine D_4 receptor gene (*DRD4*), have been shown to be associated with risk-taking behaviors (Benjamin et al. 1996; Ebstein et al. 1996). These behaviors are common in individuals with Tourette syndrome and ADHD. Thus, it was not surprising that the same *DRD4* gene markers were reported to be increased in subjects with ADHD (Lahoste et al. 1996) and in subjects with Tourette syndrome (Grice et al. 1996).

A second hypothesis for the cause of both Tourette syndrome (D. E. Comings 1990b) and ADHD (Brase and Loh 1975; D. E. Comings 1990b) is that of a defect in serotonin metabolism. Since blood levels of both serotonin and tryptophan are decreased in Tourette syndrome and ADHD probands and their relatives (D. E. Comings 1990a), we proposed that a genetic defect in the tryptophan 2,3-dioxygenase gene (*TDO2*) may be involved (D. E. Comings 1990a, 1990b, 1996). The results of studies of polymorphisms at *TDO2* are consistent with this proposal (D. E. Comings et al. 1996a).

We recently identified 27 different genes affecting dopamine, serotonin, norepinephrine, γ-aminobutyric acid (GABA), and other neurotransmsitters in Tourette syndrome subjects with ADHD (D. E. Comings, R. Gade-Andavolu, N. Gonzalez N, et al., submitted). This work supported the hypothesis that Tourette syndrome and ADHD, as well as oppositional defiant disorder, conduct disorder, and other comorbid behaviors, are polygenic and share genes in common. The presence of defects in these dopaminergic, noradrenergic, and serotonergic genes helps to explain why dopamine agonists such as methylphenidate, dextroamphetamine sulfate, and pemoline; norepinephrine-acting medications such as clonidine and guanfacine; and selective serotonin reuptake inhibitors such as fluoxetine, sertraline, paroxetine, and fluvoxamine are so effective in the treatment of ADHD or Tourette syndrome and its comorbid behaviors. The presence of such defects also contradicts those who claim there is no biological or genetic basis to ADHD and that this is a mythical "disorder" concocted by teachers and parents simply as an excuse to medicate their rambunctious offspring.

Similarities in the Treatment of Tourette Syndrome and ADHD

Both ADHD and Tourette syndrome are treated with a similar group of medications. These include clonidine; tricyclic antidepressants such as imipramine and desipramine; stimulants such as methylphenidate, dextroamphetamine sulfate, and pemoline; anticonvulsants such as carbamazepine (D. E. Comings 1990b) and valproic acid (Monroe 1975); and serotonin reuptake inhibitors such as fluoxetine (D. E. Comings 1990b; Riddle et al. 1988), clomipramine (Leonard et al. 1989; Yaryura-Tobias and Neziroglu 1977), sertraline, and paroxetine. I will not cover here the details of the use of these medications but only compare the ways some are used in the treatment of ADHD and Tourette syndrome.

Clonidine

Clonidine has been found to be useful in the treatment of both ADHD (Hunt et al. 1985) and tics (Cohen et al. 1980). Consequently, it is an ideal medication for the treatment of Tourette syndrome patients with concomitant ADHD or for ADHD patients with tics. It avoids the concern, discussed below, about the potential for stimulants to exacerbate tics in Tourette syndrome patients or to elicit the appearance of tics in patients with ADHD.

We have found transdermal clonidine to be generally superior to oral clonidine (D. E. Comings 1990b; D. E. Comings et al. 1990a). In some cases it is effective when oral clonidine is ineffective. Because of the more even delivery of the drug, transdermal clonidine is often associated with much less sedation than oral clonidine. In my experience it is effective for controlling both the tics and the ADHD, especially the symptoms of motor hyperactivity. Attention span may also improve significantly, with resultant improvement in grades. In some cases, however, supplemental methylphenidate or dextroamphetamine sulfate is necessary to optimally treat the ADHD. The combination of clonidine and a stimulant medication can be particularly useful, with the clonidine controlling the tics and enough of the motor hyperactivity such that lower doses of stimulants are required to fully control the ADHD. Clonidine can also improve or diminish some of the other comorbid conditions and behaviors such as anxiety, phobias, panic attacks, oppositional defiant disorder, conduct disorder, inappropriate sexual behaviors, and sleep problems. Clonidine can be particularly helpful for sleep problems. Parents often report that one of the first positive effects of the medication is that their child can get to sleep and stay asleep. Occasionally, a bedtime supplementation of the patch with a small oral dose of clonidine controls severe sleep problems.

A common complication of the use of the clonidine patch is the development of contact dermatitis. Having a compounding pharmacist make a clonidine cream (0.1–0.4 mg/mL) eliminates this problem, since the allergy is almost always to the patch and not to the medication. In my experience the cream works best when applied to the chest each morning. If it is allowed to dry for 20 minutes before being covered with clothing, it usually is not necessary to cover it with a bandage. Clonidine cream is also useful in the summer when children are sweating or swimming. The cream can be applied after swimming instead of in the morning.

Although there have been some reports of deaths of children on the combination of methylphenidate and clonidine, analyses of these cases indicate that other serious physical disorders probably accounted for most of the deaths and that this combination is generally safe. I have treated more than 1,000 children with this combination without problems.

Imipramine and Desipramine

Imipramine and desipramine have both been shown to be effective in the treatment of ADHD (Greenberg et al. 1975; Gualtieri et al. 1991; Rapoport 1965). They can be particularly useful in the treatment of ADHD in patients with Tourette syndrome (D. E. Comings 1990b) because they can also be effective in the treatment of tics and are less likely than stimulants to exacerbate the tics. They can also be effective in the treatment of comorbid depression, irritability, oppositional defiant disorder, conduct disorder, anxiety, sleep disorders, and elimination disorders (especially enuresis and, in some cases, encopresis). Rare reports of deaths in children on desipramine have also been reported, and electrocardiographic screening is recommended when this medication is used.

Stimulant Medications

One of the most controversial aspects of the treatment of ADHD and Tourette syndrome has been the question of whether to treat ADHD in patients with Tourette syndrome with stimulants and whether to continue stimulant treatment of children with ADHD if they develop tics following treatment with these agents.

It has been noted in numerous reports that stimulant medications can either produce or exacerbate tics in ADHD and Tourette syndrome subjects (for review, see Robertson and Eapen 1992). These reports led the manufacturers of Ritalin to put a note in the package insert and the *Physicians' Desk Reference* warning against the use of methylphenidate for subjects with Tourette syndrome or for ADHD subjects with tics. However, what was left virtually unreported was the fact that just as stimulants can reduce motor hyperactivity, they can also reduce motor and vocal tics. For example, in our series of Tourette syndrome cases, stimulants improved or eliminated the tics in 13% of the patients (D. E. Comings and Comings 1987a). In a study by Erenberg et al. (1985), stimulants decreased the tics in 5% of the patients. In addition, parents often report that the tics disappear while the stimulants are in effect but return after the medication has worn off. Some have even reported giving their child an afternoon dose of methylphenidate or dextroamphetamine sulfate just to eliminate the tics.

The effectiveness of methylphenidate and absence of troublesome exacerbation of tics were well documented in double-blind studies by Sverd and colleagues (Gadow et al. 1992; Sverd et al. 1992). These authors reported cases in which the tics were moderately increased at lower doses of methylphenidate but decreased over baseline levels at higher doses (Gadow et al. 1992; Sprafkin and Gadow 1993; Sverd et al. 1992). For the series as a whole there was a trend for modest decreases in tic ratings at the higher doses of methylphenidate.

The ability of stimulants to decrease the severity of tics in some cases makes physiological sense. If the tics and motor hyperactivity are the result of hypersensitivity of dopamine receptors in the striatum due to a relative dopamine deficiency in the limbic system and frontal lobes, alleviation of the dopamine deficiency after treatment with dopaminergic agonists would decrease that receptor hypersensitivity and alleviate the tics and hyperactivity (D. E. Comings 1990b, 1987).

It is important to place the use of stimulants in the treatment of Tourette syndrome in a proper perspective. These agents are not alone in their potential to exacerbate tics. In my experience, all the medications classically used for the treatment of tics—clonidine, haloperidol, pimozide, and clonazepam—can in some cases lead to a significant exacerbation of the tics.

The development of tics after stimulant treatment is a frequent problem in the care of children with ADHD. Among patients referred to me because of this problem, I have usually found that the tics were actually present before the initiation of stimulant treatment. The parents, and sometimes their physician, simply were not aware of the tics or did not realize what they were until they got more severe. This experience has also been reported by Sprafkin and Gadow (1993).

Unfortunately, when the tics increase, a common response of the physician is to stop the stimulants and refuse to further treat the ADHD. Since the most incapacitating aspect of Tourette syndrome is often the comorbid ADHD, not the tics, this approach results in the child essentially not being treated at all.

There are several straightforward solutions to this clinical problem. The easiest one to effect is to continue the stimulants and add a medication, such as clonidine or a neuroleptic, to control the tics. An alternative is to discontinue the stimulants and treat both the tics and the ADHD with clonidine. If oral clonidine is not effective, the trial should not be considered complete until transdermal clonidine has also been tried (D. E. Comings 1990b; D. E. Comings et al. 1990a). A common cause of a clonidine patch's "failure" is the assumption that if a single TTS-1 patch was not effective, the medication did not work. I recommend increasing the dose until it is a) effective, b) produces too much sedation or other side effects, or c) a dose of two TTS-2 patches has been reached. In some cases, imipramine or desipramine can also be used to treat both the tics and the ADHD (Caine et al. 1979; D. E. Comings 1990b). I prefer imipramine because of the higher incidence of cardiotoxicity with desipramine (Gualtieri et al. 1991).

CLINICAL IMPORTANCE OF RECOGNIZING THE SIMILARITY BETWEEN ADHD AND TOURETTE SYNDROME

The clinician may ask, So what? Why is it important to recognize that ADHD and Tourette syndrome are essentially the same disorder? There are several reasons why such a recognition is important.

Importance in Medical Treatment

As discussed earlier in this chapter, for many years it was felt that stimulants such as methylphenidate and dextroamphetamine sulfate were absolutely contraindicated in the treatment of ADHD in patients with Tourette syndrome and that these drugs could "cause" Tourette syndrome. As a result, in many cases, if a child with ADHD being treated with stimulants developed significant tics, the clinician would, as part of a knee-jerk reaction, stop the stimulants. Unfortunately, as another part of this reaction, the clinician often would discharge the patient with a statement like "Your child has Tourette syndrome. I am not comfortable with treating that disease, and you will have to find another doctor." Unfortunately, the doctor making such a statement was often the regional specialist in treating ADHD, and there was no other doctor for the family to go to. The result was an untreated, out-of-control child who often ended up in institutional care.

The recognition that Tourette syndrome and ADHD are basically the same disorder should help to eliminate such clinical reactions. As discussed earlier, the proper course would be either to switch to a drug such as clonidine or imipramine or to add clonidine or a neuroleptic to treat the tics—and to continue to care for the patient.

Importance in Psychiatric Treatment

Recognizing that ADHD and Tourette syndrome are related and that both are associated with a very high frequency of comorbid conditions, such as obsessive-compulsive disorder, oppositional defiant disorder, conduct disorder, anxiety, depression, sexual disorders, and sleep disorders, is critical for the proper total treatment of patients. Another statement parents often relate having been told is "Your child's behavioral problems are unrelated to Tourette syndrome (or ADHD)." This is often followed by statements suggesting that the problems are attributable to poor parenting skills, marital problems, divorce, or abuse. In fact, as described above and throughout this book, these comorbid disorders are often the result of the same genetic-biochemical defects that cause the ADHD and Tourette syndrome. As such, these conditions often respond well to an appropriate medication. Although psychotherapy can also be very valuable, it often works best when it is part of a combined medical-psychotherapeutic approach.

REFERENCES

American Psychiatric Association: Diagnostic and Statistical Manual of Mental Disorders, 3rd Edition, Revised. Washington, DC, American Psychiatric Association, 1987

Benjamin J, Li L, Patterson C, et al: Population and familial association between the D4 dopamine receptor gene and measures of novelty seeking. Nature Genet 12: 81–84, 1996

Biederman J, Newcorn J, Sprich S: Comorbidity of attention-deficit/hyperactivity disorder with conduct, depressive, anxiety, and other disorders. Am J Psychiatry 148: 564–577, 1991

Biederman J, Faraone SV, Keenan K, et al: Further evidence for family-genetic risk factors in attention deficit hyperactivity disorder: pattern of comorbidity in probands and relatives of psychiatrically and pediatrically referred samples. Arch Gen Psychiatry 49:728–738, 1992

Blum K, Noble EP, Sheridan PJ, et al: Allelic association of human dopamine D2 receptor gene in alcoholism. JAMA 263:2055–2059, 1990

Brase DA, Loh HH: Possible role of 5-hydroxytryptamine in minimal brain dysfunction. Life Sci 16:1005–1015, 1975

Bruun RD: The natural history of Tourette's syndrome, in Tourette's Syndrome and Tic Disorders: Clinical Understanding and Treatment. Edited by Cohen DJ, Bruun RD, Leckman JF. New York, Wiley, 1988, pp 21–39

Burd L, Kerbeshian J, Wikenheiser M, et al: Prevalence of Gilles de la Tourette's syndrome in North Dakota adults. Am J Psychiatry 143:787–788, 1986a

Burd L, Kerbeshian J, Wikenheiser M, et al: A prevalence study of Gilles de la Tourette syndrome in North Dakota school-age children. Journal of the American Academy of Child Psychiatry 25:552–553, 1986b

Caine ED, Polinsky RJ, Ebert MH, et al: Trial of chlorimipramine and desipramine for Gilles de la Tourette syndrome. Ann Neurol 5:305–306, 1979

Caine ED, McBride MC, Chiverton P, et al: Tourette's syndrome in Monroe County school children. Neurology 38:472–475, 1988

Carter AS, Pauls DL, Leckman JF, et al: A prospective longitudinal study of Gilles de la Tourette's syndrome. J Am Acad Child Adolesc Psychiatry 33:377–385, 1994

Chase TN, Geoffrey V, Gillespie M, et al: Structural and functional studies of Gilles de la Tourette syndrome. Rev Neurol (Paris) 142:851–855, 1986

Cohen DJ, Detlor J, Young JG, et al: Clonidine ameliorates Gilles de la Tourette syndrome. Arch Gen Psychiatry 37:1350–1357, 1980

Comings BG, Comings DE: A controlled study of Tourette syndrome, V: depression and mania. Am J Hum Genet 41:804–821, 1987

Comings DE: A controlled study of Tourette syndrome, VII: summary: a common genetic disorder causing disinhibition of the limbic system. Am J Hum Genet 41:839–866, 1987

Comings DE: Blood serotonin and tryptophan in Tourette syndrome. Am J Med Genet 36:418–430, 1990a

Comings DE: Tourette Syndrome and Human Behavior. Duarte, CA, Hope Press, 1990b

Comings DE: Genetic factors in substance abuse based on studies of Tourette syndrome and ADHD probands and relatives, I: drug abuse. Drug Alcohol Depend 35:1–16, 1994a

Comings DE: Genetic factors in substance abuse based on studies of Tourette syndrome and ADHD probands and relatives, II: alcohol abuse. Drug Alcohol Depend 35:17–24, 1994b

Comings DE: The role of genetic factors in human sexual behavior based on studies of Tourette syndrome and ADHD probands and their relatives. Am J Med Genet (Neuropsychiatric Genetics) 54:227–241, 1994c

Comings DE: Genetic factors in depression based on studies of Tourette syndrome and ADHD probands and relatives. Am J Med Genet (Neuropsychiatric Genetics) 60:111–121, 1995a

Comings DE: The role of genetic factors in conduct disorder based on studies of Tourette syndrome and ADHD probands and their relatives. J Dev Behav Pediatr 16:142–157, 1995b

Comings DE: Search for the Tourette Syndrome and Human Behavior Genes. Duarte, CA, Hope Press, 1996

Comings DE, Comings BG: Tourette's syndrome and attention deficit disorder with hyperactivity: are they genetically related? Journal of the American Academy of Child Psychiatry 23:138–146, 1984

Comings DE, Comings BG: A controlled study of Tourette syndrome, I: attention-deficit disorder, learning disorders, and school problems. Am J Hum Genet 41: 701–741, 1987a

Comings DE, Comings BG: A controlled study of Tourette syndrome, II: conduct. Am J Hum Genet 41:742–760, 1987b

Comings DE, Comings BG: A controlled study of Tourette syndrome, III: phobias and panic attacks. Am J Hum Genet 41:761–781, 1987c

Comings DE, Comings BG: A controlled study of Tourette syndrome, IV: obsessions, compulsions, and schizoid behaviors. Am J Hum Genet 41:782–803, 1987d

Comings DE, Comings BG: A controlled study of Tourette syndrome, VI. Early development, sleep problems, allergies, and handedness. Am J Hum Genet 41:822–838, 1987e

Comings DE, Comings BG: Tourette's syndrome and attention deficit disorder, in Tourette's Syndrome and Tic Disorders: Clinical Understanding and Treatment. Edited by Cohen DJ, Bruun RD, Leckman JF . New York, Wiley, 1988, pp 120–135

Comings DE, Comings BG: Comorbid behavioral disorders, in Handbook of Tourette's Syndrome and Related Tic and Behavioral Disorders. Edited by Kurlan R. New York, Marcel Dekker, 1993, pp 111–147

Comings DE, Comings BG, Tacket T, et al: The clonidine patch and behavioral problems. J Am Acad Child Adolesc Psychiatry 29:667–668, 1990a

Comings DE, Himes JA, Comings BG: An epidemiological study of Tourette syndrome in a single school district. J Clin Psychiatry 51:463–469, 1990b

Comings DE, Comings BG, Muhleman D, et al: The dopamine D2 receptor locus as a modifying gene in neuropsychiatric disorders. JAMA 266:1793–1800, 1991

Comings DE, Muhleman D, Ahn C, et al: The dopamine D2 receptor gene: a genetic risk factor in substance abuse. Drug Alcohol Depend 34:175–180, 1994

Comings DE, Muhleman D, Gade R, et al: Exon and intron mutations in the human tryptophan 2,3-dioxygenase gene and their potential association with Tourette syndrome, substance abuse and other psychiatric disorders. Pharmacogenetics 6:307–318, 1996a

Comings DE, Wu H, Chiu C, et al: Polygenic inheritance of Tourette syndrome, stuttering, ADHD, conduct and oppositional defiant disorder: the additive and subtractive effect of the three dopaminergic genes—DRD2, DβH and DAT1. Am J Med Genet (Neuropsychiatric Genetics) 67:264–288, 1996b

Cook EH, Stein MA, Krasowski MD, et al: Association of attention-deficit disorder and the dopamine transporter gene. Am J Hum Genet 56:993–998, 1995

Devinsky O: Neuroanatomy of Gilles de la Tourette's syndrome: possible midbrain involvement. Arch Neurol 40:508–514, 1983

Ebstein RP, Novick O, Umansky R, et al: Dopamine D4 receptor (D4DR) exon III polymorphism associated with the human personality trait of novelty seeking. Nature Genet 12:78–80, 1996

Erenberg G, Cruse RP, Rothner AD: Gilles de la Tourette's syndrome: effects of stimulant drugs. Neurology 35:1346–1348, 1985

Erenberg G, Cruse RP, Rothner AD: The natural history of Tourette syndrome: a follow-up study. Ann Neurol 22:383–385, 1987

Gadow KD, Nolan EE, Sverd J: Methylphenidate in hyperactive boys with comorbid tic disorder, II: short-term behavioral effects in school setting. J Am Acad Child Adolesc Psychiatry 31:462–471, 1992

Gittelman R, Mannuzza S, Shenker R, et al: Hyperactive boys almost grown up, I: psychiatric status. Arch Gen Psychiatry 42:937–947, 1985

Greenberg L, Yellin A, Spring C, et al: Clinical effects of imipramine and methylphenidate in hyperactive children. International Journal of Mental Health 4:144–156, 1975

Grice DE, Leckman JF, Pauls DL, et al: Linkage disequilibrium of an allele at the dopamine D4 receptor locus with Tourette's syndrome by TDT. Am J Hum Genet 59: 644–652, 1996

Gualtieri CT, Keenan PA, Chandler M: Clinical and neuropsychological effects of desipramine in children with attention-deficit/hyperactivity disorder. J Clin Psychopharmacol 11:155–159, 1991

Hunt RD, Minderaa RB, Cohen DJ: Clonidine benefits children with attention-deficit disorder and hyperactivity: report of a double-blind placebo-crossover therapeutic trial. Journal of the American Academy of Child Psychiatry 24:617–629, 1985

Knell E, Comings DE: Tourette syndrome and attention deficit hyperactivity disorder: evidence for a genetic relationship. J Clin Psychiatry 54:331–337, 1993

Kurlan R, Behr J, Medved L, et al: Familial Tourette's syndrome: report of a large pedigree and potential for linkage analysis. Neurology 36:772–776, 1986

Lahoste GJ, Swanson JM, Wigal SB, et al: Dopamine D4 receptor gene polymorphism is associated with attention-deficit/hyperactivity disorder. Mol Psychiatry 1:121–124, 1996

Leonard HL, Swedo SE, Rapoport JL, et al: Treatment of obsessive-compulsive disorder with clomipramine and desipramine in children and adolescents. Arch Gen Psychiatry 46:1088–1092, 1989

Malison RT, McDougle CJ, van Dyck CH, et al: [^{123}I]β-CIT SPECT imaging of striatal dopamine transporter binding in Tourette's disorder. Am J Psychiatry 152:1359–1361, 1995

Mannuzza S, Klein RG, Bonagura N, et al: Hyperactive boys almost grown up, V: replication of psychiatric status. Arch Gen Psychiatry 48:77–83, 1991

McCracken JT: A two-part model of stimulant action on attention-deficit/hyperactivity disorder in children. J Neuropsychiatry Clin Neurosci 3:201–209, 1991

Mefford IN, Potter WZ: A neuroanatomical and biochemical basis for attention deficit disorder with hyperactivity in children: a defect in tonic adrenaline mediated inhibition of locus coeruleus stimulation. Med Hypotheses 29:33–42, 1989

Monroe RR: Anticonvulsants in the treatment of aggression. J Nerv Ment Dis 160: 119–126, 1975

Noble EP: The D2 dopamine receptor gene: a review of association studies in alcoholism. Behav Genet 23:119–129, 1993

Noble EP, Blum K, Khalsa ME, et al: Allelic association of the D_2 dopamine receptor gene with cocaine dependence. Drug Alcohol Depend 33:271–285, 1993

Pauls DL, Hurst CR, Kruger SD, et al: Gilles de la Tourette's syndrome and attention-deficit disorder with hyperactivity: evidence against a genetic relationship. Arch Gen Psychiatry 43:1177–1179, 1986

Pauls DL, Leckman JF, Raymond CL, et al: A family study of Tourette's syndrome: evidence against the hypothesis of association with a wide range of psychiatric phenotypes (abstract). Am J Hum Genet 43:A64, 1988

Pauls DL, Leckman JF, Cohen DJ: Familial relationship between Gilles de la Tourette syndrome, attention-deficit disorder, learning disabilities, speech disorders, and stuttering. J Am Acad Adolesc Child Psychiatry 32:1044–1050, 1993

Rapoport JL: Childhood behavior and learning problems treated with imipramine. International Journal of Neuropsychiatry 1:635–642, 1965

Riddle MA, Leckman JF, Hardin MT, et al: Fluoxetine treatment of obsessions and compulsions in patients with Tourette's syndrome. Am J Psychiatry 145:1173–1174, 1988

Robertson MM, Eapen V: Pharmacologic controversy of CNS stimulants in Gilles de la Tourette syndrome. Clin Neuropharmacol 15:408–425, 1992

Robins LN, Helzer J, Croughan J, et al: National Institute of Mental Health Diagnostic Interview Schedule: its history, characteristics, and validity. Arch Gen Psychiatry 38:381–389, 1981

Shapiro AK, Shapiro ES, Young JG, et al: Gilles de la Tourette Syndrome, New York, Raven, 1988

Shaywitz BA, Klopper JH, Yager RD, et al: Paradoxical response to amphetamine in developing rats treated with 6-hydroxydopamine. Nature 261:153–155, 1976a

Shaywitz BA, Yager RD, Klopper JH: Selective brain dopamine depletion in developing rats: an experimental model of minimal brain dysfunction. Science 191:305–307, 1976b

Singer HS, Rosenberg LA: Development of behavioral and emotional problems in Tourette syndrome. Pediatr Neurol 5:41–44, 1989

Smith SS, O'Hara BF, Persico AM, et al: Genetic vulnerability to drug abuse. The D2 dopamine receptor Taq I B1 restriction fragment length polymorphism appears more frequently in polysubstance abusers. Arch Gen Psychiatry 49:723–727, 1992

Sprafkin J, Gadow KD: Four purported cases of methylphenidate-induced tics exacerbation: methodological and clinical doubts. J Child Adolescent Psychopharmacol 3:231–244, 1993

Sverd J, Gadow KD, Nolan EE, et al: Methylphenidate in hyperactive boys with comorbid tic disorder, in Tourette Syndrome: Genetics, Neurobiology and Treatment. Edited by Chase TN, Friedhoff AJ, Cohen DJ. New York, Raven, 1992, pp 271–281

Yaryura-Tobias JA, Neziroglu FA: Gilles de la Tourette syndrome: a new clinico-therapeutic approach. Progress in Neuro-psychopharmacology 1:335–338, 1977

12 Attention-Deficit/Hyperactivity Disorder and Developmental Coordination Disorder

Christopher Gillberg, M.D., Ph.D.
Björn Kadesjö, M.D.

Most clinicians and researchers are, by now, well aware that attention-deficit disorders are often comorbid with psychiatric disorders, such as affective and anxiety disorders (Biederman et al. 1997), illicit drug use (Hechtman 1996), antisocial behavior (Taylor 1986), tics, and learning disorders (Barkley 1990). It is much less well known that they are also associated with motor control dysfunction, "clumsiness," and developmental coordination disorder (DCD) (American Psychiatric Association 1994). Motor clumsiness and DCD have been considered to be the territory of child neurologists and developmental pediatricians, whereas attention-deficit disorders, including attention-deficit/hyperactivity disorder (ADHD), have been conceptualized as falling within the domain of child psychiatry. It is possibly this "split" that accounts for the fact that few psychiatrists are aware of, much less appreciate, the implications of and, sometimes, the need to do something about the motor and perceptual problems that are so often comorbid with childhood ADHD. Conversely, child neurologists often fail to appreciate the impact of attention deficits on the lives of the clumsy children referred to them for diagnosis and workup.

In this brief review, we aim to demonstrate that the links between ADHD and DCD are quite strong and need to be taken into account both in clinical practice and in research. To demonstrate this, we need to acquaint the reader with basic concepts in the field of DCD and to briefly review the literature on mild-to-moderate motor impairment as a kind of neurodevelopmental dysfunction.

MOTOR IMPAIRMENT AS A REFLECTION OF NEURODEVELOPMENTAL DYSFUNCTION

Interest in mild-to-moderate motor control problems in children grew out of the study of so-called minimal brain dysfunction (MBD) syndromes. MBD was a diagnostic term for children having normal (or near-normal) intelligence but who nevertheless showed varying degrees of learning and behavior problems associated with brain dysfunction (Clements 1966). These MBD problems were thought of as manifesting themselves in various combinations of deficits in attention, motor control, perception, impulse control, and language and memory (to mention the most important). The diagnosis of MBD relied on the documentation of these deficits, particularly motor control and perception problems, or on the demonstration of "soft neurological signs" or motor deficits that were believed to reflect brain dysfunction but for which structural neurological correlates had not been identified (Tupper 1987). Deficits in motor control or the presence of neurological soft signs was regarded as a more reliable reflection of the integrity of the central nervous system than more "pure" behavior variables. Clumsiness and poor motor coordination were seen as clear markers of neurological dysfunction (Denckla and Rudel 1978).

As a means of studying these neurological dysfunctions more reliably, various "neurodevelopmental" tests, as complements to classical neurological examination, were developed (Henderson 1987). The majority of these tests consist of a battery of items intended to measure children's neuromotor maturity. Many of the tests in use are fairly comprehensive and include items that measure not only pure "motor" function but also perceptual, intellectual, and language functions (Bax and Whitmore 1987; Michelsson et al. 1981; Rasmussen et al. 1983). Some, however, are more specifically focused on the child's neuromotor performance (Hadders-Algra et al. 1988). A large battery of tests for screening has been developed (C. Gillberg 1983; Glascoe et al. 1990). These tests are fairly condensed and easy to apply in clinical practice. The screening device for motor dyscoordination developed in a Swedish longitudinal study of perceptual, motor, and attention deficits (C. Gillberg et al. 1983) is shown in Table 12–1. For final diagnosis, however, other, more elaborate tests have been developed (Drillien and Drummond 1983; Rasmussen et al. 1983; Touwen 1979).

The association between motor control problems and behavior disturbance/learning disorder has long been recognized (Ayres 1972; Kephart 1970). Conclusions about causal relationships were drawn on the basis of association studies. A "movement" grew out of this approach, focusing on motor training programs aimed at alleviating learning and behavior problems. A meta-analysis of 180 studies of perceptual-motor training (Kavale and Mattson 1983) revealed, however, that such training will not affect "academic, cognitive or perceptual-motor variables" other than those functions being trained.

Table 12–1. Brief neurodevelopmental screening for developmental coordination disorder

A. Age-inappropriate performance on items included under B. Child allowed only one attempt per item. Test developed for 6- to 7-year-olds. In this age group, abnormality on two or more of the six items suggests presence of developmental coordination disorder. Other cutoffs apply in younger (higher cutoff) and older (lower cutoff) children.

B. The six items of the brief neurodevelopmental screening are as follows:

1. Jumping up and down 20 times on one foot, left and right scored separately. Abnormality: (a) >12 seconds or (b) two or more interruptions on any one foot.
2. Standing on one foot, left and right scored separately. Abnormality: <10 seconds on any one foot.
3. Walking on lateral aspects of feet for 10 seconds (also referred to as the Fog test) with hands hanging down (swing allowed). Abnormality: (a) elbow flexed 60 degrees or more, (b) abduction of shoulder, (c) significant associated movements of lips or tongue, or (d) significant asymmetry.
4. Diadochokinesis 10 seconds, each hand separately. Abnormality: (a) 10 or fewer prosupinations on either side, (b) significant "dysfluency," or (c) lateral elbow movements of 15 cm or more.
5. Cutting out a paper circle (10 cm in diameter) from a rectangular sheet. Abnormality: (a) 20% or more of paper circle cut "away," (b) 20% or more of extra material remaining outside paper circle, or (c) 2 minutes or more used for task.
6. Tracing task using pencil and paper. Abnormality: according to specific test used.

Source. Gillberg et al. 1983.

Studies have differed in their delineation and terminology in the field of "minor neurodevelopmental deviations." Some of the terms that have been used are "soft neurological signs" (Tupper 1987) and "minor neurological dysfunction" (Hadders-Algra and Touwen 1992). The prevalence of minor neurodevelopmental deviations varies (Duel and Robinson 1987) but is often estimated at about 5%. Some studies have reported a much higher rate. In a Dutch study (Hadders-Algra and Touwen 1992), 15% of the school-age population were judged to have mild minor neurodevelopmental deviations, and in another 6% the minor neurodevelopmental deviations were severe (occurring in boys twice as often as in girls). Minor neurodevelopmental deviations in that study referred to neurological deviance that does not result in obvious disability (e.g., minor dyscoordination, fine motor deviance, choreiform movements, and abnormalities of muscular tone). Researchers and clinicians working within the tradition of minor neurodevelopmental deviations regard the motor dysfunction as a sign of neurological disorder that may cause other problems such as language and perception dysfunction.

DEVELOPMENTAL COORDINATION DISORDER

A slightly different tradition antedates the emergence of the concept of the "clumsy child" (Gordon and McKinlay 1980) and DCD concepts. Some children lack the motor skills required for everyday activities such as play, sports, and schoolwork. The children do not generally experience developmental delay, and usually they do not have an easily identifiable neurological disorder. The motor difficulties as such are regarded as important, regardless of whether they are interpreted as a sign of neurological disorder. The DSM system acknowledged this group of children in DSM-III-R (American Psychiatric Association 1987), in which DCD was defined as motor coordination performance markedly below the expected level (i.e., inappropriate for age and IQ) that causes significant interference with academic achievement or activities of daily living. The DSM-IV definition of DCD (Table 12–2) is very similar. Before the introduction of the DSM definitions of DCD, children with this condition were described as "motor impaired," as "motor delayed," as "physically awkward," as having "perceptuo-motor dysfunction" or "motor-perceptual dysfunction," as "developmentally agnostic/apractic," or as having "clumsy child syndrome" (C. Gillberg and Rasmussen 1982; Gordon and McKinlay 1980; Gubbay 1975).

The DSM definitions do not provide clear cutoffs vis-à-vis normality.

Table 12–2. DSM-IV diagnostic criteria for developmental coordination disorder

A. Performance in daily activities that require motor coordination is substantially below that expected given the person's chronological age and measured intelligence. This may be manifested by marked delays in achieving motor milestones (e.g., walking, crawling, sitting), dropping things, "clumsiness," poor performance in sports, or poor handwriting.

B. The disturbance in Criterion A significantly interferes with academic achievement or activities of daily living.

C. The disturbance is not due to a general medical condition (e.g., cerebral palsy, hemiplegia, or muscular dystrophy) and does not meet criteria for a pervasive developmental disorder.

D. If mental retardation is present, the motor difficulties are in excess of those usually associated with it.

Coding note: If a general medical (e.g., neurological) condition or sensory deficit is present, code the condition on Axis III.

Source. Reprinted from American Psychiatric Association: *Diagnostic and Statistical Manual of Mental Disorders,* 4th Edition. Washington, DC, American Psychiatric Association, 1994.

Children's environments are variable with regard to demands and expectations of motor performance. Tradition and culture determine the experience that children have of motor activities. DCD is often stated to occur in about 5% of the general child population, but Henderson (Henderson and Hall 1982) is of the opinion that another 10% have similar but milder problems. "Poor coordination" was found in 8.1% of about 30,000 7-year-olds followed in the Perinatal Collaborative Project (Nichols 1987). In another study, among 1,443 children aged 6–12 years, the rate of such problems varied from 5.4% at age 6 years to 1.3% at age 10 years (van Dellen et al. 1990).

Children with DCD differ with regard to 1) severity and type of motor difficulties (Hoare 1994), 2) the pattern of performance in other domains (intellectual, educational, and behavioral) (Henderson and Hall 1982), and 3) background factors such as genetic and perinatal problems (C. Gillberg and Rasmussen 1982; Hadders-Algra and Touwen 1992).

Henderson (1987) has developed descriptive and functional assessment methods for the evaluation of DCD that can be carried out by nonmedical staff. The focus of the examination in such approaches is on *how* the child performs a task that is meaningful to him or her, regardless of underlying cause. These methods are the Test of Motor Impairment (Stott et al. 1984) and its successor, the Movement Assessment Battery for Children (Henderson and

Sugden 1992). Results on the Test of Motor Impairment correspond to teacher ratings of clumsiness (estimated to occur in about 5% of children in a non–special education classroom) (Henderson and Hall 1982).

Attempts to find the cause of DCD have resulted in theories positing that "processing deficits" are at the root of poor motor performance (Schoemaker and Kalverboer 1990; Schellekens 1990). These deficits could either represent a general deficit in information processing, involving a reduced rate of processing, or be more specific deficits in handling spatial information relevant to the control of movement (Henderson et al. 1994).

In a series of studies, Hulme and co-workers have shown an increased rate of visuospatial discrimination impairment in children with clumsiness (Lord and Hulme 1987). Henderson et al. (1994) were unable to find any straightforward relationship between perceptual and motor impairments. They concluded, contrary to Hulme, "that the defective processes are not essentially visual but involve strategic processes which may not be modality specific" (p. 968).

Other authors have reported an increased rate of kinesthetic perceptual difficulties in clumsy children (Laszlo et al. 1988; Piek and Coleman-Carman 1995; Sugden and Wann 1987). Dysfunction of kinesthetic perception has been forwarded as an underlying primary deficit that can account for secondary motor-control problems (Laszlo et al. 1988; Piek and Coleman-Carman 1995). However, Sims et al. (1996a, 1996b) showed that motor performance improved after "kinaesthetic training" as well as after motor training that did not include kinesthetic elements. They suggested that in designing remediation programs for clumsy children, the *way* that training is presented may be as important as the actual content of the training.

ADHD AND CLUMSINESS

Several studies by Denckla (Denckla and Rudel 1978; Denckla et al. 1985), Wolff et al. (1990), and C. Gillberg (C. Gillberg et al. 1982; I. C. Gillberg et al. 1993; Kadesjö and Gillberg 1998; Landgren et al. 1996) have shown that there is a strong relationship between ADHD and DCD, dyscoordination, or motor-perceptual dysfunction. Other authors (Szatmari et al. 1989; Witmont and Clark 1996) have reported similar findings.

In several Swedish studies, investigators demonstrated that about one in two children with ADHD also had DCD. In a study of a total population of 7-year-olds in the city of Karlstad in middle Sweden in the mid-1990s, 47% of children meeting the full DSM-III-R criteria for ADHD also met operationally defined criteria for DCD (Kadesjö and Gillberg 1998). DCD was found in almost 50% of the children with five or more ADHD symptoms but in less than 10% of those with four or fewer ADHD symptoms. Very similar rates of comorbidity were found in a population study of 3,448 6- and 7-year-olds performed in the city of Göteborg in western Sweden 20 years earlier (C. Gillberg et al. 1983). Extrapolation of the findings from that study indicates that 50% of children meeting operationally defined criteria for "attention-deficit disorder" also met the strict criteria for motor-perceptual dysfunction. The rate of comorbidity of ADHD and motor-perceptual dysfunction was closely similar in another population-based study from Sweden, performed in the early 1990s, in which roughly half of all 6-year-olds with ADHD met the criteria for motor-perceptual dysfunction (which, as defined in this study, was almost identical to DCD) (Landgren et al. 1996).

In a study designed to determine whether hyperactive children who had neither learning disability nor subtle traditional neurological soft signs might have measurable anomalies for their age on a brief examination of motor coordination, Denckla and Rudel (1978) found that this was indeed the case. Some of the measures used in this study were similar to those employed in the Swedish studies, but Denckla and Rudel included more tests of rapid alternating coordination (toe-taps, heel-toe, finger repetition, diadochokinesis, hand-pats, and finger to thumb). Associated movements and "motor overflow" were also evaluated and were found to be the strongest discriminators between boys with hyperactivity and those without. In other words, there was serious impairment in the ability to carry out discrete isolated movements (e.g., activating a flexor muscle in one finger while at the same time inhibiting the flexor muscles of the other fingers). Denckla and Rudel interpreted the overflow movements as a sign of deficient motor inhibition or motor control and considered this to be a crucial deficit in the syndrome of hyperactivity. It is interesting that Barkley—who estimated that more than 50% of children with ADHD have poor motor coordination (Barkley 1990)—has proposed that the decreased ability to delay responding may be a core feature of ADHD (Barkley 1997). This symptom seems to be very similar to that described by Denckla and Rudel.

Denckla et al. (1985) examined groups of children with dyslexia with or without comorbid attention-deficit disorder and found that those with comorbidity had deficient precision and rhythm, overflow movements, and slowness, in spite of having slightly higher IQs than those with "simply dyslexia." Denckla et al. concluded that motor speed and inhibition appear to be useful as objectively observable and less environmentally influenced, examinable "neigbourhood signs" of behavioral control. They further stated that "history and questionnaire data constitute primary criteria for a diagnosis of ADD [attention-deficit disorder], but motor developmental status may provide a valuable link to understanding underlying mechanisms or physiological components of the elusive mental state" (Denckla et al. 1985, pp. 230–231).

Similar views seem to be held by van der Meere and co-workers (1991), who concluded that input processing is not disturbed in ADHD but that motor output is dysfunctional. Timing, pacing (e.g., ability to slow down to become more thorough when solving a task after making an error), and preparation to act are all deficient. There is, in fact, a remarkable association between ADHD and motor control/motor output problems, such that it seems reasonable to postulate that ADHD may be primarily a failure in the areas of intention, inhibition, and capacity to delay responding or a "motor state regulation problem" (Denckla 1996).

DEVELOPMENTAL COORDINATION DISORDER AND ATTENTION DEFICITS

Few studies have looked in detail at the comorbidity of attentional or behavioral problems in DCD. In fact, apart from the Swedish studies reviewed in the previous section, ADHD, as such, has not been examined in direct relation to DCD.

In a study by Kadesjö and Gillberg (1998), "subclinical or clinical AD/HD" was found in 55% of individuals with "clinical DCD." Whitmore and Bax (1990) studied 5-year-old children and followed them up 2 and 5 years later. They found that of the children with deviant neurodevelopmental scores at age 5 years, 25%–46% had learning disorder or behavior problems at follow-up, compared with 4%–8% of the children without abnormal neurodevelopmental scores at age 5. I. C. Gillberg et al. (1989; I. C. Gillberg and Gillberg 1989) found that 65% of the children with motor-perceptual dysfunction in their sample had attention-deficit disorder. When this finding is taken together with the high rate (50%) of motor-perceptual dysfunction among children with attention-deficit disorder and the prevalence of comorbid attention-deficit disorder and motor-perceptual dysfunction in the general population, it seems blatantly clear that the association between attention deficits and clumsiness is very much stronger than would be predicted by chance alone.

Increased rates of behavior problems, affective disorders, school adjustment difficulties, and other social problems have been reported in children with motor control problems (Cantell et al. 1994; C. Gillberg and Gillberg 1989; Geuze and Börger 1993; Losse et al. 1991; Michelsson and Lindahl 1993).

Clumsy children have been reported to be more introverted and to have less self-confidence regarding physical and social skills (Schoemaker and Kalverboer 1990). They often have a feeling of inferiority (Gordon and McKinlay 1980) and are less well liked in their peer group (Gubbay 1975).

THE CONCEPT OF DEFICITS IN ATTENTION, MOTOR CONTROL, AND PERCEPTION

Because of the documented strong association between attention and motor control problems in research and clinical practice, and because of the difficulty of determining which domain (attention or motor-perceptual) should be regarded as primary, the concept of *deficits in attention, motor control, and perception,* or DAMP, was launched in the Nordic countries in the early 1980s (C. Gillberg et al. 1982). DAMP was conceptualized as the interface between attention-deficit disorder and motor-perceptual disorder (or, in more modern terminology, ADHD and DCD). Population studies of prevalence, descriptive studies, and etiological studies were performed in many centers in the Nordic countries. Follow-up and follow-back studies (e.g., C. Gillberg et al. 1983; Hellgren et al. 1993, 1994; Kadesjö and Gillberg 1998) revealed that DAMP had stronger validity in terms of common background factors and poorer psychosocial/academic outcome than either ADHD or DCD. The DAMP construct has now been in widespread use in the Nordic countries for about 10 years and is the preferred terminology there according to consensus agreement (Airaksinen et al. 1990). It has replaced the concept of minimal brain dysfunction. Although there is ongoing discussion of whether ADHD or DCD might be preferred diagnostic terms for reasons of diagnostic "purity," there is a widespread realization that ADHD is so often associated with motor control problems that a term acknowledging both types of deficit is needed in clinical practice.

On the basis of the literature review presented in this chapter, we feel that DAMP is a useful concept in both research and clinical practice and that, in the wake of follow-up studies demonstrating better validity for the DAMP concept than for ADHD, it should be seriously considered in other parts of the world as well. The term in itself suggests to the clinician that areas other than "attention-related" problems have to be explored before the problems faced by each individual child can be more fully understood.

CLINICAL IMPLICATIONS OF DEVELOPMENTAL COORDINATION DISORDER IN ADHD

ADHD is associated with DCD in about half of all cases. If less stringent criteria for diagnosing ADHD are applied, then the rate of associated clumsiness increases. Therefore, clinicians working with patients with ADHD need to be aware of the very strong association with motor impairment and to be able to diagnose motor control problems. Several well-researched screening instruments—in particular, the Test of Motor Impairment, the Movement Assessment Battery for Children, and the screening devices designed by the Swedish group (see, e.g., Table 12–1)—are suitable for clinical purposes.

Some children with ADHD have such severe problems with motor functions that individually designed training programs are required. Others can be helped through recognition of the problems and provision of educational and psychological support, along with a change of attitude among teachers and peers. It is unknown to what extent, if any, treatment of ADHD (e.g., with stimulants) might affect the course of the associated DCD. Motor training programs do not appear to affect the outcome of ADHD or other behavior problems.

In the light of current knowledge, it is more prudent to conclude that attentional problems and motor control deficits need to be addressed separately, even though some studies do suggest that the two are intrinsically entwined and that, therefore, treatment of an underlying deficit might help alleviate both types of problems. However, we still have but rudimentary evidence in this field, and intensified research efforts are needed. What is beyond any reasonable doubt is the fact that attention deficits are strongly associated with DCD and that the association may be stronger than any other in the context of ADHD. The strength of this association needs to be appreciated by child psychiatrists and developmental pediatricians alike so that affected children can benefit from state-of-the-art evaluation and intervention.

REFERENCES

Airaksinen E, Bille B, Carlström G, et al: Barn och ungdomar med DAMP/MBD (Children and adolescents with DAMP/MBD). Läkartidningen 88:713–717, 1990

American Psychiatric Association: Diagnostic and Statistical Manual of Mental Disorders, 3rd Edition, Revised. Washington, DC, American Psychiatric Association, 1987

American Psychiatric Association: Diagnostic and Statistical Manual of Mental Disorders, 4th Edition. Washington, DC, American Psychiatric Association, 1994

Ayres J: Sensory Integration and Learning Disorders. Los Angeles, Western Psychological Services, 1972

Barkley RA (ed): Attention Deficit Hyperactivity Disorder: A Handbook for Diagnosis and Treatment. New York, Guilford, 1990

Barkley R: ADHD and the Nature of Self-Control. New York, Guilford, 1997

Bax M, Whitmore K: The medical examination of children on entry to school. The results and use of neurodevelopmental assessment. Dev Med Child Neurol 29: 40–55, 1987

Biederman J, Faraone SV, Baldessarini RJ, et al: Predicting desipramine levels in children and adolescents: a naturalistic clinical study. J Am Acad Child Adolesc Psychiatry 36:384–389, 1997

Cantell MH, Smyth MH, Ahonen TP: Clumsiness in adolescence: educational, motor and social outcomes of motor delay detected at 5 years. Adapted Physical Activity Quarterly 11:113–129, 1994

Clements SD: Task Force One: Minimal Brain Dysfunction in Children. Washington, DC, U.S. Public Health Service, 1966

Denckla M: Biological correlates of learning and attention: what is relevant to learning disability and ADHD. J Dev Behav Pediatr 17:114–119, 1996

Denckla M, Rudel R: Anomalies of motor development in hyperactive boys. Ann Neurol 3:231–233, 1978

Denckla M, Rudel R, Chapman C, et al: Motor proficiency in dyslexic children with and without attentional disorders. Arch Neurol 42:228–231, 1985

Drillien C, Drummond M: Developmental Screening and the Child With Special Needs (Clinics in Developmental Medicine No 86). London, SIMP/Heinemann, 1983

Duel R, Robinson D: Developmental soft signs, in Soft Neurological Signs. Edited by Tupper D. Orlando, FL, Grune & Stratton, 1987, pp 95–130

Geuze R, Börger H: Children who are clumsy: five years later. Adapted Physical Activity Quarterly 10:10–21, 1993

Gillberg C: Perceptual, motor and attentional deficits in Swedish primary school children. Some child psychiatric aspects. J Child Psychol Psychiatry 24:377–403, 1983

Gillberg C, Gillberg IC: Six-year-old children with perceptual, motor and attentional deficits: outcome in the six-year perspective, in Attention Deficit Disorder: Clinical and Basic Research. Edited by Sagvolden T, Archer T. Hillsdale, NJ, Lawrence Erlbaum, 1989, pp 93–103

Gillberg C, Rasmussen P: Perceptual, motor and attentional deficits in seven-year-old children: background factors. Dev Med Child Neurol 24:752–770, 1982

Gillberg C, Rasmussen P, Carlström, et al: Perceptual, motor and attentional deficits in six-year-old children. Epidemiological aspects. J Child Psychol Psychiatry 23: 131–144, 1982

Gillberg C, Carlström G, Rasmussen P, et al: Perceptual, motor and attentional deficits in seven-year-old children. Neurological screening aspects. Acta Paediatrica Scandinavica 72:119–124, 1983

Gillberg IC, Gillberg C: Children with preschool minor neurodevelopmental disorders, IV: behaviour and school achievement at age 13. Dev Med Child Neurol 31:3–13, 1989

Gillberg IC, Gillberg C, Groth J: Children with preschool minor neurodevelopmental disorders, V: neurodevelopmental profiles at age 13. Dev Med Child Neurol 31:14–24, 1989

Gillberg IC, Winnergård I, Gillberg C: Screening methods, epidemiology and evaluation of intervention in DAMP in preschool children. Eur Child Adolesc Psychiatry 2:121–135, 1993

Glascoe F, Martin E, Humphrey S: A comparative review of developmental screening tests. Pediatrics 86:547–554, 1990

Gordon N, McKinlay I: Helping Clumsy Children. New York, Churchill Livingstone, 1980

Gubbay S: The Clumsy Child—A Study of Developmental Apraxia and Agnosic Ataxia. London, WB Saunders, 1975

Hadders-Algra M, Touwen B: Minor neurological dysfunction is more closely related to learning difficulties than to behavioral problems. Journal of Learning Disabilities 25:649–657, 1992

Hadders-Algra M, Huisjes H, Touwen B: Perinatal correlates of major and minor neurological dysfunction in school age: a multivariate analysis. Dev Med Child Neurol 30:472–481, 1988

Hechtman L: Adolescent and adult outcome in ADHD. Paper presented at the Fourth Nordic Symposium on MBD/DAMP, Aarhus, Denmark, October 1996

Hellgren L, Gillberg C, Gillberg IC, et al: Children with deficits in attention, motor control and perception (DAMP) almost grown up. General health at age 16 years. Dev Med Child Neurol 35:881–892, 1993

Hellgren L, Gillberg IC, Bågenholm A, et al: Children with deficits in attention, motor control and perception (DAMP) almost grown up: psychiatric and personality disorders at age 16 years. J Child Psychol Psychiatry 35:1255–1271, 1994

Henderson SE: The assessment of "clumsy" children: old and new approaches. J Child Psychol Psychiatry 28:511–527, 1987

Henderson S, Hall D: Concomitants of clumsiness in young school-children. Dev Med Child Neurol 24:448–460, 1982

Henderson S, Sugden D: Movement Assessment Battery for Children: Manual. San Antonio, TX, Psychological Corporation, 1992

Henderson S, Barnett A, Henderson L: Visuospatial difficulties and clumsiness. On the interpretation of conjoined deficits. J Child Psychol Psychiatry 35:961–969, 1994

Hoare D: Subtypes of developmental coordination disorders. Adapted Physical Activity Quarterly 11:158–169, 1994

Kadesjö B, Gillberg C: Attention deficits and clumsiness in Swedish 7-year-olds. Dev Med Child Neurol 40:796–804, 1998

Kavale K, Mattson D: 'One jumped off the balance beam': Metanalysis of perceptual-motor training. Journal of Learning Disabilities 16:165–173, 1983

Kephart N: The Slow Learner in the Classroom. Columbus, OH, Charles E Merrill, 1970

Landgren M, Pettersson R, Kjellman B, et al: ADHD, DAMP and other neurodevelopmental/neuropsychiatric disorders in six-year-old children. Epidemiology and comorbidity. Dev Med Child Neurol 38:891–906, 1996

Laszlo J, Bairstow P, Bartrip J, et al: Clumsiness or Perceptuo-motor Dysfunction? Amsterdam, Elsevier, 1988

Lord R, Hulme C: Perceptual judgements of normal and clumsy children. Dev Med Child Neurol 33:250–257, 1987

Losse A, Henderson SE, Elliman D, et al: Clumsiness in children—do they grow out of it? A 10-year follow-up study. Dev Med Child Neurol 33:55–68, 1991

Michelsson K, Ylinen A, Donner M: Neurodevelopmental screening at five years of age of children who are "at risk" neonatally. Dev Med Child Neurol 23:427–433, 1981

Michelsson K, Lindahl E: Relationship between perinatal risk factors and motor development at ages of 5 and 9 years, in Motor Development in Early and Later Childhood: Longitudinal Approaches. Edited by Kalverboer A, Hopkins B, Geuze R. Cambridge, UK, Cambridge University Press, 1993, pp 266–285

Nichols P: Minimal brain dysfunction and soft signs. The Collaborative Perinatal Project, in Soft Neurological Signs. Edited by Tupper D. Orlando, FL, Grune & Stratton, 1987, pp 179–199

Piek J, Coleman-Carman R: Kinesthetic sensitivity and motor performance of children with developmental co-ordination disorder. Dev Med Child Neurol 37: 976–984, 1995

Rasmussen P, Gillberg C, Waldenström E, Svenson B: Perceptual, motor and attentional deficits in seven-year-old children: neurological and neurodevelopmental aspects. Dev Med Child Neurol 25:315–333, 1983

Schellekens J: Normal and deviant motor development: motor control and information processing mechanisms, in Developmental Biopsychology: Experimental and Observational Studies in Children at Risk. Edited by Kalverboer A. Ann Arbor, University of Michigan Press, 1990, pp 153–185

Schoemaker M, Kalverboer A: Treatment of clumsy children, in Developmental Biopsychology: Experimental and Observational Studies in Children at Risk. Edited by Kalverboer A. Ann Arbor, University of Michigan Press, 1990, pp 241–256

Sims K, Henderson S, Hulme C, et al: The remediation of clumsiness, I: an evaluation of Laszlo's kinesthetic approach. Dev Med Child Neurol 38:976–987, 1996a

Sims K, Henderson S, Morton J, et al: The remediation of clumsiness, II: is kinaesthesis the answer? Dev Med Child Neurol 38:988–997, 1996b

Stott D, Moyes S, Henderson S: The Test of Motor Impairment. San Antonio, TX, Psychological Corporation, 1984

Sugden D, Wann C: The assessment of motor impairment in children with moderate learning difficulties. Br J Educ Psychol 57:225–236, 1987

Szatmari P, Offord DR, Boyle MH: Correlates, associated impairments and patterns of service utilization of children with attention deficit disorder. Findings from the Ontario Child Health Study. J Child Psychol Psychiatry 30:205–217, 1989

Taylor EA: The Overactive Child. Oxford, UK, Blackwell Scientific, 1986

Touwen BCL: Examination of the Child With Minor Neurological Dysfunction, 2nd Edition. London, SIMP/Heinemann, 1979

Tupper D: The Issues With "Soft Signs." Orlando, FL, Grune & Stratton, 1987

van Dellen T, Vaessen W, Schoemaker M: Clumsiness: Definition and Selection of Subjects. Ann Arbor, University of Michigan Press, 1990

van der Meere J, Wekking E, Sergeant J: Sustained attention and pervasive hyperactivity. J Am Acad Child Adolesc Psychiatry 32:275–284, 1991

Whitmore K, Bax M: Checking the health of school entrants. Arch Dis Child 65: 320–326, 1990

Witmont K, Clark C: Kinaesthetic acuity and fine motor skills in children with attention deficit hyperactivity disorder: a preliminary report. Dev Med Child Neurol 38:1091–1098, 1996

Wolff PH, Michel GF, Ovrut M, et al: Rate and timing of motor coordination in developmental dyslexia. Dev Psychol 26:349–359, 1990

13 Attention-Deficit/Hyperactivity Disorder and the Preschool Child

Beth A. Shepard, Ph.D.
Alice S. Carter, Ph.D.
Jennifer E. Cohen, M.A.

Clinicians, diagnosticians, and educators generally agree that some symptoms of attention-deficit/hyperactivity disorder (ADHD) (i.e., impulsivity, hyperactivity, and noncompliance) characteristically emerge during the preschool and toddler years (August and Stewart 1981; Barkley 1990; Barkley et al. 1990; Campbell 1995; Mash and Johnston 1982; Palfrey et al. 1985; Ross and Ross 1982; Towbin and Leckman 1991). Yet clinical diagnosis does not typically occur until the elementary school years (Henker and Whalen 1989), when prevalence rates for ADHD reach between 3% and 5% for school-age children in the United States (American Psychiatric Association 1994). Despite the difficulties inherent in identifying ADHD in younger, preschool-age children, there is a great need to extend our understanding of the disorder to this age group. Earlier identification and intervention could minimize later difficulties commonly observed in children diagnosed with ADHD, including problems with peer relations and self-esteem, conduct disorders, and diminished academic and vocational performance (Ross and Ross 1982).

Given the consensus regarding the early onset of ADHD symptoms, the limited empirical attention this younger age group has received is surprising. Studies that have focused on preschoolers suggest that young children who manifest early symptoms and problem behaviors associated with ADHD continue to exhibit these problems into the elementary school years and beyond (Campbell and Ewing 1990; Campbell et al. 1982, 1986; McGee et al. 1991). For example, Beitchman et al. (1987) reported that preschool-age children diagnosed with ADHD were more likely to receive the same diagnosis 5 years later than were their same-age peers whose diagnoses included conduct-type disorders and emotional disorders. Similarly, Richman et al. (1982) found that 60% of 3-year-olds described as overactive, noncompliant, and difficult to manage continued to exhibit these externalizing symptoms at age 8.

Although these limited number of investigations support the stability of attentional difficulties that emerge in the preschool years, it is not clear what percentage of preschoolers who evidence symptoms of ADHD would receive a similar diagnosis at long-term follow-up (i.e., after entering primary or secondary school). Further, the proportion of children who exhibit attentional problems during the preschool years who later develop other, non-ADHD psychiatric diagnoses (e.g., bipolar disorder, schizophrenia, Tourette syndrome, anxiety disorder) is not known. Evidence from studies of children at high risk for developing psychopathology suggests that offspring of individuals with bipolar disorder and schizophrenia often exhibit attentional difficulties in the preschool years (Zahn-Waxler et al. 1988). Different patterns of attentional difficulties (i.e., sustained attention, response inhibition, perseveration, and symptom cluster) may be evident early in the course of development, and these early patterns may distinguish later psychopathological outcomes. Thus, increased study of patterns of attentional difficulties and associated problem behaviors and competencies in the preschool period may inform our understanding of the developmental trajectories of not only ADHD but also other psychopathological conditions that emerge independently or in the context of ongoing ADHD symptoms. Finally, because symptoms of ADHD in preschoolers are influenced by both constitutional and environmental factors, efforts to predict later psychopathology may be improved by addressing social and familial contexts.

In this chapter, we discuss issues germane to ADHD during the preschool years from a developmental perspective of psychopathology; from this perspective, childhood dysfunction and disorders are framed within the context of normal maturation, development, and adjustment (Cicchetti 1984; Cicchetti and Cohen 1995; Kazdin 1989; Sroufe and Rutter 1984). We also consider the behaviors of children within the multiple contexts of their daily experiences. The social ecology of preschool-age children is changing rapidly, often the result of increased numbers of families in which both parents or a single parent is working outside of the home (Hofferth and Phillips 1991). Indeed, the percentage of children under 6 years of age whose mothers are employed outside of the home nearly doubled in the last two decades, from 29% in 1970 to 54% in 1990, and 48% of these children were being cared for in some type of day-care facility (Hofferth et al. 1991). With enrollment in day care predicted to continue rising, more young children are increasingly required to adapt to a variety of settings and to different individuals on a daily basis.

Although it has been suggested that children in the preschool age group are rarely required to participate in activities requiring sustained attention (American Psychiatric Association 1994), the more structured environments of day care and preschool settings place more stringent demands on young children to regulate their attention and behaviors to meet situational expectations (e.g., group circle-time activities, peer negotiations). The day-care or preschool setting may also bring the child to the attention of adults who may have more experience with the range of typical development than do many parents who may accept extreme behaviors as developmentally appropriate. As the number of preschool-age children entering day-care or preschool settings continues to rise (Hofferth and Phillips 1991), we might anticipate an increase in the identification of younger preschool children with ADHD who would not otherwise be noticed until they enter primary school. However, before attributing a child's failure to comply with situational demands as indicative of a problem, it is critical to consider the developmental appropriateness of the demands that are being placed on preschool children.

Our purpose in this chapter is to consider from a developmental perspective issues relevant to identification and diagnosis of and appropriate interventions for children with ADHD in the preschool years. We review 1) diagnostic issues relevant to the preschool period; 2) etiological pathways for the development of ADHD, including the role of genetics, pre- and perinatal risk, and neurobiological and environmental risk factors; 3) comorbidity of ADHD with other disorders, including anxiety, depression, conduct disorder, and learning problems; 4) the role of attention regulation in typically developing preschool children and preschool children with ADHD; 5) normative social relationships during preschool age and the impact of ADHD symptoms on those relationships; and 6) assessment and early intervention for young children with ADHD.

DIAGNOSTIC ISSUES

The average age at onset of ADHD is between ages 4 and 5 years (American Psychiatric Association 1994). Yet most children are not formally diagnosed until the elementary school years, when difficulties with school performance and social functioning distinguish children with ADHD from their typically developing peers. The diagnostic criteria for ADHD have undergone considerable revision in the three most recent editions of DSM: DSM-III (American Psychiatric Association 1980), DSM-III-R (American Psychiatric Association 1987), and DSM-IV (American Psychiatric Association 1994). These changes have focused on specific inclusion criteria for ADHD and on the constructs viewed as central to the disorder.

DSM-IV provides a multifactorial model for defining the diagnostic criteria for ADHD. Inattention is considered the first factor, and impulsivity and hyperactivity are incorporated as a second factor. For the DSM-IV diagnostic criteria for ADHD to be met, six (or more) of the nine symptoms of inattention and/or six (or more) of the nine symptoms of impulsivity/hyperactivity must be present for at least 6 months in a manner that is inappropriate to the child's developmental level. The following three diagnoses are possible when these criteria are used:

1. Attention-deficit/hyperactivity disorder, predominantly hyperactive-impulsive type (symptoms of hyperactivity/impulsivity only)
2. Attention-deficit/hyperactivity disorder, predominantly inattentive type (symptoms of inattention only)
3. Attention-deficit/hyperactivity disorder, combined type (symptoms of both inattention and hyperactivity/impulsivity)

DSM-IV emphasizes the importance of considering the child's age and developmental level, as well as the consistency of symptoms across a variety of situations, when a diagnosis of ADHD is being considered. Thus, targeted problem behaviors need to be extreme in light of the child's developmental level, since inattention, impulsivity, and hyperactivity are expected to be present in early development. Further, the criteria take into account the variability of children's behavior across contexts. Many children may respond to a particular situation or context with inattentive or impulsive behaviors. These symptomatic behaviors may be more a reflection of the environmental contingencies than a reflection of stable characteristics of the child. Therefore, evidence of significant and marked impairment across at least two contextual situations is necessary before a diagnosis of ADHD can be assigned (American Psychiatric Association 1994).

Some concern has been expressed about the validity of the hyperactive-impulsive type of ADHD (Lahey et al. 1998). During the DSM-IV field trials, it was noted that "only 24% of children who met criteria for the HI [hyperactive-impulsive] type were older than 6 years, compared with more than 70% of the children who met criteria for the combined and inattentive types" (Lahey et al. 1998, p. 696). Lahey and colleagues suggested that, given the disproportionate number of younger children who met the diagnostic criteria for the hyperactive-impulsive type, the potential exists for misdiagnosis to occur. To test the validity of this diagnosis with younger children, Lahey et al. (1998) completed diagnostic interviews with parents of 4- to 6-year-old children, and teachers of these children completed a DSM-IV checklist. The 126 children who met the diagnostic criteria were matched with comparison children. Results indicate that when diagnostic interviewing was the method used for diagnosis of the three subtypes of ADHD, the validity of the diagnosis could be demonstrated with this younger age group (Lahey et al. 1998).

DSM-III (American Psychiatric Association 1980) also employed a multifactorial model for diagnosis of ADHD. Instead of impulsivity and hyperactivity being combined as a single factor, three separate symptom constructs were presented: 1) inattention (five symptoms), 2) impulsivity (five symptoms), and 3) hyperactivity (four symptoms) (D. R. Pillow, W. E. Pelham, B. Hoza, unpublished manuscript, 1992; McBurnett et al. 1993). The combinations of these factors made two diagnoses possible: attention deficit disorder with hyperactivity and attention deficit disorder without hyperactivity. Evidence of all three factors was necessary for a diagnosis of attention deficit disorder with hyperactivity, whereas the hyperactivity factor was excluded for attention deficit disorder without hyperactivity. At least three symptoms from both the inattention and impulsivity factors were required to meet the criteria for a diagnosis of attention deficit disorder without hyperactivity.

DSM-III-R (American Psychiatric Association 1987), instead of incorporating a multifactorial model, collapsed the three factors from DSM-III—inattention, impulsivity, and hyperactivity—into a single factor conceptualized as a hyperactivity dimension. Symptoms were organized in a severity hierarchy, with fidgeting, squirming, and difficulty remaining seated at the top of the list and losing things and "engaging in physically dangerous behaviors" at the bottom. Children were required to exhibit 8 of 14 symptoms designated as criteria for the unitary disorder.

The DSM-III-R diagnostic criteria for ADHD have been considered controversial by many (August and Garfinkel 1989; Cantwell and Baker 1992; Frick and Lahey 1991; Hynd et al. 1991; Newcorn et al. 1989; Shaywitz and Shaywitz 1988). Numerous studies have revealed that, compared with the use of DSM-III criteria, the use of DSM-III-R criteria resulted in larger numbers of school-age children meeting the diagnostic criteria for ADHD (Lahey et al.

1990; Newcorn et al. 1989). A similar outcome was particularly pronounced for preschool-age children. When the eight DSM-III-R symptom criteria for preschool ADHD were used, the rate of diagnosis in a community sample was found to be 15%, which is three times the rate of diagnosis among school-age children found in the same study (Ott et al., in press). However, when the diagnostic criteria were made more restrictive, with 11 symptoms used for the preschool population, the diagnostic rate of ADHD was reduced to 5%, a rate more congruent with that obtained among older children (Ott et al., in press). These results suggest that higher thresholds of symptomatic behaviors may be necessary in diagnosing younger children with ADHD and further emphasize the importance of considering developmental level.

Along with investigators who argue for more stringent criteria in the diagnosis of ADHD in preschool-age children, other researchers have observed behaviors and looked for differences among preschool children considered to be at risk for developing ADHD. Schleifer et al. (1975) considered whether the higher activity levels typically observed in young children are symptomatic of ADHD or simply reflect age-appropriate behaviors. Children between 3 and 4 years of age (n = 28) with suspected ADHD and their matched nonaffected peers were observed by a trained teacher and volunteer in two contexts: an unstructured, free-play situation and a structured, school-like activity. Aggressive acts, amount of time "up" (child got up but remained near chair), and amount of time "away" (child left table and required retrieval) were noted during both contexts. No significant differences were found between the groups during the unstructured, free-play situation. However, during the structured activity, the group suspected of having ADHD exhibited significantly more aggressive behaviors, time "up," and time "away" than did their nonaffected peers, which suggests that overactivity can be identified in this age group.

It is possible to identify children in the preschool years who meet the diagnostic criteria for ADHD. However, to avoid inflated diagnostic rates, longitudinal, prospective research is needed that examines the influence of developmental level and measurement issues in the assignment of ADHD diagnoses. Early diagnosis can inform intervention and may also begin to foster a better understanding of the early course of the disorder and associated difficulties. Diagnostic caution is urged, however, because a misdiagnosis of ADHD may lead to attributions of problems in a child who may be responding adaptively to a maladaptive environment. Moreover, a misdiagnosis of ADHD may reflect a failure to recognize difficulties with anxiety and emotion regulation that can have some of the same symptoms as ADHD in the preschool years.

ETIOLOGICAL FACTORS

The consensus among researchers and clinicians is that ADHD is a heterogeneous disorder whose etiology involves multiple factors, including genetic, neurobiological, perinatal and prenatal, and biopsychosocial factors. Although at present no clear direct or causative etiological pathways for the development and expression of ADHD have been identified, this disorder clearly involves a complex interweaving of biological and psychosocial factors.

Genetic Risk Factors

Family, adoption, and twin studies have provided support for the heritability of ADHD (Biederman et al. 1991b; Cantwell 1972; Faraone and Biederman 1994; Faraone et al. 1991, 1994; Gilger et al. 1992; Gillis et al. 1992; Hechtman 1994; Hudziak, Chapter 2, this volume; Levy et al. 1997; Pauls 1991). School-age children, for example, who have first-degree biological relatives diagnosed with ADHD are more likely to be diagnosed themselves (American Psychiatric Association 1994; Biederman et al. 1991b). Frick et al. (1991) found that 80% of their sample of children with ADHD had at least one first-degree biological relative who reported symptoms of ADHD during childhood.

Familial associations may not be restricted to ADHD symptoms. For example, Biederman et al. (1991a) found that children whose parents had a mood disorder displayed high rates of ADHD. Epidemiological family studies have documented significantly higher rates of mood disorders in parents and first-degree relatives of children with ADHD (Biederman et al. 1991a).

Although genetic factors contribute to the expression of ADHD symptoms, genetic vulnerability is not the only determinant of whether a child will manifest symptoms of and meet the full criteria for ADHD. Pauls (1991) noted that some children with ADHD appear to have no familial history and suggested that longitudinal prospective studies focusing on the early course of symptoms and on aspects of family environment are needed to unravel the co-contributions of genes and environment in ADHD.

Neurobiological Risk Factors

Several neuroanatomic structures have been implicated in ADHD. One of the earliest hypotheses was put forth by Laufer et al. (1957), who suggested that ADHD was the result of diencephalic dysfunction in the thalamus and hypothalamus. Satterfield and Dawson (1971) argued for decreased excitation in the reticular activating system. More recently, Weinberg and Harper (1993) argued that ADHD is a disorder of vigilance and implicated the right inferior parietal lobule and posterior parietal cortices. Several contemporary studies suggest frontal lobe involvement on the basis of an association with impairment in executive function tasks in school-age children (e.g., Barkley et al. 1992; Chelune et al. 1986; Everett et al. 1991; Gorenstein et al. 1989; Gualtieri and Hicks 1985; Lou et al. 1984; Mattes 1980; Tannock et al. 1989). Frontal lobe functions include regulation of motor output, planning, and the inhibition of behaviors that interfere with goal-directed behavior (Hynd et al. 1991). Schachar et al. (1993) suggested that the ability to inhibit responding is the basis of ADHD and that this inhibitory deficit represents the impulsivity aspect of the diagnostic criteria for ADHD.

Neuroimaging studies of school-age children have provided important information for understanding brain involvement in ADHD. However, none of the investigations to date have included preschool-age children. Studies using computed tomography have revealed that school-age children with ADHD show differences in the caudate area of the brain, a subcortical area known for motor activity that projects into the frontal lobes (Lou et al. 1984). When these children were given methylphenidate, metabolic activity in the caudate was no longer abnormal. Thus, the pattern of differences may be in response to ADHD behaviors rather than causal. With regard to the frontal lobe hypothesis, Hynd et al. (1991), using magnetic resonance imaging, demonstrated that children with ADHD did not have the right frontal asymmetry typically found in children with ADHD.

Positron emission tomography studies have demonstrated that glucose utilization is reduced in adults with ADHD, particularly in the right frontal area (Zametkin et al. 1990). Thus, it may be that decreased blood flow and reduced metabolic activity in the caudate and frontal lobes are characteristic of individuals with ADHD (Lou et al. 1989), although it would be premature to draw firm conclusions, since the number of neuroanatomic studies is currently limited. As neuroimaging methods become less invasive, it may become possible to examine developmental differences in brain structure and function. From ascertainment of samples of children at risk for developing ADHD, it may be possible to determine whether structure or functional differences precede, are concurrent with, or follow the emergence of ADHD symptoms.

Perinatal and Prenatal Risk Factors

In an early investigation exploring perinatal risk, Pasamanick et al. (1956) reported that mothers of children with ADHD experienced significantly higher numbers of complications throughout their pregnancies. Minde et al. (1968) found that mothers of children with ADHD, compared with mothers of children without ADHD, were more likely to have very long or very short labors and high rates of toxemia (Conners 1975). Sprich-Buckminster et al. (1993) found that mothers of children with ADHD were almost four times more likely than unaffected control subjects to have had a delivery complication, six times more likely to have had an infancy complication, and twice as likely to have had any pregnancy, delivery, or infancy complication. In contrast, Chandola et al. (1992) reported only modest relationships between pre- and perinatal factors and hyperactivity in their longitudinal study. These authors suggested, alternatively, that social class, maternal age, length of second stage labor, antepartum hemorrhage, 1-minute Apgar, and child gender are important factors in the later expression of ADHD, although the predictive powers of these factors are, at best, limited. These inconclusive findings are representative of those from studies attempting to determine perinatal risk factors for ADHD.

Prenatal risk factors that have been associated with a later diagnosis of ADHD include in utero exposure to alcohol, cocaine, and/or heroin (Towbin and Leckman 1991); prolonged oxygen deprivation during the birth process; extreme prematurity; hydrocephalus; and interventricular hemorrhages (Hynd et al. 1991).

Biopsychosocial Models

We have provided evidence to suggest the involvement of genetic, neurobiological, and perinatal and prenatal factors in the etiology of ADHD. It is important, however, to also consider parent-child interactions as a mechanism for influencing the symptoms of ADHD. Recent studies have emphasized the contributions made by each member of the dyad in an interaction; interactions between children with ADHD and their parents can be particularly complex and stressful, often characterized by negatively charged, controlling exchanges that typically include minimal amounts of positive mutuality (Barkley et al. 1990; Bugental et al. 1980; Campbell 1975; Lyman and Hembree-Kigin 1994; Mash and Johnston 1982). Investigations have often attempted to determine whether parents are responding to annoying and frustrating child behaviors with increased demandingness, overintrusiveness, inconsistent punishment, and overly harsh reactions or, alternatively, whether children increase their annoying and frustrating behaviors in response to the parental behaviors just described. Clearly, by the time children reach preschool age, these interactions have evolved to include bidirectional elements.

Mash and Johnston (1983) proposed a model for understanding parent-child interaction that focuses on how existing child attributes are mediated by parents and the broader environment. Child attributes include behavior problems, temperament, and physical and cognitive traits. Maternal cognitions are also incorporated as variables that contribute to the quality of the parent-child interaction. These variables include attitudes and beliefs about the child (Mash and Johnston 1983; Sobol et al. 1989), attributions for child problems (Dix et al. 1989), and parents' expectations of their own parenting skills and of their ability to influence the child's behavior (George and Solomon 1989; Mash and Johnston 1983).

Mash and Johnston (1982) found that mothers of hyperactive children, particularly mothers of younger hyperactive children, were more controlling, directive, and negative in their interactions than mothers of nonhyperactive children, and these differences could be observed in the behaviors of both the child and the mother (Mash and Johnston 1982). Similarly, Schleifer and colleagues (1975) demonstrated that in homes where there was a hyperactive preschool-age child, mother-child interactions were rated as more tense and less talkative and playful when compared with mother's interactions with nonhyperactive siblings. Mothers of hyperactive preschoolers were also found to use more physical punishment and to exhibit more frustration. In a study comparing mother-child interactions among several groups of school-age boys with ADHD, O'Connor et al. (1993) found that mothers of sons diagnosed as having "ADHD only" were more positive, more supportive, and more involved than mothers of boys with comorbid diagnoses—a finding which suggests that ADHD alone cannot account for the difficulties in mother-child interactions in this group. Rather, it may be the comorbid diagnoses that differentiate the interactional styles of the groups. Anastopoulos et al. (1992) obtained similar results with a comparable methodology.

In addition to parenting style and child characteristics, parental psychopathology and problems in marital and family functioning have been associated with the presence of ADHD in children. Specifically, associated difficulties include a higher incidence of maternal depression (Anastopoulos et al. 1992; Cunningham et al. 1988; Griest et al. 1979; Lahey et al. 1998; Mash and Johnston 1982), reduced marital satisfaction (Barkley et al. 1990; Befera and Barkley 1985; Johnson and Lobitz 1974), and parents' perceptions of their interactions with their children as more stressful and less rewarding (Barkley 1981; Breen and Barkley 1988; Mash and Johnston 1983). Anastopoulos et al. (1992) proposed that parental factors (maternal psychopathology in particular) may "introduce unrealistic, negative bias into parental perceptions of child behavior or alter parental cognitions in other ways, thus exacerbating parenting stress" (p. 517). It has been further suggested that because of increased stress, parents may not be as aware of the child's positive behavior and may unintentionally overreact to negative behaviors or respond to the child inconsistently (Anastopoulos et al. 1992). This style of interaction may, in turn, increase the child's negative behavior, resulting in increased parental stress. Thus, it appears a negative spiraling may be occurring in these parent-child interactions and that each member of the dyad contributes to the difficulties.

Hartsough and Lambert (1985) proposed a biopsychosocial model for the development and expression of ADHD, arguing that although some perinatal, prenatal, neurobiological, and genetic factors may predispose a child to ADHD, the disorder will not be expressed unless environmental conditions interact with psychological and biological factors. In a large, epidemiological prospective and longitudinal study, Hartsough and Lambert (1985) annually collected data on ADHD symptoms from several reporting sources (e.g., parents, teachers, physicians). Perinatal and prenatal factors found to increase risk for ADHD included 1) evidence of fetal distress during labor or birth, 2) congenital problems, 3) health problems in infancy, 4) poor maternal health during pregnancy, 5) presence of toxemia or eclampsia in pregnancy, 6) maternal youth, 7) long labor, and 8) being a first-born. Child factors that were found to increase risk for ADHD included 1) delayed speech, 2) delayed bowel control, 3) difficulty with coordination and speech, and 4) four or more serious accidents during infancy and early childhood. Family environmental risk factors included family stressors and parenting style (Hartsough and Lambert 1985). A major contribution of Hartsough and Lambert's epidemiological study is the identification of multiple sources of risk and their transactions in the family context.

COMORBIDITY

Examining issues of comorbidity is important to understanding the etiology and treatment of childhood disorders from the perspective of developmental psychopathology (Pennington et al. 1993). Several investigations have confirmed that children with ADHD are at greater risk for developing other mental disorders, including oppositional defiant disorder, conduct disorder, and depression (Biederman et al. 1991b; Henker and Whalen 1989). Indeed, the diagnoses of ADHD, oppositional defiant disorder, and conduct disorder have often been considered a triad of disruptive behavior disorders (Henker and Whalen 1989) or "undercontrolled disorders" (Barkley 1990; Cicchetti and Cohen 1995; Henker and Whalen 1989; Kazdin 1989). Lyman and Hembree-Kigin (1994) reported that up to 70% of school-age children with ADHD referred to child guidance clinics also have problems with conduct and aggression. Overlap of these diagnoses among school-age children is reported to be as high as 50% (Henker and Whalen 1989; Lyman and Hembree-Kigin 1994). However, these unusually high numbers may be the result of ascertainment biases in clinical samples. That is, the greater the number of comorbid conditions a child has, the more likely a family is to seek treatment. Thus, children with ADHD and comorbid diagnoses generally experience more behavioral and emotional difficulties and are more likely to be identified and referred for clinical intervention.

Studying the comorbidity of ADHD with other psychiatric disorders is particularly challenging during the preschool years. For example, transient oppositional behavior is considered age-appropriate in preschool children (Henker and Whalen 1989). Indeed, approximately 50% of a sample of preschool children without ADHD were rated by their mothers as situationally overly oppositional and disobedient (Campbell and Breaux 1983). Thus, for oppositional defiant disorder to be a diagnostic consideration for preschool-age children, noncompliance and oppositionality need to be sufficiently severe. Futhermore, conduct disorder is not a relevant diagnostic category for preschool-age children.

In an attempt to clarify the often complex results of investigations of ADHD and comorbidity, Biederman and colleagues (1991b) completed a meta-analytic study. However, generalization of these findings to the preschool-age child should be done judiciously: only 3 of the 46 studies used in the meta-analysis included children under 5 years of age. To be inclusive in consideration of nomenclature for attentional problems, Biederman et al. included both current and historical diagnostic terms: "hyperactivity, hyperkinesis, attention deficit disorder, and attention deficit hyperactivity disorder" (p. 565). Terms were cross-referenced with "anti-social disorder (aggression, conduct disorder, anti-social disorder), depression (depression, mania, depressive disorder, bipolar), anxiety (anxiety disorder, anxiety), learning problems (learning, learning disabilities, academic achievement), substance abuse (alcoholism, drug abuse), and Tourette's disorder" (p. 565). Comorbidity rates for both clinical and epidemiological samples were 30%–50% for ADHD and conduct disorder, approximately 35% for ADHD and oppositional defiant disorder (although the number of studies was limited),

15%–75% for ADHD and mood disorders, and 25% for ADHD and anxiety disorders. There is a need for more epidemiological research that uses current diagnostic criteria and multiple methods (i.e., interview, questionnaire, observation) and informants (i.e., parents, teachers, children) so that more stable estimates of comorbidity can be obtained.

In a prospective study of a sample of 803 children, McGee et al. (1992) identified 45 children (40 boys and 5 girls) who met the DSM-III-R criteria for ADHD. Unfortunately, because of the small number of girls with ADHD in this sample, analyses were limited to boys with ADHD. Of the 40 boys identified, 20 had one or more additional diagnoses. Nineteen boys with ADHD also met the diagnostic criteria for conduct disorder or oppositional defiant disorder. Nine of these 19 also met the criteria for anxiety and/or depression. Comorbidity was more likely when the onset of ADHD was at preschool age (i.e., ages 3–5 years) than at age 6 years (McGee et al. 1992).

Thus, ADHD is a multifactorial disorder with significant and multiple comorbidity. Distinct subgroups of ADHD may exist (Biederman et al. 1991b; Barkley et al. 1992; Schleifer et al. 1975), each with unique symptom clusters, neurobiology, response to pharmacological intervention, and prognosis. It is also possible that different subgroups of children with ADHD may differ in their risk for specific comorbid conditions. Future research should attempt to identify subgroups and must address heterogeneity within ADHD, as well as the role of comorbid diagnoses. Studies that assess relatives may be particularly illuminating. For example, children with ADHD with first-degree family members with affective disorders (Biederman et al. 1991a) may evidence greater comorbidity for depression. In addition to genetic risk for specific comorbid conditions, family functioning may be particularly relevant in disentangling comorbid adaptive as well as maladaptive behaviors (Carter et al. 1994).

ATTENTION

The diagnostician must be familiar with normative patterns of attention, emotion, and behavior regulation in the preschool years to recognize symptoms that warrant a diagnosis of ADHD. Unfortunately, measurement instrumentation for assessing ADHD in the preschool years is more limited than that available for school-age children. The vast majority of measures are not appropriate for 3-year-olds. Given the current limits of available standardized assessment instruments, clinicians must rely almost exclusively on their knowledge of the range of normative behaviors. Therefore, we now present a brief review of studies of attention regulation in typically developing preschool children.

The ability to pay attention and focus is central to information processing. learning, cognition, and memory. As Ruff et al. (1990) noted, "Attention involves processes that allow individuals to focus on particular aspects of the environment and to mobilize sufficient effort for learning and problem solving" (p. 60). By the preschool years, children have been observed to engage in a single activity for up to 30 minutes (Anderson and Levin 1976), a period of time that enables children of this age to focus and attend to environmental stimuli.

Although inappropriate as diagnostic tests for ADHD, computerized continuous performance tasks (CPTs) are the most frequently used method for assessing sustained attention in school-age children (Aman and Turbott 1986; Gordon 1986; Rosvold et al. 1956). Children are required to watch a computer screen and to respond (e.g., by pressing a button or computer key) when a target letter or number appears on the screen. These tasks assess the duration of a child's ability to attend, whereas reaction time tasks, in which a similar method is used, focus on how quickly children respond to target stimuli. School-age children with ADHD demonstrate lowered sensitivity to stimuli (errors of omission; nonresponse to stimuli) as well as more impulsive responding (errors of commission; response to nontarget stimuli). Studies of school-age children using methylphenidate and amphetamine have demonstrated improved performance on both CPTs and reaction time tasks (Aman et al. 1991; Levy and Hobbes 1988; Sostek et al. 1980; Sykes et al. 1972, 1977).

There has been very limited work using this methodology with preschool-age children. Most existing CPTs are developmentally too advanced for preschool-age children. The preschool years are a particularly challenging period during which to assess attention regulation, because there is significant individual variability and situational specificity within which to observe sustained attention in this age group. However, a limited number of investigations have been completed that assess attention during free play or television viewing as age-appropriate tasks. For example, Anderson and Levin (1976) found that from 1 to 4 years of age, children's attention while viewing *Sesame Street* increased in both frequency and duration. Allesandri (1992) found that preschoolers with ADHD, compared with their non-ADHD counterparts, demonstrated more off-task behaviors and had significantly more difficulty with structured tasks that require prolonged, focused attention.

Other attempts to measure attention regulation in preschool-age children have focused on the modification of CPTs to make them more age-appropriate. Levy (1980), for example, using a letter-based CPT, found that attention regulation improved between the ages of 4 and 6 years. In this sample, 73% of the 3- to 3.5-year-old children were unable to complete this task, compared with 29% of the 4-year-olds. Several studies in which Levy's task was modified by replacing letters with pictures found that preschool-age children are better able to complete the picture-based task (Boyd et al. 1991; Kristjansson et al. 1989). Reaction time also improved in 2.5- to 4.5-year-old children when a picture CPT was used (Weissberg et al. 1990), with the most significant increase in attention occurring between the ages of 3.5 and 4.5.

Hartup (1983) proposed that regulation of attention and increased control over disruptive behaviors represent early components of social competence, which has important implications for the development of satisfactory peer relationships, as discussed below.

PEER RELATIONSHIPS AND SOCIABILITY

Despite the early onset of ADHD and evidence of enduring patterns of social and interpersonal difficulties, few studies have examined the behavioral and emotional correlates of ADHD from a developmental perspective during the preschool years. This is surprising given the central role that developmental psychologists attribute to effective peer relations and social functioning during this developmental epoch (Sroufe and Rutter 1984). Indeed, the establishment and negotiation of peer contacts has been described as one of the more important issues of development during the preschool years (Sroufe and Rutter 1984). Hartup (1983) referred to the preschool years as a time when qualitative changes occur in relationships with the emergence of "friendships" and a deeper understanding of reciprocity. Thus, considered along a developmental trajectory, problems with attention and behavior regulation in the preschool years may lead to difficulties in acquiring the requisite skills necessary for effective social functioning and may increase risk for delays and potential difficulties in future social relationships.

Although the number of children with ADHD who exhibit peer problems is unknown, Pelham and Bender (1982) have estimated that over 50% of school-age children with ADHD experience significant peer and interpersonal difficulties. These children have been observed to be consistently more aggressive, noisier, and more off-task and "on the go" than their same-age peers, regardless of setting and method of measurement (Pelham and Bender 1982; Whalen and Henker 1985). Boys rated by their peers as hyperactive are also more likely to be rated as rejected by peers (Henker and Whalen 1989; Whalen and Henker 1985). When first-graders were asked what makes a child "popular," responses included greater altruism, more acceptance of others' invitations to play, better conversational skills, and participation in play. In contrast, "unpopular children" were described as more aggressive and less likely to play (Dygdon et al. 1987). It is apparent from these findings that establishing a role in the school peer hierarchy begins early.

Studies of sociability in preschool-age children, although limited in number, have found associations between hyperactive behavior, deficits in social skills, and aggression toward peers (Allesandri 1992; Campbell 1990; Campbell and Cluss 1982; Schleifer et al. 1975). Specific cognitive and behavioral skills emerging during the preschool years that have an impact on the ability to maintain and negotiate friendships include the ability to differentiate self from other, the ability to take another's perspective, and an increasing capacity to regulate behavior and emotions (Eisenberg and Fabes 1991; Iannotti 1985). The role of sustained attention deficits and nonaggressive impulsivity in the development of peer relations is less clear. When children are highly distractible and impulsive, it may be more difficult to acquire age-appropriate perspective-taking skills. Clearly, many children with ADHD evidence problems in regulating behavior (i.e., hyperactivity) and emotions.

Investigations have found that children with ADHD can exhibit socially appropriate behaviors, depending on the level of structure and the complexity of the situation. The more complicated the task, and hence the greater its demand for planning, organization, and executive regulation of behavior, the greater the likelihood that children with ADHD will evidence difficulties compared with non-ADHD children (Barkley 1990; Douglas 1983; Luk 1985). For example, Tannock et al. (1993) used a story retelling task to assess the narrative abilities of school-age children with ADHD compared with those of their non-ADHD peers. No differences were found in the two groups' ability to comprehend and extract main ideas from the stories. However, the children with ADHD provided less information overall, were more disorganized, produced less cohesive stories in retelling, and had more inaccuracies in recall (Tannock et al. 1993). Similarly, adults with ADHD reported experiencing more difficulty when presented with social tasks requiring generative skills (i.e., free-response questionnaire) and having better performance when the task required selective processes (i.e., multiple-choice questionnaire) (Hechtman et al. 1980). These results suggest that individuals with ADHD may indeed know the right answer when presented with socially appropriate response choices, but that difficulties emerge when they must generate a social solution independently (Whalen and Henker 1985).

Whereas investigators in several studies reported findings of social skills deficits in children with ADHD, other investigators found no significant differences in social knowledge and perspective taking when children with ADHD were compared with their non-ADHD peers (Ackerman et al. 1979; Campbell and Paulauskas 1979; Whalen and Henker 1985). Hypotheses to account for these contradictory findings include the proposal that the deficits that children with ADHD exhibit may not be in the knowledge of appropriate social actions, but rather in the production of solutions (Hechtman et al. 1980; Tannock et al. 1993; Whalen and Henker 1985; Zentall 1988). This production deficit interferes with the integrated processes in the evaluation, generation, and implementation of appropriate actions in social situations.

Although not directly addressing children with ADHD, Zahn-Waxler et al. (1994), using a set of scripted structured and unstructured narrative situations that present conflict and distress, compared at-risk and low-risk preschool children to explore their ability to resolve interpersonal dilemmas and their social problem-solving abilities and social competences. The authors found that the at-risk children seemed to understand that prosocial, reparative, affiliative solutions were expected, and their answers were not significantly different from those of the low-risk children. Perhaps, when provided with scripted, hypothetical conflicts, the at-risk child has enough time to make more socially appropriate decisions; when facing real-life situations with social demands requiring the need for rapid decision making, such as requests for compliance, sharing, and cooperation, the at-risk child is overwhelmed by impulsivity, inattentiveness, noncompliance, and hyperactivity, which preclude his or her making the socially appropriate choice.

ASSESSMENT

Preschool-age children suspected of having attentional problems require careful and thorough assessment involving multimodal and multidimensional methods of evaluation (Barkley 1990; Lyman and Hembree-Kigin 1994; Schaughency and Rothlind 1991). Because children vary in their behaviors and performance across settings and tasks, it is imperative that assessments be completed in multiple domains, with input from multiple informants. Methods that are particularly useful include standardized questionnaires, naturalistic observations, and psychological testing. It is critical to gather questionnaire data from multiple informants (e.g., mother, father, teacher) and to assess multiple domains of problem behaviors and competencies.

When possible, child observations should be completed in several settings, including at home and in structured situations outside of the home, such as preschool, day care, or library (during storytelling time). Optimally, children should be observed with parents, other adult authority figures (e.g., teachers, babysitters), siblings, peers, and unfamiliar persons. Observations should be conducted over several days and at different times of the day.

Children with ADHD can vary in their overactive and inattentive behaviors. Indeed, even when engaged in the same task, children with ADHD often perform erratically, employing focused attention during one episode, yet appearing as though the task were never learned the next time the task is attempted. This lack of predictability can lead parents and teachers to conclude that the child is lazy or stubborn (e.g., "I know he can do it if he wants to—I've seen him do it before"). Erratic performance is one of the hallmarks of ADHD; performance, activity level, and focused attention can fluctuate within days and even hours (Barkley 1990).

Assessments of parent-child interactions and family functioning may be particularly important for the preschool child. The presence of maladaptive interactional patterns or of stress in the family does not imply that family factors are causing the child's attentional difficulties. Parenting a child with ADHD can create unique stressors in the family. Thus, the family's adaptation to the symptoms of ADHD in the child should not be confused with the family's general level of functioning.

In addition to observational methods and paper-and-pencil measures, psychological testing can provide useful and important information. Domains to be assessed should include overall cognitive ability, visual-motor integration, and attention. Evaluation of formal learning disabilities in preschool children is difficult because children in this age group are not expected to read or perform mathematical operations. Measures of academic readiness, however, can and should be used with children in this age group.

Multisession, multimodal data collection is complex and time-consuming. It can, however, provide a comprehensive picture of the preschool child, which is important for diagnosis and treatment planning.

INTERVENTION

Although it is clear that interactions between children with ADHD and their parents can be frustrating and stressful, comprehensive behavioral intervention programs focused on helping parents understand their child's behaviors as well as teaching effective parenting strategies have been useful with school-age children (Pisterman et al. 1989). The ideal intervention for preschool-age children, much like the ideal assessment, is both multimodal and multifocused. Parent education and counseling are imperative. The overall goal of most parent training interventions is to help the parent assist the child in managing his or her behaviors. Long-term goals include parents' helping their child acquire greater awareness of and control over his or her own behaviors. Parents may also need assistance in educating school personnel about their child's educational needs.

Pisterman et al. (1989) developed a compliance-based parent intervention program specifically designed for preschool children and their parents. Families participating in the program included parents with children (ages 3–6 years) who met the DSM-III criteria for attention deficit disorder (American Psychiatric Association 1980). The parent training program consisted of 12 weekly sessions. In sessions 1 through 3 the focus was on educating parents about the etiology and course of ADHD, behavior management principles, and the interactive aspects of the parent-child relationship. In sessions 4 through 11 the focus was on parenting skill development, by which parents were taught "how to give differential attention to appropriate behavior, how to issue appropriate commands and how to use time-outs for noncompliance" (Pisterman et al. 1989, p. 630). Instructional methods included role taking, modeling, and rehearsal.

The multimodal approach of Pisterman and colleagues appears to be an efficacious and effective strategy for preschool-age children and their parents. Preschool children exhibited a significant reduction in noncompliant behaviors following the 12-week treatment. In addition, parents became more directive and more consistent in their requests of their children. Parental reinforcement of their children's compliant behaviors also increased significantly. In turn, children's compliance increased. Unfortunately, however, these effects were evident only with targeted behaviors and could not be generalized to other aspects of the parent-child relationship (Pisterman et al. 1989).

Studies with similar methodologies have found that preschool children's attention to tasks can be increased (Pisterman et al. 1992) and that with improvement in the quality of family relationships and child behavior, parents reported reduced parent stress, improved self-esteem, and more marital satisfaction (Anastopoulos et al. 1993). In a long-term follow-up study, 14 years after participating in a parent training program, children who had been diagnosed with ADHD had functioning comparable to that of children in a nonclinical sample (Long et al. 1994).

In a more recent study from Pisterman's laboratory (Musten et al. 1997), it was found that when parent training was not included as a form of intervention (medication was the only intervention), preschool-age children who met the diagnostic criteria for ADHD did not show improvements in their compliance to parents' requests, though other improvements were noted.

Clearly, results such as these strongly suggest that parents and children can benefit from parent training. The positive results of such interventions, like the escalating stress in parent-child interactions in families with children with ADHD, are bidirectional: reducing the number of problematic behaviors observed in children with ADHD increases child self-esteem, which has an impact on parents by reducing stress and increasing parent self-esteem, which in turn improves the overall quality of interaction between parents and children. When positive effects of stimulant medication were evident in child behaviors, such as reduced numbers of negative, defiant, impulsive, and inattentive behaviors, concomitant changes in the mother's behavior were also observed. Mothers of children of all ages, including preschool children, became less directive, more positive, and less controlling in their interactions with their child (Barkley et al. 1984). However, the use of psychostimulant medications with preschooler children is controversial.

Psychopharmacology

Psychostimulant medication is the most frequently prescribed treatment for school-age children with ADHD; it has been variously estimated that between 2% (750,000 children) (Safer and Krager 1988) and 6% (1,600,000 children) (Safer and Krager 1988; Wilens and Biederman 1992) of the school-age population in the United States take these medications. Effectiveness rates are reported to range from 50% to 95% for this age group. The positive effects of psychostimulants include improved attention regulation (Abikoff and Gittelman 1985; DuPaul and Rapport 1993), better learning and academic performance, and less aggressive social interactions. Until recently, only a very limited number of studies evaluating the effects of psychostimulant medications in preschool-age children were available, and the results were equivocal.

Schleifer et al. (1975) found that preschool-age children taking psychostimulant medication exhibited significantly reduced amounts of hyperactivity as assessed by maternal report. These results could not be corroborated on the basis of nursery school observations and psychological assessments. Indeed, in school these children were observed to exhibit an increase in negative mood and difficulties with irritability, more aggressive peer interactions, excessive hugging, and increased solitary play.

Cohen et al. (1981) compared the efficacy of medication with that of a behavior modification program for kindergarten children diagnosed with ADHD. As in Schleifer et al.'s study, parental ratings suggested that children receiving medication displayed greater behavior change at post-treatment assessment than the children participating in the behavior modification program only. Parental reports were not consistent with observational data or results on teacher rating scales; no positive effects were found by either assessment method with medication alone or behavior modification with medication. Although the inconsistency of parental ratings with other measures does not negate the validity of parental reports, the magnitude and generalizability of possible positive effects that parents are reporting come into question. Of note, both of these studies found that although parents rated their children's behavior as improved, most parents made the decision to discontinue medication at the study's conclusion.

One of the more recent studies, and one that is arguably methodologically the most rigorous, found that the use of methylphenidate with 4- to 6-year-olds can be helpful in the reduction of ADHD symptoms (Musten et al. 1997). Thirty-one children (28 boys) and their parents participated in a double-blind, placebo-controlled study that used two different doses of methylphenidate and placebo. Each child received all three conditions in randomized order, and multiple assessments were completed in each condition. The investigators demonstrated improvements in cognitive functioning, ability to pay attention, and reductions in impulsive behaviors when the higher dose of medicine was used (0.5 mg/kg) compared with when a lower dose (0.3 mg/kg) or placebo was used. In an assessment of mother-child interactions, when children were on the higher dose of medicine, they were able to work with significantly greater productivity and were more able to remain focused. It was proposed that the use of medicines to improve the functioning of preschool-age children has "expanded the treatment repertoire for very young children with ADHD" (Musten et al. 1997, p. 1415).

Despite these results, decisions regarding the use of psychostimulant medication should be carefully made when preschool-age children are involved. Barkley (1990) has cautioned against using psychostimulants with children under 4 years of age. The probability of these drugs being effective decreases below age 5 years, and it has been hypothesized that the prefrontal cortex, the brain area that is the primary site of action of psychostimulants, is not fully mature at this young age (Barkley et al. 1990). Other organ systems responsible for the breakdown and secretion of psychostimulants are also immature at this age (Barkley et al. 1989). Moreover, it is important to consider that the primary reason for prescribing psychostimulant medication is to help a school-age child focus more clearly and complete schoolwork. Since preschool children do not typically engage in these activities, the primary use for stimulant medication with this population would be behavior control, unless, as is the case for children attending preschool, the child is placed in a structured environment with the expectation of behavior regulation. However, even in more structured environments, medication use should be judicious and assessed on a child-by-child basis, since several investigations have demonstrated that parent training interventions can be quite effective in improving compliance and reducing aggression in this age group.

CONCLUSION

It is both possible and very important to identify the early symptoms of ADHD when they first emerge in the preschool years. Specifically, early identification creates opportunities for early intervention. At the present time, the most efficacious intervention in the preschool period focuses on improving parenting interactions and educating parents about ADHD (e.g., Pisterman et al. 1992). It is possible that early identification and intervention will reduce some of the associated symptoms and comorbid diagnoses that children with ADHD often exhibit (e.g., aggression, problems in peer relations, conduct disorder). Furthermore, improved understanding of the disorder, as well as the availability of strategies and support for coping with the impact of the disorder in the family, will likely result in diminished family and parenting stress.

Developmental considerations in the preschool period suggest that more stringent criteria may need to be used when making a diagnosis of ADHD (Ott et al., in press). Specifically, the preschool period is marked by dramatic gains in attention and behavior regulation (Anderson and Levin 1976; Sroufe and Rutter 1984). Many young preschool-age children may engage in age-appropriate behaviors that would be considered problematic or hyperactive in older children. Multimodal assessment involving multiple informants is particularly critical in the evaluation of preschool children.

Future research that would be particularly informative for understanding ADHD among preschool-age children could involve longitudinal prospective studies of children at risk for ADHD by virtue of having a first-degree relative with ADHD. In this design, the etiological role of heritability, pre- and perinatal complications, early child temperament, and family environment (e.g., parenting interactions, marital relations, stress) could be incorporated to address a biopsychosocial model that could help begin to unravel the complexities of ADHD.

REFERENCES

Abikoff H, Gittelman R: The normalizing effects of methylphenidate on the classroom behavior of ADDH children. J Abnorm Child Psychol 13:33–44, 1985

Ackerman PT, Elardo PT, Dykman RA: A psychosocial study of hyperactive and learning-disabled boys. J Abnorm Child Psychol 7:91–99, 1979

Allesandri SM: Attention, play, and social behavior in ADHD preschoolers. J Abnorm Child Psychol 20:289–302, 1992

Aman MG, Turbott SH: Incidental learning, distraction, and sustained attention in hyperactive and control subjects. J Abnorm Child Psychol 14:441–455, 1986

Aman MG, Marks RE, Turbott SH, et al: Methylphenidate and thioridazine in the treatment of intellectually subaverage children: effects on cognitive-motor performance. J Am Acad Child Adolesc Psychiatry 30:816–824, 1991

American Psychiatric Association: Diagnostic and Statistical Manual of Mental Disorders, 3rd Edition. Washington, DC, American Psychiatric Association, 1980

American Psychiatric Association: Diagnostic and Statistical Manual of Mental Disorders, 3rd Edition, Revised. Washington, DC, American Psychiatric Association, 1987

American Psychiatric Association: Diagnostic and Statistical Manual of Mental Disorders, 4th Edition. Washington, DC, American Psychiatric Association, 1994

Anastopoulos AD, Guevremont DC, Shelton TL, et al: Parenting stress among families of children with attention deficit hyperactivity disorder. J Abnorm Child Psychol 20:503–520, 1992

Anastopoulos AD, Shelton TL, DuPaul GJ, et al: Parent training for attention-deficit hyperactivity disorder: its impact on parent functioning. J Abnorm Child Psychol 21:581–595, 1993

Anderson DR, Levin SR: Young children's attention to Sesame Street. Child Dev 47:806–811, 1976

August GJ, Garfinkel BD: Comorbidity of ADHD and reading disability among clinic referred children. J Abnorm Child Psychol 18:29–45, 1989

August GJ, Stewart MA: Is there a syndrome of pure hyperactivity? Br J Psychiatry 140:305–311, 1981

Barkley RA: Hyperactive Children. New York, Guilford, 1981

Barkley RA: Attention Deficit Hyperactivity Disorder: A Handbook for Diagnosis and Treatment. New York, Guilford, 1990

Barkley RA, Karlsson J, Strzelecki E, et al: Effects of age and Ritalin dosage on mother-child interactions of hyperactive children. J Consult Clin Psychol 52:750–758, 1984

Barkley RA, McMurray MB, Edelbrock CS, et al: The response of aggressive and nonaggressive ADHD children to two doses of methylphenidate. J Am Acad Child Adolesc Psychiatry 28:873–881, 1989

Barkley RA, Fischer M, Edelbrock CS, et al: The adolescent outcome of hyperactive children diagnosed by research criteria, I: an 8-year prospective follow-up study. J Am Acad Child Adolesc Psychiatry 29:546–557, 1990

Barkley RA, Grodzinsky G, DuPaul GJ: Frontal lobe functions in attention deficit disorder with and without hyperactivity: a review and research report. J Abnorm Child Psychol 20:163–188, 1992

Befera M, Barkley RA: Hyperactive and normal girls and boys: mother-child interactions, parent psychiatric status, and child psychopathology. J Child Psychol Psychiatry 26:439–452, 1985

Beitchman JH, Wekerle C, Hood J: Diagnostic continuity from preschool to middle childhood. J Am Acad Child Adolesc Psychiatry 26:694–699, 1987

Biederman J, Faraone SV, Keenan K, et al: Evidence of familial association between attention deficit disorder and major affective disorders. Arch Gen Psychiatry 48: 633–642, 1991a

Biederman J, Newcorn J, Sprich S: Comorbidity of attention-deficit hyperactivity disorder with conduct, depressive, anxiety, and other disorders. Am J Psychiatry 148:564–577, 1991b

Boyd TA, Ernhart CB, Greene TH, et al: Prenatal alcohol exposure and sustained attention in the preschool years. Neurotoxicol Teratol 13:49–55, 1991

Breen MJ, Barkley RA: Child psychopathology and parenting stress in girls and boys having attention deficit disorder with hyperactivity. J Pediatr Psychol 13:265–280, 1988

Bugental DB, Caporeal L, Shennum WA: Experimentally produced child uncontrollability: effects of the potency of adult communication patterns. Child Dev 51: 520–528, 1980

Campbell SB: Mother-child interaction: a comparison of hyperactive, learning disabled and normal boys. Am J Orthopsychiatry 45:51–57, 1975

Campbell SB: Behavior Problems in Preschool Children: Clinical and Developmental Issues. New York, Guilford, 1990

Campbell SB: Behavior problems in preschool age children: a review of recent research. J Child Psychol Psychiatry 36:113–149, 1995

Campbell SB, Breaux AM: Maternal ratings of activity level and symptomatic behavior in a non-clinical sample of young children. J Pediatr Psychol 8:73–82, 1983

Campbell SB, Cluss P: Peer relationships of young children with behavior problems, in Peer Relationships and Social Skills in Childhood. Edited by Rubin K, Ross H. New York, Springer-Verlag, 1982, pp 323–351

Campbell SB, Ewing LJ: Follow-up of hard-to-manage preschoolers: adjustment at age 9 and predictors of continuing symptoms. J Child Psychol Psychiatry 31:871–889, 1990

Campbell SB, Paulauskas S: Peer relations in hyperactive children. J Child Psychol Psychiatry 20:233–246, 1979

Campbell SB, Szumowski EK, Ewing LJ, et al: A multidimensional assessment of parent identified behavior problem toddlers. J Abnorm Child Psychol 10:569–592, 1982

Campbell SB, Ewing LJ, Breaux LM, et al: Parent-referred problem three-year-olds: follow-up at elementary entry. J Child Psychol Psychiatry 27:473–488, 1986

Cantwell DP: Psychiatric illness in the families of hyperactive children. Arch Gen Psychiatry 27:414–417, 1972

Cantwell DP, Baker L: Attention deficit disorder with and without hyperactivity: a review and comparison of matched groups. J Am Acad Child Adolesc Psychiatry 31:432–438, 1992

Carter AS, Pauls DL, Leckman JF, et al: A prospective longitudinal study of Gilles de la Tourette's syndrome. J Am Acad Child Adolesc Psychiatry 33:377–385, 1994

Chandola CA, Robling MR, Peters TJ, et al: Pre- and perinatal factors and the risk of subsequent referral for hyperactivity. J Child Psychol Psychiatry 33:1077–1090, 1992

Chelune GJ, Ferguson W, Koon R, et al: Frontal lobe disinhibition in attention deficit disorder. Child Psychiatry Hum Dev 16:221–234, 1986

Cicchetti D: The emergence of developmental psychopathology. Child Dev 55:1–7, 1984

Cicchetti D, Cohen DJ (eds): Developmental Psychopathology, Vol 1: Theory and Methods. New York, Wiley, 1995

Cohen NJ, Sullivan J, Minde K, et al: Evaluation of the relative effectiveness of methylphenidate and cognitive behavior modification in the treatment of kindergarten-aged children. J Abnorm Child Psychol 9:43–54, 1981

Conners CK: Controlled trial of methylphenidate in pre-school children with minimal brain dysfunction. International Journal of Mental Health 4:61–74, 1975

Cook EH, Stein MA, Krasowski MD: Association of attention deficit disorder and the dopamine transporter gene. Am J Hum Genet 56:993–998, 1995

Cunningham CE, Benness BB, Siegel LS: Family functioning, time allocation, and parental depression in the families of normal and ADHD children. J Clin Child Psychol 17:169–177, 1988

Dix T, Ruble DN, Zambarano RJ: Mothers' implicit theories of discipline: child effects, parent effects, and the attribution process. Child Dev 60:1363–1391, 1989

Douglas VI: Attention and cognitive problems, in Developmental Neuropsychiatry. Edited by Rutter M. New York, Guilford, 1983, pp 280–329

DuPaul GJ, Rapport MD: Does methylphenidate normalize the classroom performance of children with attention deficit disorder? J Am Acad Child Adolesc Psychiatry 32:190–198, 1993

Dygdon JA, Conger AJ, Keane SP: Children's perceptions of the behavioral correlates of social acceptance, rejection, and neglect in their peers. J Clin Child Psychol 16:2–8, 1987

Eisenberg N, Fabes RA: Prosocial behavior and empathy: a multimethod, developmental perspective, in Review of Personality and Social Psychology, Vol 12. Edited by Clark M. Newbury Park, CA, Sage, 1991, pp 34–61

Everett J, Thomas J, Cote F: Cognitive effects of psychostimulant medication in hyperactive children. Child Psychiatry Hum Dev 22:79–87, 1991

Faraone SV, Biederman J: Is attention deficit hyperactivity disorder familial? Harv Rev Psychiatry 1:271–287, 1994

Faraone SV, Biederman J, Keenan K, et al: Separation of DSM-III attention deficit disorder and conduct disorder: evidence from a family genetic study of American child psychiatric patients. Psychol Med 21:109–121, 1991

Faraone SV, Biederman J, Milberger S: An exploratory study of ADHD among second-degree relatives of ADHD children. Biol Psychiatry 35:398–402, 1994

Frick PJ, Lahey BB: The nature and characteristics of attention deficit hyperactivity disorder. School Psychology Review 20:163–173, 1991

Frick PJ, Lahey BB, Christ MAG, et al: History of childhood behavior problems in biological parents of boys with attention-deficit hyperactivity disorder and conduct disorder. J Clin Child Psychol 20:445–451, 1991

George C, Solomon J: Internal working models of caregiving and security of attachment at age six. Paper presented at the biennial meeting of the Society for Research in Child Development, Kansas City, MO, April 1989

Gilger JW, Pennington BF, DeFries JC: A twin study of the etiology of comorbidity: attention deficit hyperactivity disorder and dyslexia. J Am Acad Child Adolesc Psychiatry 31:343–348, 1992

Gillis WJ, Gilger JW, Pennington BF, et al: Attention deficit disorder in reading-disabled twins: evidence for a genetic etiology. J Abnorm Child Psychol 20: 303–315, 1992

Gordon M: Microprocessor-based assessment of attention deficit disorders. Psychopharmacol Bull 22:288–290, 1986

Gorenstein EE, Mammato CA, Sandy JM: Performance of inattentive-overactive children on selected measures of prefrontal-type function. J Clin Psychol 45:619–632, 1989

Griest DL, Wells KC, Forehand R: An examination of predictors of maternal perceptions of maladjustment in clinic-referred children. J Abnorm Psychol 88:277–281, 1979

Gualtieri CT, Hicks RE: Neuropharmacology of methylphenidate and a neural substrate for childhood hyperactivity. Psychiatr Clin North Am 8:875–892, 1985

Hartsough CS, Lambert NM: Medical factors in hyperactive and normal children: prenatal, developmental and health history findings. Am J Orthopsychiatry 55: 190–201, 1985

Hartup W: Peer relations, in Carmichael's Manual of Child Psychology, Vol 4: Social and Personality Development. Edited by Hetherington E M. New York, Wiley, 1983, pp 103–196

Hechtman L: Genetic and neurobiological aspects of attention deficit hyperactivity disorder: a review. J Psychiatry Neurosci 19:193–201, 1994

Hechtman L, Weiss G, Perlman T: Hyperactives as young adults: self-esteem and social skills. Can J Psychiatry 25:478–483, 1980

Henker B, Whalen CK: Hyperactivity and attention deficits. Am Psychol 44:216–223, 1989

Hofferth SL, Phillips DA: Child care social policy. Journal of Social Issues 47:1–13, 1991

Hofferth SL, Brayfield A, Deich S, et al: The National Child Care Survey, 1990. Washington, DC, Urban Institute, 1991

Hynd GW, Hern KL, Voeller KK, et al: Neurobiological basis of attention deficit hyperactivity disorder (ADHD). School Psychology Review 20:174–186, 1991

Iannotti RJ: Naturalistic and structured assessments of prosocial behavior in preschool children: the influence of empathy and perspective taking. Dev Psychol 21:46–55, 1985

Johnson SM, Lobitz GK: Parental manipulation of child behavior in home observations. J Appl Behav Anal 7:23–31, 1974

Kazdin AE: Developmental psychopathology. Am Psychol 44:180–187, 1989

Kristjansson EA, Fried PA, Watkinson B: Maternal smoking during pregnancy affects children's vigilance performance. Drug Alcohol Depend 24:11–19, 1989

Lahey BB, Loeber R, Stouthamer-Loeber M, et al: Comparison of DSM-III and DSM-III-R diagnoses for prepubertal children: changes in prevalence and validity. J Am Acad Child Adolesc Psychiatry 29:620–626, 1990

Lahey BB, Pelham WE, Stein MA, et al: Validity of DSM-IV attention-deficit/hyperactivity disorder for younger children. J Am Acad Child Adolesc Psychiatry 37: 695–702, 1998

Laufer MW, Denhoff E, Solomons G: Hyperkinetic impulsive disorder in children's behavior problems. Psychosom Med 19:38–49, 1957

Levy F: The development of sustained attention (vigilance) and inhibition in children: some normative data. J Child Psychol Psychiatry 21:77–84, 1980

Levy F, Hobbes G: The action of stimulant medication in attention deficit disorder with hyperactivity: dopaminergic, noradrenergic, or both? J Am Acad Child Adolesc Psychiatry 27:802–805, 1988

Levy F, Hay D, McStephen M, et al: Attention deficit hyperactivity disorder: a category or a continuum? Genetic analysis of a large-scale twin study. J Am Acad Child Adolesc Psychiatry 36:737–744, 1997

Long P, Forehand R, Wierson M, et al: Does parent training with young noncompliant children have long term effects? Behav Res Ther 32:101–107, 1994

Lou HC, Henriksen L, Bruhn P: Focal cerebral hypoperfusion in children with dysphasia and/or attention deficit disorder. Arch Neurol 41:825–829, 1984

Lou HC, Henriksen L, Bruhn P, et al: Striatal dysfunction in attention deficit and hyperkinetic disorder. Arch Neurol 46:48–52, 1989

Luk S: Direct observation studies of hyperactive behaviors. Journal of the American Academy of Child Psychiatry 24:338–344, 1985

Lyman RD, Hembree-Kigin TL: Conduct and attentional problems, in Mental Health Interventions With Preschool Children. New York, Plenum, 1994, pp 143–161

Mash EJ, Johnston C: A comparison of the mother-child interactions of younger and older hyperactive and normal children. Child Dev 53:1371–1381, 1982

Mash EJ, Johnston C: Parental perceptions of child behavior problems, parenting self-esteem, and mothers' reported stress in younger and older hyperactive and normal children. J Consult Clin Psychol 51:86–99. 1983

Mattes JA: The role of frontal lobe dysfunction in childhood hyperkinesis. Compr Psychiatry 21:358–369, 1980

McBurnett K, Lahey BB, Pfiffner LJ: Diagnosis of attention-deficit disorders in DSM-IV: scientific basis and implications for education. Exceptional Children 60:108–117, 1993

McGee R, Partridge F, Williams S, et al: A twelve-year follow-up of preschool hyperactive children. J Am Acad Child Adolesc Psychiatry 30:224–232, 1991

McGee R, Williams S, Feehan M: Attention deficit disorder and age of onset of problem behaviors. J Abnorm Child Psychol 20:487–501, 1992

Minde K, Webb G, Sykes D: Studies on the hyperactive child, VI: prenatal and perinatal factors associated with hyperactivity. Dev Med Child Neurol 10:355–363, 1968

Musten LM, Firestone P, Pisterman S, et al: Effects of methylphenidate on preschool children with ADHD: cognitive and behavioral functions. J Am Acad Child Adolesc Psychiatry 36:1407–1415, 1997

Newcorn JH, Halperin JM, Healey JM, et al: Are ADDH and ADHD the same or different? J Am Acad Child Adolesc Psychiatry 28:734–738, 1989

O'Connor E, Crowell JA, Sprafkin J: Mother-child interaction in ADHD boys and its relation to secondary symptoms. Paper presented at the biennial meeting of the Society for Research in Child Development, New Orleans, LA, March 1993

Ott J, Eisenstadt TH, Eugrin C, et al: DSM-III-R and DSM-IV criteria for attention deficit disorders: applicability to young children. J Child Psychol Psychiatry (in press)

Palfrey JS, Levine MD, Walker DK, et al: The emergence of attention deficits in early childhood: a prospective study. J Dev Behav Pediatr 6:165–174, 1985

Pasamanick B, Rogers ME, Lillienfeld AM: Pregnancy experience and the development of behavior disorder in children. Am J Psychiatry 112:613–618, 1956

Pauls DL: Genetic factors in the expression of attention deficit hyperactivity disorder. J Child Adolesc Psychopharmacol 1:353–360, 1991

Pelham WE, Bender ME: Peer relationships in hyperactive children: description and treatment, in Advances in Learning and Behavioral Disabilities: A Research Annual, Vol 1. Edited by Gadow KD, Bailer I. Greenwich, CT, JAI Press, 1982, pp 365–436

Pennington BF, Groisser D, Welsh MC: Contrasting cognitive deficits in attention deficit hyperactivity disorder versus reading disability. Dev Psychol 29:511–523, 1993

Pisterman S, McGrath P, Firestone P, et al: Outcome of parent-mediated treatment of preschoolers with attention deficit disorder with hyperactivity. J Consult Clin Psychol 5:628–635, 1989

Pisterman S, Firestone P, McGrath P, et al: The role of parent training in treatment of preschoolers with ADDH. Am J Orthopsychiatry 62:397–407, 1992

Richman SL, Stevenson J, Graham PJ: Preschool to School: A Behavioral Study. London, Academic Press, 1982

Ross DM, Ross SA: Hyperactivity: Current Issues, Research, and Theory, 2nd Edition. New York, Wiley, 1982

Rosvold H, Mirsky A, Sarason I, et al: A continuous performance test of brain damage. Journal of Consulting Psychology 20:343–352, 1956

Ruff HA, Lawson KR, Parrinello R, et al: Long-term stability of individual differences in sustained attention in the early years. Child Dev 61:60–75, 1990

Safer DJ, Krager JM: A survey of medication treatment for hyperactive/inattentive students. JAMA 260:2256–2258, 1988

Satterfield JH, Dawson ME: Electrodermal correlates of hyperactivity in children. Psychophysiology 8:191–197, 1971

Schachar RJ, Tannock R, Logan G: Inhibitory control, impulsiveness, and attention deficit hyperactivity disorder. Clin Psychol Rev 13:721–739, 1993

Schaughency EA, Rothlind J: Assessment and classification of attention deficit hyperactivity disorders. School Psychology Review 20:187–202, 1991

Schleifer M, Weiss G, Cohen N, et al: Hyperactivity in preschoolers and the effect of methylphenidate. Am J Orthopsychiatry 45:38–50, 1975

Shaywitz SE, Shaywitz BA: Increased medication use in attention deficit hyperactivity disorder: regressive or appropriate? JAMA 260:2270–2272, 1988

Sobol MP, Ashbourne DT, Earn BM, et al: Parents' attributions for achieving compliance from attention-deficit-disordered children. J Abnorm Child Psychol 17:359–369, 1989

Sostek AJ, Buchsbaum MS, Rapoport JL: Effects of amphetamine on vigilance performance in normal and hyperactive children. J Abnorm Child Psychol 8:491–500, 1980

Sprich-Buckminster S, Biederman J, Milberger S, et al: Are perinatal complications relevant to the manifestation of ADD? Issues of comorbidity and familiality. J Am Acad Child Adolesc Psychiatry 32:1032–1037, 1993

Sroufe LA, Rutter M: The domain of developmental psychopathology. Child Dev 55:17–29, 1984

Sykes DH, Douglas VI, Morganstern G: The effect of methylphenidate (Ritalin) on sustained attention in hyperactive children. Psychopharmacologia 25:262–274, 1972

Sykes DH, Douglas VI, Weiss G, et al: Attention in hyperactive children and the effect of methylphenidate (Ritalin). J Child Psychol Psychiatry 12:129–139, 1977

Tannock R, Schachar RJ, Carr RP: Effects of methylphenidate on inhibitory control in hyperactive children. J Abnorm Child Psychol 17:473–491, 1989

Tannock R, Purvis KL, Schachar RJ: Narrative abilities in children with attention deficit hyperactivity disorder and normal peers. J Abnorm Child Psychol 21:103–117, 1993

Towbin KE, Leckman JF: Attention deficit hyperactivity disorder, in Rudolph's Pediatrics, 19th Edition. Edited by Rudolph AM. Norwalk, CT, Appleton & Lange, 1991, pp 115–116

Warren RP, Odell JD, Warren LW, et al: Reading disability, attention-deficit hyperactivity disorder and the immune system. Science 268:786–787, 1995

Weinberg WA, Harper CR: Vigilance and its disorders. Behav Neurol 11:59–78, 1993

Weissberg R, Ruff HA, Lawson KR: The usefulness of reaction time tasks in studying attention and organization of behavior in young children. J Dev Behav Pediatr 11:59–64, 1990

Whalen CK, Henker B: The social worlds of hyperactive children. Clin Psychol Rev 5:1–32, 1985

Wilens TE, Biederman J: The stimulants. Psychiatr Clin North Am 15:191–222, 1992

Zahn-Waxler C, Mayfield A, Radke-Yarrow M, et al: A follow-up investigation of offspring of parents with bipolar disorder. Am J Psychiatry 145:506–509, 1988

Zahn-Waxler C, Cole PM, Richardson DT, et al: Social problem solving in disruptive preschool children: reactions to hypothetical situations of conflict and distress. Merrill-Palmer Quarterly 40:98–119, 1994

Zametkin AJ, Nordahl TE, Gross M, et al: Cerebral glucose metabolism in adults with hyperactivity of childhood onset. N Engl J Med 323:1361–1366, 1990

Zentall SS: Production deficiencies in elicited language but not in spontaneous verbalizations of hyperactive children. J Abnorm Child Psychol 16:657–673, 1988

14 Subgroups of Adult Outcome of Attention-Deficit/ Hyperactivity Disorder

Lily Hechtman, M.D., F.R.C.P.

It is interesting to be discussing subgroups of *adult* attention-deficit/hyperactivity disorder (ADHD), because not very long ago ADHD was seen as a disorder of childhood, and symptoms were thought to disappear with onset of puberty (Munoz-Millan and Casteel 1989). More recently, however, follow-up studies have shown that 30%–70% of children with ADHD continue to have symptoms of ADHD in adolescence and adulthood (Gittelman et al. 1985; Mannuzza et al. 1989, 1998; Weiss and Hechtman 1993).

The picture of various adult subgroups of ADHD is drawn from a number of different sources: 1) studies of childhood subgroups, 2) studies of comorbid conditions and their effects on outcome, 3) family studies, 4) adult treatment studies, and 5) long-term follow-up studies.

STUDIES OF CHILDHOOD SUBGROUPS

DSM-III had two diagnostic subgroups of attention deficit disorder: one with and the other without hyperactivity. In DSM-III-R, with the diagnosis of attention-deficit hyperactivity disorder, this distinction was dropped and no differentiation was made between the two subtypes. The DSM-IV diagnosis of ADHD has two symptom groups: hyperactive/impulsive symptoms and inattentive symptoms. Thus, subjects can receive an ADHD diagnosis with symptoms in both groupings (combined type) or with symptoms in only one grouping (e.g., inattentive or hyperactive/impulsive).

Considerable controversy has ensued regarding the importance and distinction of these two subgroups (i.e., with and without hyperactivity). A number of authors (August and Garfinkel 1993; Mauer and Stewart 1980; Rubenstein and Brown 1984) have reported no significant differences between the subtypes of attention-deficit disorder on a number of parameters. However, a greater number of researchers—for example, Barkley et al. (1990a), Edelbrock et al. (1984), King and Young (1982), Lahey et al. (1984, 1987), to name just a few—have demonstrated significant differences in these two groups. Generally, subjects with attention-deficit disorder with hyperactivity are found to be more impulsive, distractible, socially rejected, aggressive, and oppositional, whereas the subjects with attention-deficit disorder without hyperactivity are more sluggish and lethargic, daydream more, and tend to be more shy and anxious.

Some authors (Edelbrock et al. 1984; Lahey et al. 1984) showed that subjects with attention-deficit disorder without hyperactivity had poorer academic achievement than subjects with attention-deficit disorder with hyperactivity. However, Carlson et al. (1986) showed that there was no significant difference between the two groups with respect to academic achievement. Frank and Ben-Nun (1988) suggested that subjects with attention-deficit disorder without hyperactivity have a history of more pre- and perinatal problems than subjects with attention-deficit disorder with hyperactivity. However, Barkley et al. (1990b) found no significant difference between the two groups on this measure. Barkley et al. (1990b) did, however, show that the two groups differed in terms of parental pathology, with attention-deficit disorder subjects with hyperactivity having parents with problems of aggression and substance abuse, and attention-deficit disorder subjects without hyperactivity having parents with more anxiety problems. Frank and Ben-Nun (1988), however, found no differences in parental pathology in the two groups.

Finally, with regard to medication response, Barkley et al. (1991) found the subjects with attention-deficit disorder without hyperactivity more often to be nonresponders to methylphenidate than were the subjects with attention-deficit disorder with hyperactivity, and when they did respond they did best on lower dosages when compared with the hyperactive subjects. Pliszka (1989) also found the subjects with attention-deficit disorder without hyperactivity, as a group, to be more anxious and to respond less well to stimulants.

We thus see that these two childhood subgroups present different clinical pictures, different family pictures, and different response to medication treatment. It is therefore very likely that in adulthood they will constitute different subgroups with different outcomes. Later in life, as adults, children with attention-deficit disorder with hyperactivity will probably have more antisocial problems, whereas children with attention-deficit disorder without hyperactivity will have more internalization problems, with continuity of anxiety and possibly depression.

COMORBIDITY STUDIES

It is clear that if ADHD is comorbid with various other conditions, the particular combinations of ADHD and these comorbid conditions will constitute particular subgroups, both in childhood and in adulthood. Evidence that ADHD is often comorbid with various other psychiatric disorders comes from two types of studies; epidemiological studies in New Zealand (Anderson et al. 1987), Puerto Rico (Bird et al. 1988), and Canada (Szatmari et al. 1989); and clinical studies (August and Garfinkel 1989; Biederman et al. 1991; Munir et al. 1987; Pliszka 1989). Although rates vary considerably in different studies, generally the authors found that the rates of comorbidity of ADHD with other psychiatric disorders are as follows: ADHD and conduct disorder, 30–50%; ADHD and oppositional defiant disorder, 35%–60%; ADHD and anxiety disorder, 20%–30%; ADHD and mood disorder (depression), 20%–30%; and ADHD and specific learning disabilities, 20%–30%.

It should be noted that 20% of ADHD subjects may have two or more comorbid conditions (Biederman et al. 1992). Furthermore, one needs also to keep in mind that, as Biederman et al. (1992) have pointed out, close to 50% of ADHD children do *not* have comorbid conditions.

The number, type, and particular combination of comorbid conditions have significant implications for etiology (Biederman et al. 1987; Szatmari et al. 1989), course (Gittelman et al. 1985; Weiss et al. 1985), and treatment (Barkley et al. 1991; Pliszka 1989).

Some subgroups of subjects with comorbid disorders have been extensively studied and have been shown to be particularly vulnerable (Table 14–1). Thus, subjects with ADHD and comorbid oppositional defiant disorder or conduct disorder have been found at follow-up to more often still have ADHD (August et al. 1983; Barkley et al. 1990b; Mannuzza et al. 1998; Moffitt 1990) and significant antisocial pathology (August et al. 1983; Barkley et al. 1990b; Farrington 1990; Mannuzza et al. 1998; Moffitt 1990). This subgroup also has more drug and alcohol use (August et al. 1983; Barkley et al. 1990b), more parental and family pathology (Barkley et al. 1990b; Lahey et al. 1988; Moffitt 1990), and more academic underachievement (Hinshaw 1992; Moffitt 1990).

Table 14–1. Vulnerabilities in outcome for subjects with ADHD and comorbid oppositional defiant disorder or conduct disorder

Vulnerability at follow-up	Reference(s)
More still having ADHD	August et al. 1983; Barkley et al. 1990b; Mannuzza et al. 1998; Moffitt 1990
More still exhibiting antisocial behavior	August et al. 1983; Barkley et al. 1990b; Farrington 1990; Mannuzza et al. 1998; Moffitt 1990
More drug and alcohol use	August et al. 1983; Barkley et al. 1990b
More family pathology	Barkley et al. 1990b; Lahey et al. 1988; Moffitt 1990
More academic underachievement	Hinshaw 1992; Moffitt 1990

The group of subjects with ADHD and comorbid oppositional defiant disorder or conduct disorder most probably corresponds to the negative adult outcome group reported by Hechtman et al. (Hechtman and Weiss 1988; Hechtman et al. 1981, 1984a, 1984b), Gittelman et al. (1985), Mannuzza et al. (1989), and Loney et al. (1983). The individuals in this subgroup continue to have significant antisocial and psychiatric problems in adulthood.

Another subgroup of comorbidity that has received some attention is that of ADHD and learning disorder. Subjects with this comorbidity again show more delinquency, poorer self-esteem, and greater academic underachievement than do groups of subjects with learning disability (Ackerman et al. 1977) or ADHD only. This subgroup may constitute a lower academic and work status group in adulthood, and the individuals in this group may be more prone to anxiety and depression.

There has been relatively little research on other comorbidities with ADHD—for example, that with anxiety and depression—in childhood and adulthood. There also appears to be some controversy about the comorbid prevalence of mood disorders (anxiety and depression) in children and adults with ADHD. Biederman et al. (1992) suggested that 20%–30% of subjects with ADHD have comorbid anxiety and depression and that 20%–30% of the relatives of ADHD children also have affective disorders. However, prospective longitudinal studies by Weiss and Hechtman (1993), Gittelman et al. (1985), and Mannuzza et al. (1989, 1998) have found few subjects with affective disorders. Gittelman et al. (1985) suggested that relatives and parents of ADHD children may have skewed memories when interviewed shortly after their child is diagnosed with ADHD. In any event, this remains an area requiring more careful research.

Biederman et al. (1996) reported very high rates (11%–21%) of comorbid bipolar disorder in children with ADHD. This report has met with a great deal of controversy, because no other researchers have confirmed this finding. In a review of juvenile onset of bipolar disorder, Hechtman and Greenfield (1997) tried to explain this discrepancy. The high rate of comorbidity may be an artifact of the fact that the four ADHD symptoms required by DSM-IV for diagnosis are similar to the symptoms required for mania (i.e., increased talkativeness, distractibility, increased goal-directed activity, and excessive involvement in pleasurable activities with high potential for painful consequences). Given that these four symptoms, coupled with irritable mood, can give a child the diagnosis of mania, one can readily see how a high rate of comorbidity of ADHD with bipolar disorder can appear. This diagnostic overlap is clearly a weakness of DSM-IV and does not necessarily reflect high comorbidity of ADHD and bipolar disorder. Clearly, children with ADHD and comorbid bipolar disorder would have significant problems in adulthood secondary to their bipolar condition, with possible repeated breakdowns and hospitalizations.

FAMILY STUDIES

There is a presupposition that by examining adult relatives of children with ADHD, one gets some view of the adult outcome of this condition. Some of these family studies were comprehensively reviewed by Weiss and Hechtman (1993) in the context of their discussion of families of hyperactive children. Early family studies by Morrison and Stewart (Morrison 1980; Morrison and Stewart 1971, 1973), Stewart and Morrison (1973), and Cantwell (1972) suggested that biological parents of hyperactive children had higher rates of sociopathy (antisocial behavior or antisocial personality disorder, alcoholism, and hysteria). Stewart and Morrison (1973) also reported higher incidence of unipolar, but not bipolar, affective disorders in second-degree relatives of hyperactive children as a group.

Early studies did not focus on comorbid conditions in hyperactive children. Recent work suggests, however, that children with ADHD and different comorbid conditions may have significantly different family patterns than children with only ADHD. Thus, Biederman et al. (1987) showed that families of hyperactive children with conduct or oppositional disorder had significantly higher rates of antisocial disorder, oppositional disorder, antisocial personality disorder, nonbipolar depressive disorder, and overanxious disorder compared with relatives of psychiatrically healthy control subjects and hyperactive children without coexisting conduct or oppositional disorder. The rates of ADHD did not differ in relatives of children with ADHD alone, ADHD without conduct disorder, and ADHD without oppositional disorder, with the rates being high (34%) in all three groups. There were no differences in the rates of drug or alcohol abuse or dependence in the three groups. Lahey et al. (1988) and Barkley et al. (1990b) also found higher rates of parental pathology in parents of hyperactive children with conduct disorder. This pathology included antisocial personality disorder and antisocial behavior, particularly among the fathers.

We see, then, that relatives of hyperactive children may be categorized into various subgroups: those with little or no pathology (these are usually relatives of ADHD children with no other comorbid conditions) (10%–20%); those with antisocial or drug substance abuse symptoms (30%–40%) (of these relatives, 20%–34% may also have continuing ADHD symptoms); and, finally, those with affective disorders (depression and anxiety) (20%–30%). There is obviously overlap in these subgroupings, because family members can have both antisocial and affective symptoms. However, this broad outline provides some subgroupings of possible adult pathology in this familial condition.

TREATMENT STUDIES OF ADULT ADHD PATIENTS

A number of authors (Gualtieri et al. 1985; Mattes et al. 1984; Wender et al. 1981; Wood et al. 1976) have described studies in which they identified and treated adults with ADHD symptoms. However, the clinical picture and treatment results suggest that the patient populations in these studies were quite different. Wood et al. and Wender et al. treated an outpatient, clinic, and/or community sample of patients who responded fairly well to stimulants with little additional treatment. Mattes et al., however, treated a veterans' hospital outpatient population. The patients seemed to have comorbid conditions such as affective disorders and substance abuse disorders, and the treatment efficacy was thus limited.

Adult treatment studies suggest at least two subgroups: a less disturbed group of individuals with less comorbidity who are more responsive to stimulant treatment (Wender et al. 1981; Wood et al. 1976) and a more disturbed group of individuals with more comorbidity who are less responsive to such treatment (Mattes et al. 1984).

LONG-TERM FOLLOW-UP STUDIES

Adolescent Follow-Up

Follow-up studies of children with ADHD into adolescence (Barkley et al. 1990b; Cantwell and Baker 1989; Gittelman et al. 1985; Satterfield et al. 1982; Weiss et al. 1971) have identified three subgroups:

- Subjects with few problems. This is a small subgroup, accounting for 10%–20% of ADHD subjects.
- Subjects who continue to have symptoms of the syndrome, along with social, academic, and emotional problems. Most ADHD subjects (about 70%) fall into this group.
- Subjects with antisocial behavior, as well as continuing symptoms of the syndrome. This subgroup accounts for about 25% of ADHD subjects.

Lambert et al. (1987) followed children with ADHD into adolescence and identified three groups:

- Subjects with no problems (20%). This group is characterized by cognitive and behavioral maturity.
- Subjects with persistent learning, behavioral, or emotional problems who are no longer on medication (37%). This group is characterized by cognitive immaturity but behavioral maturity.
- Subjects with hyperactivity and learning, behavioral, and emotional difficulties who are still being treated for ADHD (43%). This group is characterized by cognitive and behavioral immaturity.

Controlled Prospective Follow-Up

For several reasons, the controlled prospective follow-up study provides the clearest, most reliable picture of adult outcome of ADHD. First, the diagnosis is made in childhood by directly assessing the child and obtaining information from parents and teachers. Second, the hyperactive subjects and, generally, a matched control group are followed and periodically reassessed with standardized measures. Thus, prospective studies are not limited by sketchy old charts (as in, e.g., retrospective studies) or selective patient and parental memories (as in, e.g., adult patient or family studies). In addition, adults who are well but who were affected in childhood are also seen, and this provides a more comprehensive and less negatively biased picture. Unfortunately, to date, few controlled prospective follow-up studies have followed hyperactive subjects into adulthood, and these have all followed only individuals whose ADHD symptoms included hyperactivity in childhood.

Gittelman et al. (1985) conducted a comprehensive prospective study of 101 hyperactive individuals and 100 matched control subjects. The mean ages at the first and second follow-ups were 18 years and 26 years, respectively (Mannuzza et al. 1998). The subjects could be generally divided into three outcome groups.

- Subjects with a fairly normal outcome and with no significant disabling problems.
- Subjects with continuing problems with symptoms of the syndrome and with general social, emotional, and work difficulties.
- Subjects with significant problems. Antisocial behavior was reported in 27% at age 18 and 18% at age 26. Drug use disorder was reported in 16% at age 18 and 16% at age 26. Multiple arrests were reported in 23%, and 9% had been incarcerated by age 18.

These negative outcomes were often linked to continuity and persistence of ADHD symptoms. The combination of continuing ADHD symptoms, antisocial personality disorder, and substance abuse tended to congregate in the same individuals.

Weiss and Hechtman (1993) carried out a controlled prospective follow-up study of 103 children who were initially assessed at 6–12 years of age. Ninety-one were reassessed at 5-year follow-up (mean age = 13.3 years), 75 were seen again at 10-year follow-up (mean age = 19 years), and 64 were seen at 15-year follow-up (mean age = 25). In adolescence, a control group matching the hyperactive children in age, sex, IQ, and socioeconomic status was selected and followed with the hyperactive group. Half the subjects lost to follow-up could not be traced and probably constituted a somewhat negative outcome group. The other half, when contacted by telephone, described in detail that they were doing well but explained that they did not wish to come in to be reevaluated and be reminded of past problems. These subjects reflected a more positive outcome group. The comprehensive assessments included demographic, academic, occupational, psychiatric, psychological, social (including antisocial behavior and drug and alcohol abuse), and physiological parameters. Data were obtained from direct interviews with subjects and parents and via reports from schools, employers, and the court system.

Three outcome groups (mean age = 19–25 years) could again be identified (Weiss et al. 1978, 1985):

- Subjects with fairly normal outcome (30%–40%)
- Subjects with continuing symptoms of the syndrome (50%–60%)
- Subjects with severe problems, involving psychiatric disturbance (10%) and/or antisocial disturbance (10%)

The first group comprises individuals who function fairly well and are not significantly differently from a matched normal control group. The second group is composed of adults who continue to have significant concentration, social, emotional, and impulsive problems. These symptoms often result in difficulties with work, interpersonal relationships, poor self-esteem, impulsivity, irritability, anxiety, and emotional lability. The vast majority of young hyperactive adults fall into this group. Finally, the third group comprises hyperactive adults with significant psychiatric and/or antisocial pathology. These adults may be seriously depressed, even suicidal, and heavily involved in drug/alcohol abuse. They may exhibit significant antisocial behavior (e.g., assault, armed robbery, breaking and entering, or drug dealing). This negative adult outcome is seen in a relatively small proportion of hyperactive children.

Herrero et al. (1994) looked at individual pathways of antisocial outcome in hyperactive adults by tracing antisocial problems at each developmental stage. The authors discovered four fairly distinct groupings with regard to pathways of antisocial outcome.

- Subjects who never presented with any antisocial behavior or antisocial personality disorder (26%)
- Subjects who presented with antisocial behavior or antisocial personality disorder at 15-year follow-up and previously (30%)
- Subjects who presented with behavioral problems or antisocial problems at initial intake but not at 5-, 10-, or 15-year follow-ups (18%)
- Subjects who did not present with antisocial behavior at 15-year follow-up but had a history of antisocial behavior or behavioral problems, either initially or at 5- or 10-year follow-up (26%)

It appears that boys are at greater risk for antisocial outcome than are girls. All the girls in the sample (n = 5) were in the first group (i.e., never presented with antisocial behavior).

The absence of behavioral problems at initial intake is predictive of the absence of antisocial disorders in adulthood. However, the presence of such problems at intake is not predictive of an antisocial outcome. It appears that in aggressive hyperactive children with behavioral problems, the mental health of family members and a positive emotional climate at home may be protective factors against later antisocial outcome (e.g., group 3).

As with groupings from other follow-up studies, three subgroups may be distinguished: subjects with fairly normal outcome, subjects with some cognitive and behavioral disturbance, and subjects with significant antisocial behavior.

FACTORS INFLUENCING ADULT OUTCOME

One can well ask what factors determine or influence adult outcome of ADHD. Some of these factors are related to the initial characteristics of the patients themselves (Table 14–2). For example, Herrero et al. (1994) clearly showed that hyperactive boys and girls have different risks for antisocial outcome. Similarly, Mannuzza and Gittelman (1984) did not find the expected risk of more negative outcome in the hyperactive girls they followed. Again, their sample, like ours, was relatively small ($N = 12$). However, boys appear to be at greater risk than girls for negative outcome.

Initial subtype of attention-deficit disorder—that is, with or without hyperactivity—may also predict different outcomes, with the hyperactive group having more long-term conduct and antisocial problems, and the group without hyperactivity having more learning disorders and affective difficulties, particularly anxiety disorders.

Other initial symptoms also appear to predict later outcome. Noteworthy among these is aggression, which was first shown by Loney et al. (1983) to be associated with negative outcome. Hechtman et al. (1984a) showed that emotional lability, which was highly correlated with aggression, was also predictive of adult outcome. Most recently, Fischer et al. (1993) showed that childhood defiance was predictive of later arrests. IQ was found to be an important predictor of outcome, particularly for academic achievement (Hechtman et al. 1984a) and drug and alcohol abuse (Loney et al. 1983).

It is also clear that outcome is significantly affected by various comorbid conditions. Specifically, comorbid conduct and oppositional defiant disorder seem to result in more negative outcome, particularly adult antisocial behavior and antisocial personality disorder (August et al. 1983; Barkley et al. 1990b; Gittelman et al. 1985). Comorbid learning disability with associated poor academic performance also increases the risk for more negative outcome (Ackerman et al. 1977; Moffitt 1990).

Many studies have shown that parental psychopathology can contribute to more negative adult outcome (Hechtman et al. 1984a; Offord et al. 1992),

Table 14–2. Factors influencing adult outcome of ADHD

Initial patient characteristic	Reference(s)
Sex (males vs. females)	Herrero et al. 1994; Mannuzza and Gittelman 1984
ADHD vs. ADD	
Other symptoms	
Aggression	Loney et al. 1983
Emotional lability	Hechtman et al. 1984a
Defiance	Fischer et al. 1993
IQ	Hechtman et al. 1984a; Loney et al. 1983
Comorbidity	Ackerman et al. 1977; Moffitt 1990
Conduct and oppositional defiant disorders	
Anxiety	
Depression	
Learning disability	
Parental pathology	Fischer et al. 1993; Hechtman et al. 1984a; Herrero et al. 1994; Offord 1992
SES	Cadoret and Stewart 1991; Hechtman et al. 1984a; Offord et al. 1992

Note. ADD = attention-deficit disorder; ADHD = attention-deficit/hyperactivity disorder; SES = socioeconomic status.

while parental mental health can effect a more positive outcome (Fischer et al. 1993; Herrero et al. 1994).

Finally, socioeconomic status may also influence adult outcome of ADHD. There is considerable risk for more negative outcome associated with lower socioeconomic status (Cadoret and Stewart 1991; Hechtman et al. 1984a; Offord et al. 1992).

CONCLUSION

The review of studies in this chapter suggests that at least three distinct adult outcome subgroups for children with ADHD can be identified: 1) subjects with few problems; 2) subjects who continue to have symptoms of the syndrome and associated social, emotional, and work problems (many hyperactive adults fall into this subgroup); and 3) subjects with significant antisocial and/or psychiatric pathology (a relatively small proportion of the hyperactive adult population).

Various factors influence membership in these various subgroups—for example, initial characteristics of the subjects such as sex, IQ, type of attention-deficit disorder (i.e., with or without hyperactivity), and particular symptoms such as aggression and defiance. In addition, the presence of various comorbid conditions also affects outcome, with comorbid conduct and oppositional defiant disorders, in particular, effecting negative outcome. Parental psychopathology and socioeconomic status also influence adult outcome of childhood ADHD.

We are left with the important challenge of developing more effective prevention and treatment interventions that will decrease the risk factors outlined in this chapter and result in more positive long-term outcome in adulthood. Such interventions are currently being explored.

REFERENCES

Ackerman PT, Dykman RA, Peters JE: Teenage status of hyperactive and nonhyperactive learning disabled boys. Am J Orthopsychiatry 47:577–596, 1977

Anderson JC, Williams S, McGee R, et al: DSM-III disorders in preadolescent children: prevalence in a large sample from the general population. Arch Gen Psychiatry 44:69–76, 1987

August GJ, Garfinkel BD: Behavioral and cognitive subtypes of ADHD. J Am Acad Child Adolesc Psychiatry 28:739–748, 1989

August GJ, Garfinkel BD: The nosology of attention-deficit hyperactivity disorder. J Am Acad Child Adolesc Psychiatry 32:155–165, 1993

August GJ, Steward MA, Holmes CS: A four year follow-up of hyperactive boys with and without conduct disorder. Br J Psychiatry 143:192–198, 1983

Barkley RA, DuPaul GJ, McMurray MB: Comprehensive evaluation of attention deficit disorder with and without hyperactivity as defined by research criteria. J Consult Clin Psychol 58:775–789, 1990a

Barkley RA, Fischer M, Edelbrock CS, et al: The adolescent outcome of hyperactive children diagnosed by research criteria, I: an 8-year prospective follow-up study. J Am Acad Child Adolesc Psychiatry 29:546–557, 1990b

Barkley RA, DuPaul GJ, McMurray MB: Attention deficit disorder with and without hyperactivity: clinical response to three dose levels of methylphenidate. Pediatrics 87:519–531, 1991

Biederman J, Munir K, Knee D: Conduct and oppositional disorders in clinically referred children with attention deficit disorder: a controlled family study. J Am Acad Child Adolesc Psychiatry 26:724–727, 1987

Biederman J, Newcorn J, Sprich SE: Comorbidity of attention-deficit hyperactivity disorder with conduct, depressive, anxiety, and other disorders. Am J Psychiatry 148:564–577, 1991

Biederman J, Faraone SV, Lapey K: Comorbidity of diagnosis in attention deficit hyperactivity disorder. Child Adolesc Psychiatr Clin N Am 2:335–361, 1992

Biederman J, Faraone S, Mick E, et al: Attention deficit hyperactivity disorder and juvenile mania: an overlooked comorbidity? J Am Acad Child Adolesc Psychiatry 35:997–1008, 1996

Bird HR, Canino G, Rubio-Stipec M, et al: Estimates of the prevalence of childhood maladjustment in a community survey in Puerto Rico: The use of combined measures. Arch Gen Psychiatry 45:1120–1126, 1988

Cadoret RJ, Stewart MA: An adoption study of attention deficit/hyperactivity/aggression and their relationship to adult antisocial personality. Compr Psychiatry 32: 73–82, 1991

Cantwell DP: Psychiatric illness in families of hyperactive children. Arch Gen Psychiatry 27:414–417, 1972

Cantwell DP, Baker L: Stability and natural history of DSM-III childhood diagnoses. J Am Acad Child Adolesc Psychiatry 28:691–700, 1989

Carlson CL, Lahey BB, Neeper R: Direct assessment of the cognitive correlates of attention deficit disorder with and without hyperactivity. Journal of Behavior Assessment and Psychopathology 8:69–86, 1986

Edelbrock CS, Costello A, Kessler MD: Empirical corroboration of attention deficit disorder. Journal of the American Academy of Child Psychiatry 23:285–290, 1984

Farrington DP: Long-term criminal outcomes of hyperactivity-impulsivity-attention deficit (HIA) and conduct problems in childhood, in The Straight and Devious Pathways From Childhood to Adulthood. Edited by Robins LN, Rutter M. New York, Cambridge University Press, 1990

Fischer M, Barkley RA, Fletcher KE, et al: The adolescent outcome of hyperactive children: predictors of psychiatric, academic, social, and emotional adjustment. J Am Acad Child Adolesc Psychiatry 32:324–332, 1993

Frank Y, Ben-Nun Y: Toward a clinical subgrouping of hyperactive and nonhyperactive attention deficit disorder: results of a comprehensive neurological and neuropsychological assessment. Am J Dis Child 142:153–155, 1988

Gualtieri CT, Ondrusek MG, Finley C: Attention deficit disorders in adults. Clin Neuropharmacol 8:343–356, 1985

Gittelman R, Mannuzza S, Shenker R, et al: Hyperactive boys almost grown-up, I: psychiatric status. Arch Gen Psychiatry 42:937–947, 1985

Gittelman-Klein R: Prognosis of attention deficit disorder and its management. Adolescence Pediatrics in Review 8:216–223, 1987

Hechtman L, Greenfield B: Juvenile onset bipolar disorder. Curr Opin Pediatr 9:346–353, 1997

Hechtman L, Weiss G: Controlled prospective 15-year follow-up of hyperactives as adults: non-medical drug and alcohol use and antisocial behaviour. Can J Psychiatry 31:557–567, 1988

Hechtman L, Weiss G, Perlman T, et al: Hyperactives as young adults: various clinical outcomes. Adolesc Psychiatry 9:295–306, 1981

Hechtman L, Weiss G, Perlman T, et al: Hyperactives as young adults: initial predictors of adult outcome. Journal of the American Academy of Child Psychiatry 25:250–260, 1984a

Hechtman L, Weiss G, Perlman T: Hyperactives as young adults: past and current antisocial behavior (stealing, drug abuse) and moral development. Am J Orthopsychiatry 54:415–425, 1984b

Herrero ME, Hechtman L, Weiss G: Antisocial disorders in hyperactive subjects from childhood to adulthood: predictive factors and characterization of subgroups. Am J Orthopsychiatry 64:510–521, 1994

Hinshaw SP: Academic underachievement, attention deficit and aggression: comorbidity and implications for intervention. J Consult Clin Psychol 60:893–903, 1992

King C, Young R: Attention deficit with and without hyperactivity: teacher and peer perceptions. J Abnorm Child Psychol 10:463–496, 1982

Lahey BB, Schaughency E, Strauss CC, et al: Are attention deficit disorders with and without hyperactivity similar or dissimilar disorders? Journal of the American Academy of Child Psychiatry 23:302–309, 1984

Lahey BB, Shaughnecy EA, Hynd GW, et al: Attention deficit disorder with and without hyperactivity: comparison of behavior characteristics of clinic referred children. J Am Acad Child Adolesc Psychiatry 26:718–723, 1987

Lahey BB, Piacentini JC, McBurnett K, et al: Psychopathology in the parents of children with conduct disorder and hyperactivity. J Am Acad Child Adolesc Psychiatry 27:163–170, 1988

Lambert NM, Hartsough CS, Sassone D, et al: Persistence of hyperactivity symptoms from childhood to adolescence and associated outcomes. Am J Orthopsychiatry 57:22–32, 1987

Loney J, Whaley-Klahn MA, Kosier T, et al: Hyperactive boys and their brothers at 21: predictors of aggressive and antisocial outcomes, in Prospective Studies of Crime and Delinquency. Edited by Van Dusen KT, Mednick SA. Boston, MA, Kluwer-Nijhoff, 1983, pp 181–206

Mannuzza S, Gittelman R: The adolescent outcome of hyperactive girls. Psychiatry Res 113:19–29, 1984

Mannuzza S, Gittelman-Klein R, Horowitz-Konig P, et al: Hyperactive boys almost grown-up, IV: criminality and its relationship to psychiatric status. Arch Gen Psychiatry 46:1073–1079, 1989

Mannuzza S, Klein RG, Bessler A, et al: Adult psychiatric status of hyperactive boys grown up. Am J Psychiatry 155:493–498, 1998

Mattes J, Boswell L, Oliver H: Methylphenidate effects on symptoms of attention deficit disorder in adults. Arch Gen Psychiatry 41:1059–1063, 1984

Mauer RG, Stewart M: Attention deficit disorder without hyperactivity in a child psychiatry clinic. J Clin Psychiatry 41:232–233, 1980

Moffitt TE: Juvenile delinquency and attention deficit disorder: boys' developmental trajectories from age 3 to age 15. Child Dev 61:893–910, 1990

Morrison JR: Adult psychiatric disorders in parents of hyperactive children. Am J Psychiatry 137:825–827, 1980

Morrison JR, Stewart MA: A family study of the hyperactive child syndrome. Biol Psychiatry 3:189–195, 1971

Morrison JR, Stewart MA: The psychiatric status of legal families of adopted hyperactives. Arch Gen Psychiatry 28:888–891, 1973

Munir K, Biederman J, Knee D: Psychiatric comorbidity in patients with attention deficit disorder: a controlled study. J Am Acad Child Adolesc Psychiatry 26:844–848, 1987

Munoz-Millan RJ, Casteel CR: Attention-deficit hyperactivity disorder: recent literature. Hospital and Community Psychiatry 40:699–707, 1989

Offord D, Boyle M, Racine Y, et al: Outcome, prognosis and risk in a longitudinal follow-up study. J Am Acad Child Adolesc Psychiatry 31:5:916–926, 1992

Pliszka SR: Effect of anxiety on cognition, behavior, and stimulant response in ADHD. J Am Acad Child Adolesc Psychiatry 28:882–887, 1989

Rubenstein RA, Brown RT: An evaluation of the validity of the diagnostic category of attention deficit disorder. Am J Orthopsychiatry 54:398–414, 1984

Satterfield JH, Hoppe CM, Schell AM: A prospective study of delinquency in 110 adolescent boys with attention deficit disorder and 88 normal adolescent boys. Am J Psychiatry 139:795–798, 1982

Stewart MA, Morrison JR: Affective disorder among the relatives of hyperactive children. J Child Psychol Psychiatry 14:209–212, 1973

Szatmari P, Offord DR, Boyle MH: Ontario Child Health Study: prevalence of attention deficit disorder with hyperactivity. J Child Psychol Psychiatry 30:219–230, 1989

Weiss G, Hechtman L: Hyperactive Children Grown Up, 2nd Edition. New York, Guilford, 1993

Weiss G, Minde K, Werry J, et al: A five-year follow-up study of 91 hyperactive school children. Arch Gen Psychiatry 24:409–414, 1971

Weiss G, Hechtman L, Perlman T: Hyperactives as young adults: school, employers and self-rating scales obtained during 10-year follow-up evaluation. Am J Orthopsychiatry 48:438–445, 1978

Weiss G, Hechtman L, Milroy T, et al: Psychiatric studies of hyperactives as adults: a controlled prospective 15-year follow-up of 63 hyperactive children. Journal of the American Academy of Child Psychiatry 23:211–220, 1985

Wender PH, Reimherr FW, Wood DR: Attention deficit disorder ('minimal brain dysfunction') in adults: a replication study of diagnosis and drug treatment. Arch Gen Psychiatry 38:449–456, 1981

Wood DR, Reimherr FW, Wender PH, et al: Diagnosis and treatment of minimal brain dysfunction in adults: a preliminary report. Arch Gen Psychiatry 33:1453–1460, 1976

Assessment and Interventions for Attention-Deficit Disorders

15 Assessment of Attention-Deficit/Hyperactivity Disorder and Comorbidities

Donald M. Quinlan, Ph.D.

The diagnosis of attention-deficit/hyperactivity disorder (ADHD) is a clinical process—one in which the clinician weighs what the patient says about the symptoms, what teachers, parents, or spouse observes about the patient, what the clinician observes in the course of the evaluation of the patient, and what can be obtained from other sources such as school records and employment evaluations. In addition, the clinician uses structured information-gathering tools, including tests of cognitive functions covering a range of skills, abilities, and other functions.

ADHD presents a particular challenge to a clinician because, by the nature of the condition, patients frequently do not observe many of their symptoms or are not able to gauge the degree of impairment. In the diagnostic process, the clinician must judge whether the level of a particular process creates enough difficulty for the patient that it reaches the status of a "symptom," and whether the configuration of symptoms constitutes ADHD per se or another disorder. In assessing memory, for example, the clinician needs to keep in mind that almost everyone will have a less-than-perfect memory. To constitute a symptom, the memory impairment must be of such a degree that the patient's adaptation is impaired. In judging whether a particular symptom reaches a level that constitutes an "impairment," the clinician can be assisted by information from independent sources. Typically, other sources of observations include parents, teachers, or spouse. The clinician may interview these observers about the patient's behavior to assess the symptoms and degree of impairment. Added to this information is the clinician's own observation of the patient in the interview process.

The clinical interview is the core of any evaluation. In assessing ADHD, the clinician needs to explore the presenting symptoms; history of those symptoms; academic, social, and developmental history; current functioning in a variety of settings; current mental status; and presence of other disorders that may be either the principal underlying disorder or a comorbid disorder that affects the patient. With children and adolescents, the evaluation process goes beyond the patient to include one or both parents and, often, information from school. In adults, the sources of information similarly may need to be broadened to include spouse, parents, siblings, and, at times, friends, coworkers, and employers.

PSYCHOLOGICAL TESTING IN THE EVALUATION OF ADHD

Psychological testing is a valuable supplement that can provide critical information contributing to diagnosis and also to assessment of the extent and degree of the effects of the disorder on functioning. Psychological testing expands the types of data and changes the method of observing the patient to allow the gathering of more extensive data, with clear norms and known reliability. The clinician can make use of a wide variety of procedures and standardized checklists, interviews, and psychometric tests that can make the inquiry more efficient and more systematic and that involve measuring behavior in areas not readily observed or quantified by the patient, significant other, or clinician.

In this chapter I review some of the procedures for extending the range of assessment strategies and discuss the strengths and weaknesses of various approaches in the assessment of ADHD. Approaches to enhancing the information available from a clinical interview include checklists of symptoms, structured and semistructured interviews, and standardized cognitive tests, including ability testing, specialized tests of attention and concentration, and other tests derived from those used for neuropsychological assessment.

From the beginning, it must be emphasized that the diagnosis of ADHD is made by the clinician, who must gather and weigh information from many different sources and combine data from different areas of functioning to gauge the presence and severity of the disorder. The tools of psychological testing described here are designed to help the process of clinical judgment, not to replace it.

DIAGNOSIS OF ADHD

The diagnosis of ADHD follows the guidelines in DSM-IV (American Psychiatric Association 1994). Two clusters of ADHD symptoms are defined: symptoms of inattention and symptoms of hyperactivity–impulsivity. Within each DSM-IV cluster, nine criterion symptoms are listed for evaluation by the clinician. For the diagnosis to warrant further consideration, six of nine criterion symptoms within either or both (i.e., six each under both clusters) must be reported at the level that they constitute a significant problem. For the diagnosis, additional criteria must be met, including emergence of clinically significant impairment at an early age, effects of the disorder on the individual in more than one sphere of activity, and the requirement that the symptoms must not be attributable to other diagnoses. One of three diagnoses can be given: predominantly inattentive type (code 314.00), predominantly hyperactive/impulsive type (code 314.01), or combined type (also code 314.01). Another category (designated by code 314.9), that of ADHD not otherwise specified, can be used for diagnosing conditions with prominent symptoms that do not meet the strict criteria for ADHD.

These criteria mark a departure from DSM-III-R in that the predominantly inattentive type is fully defined. This change in the diagnostic criteria reflects the research into the disorder that occurred between the time of DSM-III-R (American Psychiatric Association 1987) and DSM-IV. Addition of the predominantly inattentive type brings new importance to the assessment of impairments in attention, concentration, memory, and organization. These symptoms are most readily observable by the patient, but it is not unusual to find patients who are unaware of their difficulties in these areas.

The process of diagnosis involves, but is not limited to, inquiry about whether the symptoms and other criteria are met. This process can be accomplished by asking not only the patient but also his or her parents, teachers, or spouse. With psychological checklists and tests, areas of reported and unreported impairment are assessed in other ways, with different tools for documenting the state of the patient and with different potential for biases and different sources of error. When the information from interview, observation, and testing converges, the process is simpler and more certain. When there are disagreements, the clinician must weigh the reports, observations of the patient, and the test data to tease out the underlying picture. Defenses, compensations, adaptations, and maladaptive behaviors that may arise in coping with the disorder, and the other strengths and weaknesses, all must be considered. Checklists are useful in eliciting systematic observations from patients and those around them. Psychological tests can be important supplements to the interview process because they are less vulnerable to reporting biases of the patient and significant others.

LIMITATIONS OF SELF-REPORT

One of the obstacles in assessing a patient for symptoms of ADHD is that the individual may not be a good observer of his or her own behavior (see, e.g., Wender 1987). In answering a question about a problem or symptom, it is necessary for the patient both to observe the behavior in question and to compare it with what is typical or "normal." Obstacles can emerge when a patient is not inclined to observe or think about his or her own behavior, dismisses difficulties as "normal" behavior, or, in the opposite direction, is hypervigilant to the slightest departure from optimal. Biases in reporting symptoms can both minimize and exaggerate the presence of a symptom and the degree of impairment. It is not uncommon to interview a patient who reports a minimal set of symptoms and then to interview a parent or spouse and get a much more detailed list of problems and a picture of a much more severe disorder.

When the sources of information disagree, the clinician's judgment is critical in weighing the differing perspectives. The parents may report multiple problems (e.g., focusing on or organizing for schoolwork), and yet the teachers working with the patient do not observe many of the signs. Some children have been observed to disguise their difficulties in school by maintaining eye contact, answering questions frequently to maintain their focus, and avoiding as much as possible school situations that bring out their underlying difficulties. Another type of situation can arise when teachers report to parents that their child is daydreaming, is working below potential, and does not bring in homework, but the parents, who may experience ADHD themselves, do not notice these problems or minimize or rationalize what they do see (Biggs 1995). Although many such differences of perspective arise, it is not uncommon to observe an adolescent in a tense relationship with his or her parents deny any difficulties in attending or focusing when the parents report a high degree of dysfunction; however, we have on occasion seen a reasonably well functioning adolescent brought in for evaluation for failure to meet parents' unreasonably high expectations or ambitions.

Using informants other than the patient for reporting symptoms is not without problems. Asking anyone, whether patient or relative, to make a judgment of the seriousness of a given symptom requires the person to respond in terms of his or her own "scale" for severity of a problem. Highly anxious parents, for example, may find that any but the most academically serious child is "working below potential." A teacher with many students presenting multiple behavior and emotional problems may overlook a daydreaming child who behaves well in school, even though the child may be thinking excessively of things that have nothing to do with the work of the classroom.

Self-report and observers' reports are limited by problems of reporting bias. These biases require the clinician to gauge the reporting accuracy of the source carefully and to obtain data from other sources of information. The problem of scaling imprecision arises from the fact that each person rating the patient must have an opportunity to observe the behavior in question, must be observant enough to notice the behavior, and must have a sense of the normal variation of that characteristic in order to rate severity. In research studies, a great deal of time is spent training judges to observe a behavior and to scale the judgments and check them for reliability. We give a similar task to a patient, teacher, parent, or spouse without the training and with unknown reliability. As a colleague of mine once observed: "To use self-report is to employ an untrained judge." Nevertheless, checklists are often the only way to elicit information from some sources (e.g., teachers) and can provide a valuable source of information not otherwise obtainable, but they must be used judiciously.

ASSESSMENT OF ADHD

There are many instruments to assist the clinician in assessing many of the aspects of ADHD. These instruments fall into four categories: structured interviews, checklists, psychometric tests of cognitive functioning, and specialized instruments for measuring specific critical variables associated with ADHD. These tools allow the clinician to go beyond immediate observation and judgment, to survey areas in a systematic fashion, to measure processes more precisely, and to observe in a standard and objective way how the patient functions. To be useful, any tool must give the clinician information in a consistent, predictable way: it must be repeatable under many conditions (i.e., reliable), must give information that is relevant to the diagnosis of ADHD or a particular aspect of the disorder (i.e., valid), and must do so in a way that is worth the time, effort, and expense involved (i.e., cost-effective).

No instrument, no matter how much data it generates and no matter how sophisticated it is in measuring a process, is necessary or sufficient to generate a diagnosis of ADHD. But many instruments give reliable, valid, and valuable information that can usefully be weighed in with the patient's own observations and the reports of others close to him or her.

The diagnosis of ADHD requires a clinical assessment involving not only the symptoms of the disorder but also possible other disorders that may cause similar symptoms; it requires a judgment that the effects of the disorder are significant and are in multiple areas of functioning. No test can cover all these areas, and no test can "make a diagnosis" (American Academy of Child and Adolescent Psychiatry [AACAP] 1997). But test instruments can give the clinician valuable data that make the judgment of whether a a symptom is present and the degree of impairment a more objective, quantifiable, and reliable decision. For example, although a patient can report that he or she is having a problem with short-term memory, a memory test that reveals the degree to which memory is impaired under standard conditions gives a more objective and quantifiable measure of that impairment. Test instruments go beyond the classification question of "Is the symptom present?" to give a more dimensional description of severity of the symptom and the degree of impairment relative to the general population of the same age.

One of the difficulties in selecting instruments for helping with the assessment of ADHD is that the disorder has gone through a number of shifts in conceptualization and definition. The observation of the disorder began with hyperactive children, and the early definitions of the syndrome, then referred to as "hyperkinetic disorder," emphasized the role of hyperactivity and impulsivity symptoms in the definition of the disorder. As understanding of the disorder evolved, and long-term studies of children with the disorder followed them through adolescence and into adulthood, the picture of developmental changes in the appearance of ADHD came to involve symptoms of attention, concentration, effort, and memory. The definition shifted from "hyperactivity disorder" to attention-deficit disorder. Through subsequent revisions of DSM, increasing attention was given to the symptoms of inattention. As a result of this evolution in conceptualization, ADHD has been a shifting target, with different criteria for diagnosis prevalent at different times.

Instruments for use in assessing a disorder take time and effort to construct and validate. As a result, some instruments and tests may be directed at an outdated definition of the disorder. For example, checklists generated at a time when the defining aspect of ADHD was the symptoms of hyperactivity place undue weight on restlessness and impulsivity at the expense of the attention, effort, memory, and other more recently recognized aspects of the disorder.

In using these instruments, the final judgment remains with the clinician on how much weight to place on a finding from an instrument. The decision must be made whether critical aspects of the patient's symptoms are included in the assessment and whether a given level of impairment constitutes a "disorder."

Categories of existing test instruments useful for the assessment of ADHD include structured and semistructured interviews, checklists, and psychometric tests of attention and memory, of organization and planning, of skills, of learning deficits, and of other functions frequently affected by ADHD such as reading, mathematics, persistence, and concept formation. In this section I review categories of tests for these functions. Tests for learning deficits are covered in Chapter 7 of this volume. It is impossible within the confines of a chapter such as this to review all measures that are pertinent or useful. I concentrate instead on some we at the Clinic for Attention and Related Disorders have found to be helpful and to describe the issues relevant to use of tests in each of these areas.

Interview Instruments

The first and primary tool in gathering information about a patient presenting for an evaluation of difficulties in his or her life is the interview. The interview provides not only a way to elicit information from the patient's answers to questions but also an opportunity to observe the patient in action as he or she responds to questions, interjects observations, or deflects a question. Interviews with patients with ADHD are limited to some degree in that many children, and most adolescents and adults, are able to maintain attention and focus for the course of an interview (cf. AACAP 1997), and the true extent of impaired functioning may not emerge in the clinician's office. Evaluation of ADHD routinely includes gathering information from other sources. With children and adolescents, the interview with the patient is usually supplemented with interviews with parents and observations obtained from teachers; with adults, involvement of a spouse, sibling, or, when available, parents is desirable, though not always feasible.

Structured and semistructured interviews for patients with ADHD allow the clinician to cover a broad range of issues that are easily overlooked with patients whose conversation frequently wanders from topic to topic. A degree of flexibility by the clinician is needed. The setting in which questions follow in lockstep fashion is likely to elicit inattentive behavior from the patient, regardless of whether ADHD is present or not. An outline of recommended areas for assessment is provided by the Work Group on Quality Issues (AACAP 1997). Briefly, the areas include history (including developmental history), symptoms of ADHD, symptoms of other alternative or comorbid diagnoses, history of treatments and interventions, areas of strength, medical history, family history, and a physical evaluation (including results of recent physical examinations and recent treatment). Family history includes inquiry about possible ADHD, substance abuse, and other comorbid disorders in other family members.

The Barkley Interview for ADHD (Barkley 1998) is a structured interview covering numerous signs and symptoms of ADHD. Clinical areas include not only the criterion symptoms of ADHD (from DSM-III-R) but also numerous attending symptoms, hyperactivity, and impulsivity symptoms that further document contributions to the severity of the disorder.

The Brown ADD Diagnostic Form (T. E. Brown 1996b) is a semistructured interview for the assessment of adolescents and adults suspected of attention-deficit disorder. (Separate formats for adolescents and for adults are available.) The form provides probes for eliciting presenting symptoms, school and work history, developmental history, health issues, familial patterns, leisure time, and treatment history. A set of screening questions with follow-up probes is provided for alternative and comorbid disorders, and an interview-administered checklist for the symptoms of ADHD specified in DSM-IV is provided, with provision for answers from the patient, collateral (parent, sibling, or spouse), and interviewer. Summary sections are provided to allow tabulation of data from diverse sources, and a calculation sheet for the Bannatyne indexes (discussed later in this chapter) is provided.

The Structured Clinical Interview for DSM-IV (SCID-IV) is a research instrument for systematic diagnosis on the basis of DSM-IV criteria. The interview is a comprehensive instrument for assessment of the DSM-IV diagnoses. The section on ADHD is incomplete, and supplements from the child version of the Schedule for Affective Disorders and Schizophrenia (see below) are used for assessment of ADHD in older adolescents and adults.

The child version of the SADS—the Schedule for Affective Disorders and Schizophrenia for School-Age Children—Epidemiological Version (K-SADS; Orvaschel and Puig-Antich 1987)—is a structured interview for the assessment of childhood disorders. Additions have been made (K-SADS-LP) to include probes for ADHD. Multiple adaptations have been made for different projects, building on the core diagnoses. The interview is extensive and, for most clinical purposes, too long and low in yield of new information for use with most patients. A clinician may want to be familiar with the structure and the kind of probes used, however, in order to be able to inquire about relevant comorbid disorders. Of particular note is the tendency to underdiagnose anxiety disorders. Routine inquiry into anxiety, phobias, and related symptoms is advisable, as is inquiry into levels of other dysphoric affect. The co-occurrence of dysthymia with attention-deficit disorders is quite high. In addition, as T. E. Brown (1996b) noted, specific affective symptoms of attention deficit, depressive affect, volatile temper, and sensitivity to criticism frequently occur as part of the ADHD picture. Diagnosis of ADHD needs to occur in the context of a complete evaluation for psychiatric disorders (AACAP 1997). In addition, the diagnosis of ADHD frequently requires information about current or past educational history, learning deficits, and learning styles.

Checklists

The number of checklists for symptoms of ADHD has grown rapidly. Rather than attempt to review all the checklists, I discuss some general issues in evaluating the usefulness of a checklist and review some that are in more common use.

The time at which a checklist is written has considerable influence on the content. When hyperactivity and impulsivity were the major symptoms of the disorder, the lists developed understandably included, for the most part, only items of these symptoms phrased in various ways for different settings. As the concept and extent of ADHD evolved, more and more items were added to the checklists, with many of the items involving the previously unrepresented symptoms. Many recent studies have featured factor analyses of these checklists, revealing the different dimensions represented by the different items. Most commonly, checklists report one overall score representing the cumulative number of symptoms. This summary score, however, represents the contribution of all the items. The meaning of the summary score depends on the number of items and the variation of the items in the samples studied; the representation by a checklist sum is a score weighted by the relative representation of the items both in number and in degree of variation. Many of the composite checklists consist of numerous items, but often there is an excessive weighting for the symptoms of hyperactivity and impulsivity relative to symptoms of inattention.

For critical use of a checklist, it is important to understand the composition and relative contribution of the different aspects of ADHD. It is not enough to have items representing an attention factor, for example, when these items are only a minority of the total checklist. More useful checklists incorporate subscale scores with separate norms for each subscale. As the additional symptoms included in the DSM-IV definition of ADHD become incorporated into checklists, the resulting instruments become more and more useful instruments.

Rating Scales

Rating scales useful for ADHD fall into two general types: general, or broad-spectrum, scales to screen for comorbid conditions and ADHD-specific scales. The broad-spectrum scales are many and varied (for reviews, see Barkley 1990; Klein et al. 1994). The ADHD-specific scales include a broad variety of scales for self-report, for parent and teacher report, and, in adults, for reports from the spouse or significant other.

Broad-Spectrum Rating Scales

A number of other checklist-type scales are in common use that can contribute to the understanding of the child with ADHD. Three broad-spectrum rating scales in wide use are 1) Achenbach's Child Behavior Checklist, with the accompanying self-report form, the Youth Self-Report (Achenbach 1991a); 2) Behavior Assessment System for Children (Reynolds and Kamphaus 1992); and 3) Child Symptom Inventories (Gadow and Sprafkin 1994).

The Child Behavior Checklist and Youth Self-Report provide multiple scales that are summarized in two overall scales, Internalizing symptoms and Externalizing symptoms. Three of the scales are of particular relevance in children with ADHD, the Attention symptoms scale, the Aggression symptoms scale, and the Delinquency symptoms scales. Norms from extensive national samples and specific samples are available for boys and girls, and the structure of the scales is slightly different for boys and girls. Although areas such as psychotic symptoms are not as adequately measured, the breadth of normative data and the specificity of some of the scales make these rating scales useful in many situations with children and adolescents.

A series of inventory scales from early childhood to adolescence has been provided by Gadow and colleagues (Gadow and Sprafkin 1994; Gadow et al. 1995; Sprafkin and Gadow 1996). Multiple items are provided for rating by parents and/or teachers; the items are keyed to diagnostic categories. The authors emphasize that the checklists are preliminary forms for arriving at a diagnosis and not a means of making a diagnosis. The emphasis is on careful observation of the child. This approach was carried over into the AD/HD School Observation Code (Gadow et al. 1996), which uses observations of the child in three settings: classroom, lunchroom, and playground. The manual elaborates on the different approaches for the observation of ADHD and other disorders (e.g., oppositional defiant disorder, conduct disorder).

The Behavior Assessment System for Children (Reynolds and Kamphaus 1992) also provides an integrated system for self-report, parent report, and teacher report for a broad spectrum of emotional and behavioral disorders in children aged 6 to 18 years.

Rating Scales Specific to ADHD

The number of scales for symptoms of ADHD is large and growing rapidly. Forms for children, adolescents, and adults exist with different emphases, different levels of symptom representation, and different levels of research documentation. Forms for the patient, for the parent, and for teachers are all useful in eliciting information about the functioning of the patient in different situations. Rating scales themselves cannot provide the information for a definitive diagnosis. Scales form the beginning of the diagnostic process and allow systematic collection of information from multiple sources that may not be readily available in diagnostic interviews. The clinical use of the rating scale includes review of the information with the patient, teacher, or parent, a process that can provide the basis of discussion and inquiry about the degree and level of symptoms reported.

For children, a number of rating scales are available for use with patient, parent, and teacher. The Conners Rating Scales—Revised (Conners 1997) include the Conners Teacher Rating Scales—Revised, the Conner Parent Rating Scales—Revised, and the Conners-Wells Adolescent Self-Report Scale. The Conners Rating Scales—Revised cover ages 3 to 17 years and are well-normed to provide useful assessment data regarding ADHD and related problems. They are available in both long and short forms. Barkley has adapted scales from the Child Behavior Checklist for the Child Attention Problems Checklist (Barkley 1990; Barkley et al. 1989), designed to be used as a weekly rating of both hyperactivity/impulsivity and inattention problems. He and Murphy (1998) have also published the Disruptive Behavior Rating Scale, the Home Situations Questionnaire, and the School Situations Questionnaire for assessment of children and adolescents. The IOWA Conners Teacher Rating Scale is a short form that has been found to differentiate hyperactivity/impulsivity from oppositional defiant disorder (Loney and Milich 1982; Pelham et al. 1989).

The Brown Attention Deficit Disorder Scales (T. E. Brown 1996a) is a set of rating scales that focuses on symptoms of inattention. One form is available for adolescents (ages 12–18 years), and another for adults. Forty items are responded to in a clinical interview format by the patient and/or a collateral rater (parent or teacher). Items are grouped into five clinical subareas: organizing and activating for work, sustaining attention and concentration, sustaining energy and effort, managing affective interference, and utilizing working memory and accessing recall. Norms for each of the five subareas are provided, along with cutoff scores for the overall total. Different norms are provided for adolescents ages 12–18 years and adults (high school graduates and older). A form for younger children (ages 3–12 years) is in press (T. E. Brown, in press). The Brown scales differ from other rating scales in that they focus on a wide range of symptoms of inattention and related problems. Some areas, such as managing affective interference, do not appear on the DSM-IV list of criterion symptoms but are included to reflect the appearance of such symptoms in attention-deficit disorders.

Adult scales are a relatively recent addition to the instruments for assessing ADHD. Scales for children do not readily translate into assessment of adults and older adolescents. Some pioneering work by Ward, Wender, and colleagues (1993) led to the development of the Wender Utah Rating Scale for the identification of ADHD in adults. This scale uses criteria that emphasize the early appearance of the disorder and symptoms of hyperactivity; the behaviors rated are recollections of childhood behavior. Ward and colleagues demonstrated that the scale differentiated between adults with depression and psychiatrically healthy adults from adults with childhood ADHD. The Wender Utah Rating Scale is based on a traditional approach to the identification of ADHD as a developmental disorder and emphasizes the childhood roots of the disorder rather than the current symptom picture. As noted earlier, it retains the strong historical emphasis on hyperactive and impulsive behaviors. As a result, the agreement of this scale with other scales based on contemporary expression of symptoms is lower than for most other scales for adult symptoms.

Conners has developed a scale for adults, the Conners Adult Attention Rating Scale (Conners et al. 1999). The scale consists of items written for adults with ADHD, including a number of items directed at attention and affect. Factor analysis reveals that factors differentiate along lines of inattention, hyperactivity, mood/emotional reactions, and concentration. Early results suggest that the different scales differentiate subtypes of ADHD.

Psychometric Testing

General Issues

Although psychometric testing gives the clinician an opportunity to observe and measure behavior of a patient with possible ADHD, other issues arise in the testing interaction that influence the quality of information obtained. These issues can both enhance and interfere with the performance of the patient in the testing situation. The first issue is that the tests given, to a greater or lesser degree, can re-create the experience the patient has had in academic situations where his or her performance was evaluated through tests, often to the detriment of the individual. More negativistic patients may respond to the evaluation, particularly if it is performed at the behest of a parent or spouse, as another situation designed to reveal his or her incompetence. The clinician examining the patient must keep in mind the approach the patient takes to the testing, establish a collaborative, information-seeking approach, and minimize the sense of failure the patient is all too often prone to experience when evaluated. Mixing the content and format of the tests, to provide novelty and a stimulating pace for the patient, can help to alleviate the negative expectations many patients bring to the situation.

Another issue with psychometric testing, almost opposite in effect to the first issue, is that the patient may do well in the testing and disguise the extent of his or her problems and difficulties. The testing situation presents a setting with a high degree of novelty and a high degree of feedback from the testing itself and from the examiner. A patient may see the testing as a chance to demonstrate his or her level of ability, allowing the patient to become engaged in and focused on the testing in a manner different from that exhibited in his or her day-to-day work; consequently, the testing may yield a picture of better functioning in which the underlying deficits are disguised (cf. Hallowell and Ratey 1994).

In evaluating reading, for example, tests typically involve materials, whether words, sentences, or passages, that are much briefer than those with which most patients with ADHD experience difficulty—namely, chapters, articles, and entire books. Such reading extends over a much longer duration than is used on some reading tests, and the more extended reading makes higher demands on focus and concentration. The reading difficulty for a person with ADHD may not be of the same nature as that for an individual with a learning disability. For some patients, the length of concentration required in a reading test with brief passages may be within the span of concentration that can be mustered. Yet longer passages, even half a page, may be too long for effective ability to read, comprehend, and remember the material long enough to answer questions about the content. To read such passages, the patient is required to move back and forth from question to passage—a process that slows the rate of completion and hampers the quality of the answers.

Memory testing can be another source of misleading data. Some memory tests—for example, the Digit Span subtest from the Wechsler Adult Intelligence Scale–III, assess handling of brief amounts of material with immediate recall. When energized for the evaluation, individuals with quite severe memory difficulties may be able to complete the test with a relatively high score, but they may not be able to recall what happened in the discussion with the interviewer a half hour before. Many patients with ADHD have difficulty with materials as brief as the Digit Span subtest; others may be able to recall this kind of material immediately after hearing it but report difficulties with more extended material, with more verbal content, that requires longer periods of concentration and focus.

Tests are samples of behavior used to predict other behavior (Anastasi 1988). In evaluating an individual with possible ADHD, it is important that the sampling be broad and that the kinds of material used for the evaluation include forms of behaviors more challenging for the patient as well as forms that are able to elicit the relatively intact functions. The more relevant the material sampled in the testing to the day-to-day functioning of the patient, the more likely the test will produce results that mirror the patient's strengths and weaknesses.

A number of cognitive functions are particularly affected by the symptoms of ADHD. Primary to the disorder are effects on attention, in the areas of focusing attention at will, sustaining attention, and shifting attention from one task to another at will. All three areas are potentially affected, separately or together, in any given patient. It is important to remember in assessing attention that attention comprises multiple functions, and one function may be affected while others are relatively intact, or most or all of the many attention functions may be affected in any one individual. In almost all patients, some functions of attention are intact. For example, one patient was able to compose music for hours on end but could not write the simplest sentence without distraction. Another patient was an expert chef, able to manage the preparation of multiple gourmet dishes at one time and bring them to completion at the same moment, but could not keep track of a checkbook or manage the business affairs of his restaurant. Many clinicians have observed the phenomenon of "hyperfocus," in which the individual is able to focus and maintain concentration on a given task and exclude all distractions while engaged in the task. For example, parents of a distractible child remarked to an examiner that the teachers must be observing a different child when they said their daughter was inattentive. They recounted having observed her playing a computer game, adding, "We have to get in front of her or turn off the machine to get her attention."

One of the difficult aspects of evaluating patients with ADHD is that the expression of the disorder is quite variable and often situation-specific. One patient may be able to pick up a book and read it from cover to cover, whereas another may not be able to get into the first chapter without becoming distracted and forgetting what he or she read a few pages earlier. One patient may report that daydreaming and inattention while reading has been a crippling symptom from the very beginning, whereas another may report having found refuge from abusive parents in reading and the resulting feedback from supportive teachers but having been unable to write any significant material.

Another area frequently affected in ADHD is memory. In some patients, all aspects of memory may be affected; in others, short-term and long-term memory may be intact but working memory—which we define as the ability to recall from a minute to a day, to maintain focus on an activity while attending to another, and to retrieve information previously learned—is impaired. One patient reported that his memory was excellent. He was able to recall the scenes and flow of a movie he had watched with his family on vacation 4 years earlier. He could not, however, recall what had been said 5 minutes earlier.

Attention and memory are intertwined; to remember, one must first attend to what is going on. We have seen quite a few patients who could focus on neutral material such as strings of numbers on the Digit Span subtest of the Wechsler Adult Intelligence Scale—Revised (Wechsler 1981) but could not recall paragraphs on the Logical Memory subtest of the Wechsler Memory Scale—Revised (Wechsler 1987). Some are even able to muster attention for the minute or so required for listening to brief passages but cannot sustain attention for a page of reading and recall the material on the page sufficiently well to answer multiple-choice questions immediately after reading it.

Tests of attention vary in the degree to which they require focusing of attention, shifting of attention, and sustaining focus of attention. It is important for the clinician in assessing attention to keep in mind the variable expression of attention difficulties. No one test of attention encompasses all the possible manifestations of attention difficulties. Furthermore, individuals with relatively intact attention and concentration may vary in the levels of skill in the different areas. An important criterion to keep in mind in assessing a patient is to determine not only the state of different functions of attention but also their impact on the individual's adaptation in study, work, leisure, and interpersonal relationships.

General Assessment of Cognitive Abilities

A useful base for evaluation of a patient's functioning is a general measure of overall cognitive abilities such as a general intelligence test. Although the overall IQ score is not the goal of such testing, it is helpful to know the level of functions that are not particularly affected by ADHD as well as the level of those that are more likely to be affected. In addition, knowing the patient's ability in a particular area of functioning often helps in gauging the degree of discrepancy between the individual's potential and realized intellectual capacities. Very few individuals fully actualize the full capacity of their abilities, but in patients with ADHD (as well as patients with other clinical disorders) there is frequently a large discrepancy between the indicators of potential and the accomplishments in applied academic work and, in adults, occupational achievement and functioning.

General intelligence tests typically measure a number of functions representing a broad range of abilities. Some of these abilities are heavily influenced by difficulties in attention and concentration, whereas others reflect the accumulation of knowledge through the educational process. Other areas of ability are relatively less influenced by cultural and academic exposure and provide a basis for estimating "potential." The concept of "potential" is a tricky and elusive one, but in practical clinical situations it involves the level of functioning estimated from the base of the more intact functions.

General intelligence tests commonly used in clinical practice include the Wechsler scales, the Stanford-Binet Intelligence Scale, and a number of brief tests of intelligence, such as the Kaufman Brief Intelligence Test (Kaufman and Kaufman 1990). The Wechsler scales range from preschool to adult forms and include the Wechsler Preschool and Primary Scales of Intelligence—Revised (WPPSI-R; Wechsler 1989), the Wechsler Intelligence Scale for Children–III (WISC-III; Wechsler 1991), the Wechsler Adult Intelligence Scale—Revised (WAIS-R; Wechsler 1981), and the Wechsler Adult Intelligence Scale–III (WAIS-III; Wechsler 1997a). The Wechsler scales include a number of subtests (11–14) grouped into verbal and performance domains. The WISC-III and WAIS-III include a number of index scores that facilitate comparison of clusters of related subtests. The Stanford-Binet Intelligence Scale, 4th Edition (Thorndike et al. 1986), presents a similar structure of subtests, with verbal and performance subscales and indexes within the subareas. These indexes are useful as a means of obtaining first approximations of functions with different vulnerability to the effects of ADHD. Forms of the various tests discussed above exist in other languages as well.

The WISC-III consists of 13 subtests (7 verbal and 6 performance subtests), 10 of which are used for the estimation of IQ. The Information subtest elicits information (facts about people, places, and general knowledge) that reflects cultural richness and academic background. In the Vocabulary subtest, the patient is asked to define common words. This subtest is somewhat influenced by richness of background and education, is consistently among the most reliable subtests, and has the highest correlation with overall and verbal IQ. The Comprehension subtest is used to assess commonsense social expectations and practical knowledge. Individuals with strong practical "common sense" can often do well on this subtest in spite of limited educational or cultural exposure. In the Similarities subtest, the patient is asked to provide the underlying concepts linking two words (e.g., "apple" and "orange"). This subtest reflects the tendency to think conceptually rather than in concrete or functional terms. These four subtests are combined in the Verbal Composite Index to indicate the individual's ability based on these subtests, which tend to correlate most highly with achievement in ordinary academic situations. Similar subtests with similar names appear in the WAIS-III, but the Verbal Index is based on only the Vocabulary, Similarities, and Information subtests (see the discussion of the Bannatyne Indexes later in this section for an alternative approach to assessing general cognitive abilities).

The WISC-III, WAIS-R, and WAIS-III also include a number of subtests involving short-term memory and the solution of verbally presented arithmetic word problems. The Digit Span subtest requires the patient to recall strings of verbally presented digits, initially recalling them in the forward direction, then other strings in the reverse direction. This form of memory requires brief but focused attention on neutral material with low levels of associative interference. Although this subtest is frequently included as a test of memory, the form of memory assessed is different from that assessed in most other memory tests, in that there is no expectation that the material recalled be available for later recall. This form of memory has been termed "short-term store" or "scratchpad" memory. Although this form of memory is frequently observed to be deficient in individuals with ADHD, some persons with the condition are capable of managing the brief focus and short interval before recall and yet be unable to remember the most elementary details of social interactions 5 minutes later. The Digit Span subtest is not included in the subtests used to calculate IQ in the WISC-III, and this at times leads to a shift in IQ when the patient becomes old enough for the adult Wechsler scale, which does include this subtest in estimating IQ.

The Arithmetic subtest of the Wechsler scales involves the solution of verbally presented word problems of increasing levels of difficulty. Particularly when the problem involves more than one calculation step, the subtest can be substantially affected by problems of focus and concentration. This is yet another subtest vulnerable to the effect of ADHD. Other influences may affect performance on this test, however. Individuals with a weak background in arithmetic, especially those who have an immediate reaction of anxious expectation of failure, may do poorly without any necessary implication of an attention-deficit disorder. Other individuals with an attention-deficit disorder may have overlearned their arithmetic operations to such an extent that they are able to solve the problems immediately, without invoking demands on memory, and do well on this subtest but not on others that place greater demands on memory and concentration. A pattern frequently observed in individuals with ADHD consists of rapid and efficient completion of low-level items, occasional impulsive errors as the items become more difficult, and then difficulty with the higher-level items marked by frequent requests for repetition of the question and inability to complete problems when the solution requires remembering the results of intermediate calculations, a function that clearly involves working memory at higher levels of difficulty.

The Digit Span and Arithmetic subtests are combined in the Freedom From Distractibility Index on the WISC-III, with a table of norms for conversion to an "IQ-like" index score (mean = 100, SD = 15). The WAIS-III adds a new subtest, Letter-Number Sequencing, that represents a challenging short-term memory task. The examiner reads a list of numbers and letters in scrambled order; the patient is asked to recall the numbers in ascending order and the letters in alphabetic order. This subtest is too new for evaluation studies in ADHD; preliminary experience indicates that it is sensitive to the effects of ADHD at least at the level of Digit Span and Arithmetic. Together with Arithmetic and Digit Span, this subtest is combined into a Working Memory Index on the WAIS-III and converted into an index score. The index is also too new for evaluation of its effectiveness in detecting memory problems with ADHD, but it has promise as a useful measure.

The WAIS-III adds tables for comparing the Digit Span forward and backward recall totals. The recall of numbers in the reverse direction is a more demanding task, and it is not uncommon to observe a much lower recall on the backward trials compared with that on the forward trials. This contrast illustrates a possible difference between short-term recall (which is used in digits forward trials) and working memory (which is drawn on more than short-term memory in complex digits backward trials).

Visual and visual-motor skills are assessed in the Performance sections of the Wechsler scales. Picture Completion requires the identification of missing details in pictures, a skill that is sometimes undercut by impulsivity. Block Design involves the manipulation of blocks with solid red-and-white and diagonally mixed red-and-white faces to match designs of varying complexity. This subtest correlates highly with nonverbal measures of abstraction and is one of the subtests most highly correlated with nonverbal measures of ability. Object Assembly requires the assembling of puzzlelike objects. On the

WISC-III, these three subtests are combined in the Perceptual Orientation Index. In the WAIS-III, another performance subtest, Matrix Reasoning, substituted for Object Assembly and is added to the Perceptual Orientation Index. This subtest requires the patient to identify patterns and series in a set of complex visual patterns and to identify what pattern is needed to complete the stimulus. It is an untimed test, a feature that reduces the emphasis on speed in some of the Performance subtests. It adds a measure of abstract visual reasoning. Along with Block Design, it is highly correlated with both Full Scale and Performance IQ.

The performance subtests weight rate of completion with differing emphasis. Block Design and Object Assembly allow bonus points for rapid completion; these points are weighted especially in the Object Assembly subtest. Two subtests on both the WAIS-III and the WISC-III are more direct measures of rate of work. Coding (WISC-III), Digit Symbol (WAIS-R), and Digit Symbol/Coding (WAIS-III) are subtests heavily weighting rate of work. They involve completing a digit-to-symbol code presented at the top of the page after brief practice, for 90 (WAIS-R) to 120 seconds (WISC-III, WAIS-III). Digit Symbol/Coding is a test vulnerable to a large number of influences, both from functional and from neurological sources. In ADHD, the patient may be able to muster energy and work efficiently for the brief period, or the distractibility and lack of persistence may set in, with a resulting low rate of work. Other influences that may occur include weak visuospatial or visuomotor functioning, poor motor control, and effects of neurological disorders.

On the WISC-III and WAIS-III, another subtest, Symbol Search, is added that emphasizes speed, but with reduced requirements for visuomotor coordination. The subject must scan the stimulus symbols on the left of the page and determine whether one of them is present in the set of symbols at the right of the page, checking "yes" or "no." The Digit Symbol/Coding subtest is combined with the Symbol Search subtest in the Processing Speed Index.

The Bannatyne Indexes (Bannatyne 1974) adapted by T. E. Brown (1996) are a set of three indexes of WAIS-R subtest scores that consist of three regression equations to create index scores with a mean of 100 and a standard deviation of 15 (the same as for the IQ scores). The Verbal Index is composed of estimates from the Comprehension, Vocabulary, and Similarities subtests. It differs from the Verbal Composite of the WISC-III in not including Information, and it differs from the Verbal Comprehension index of the WAIS-III in that the latter includes Information, but not Comprehension. Although comparative studies have not been performed, it may be useful to continue to use the Bannatyne Verbal Index given that Information is relatively sensitive to the cultural and educational background, at least more so than Comprehension. Preliminary results from a clinical sample show the mean Comprehension score is 1 scale-score point (1/3 SD) above that for Information.

Another Bannatyne Index is the Spatial Index, composed of Picture Completion, Block Design, and Object Assembly. These three subtests have in common an emphasis on overcoming "embedding context" (Witkin et al. 1962) and represent subtests that consistently appear on a single factor. On the WAIS-III, Object Assembly is an optional subtest and is replaced by Matrix Reasoning. The Matrix Reasoning subtest has many desirable qualities, including less reliance on motor speed. The WAIS-III index may be preferable for that reason but thus far has not been studied.

The final Bannatyne Index is the Concentration Index, composed of Digit Span, Arithmetic, and Digit Symbol/Coding. This is a more heterogeneous index, in that it combines two verbal subtests and one performance subtest and mixes attention and concentration measures with a measure of motor speed. Although all three subtests have been found to be impaired in attention-deficit disorders, mixing of such heterogeneous skills may result in false negatives and false positives in conditions in which other factors influence one or more subtests.

Patterns of Functioning on the Wechsler Scales

As we have emphasized, there is no one pattern of cognitive deficits in ADHD, but there are patterns encountered frequently in many patients that serve to indicate the nature and extent of impairment in the patient.

Digit Span. Digit Span has frequently been used as the representative of "memory" in the assessment of ADHD. It is sensitive to the process of maintaining focus in the immediate verbal interaction and requires detailed and sequenced recall. Numerous studies have found scores for Digit Span to be significantly lower than those for other verbal subtests. In our own clinic results with adolescents and adults, the age-corrected score for Digit Span is 1.4 standard deviations (22 points expressed as an index score) below the mean of the Verbal Index. Nonetheless, some patients show a false-negative pattern. They are able to focus on the neutral material of Digit Span and remember numbers adequately. Some of these patients have been involved in occupations that expose them to numbers frequently (e.g., an accountant, a case manager for a health care organization). False positive results can occur in patients with a high level of anxiety and/or depression, in whom attention and concentration are often impaired.

Arithmetic is another subtest frequently found to be impaired in patients with ADHD. The subtest requires not only attention to the question but also sustained concentration to solve the problem, particularly when more than one computational step is required. In our clinic sample of adolescents and adults, the Arithmetic subtest was 0.61 standard deviation below the mean of subtests on the Verbal Index. Again false negative results were observed in some patients who had enough familiarity with arithmetic that the problems demanded little concentration once the problem was heard, although this sometimes involved repeated reading of the problem. False positive results can also be found in patients with other conditions such as a mathematics learning disorder and in patients who are anxious about working with arithmetic problems after an experience that convinces them that they "cannot do" mathematics.

Digit Symbol/Coding. The Digit Symbol/Coding subtest is multifaceted, involving visual, spatial, motor, and sequencing abilities. This subtest is one of the more sensitive general indicators of neurological impairment. In our clinic sample, the Digit Symbol subtest was 0.85 standard deviation below the mean of subtests on the Verbal Index. Patients should be observed for indicators of impulsivity, including not observing the end of the samples, skipping around in spite of instructions to complete the items in order, and writing letters instead of symbols.

Verbal Index versus Concentration Index. The subtests Digit Span, Arithmetic, and Digit Symbol are combined in the Bannatyne Concentration Index to form an estimate of IQ. The three subtests composing this index of concentration are all sensitive to the effects of ADHD, although each of them shows somewhat different sensitivity. In our clinic sample, the Concentration Index was 10.9 index points below the Verbal Index (0.72 SD).

Verbal Index versus Spatial Index. In our clinic sample, the Spatial Index was significantly lower than the Verbal Index. The comparable figures for the Spatial Index give a mean difference of 4.67 points (0.31 SD) between the two indexes. In general, clients at the clinic scored lower on the Spatial Index than on the Verbal Index, a possible reflection of the selection factors influencing who seeks out assessment in a university-based clinic. For a number of clients, however, the Spatial Index and Performance IQ were higher than the Verbal Index and Verbal IQ. These individuals tended to have very highly developed technical skills but at times had problems with language skills or had had a negative experience with humanities subjects in high school and college, which frequently create stress for students with impaired reading skills.

Tests of Attention

The assessment of ADHD has seen the development of instruments for evaluating attention in multiple forms. The continuous performance test (CPT) was originally developed to study attention in schizophrenic patients. A number of versions, differing in presentation, modalities (visual vs. auditory), and response characteristics (e.g., response to targets vs. withholding response to targets), have been developed.

Gordon Diagnostic System. The Gordon Diagnostic System (Gordon 1986) consists of a free-standing stimulus-response unit into which multiple forms of testing have been programmed. The standard CPT is presented as a series of letters on a screen paced by the apparatus. Responses are recorded and stored within the system and retained for readout with an external microcomputer. Subjects respond only to targets, with irrelevant nontarget stimuli interspersed.

Tests of Variables of Attention. The Test of Variables of Attention (TOVA; Greenberg and Waldman 1993) is a program for an IBM-compatible personal computer with two rates of presentation of the target stimulus, rare and frequent. The test is divided into two sequences, frequent and rare targets, with the entire test taking 24 minutes. Subjects respond to a target letter interspersed among nontarget letters. Norms have been established for ages 4 to 80 years (L. M. Greenberg and R. D. Crosby, unpublished manuscript, 1992). Scores produced include errors of omission (missed targets), errors of commission (false positive responses), response time for correct trials, and anticipatory errors (response before the target stimulus appears). The pattern of errors gives information about impulsivity as well as inattention.

Conners Continuous Performance Test. The Conners Continuous Performance Test (Conners 1985) is a program for an IBM-compatible personal computer. Letters are presented one at a time, with the target letter occurring in a random sequence among one of six distracter letters. In this test, unlike other CPTs, the subject is instructed to respond to nontarget letters and to withhold response to the target (the letter *X*). The entire test takes 14 minutes. The rate of presentation varies across the test—a feature that allows for assessment of processing at different rates. The scores provided include errors of omission, errors of commission, reaction times, and variability of responses during the task. The use of an inhibited response to the target provides a more direct analog to impulsivity, or failure to inhibit a response when appropriate.

Effectiveness of continuous performance tests in the assessment of ADHD. A large number of studies, mostly with children but also with adults, have shown that individuals with ADHD perform more poorly on CPT measures. The results vary from study to study, and the degree of difference between psychiatrically healthy samples and identified ADHD patients varies with age and characteristics of the samples. In a meta-analytic study of 26 studies of children with attention-deficit disorder, Losier et al. (1996) assessed the net effect size of the difference between children with attention-deficit disorder and children without that disorder. The authors found that, in general, the children with attention-deficit disorder showed more errors of omission and errors of commission, but there was little evidence of differences in response bias (tendency to respond or to not respond). In general, the shorter the stimulus duration, the greater the difference, and the shorter the trials (time between stimuli) and the higher the proportion of target to nontarget stimuli, the lower the error rate difference for children with ADHD.

The classic CPT involves presentation of a series of visual targets. A more recent development has been the development and norming of auditory CPTs. Impairment in auditory attention is more broadly implicated in ADHD than is impairment in attention to visual stimuli (Seidman et al. 1997), so the use of the auditory modality is more likely to assess inattention in ADHD. Thus far, however, this assumption has not been confirmed to any strong degree, although the reasoning behind the use of auditory CPT is consistent with findings in other areas (e.g., memory).

Multiple studies have shown a reduction in CPT errors when children are treated, principally with methylphenidate. This finding has led to the use of the CPT by some clinicians to measure treatment response. In some of the more extreme statements about CPTs, it is asserted that the test is the definitive test for attention-deficit disorders. In commenting on the claims for neuropsychological testing in ADHD in general, Barkley (1997) points out that the correspondences between test findings and diagnosis are never close to 100%. What is not highlighted in the studies of CPTs (and other measures) in ADHD is the diagnostic efficiency of the measure used. Some affected individuals score normally on the CPT (false negative results), and some individuals without ADHD have difficulty with the test (false positive results) (Trommer et al. 1988).

The literature on use of the CPT in the assessment of ADHD has developed primarily with hyperactivity and impulsivity as the defining features of the disorder. Barkley (1990) suggested that the CPT is more sensitive to impulsive forms of ADHD, with a higher degree of variability for subjects affected by the primarily inattentive type. Caution in interpreting CPT results is warranted also for two other reasons. First, the test was originally developed and used for assessment of other conditions, primarily schizophrenia and neurological conditions. The literature on the CPT for other conditions is extensive and suggests that the test is sensitive to a broad variety of conditions in addition to ADHD. As in the diagnosis of ADHD itself, any positive test finding needs to be evaluated further for what other conditions may be present that would give rise to the result (cf. Corkum and Siegel 1993; Power 1992). Second, a number of individuals may be capable of responding to the new situation (the CPT) with increased interest and arousal and function normally even when they are experiencing problems of impulsivity and attention in their daily lives.

Behavioral observation of patients taking the CPT has been found to be a useful supplement to the scores obtained (Barkley 1991). In one study, for example, infrared measurement of activity during the CPT was combined with the scores to distinguish boys with and without ADHD from healthy control subjects (Teicher et al. 1996).

Tests of Memory

One of the functions most often affected in ADHD is verbal working memory. Memory is a complex set of functions, potentially involving events from the most immediate to those that happened long ago. The term *working memory* has evolved to include a group of memory types ranging from immediate, short-term recall to more complex and extended memory for discourse. Lezak (1995) has proposed a model of *declarative memory,* which involves registration, short-term storage, and long-term memory, each comprising substages with different characteristics in different modalities. Although there are memory components for all the senses, the two most relevant for our discussion are visual and auditory memory.

Registration, or immediate short-term sensory storage, is of limited capacity and interacts with affective, set, and attention focusing mechanisms for the registration of memory elements. *Immediate memory,* the first stage of short-term memory, can be termed the "span of attention" (Lezak 1995). It is a system of limited capacity (Watkins 1974) and typically lasts up to 30 seconds. *Active working memory* typically lasts from 30 seconds to a few minutes. This working memory functions to hold information in mind and to use that information to guide behavior in the absence of reliable external cues. With rehearsal, *short-term working memory* can last for a few hours. Translation into *long-term memory* follows a number of stages, including consolidation, long-term storage, and retrieval.

The memory most of interest in the understanding of ADHD is short-term working memory. Examination of memory tests used to assess memory in the clinical situation reveals different emphases of different aspects of these types of memory. Digit Span, the subtest of the Wechsler scales most frequently used for assessing brief memory, is qualitatively different from measures of other forms of verbal memory, such as list recall, sentence recall, and story recall (e.g., Wechsler Memory Scale—Revised Logical Memory). Some forms of memory testing make a further assessment for delayed recall (e.g., the California Verbal Learning Test, the Wechsler Memory Scale—Revised, the Wide Range Assessment of Memory and Learning, and the Children's Memory Scale). Each test type makes different demands on memory. Visual memory tests are less often used in the assessment of ADHD and appear to be less vulnerable to the disorder.

Digit Span. Digit Span appears on the various forms of the Wechsler scales, and there is a similar test on the Stanford-Binet. It is often included as part of the mental status examination. Digit Span has two components, digits forward and digits backward. In most test uses of Digit Span, the components are treated as two parts of a single scale, although there is increasing evidence that the recall of digits forward is different from the recall of digits backward. Digits forward is a "passive memory" test (Rapaport et al. 1968), requiring only that the patient recall the material heard in the same order received. As such, it comes close to a "pure" test of auditory registration, with the requirement that the patient be alert to receive the material but not to process it. By contrast, digits backward requires a manipulation of the material in working memory (Banken 1985; Black 1986; Hayslip and Kennelly 1980; Lezak 1995). The digits backward score is generally one to two numbers lower than the digits forward score (Black and Strub 1978; Kaplan et al. 1991; Lezak 1995).

Scores for Digit Span are frequently lower than those for other subtests in individuals with ADHD. Low scores on Digit Span are frequently accompanied by low scores on the other tests on the Concentration Index—namely, Arithmetic and Digit Symbol. In adults, Digit Span performance is frequently substantially below estimates of verbal ability (Quinlan and Brown 1997a, 1997b), to the point that 30%–70% of high-functioning adults have a Digit Span score a full standard deviation or more lower than Verbal Index measures.

There are, however, a number of individuals with ADHD who do not show the deficit in Digit Span but do show deficits in other areas. These individuals are able to muster attention for the brief period required for the task but are unable to hold this level of alertness for longer memory demands.

List learning. A number of tests examine the ability to learn lists of words. Tests vary in the degree to which the words are grouped by concepts. The typical list-learning test requires the patient to learn 10–15 words without specific order. A special variant of list learning is the *learning paired associates*—words learned as pairs, with the initial word used as a cue for retrieval. List learning represents an intermediate length of material for memorization, invoking working memory, but for discrete content.

The California Verbal Learning Test (Delis et al. 1987) is a list-learning test with multiple presentation that uses a standard interference procedure before eliciting a delayed recall trial. Items are selected from one of four categories: fruits, herbs and spices, articles of clothing, and tools. The instrument has been used extensively with neurological patients and with adults with ADHD (Seidman, et al., 1997). A children's version has been published (Delis et al. 1994). The children's version (the adult form is similar) involves learning two lists, an initial, "Monday" list for five trials, followed by a second, "Tuesday" list. After the second list, a free recall is made for the first list; this is followed by a cued-recall trial, in which the patient is asked to remember words from the list by category. After a delay filled with other tests, the patient is asked to repeat the first list in a free recall, then in a cued recall, and finally in a recognition recall. Scores are obtained for 21 different indexes, including indexes for the first and fifth trial; the recall of the second list; short delay free and cued recall; long delay free and cued recall; semantic and serial clustering (i.e., the degree to which the patient recalls words by content category or list position); early, middle, and late items on the list; the slope of learning (i.e., rate of increase in retention over the trials); and the consistency of recall. Intrusions, perseverations, and false positives are also indexed. Scores are also calculated for discrimination of target words from distracters. Correlations of indexes are significant in the normative sample but low in magnitude (0.30–0.40).

The List Learning subtest of the Wide Range Assessment of Memory and Learning (Adams and Sheslow 1990) provides a list of 9 or 15 items, depending on age, with up to six learning trials and a recall trial after interpolated tasks followed by a recognition trial. Age norms are presented both for initial learning on the first three trials and for delayed recall and recognition.

The Paired Associates Learning subtest of the Wechsler Memory Scale–Revised for adults presents eight pairs of words, four with common associations (e.g., "apple–pear," [not an actual item]) and four with infrequent associations (e.g., "college–supermarket," [also not an actual item]). Age-corrected norms are given for initial learning and delayed recall. The Paired Associates Learning subtest of the Wechsler Memory Scale–III (Wechsler 1997b) involves eight pairs of words, with low levels of association on four learning trials and a delayed recall trial, followed by a recognition test.

List learning is not always sensitive to the effects of ADHD. Seidman et al. (1997) found that scores on the California Verbal Learning Test in adolescent referred patients older than 17 years and the Wide Range Assessment of Memory and Learning subtest in referred patients under 17 years were not significantly different from those in psychiatrically healthy age-matched control subjects.

Sentence repetition. A longer unit of memory than that assessed by a number memory test is the sentence, and specifically sentences of varying length. Patients typically can remember semantically related material, such as meaningful sentences, in longer strings than they can unrelated material (e.g., digits). Sentence memory is used in a number of neuropsychological batteries and is sensitive to damage in the dominant (language) hemisphere (Lezak 1995; McFie 1960), to diffuse damage (Lezak 1995), and to attentional impairments (Lezak 1991; Lezak et al. 1990).

A number of tests are available for assessing sentence memory. In the neuropsychological literature, the Sentence Repetition Test from the Multilingual Aphasia Examination (Benton and Hamsher 1989) has two forms with seven different linguistic constructions. A similar test was produced by Spreen and Strauss (1991) in two forms, with both adult and child norms. Forms of the Sentence Repetition Test appear in various other subtests. Memory for Sentences appears in Stanford-Binet Intelligence Scale, 4th Edition (Thorndike et al. 1986), with norms for ages 2–23 years. The Wide Range Assessment of Learning and Memory includes a Sentence Memory subtest for ages 6–16 years. The Children's Memory Scale (Cohen 1997) also contains a section on sentence memory. The Test of Adolescent Language–3 (Hammill et al. 1994) incorporates a sentence memory assessment as the Speaking/Grammar subtest, with norms for adolescents through early adulthood.

These tests, although not equivalent in difficulty or norms, represent a readily available source of intermediate-length material for assessing memory. Memory impairments can occur across a broad spectrum of material. Patients with more severe forms can show impairment in the briefest memory test, whereas patients with more intact memory may not have difficulty in any of the memory spans typically assessed in memory testing; if they do have difficulty, it is only at the more extended durations, with greater amounts of material and longer intervals between exposure and recall.

Memory for more extended material. Strings of digits, word lists, paired associates, and sentences represent increasing demands on working memory. A form of memory assessment, present since the Babcock Story Recall (Babcock

1930), is the memory for passages, typically 150–200 words in length. The Wechsler Memory Scale—Revised includes two stories of 25 content units each, administered with an immediate recall and a 30-minute delayed recall. Since patients rarely recall elements verbatim, guidelines are given for rating a unit as correct or incorrect. Age norms for ages 16 to 70 years are given. A revision of this test has been published in the Wechsler Memory Scale—III. The procedure is modified by the addition of a second reading and recall for the second of the two stories. Delayed recall of both passages is elicited after 25—30 minutes. The length of the passages is sufficient to exceed the immediate registration memory limits, and the task requires short-term memory as well (Lezak 1995).

The form of verbal memory involved in the Logical Memory subtest appears to be quite sensitive to the problems of attention and concentration found in ADHD. We reported on the results on the Logical Memory subtest in two clinical samples of adults (Quinlan and Brown 1997b); when converted to a Logical Memory Index score, a score on a scale similar to IQ scores (mean = 100, SD = 15), the average difference between the Verbal Index and the Logical Memory Index scores was 21 points in one sample of 113 clients and 26.6 points in a second sample of 73 clients. The scores for the delayed recall did not differ significantly from those for the initial recall in either group, suggesting that the rate of memory decay was not unusual. Other investigators have found similar difficulties among clients with ADHD. Similar results are found in subsamples of individuals with superior IQ (Quinlan and Brown 1997a).

Other Neuropsychological Measures

A number of findings have found underlying differences in the neurological functioning of individuals with ADHD (Seidman et al. 1997). A variety of measures commonly used in neuropsychological assessment lend themselves to use in the assessment of ADHD. Other neuropsychological measures that are potentially useful, in addition to the measures of memory discussed previously, are those directed at executive functions and response inhibition.

Wisconsin Card Sorting Test. The Wisconsin Card Sorting Test, developed by Berg (Berg 1948; Grant and Berg 1948) and modified by Heaton (Heaton 1981; Heaton et al. 1993), is also available in a computer-administered form that allows one to avoid possible errors in the complex administration and scoring. The subject is presented with four "label" cards varying in color, shape of figure, and number of figures. Each of the 128 stimulus cards is to be matched to a label on the basis of one of the stimulus dimensions, but the subject is told only to match the card to the label at the top. The criteria are color, shape, and number. After 10 correct trials for a given criterion dimension, the criterion for correct response is shifted without informing the subject. The subject must infer the shift in criterion from the pattern of correct and incorrect answers; after 10 consecutive correct trials to the second criterion, the criterion is shifted again. After three correct criteria are completed, the principle is again shifted to the first criterion, until the subject has mastered six criteria with 10 consecutive correct responses or the 128 cards are exhausted. Scores are derived for number of criteria met, number of errors, number of perseverative errors, number of perseverative answers, learning to learn (shifting more efficiently after initial concepts), and loss of set (deviation from the correct criterion after three correct trials).

The test was originally presented as a measure of frontal lobe functioning, and a number of studies have shown that the test discriminates patients with frontal lobe dysfunction from control patients. Perseverative errors are particularly prominent in the performance of patients with frontal lobe damage (Graffman et al. 1990; Janowsky et al. 1989; Milner 1963; Robinson et al. 1980). Impaired frontal lobe functioning is strongly implicated in ADHD (Shue and Douglas 1992). Positron emission tomography (PET) scans of the brains of adults with ADHD reveal low levels of activation in prefrontal and premotor areas (Zametkin et al. 1990). In a recent study by Seidman et al. (1997), a sample of referred adolescents with ADHD were found to show more perseverative and nonperseverative errors with the Wisconsin Card Sorting Test.

Lezak (1995) has voiced some caution about the interpretation of the Wisconsin Card Sorting Test in neurological patients. Studies of its use in neurological patients have produced inconsistent evidence of lateralization of damage. Comparisons of patients with frontal lesions with patients with nonfrontal lesions showed that both had equal levels of compromise (Anderson et al. 1991; Graffman et al. 1990), while another study found similar rates of errors in patients with diffuse damage (Robinson et al. 1980). Given the potential frustration patients experience in this ambiguous test, Lezak recommends caution in employing this test.

Stroop Color-Word Interference Test. The Stroop Color-Word Interference Test (Golden 1978), referred to here as the Stroop test, has been used in various forms for over a hundred years. Formulated by Stroop in 1935, this test is based on the finding that it takes longer to say the names of colors than to read the names of colors, and when the color of the word differs from the color named in the word, even more interference appears. The phenomenon has been variously attributed to response conflict, failure of inhibition, or failure of attention (Dyer 1973; Zajano and Gorman 1986) and to difficulties in warding off distraction (Lezak 1995). Differing formats are used, but typically the patient is asked to read the names of colors on the first trial, to name the colors of nonword shapes, and then to name the colors when the names are printed in another color. The tendency to read the name is a very strong, habituated response, and even neuropsychiatrically normal subjects experience a slowing of the "interference" trial. Slowed rates of reading were found to be associated with other signs of attention problems in patients with closed head injuries (Bohnen et al. 1992).

The Stroop test is sensitive to the distractibility and impulsivity in patients with ADHD. Seidman et al. (1997) found that the word raw score was significantly different in adolescents referred for ADHD after correction was made for age, socioeconomic status, psychiatric comorbidity, and learning disability. The other scores—color raw score, color-word difference raw score, and interference score—were all significantly different in the uncorrected data, but partialling the data for learning disability caused the results to be reduced to nonsignificance. These findings alert the clinician using the Stroop to the fact that many other conditions affect performance on the test, including head injury, age, parkinsonism, and dementia. At least nine studies have used this test with children having ADHD (R. A. Barkley, personal communication, 1998). All have found that the interference portion of the test significantly differentiates ADHD children from control subjects.

Rey-Osterreith Complex Figure. The Rey-Osterreith complex figure (Osterreith 1944; Rey 1941; see also Corwin and Bylsma 1993) is a test involving copying a complex figure followed by recall after a delay period. A number of scoring systems, with a high level of reliability (at 0.90 or above) (e.g., Waber and Holmes 1985), have been developed. The test is sensitive to a variety of neurological impairments, including frontal lobe impairments (Lezak 1995). Scores are assigned for the organization of the copy, the accuracy of the copy, and the organization and accuracy of the delayed recall. In a study of adolescents referred for evaluation of ADHD, the copy organization score significantly differentiated the referred patients from control subjects after the effects of age, socioeconomic status, psychiatric comorbidity, and comorbid learning disability were partialled out. The difference in organization for the delayed trials was significant until the effects of learning disability were partialled out.

The Rey-Osterreith Complex Figure has the advantage of allowing the examiner to look at the organization of test performance that is outside the awareness of most patients. The test presents few cues to failure in most individuals who have difficulty, although some are aware of problems. The scoring system places some burden on the examiner in that it is detailed and takes time and care for accurate scoring.

Paced Auditory Serial Addition Test. The Paced Auditory Serial Addition Test (Gronwall 1977; Gronwall and Sampson 1974) is a commonly used test of working memory in adult neuropsychology (Lezak 1983) administered on computer. The test requires subjects to listen to a string of digits and to add the next digit to the one immediately preceding it, giving the sum of both digits as their response. The test involves 60 digits given in each of four trials, with each trial differing in rates of speed, ranging from 1.2 to 2.4 seconds, and each speed increasing by 0.4 second within this range. The score is the percentage correct for each trial. Tannock et al. (1995) showed that children with ADHD have difficulty with a child version of this task and display significant improvements in performance when stimulant medication is administered. This test most likely reflects verbal working memory. PET scans taken during task performance show that, compared with control subjects, adults with ADHD rely more on visual imagery systems than on verbal rehearsal and have a more shallow learning curve.

Gronwall and Wrightson (1981) concluded that the test is related to differences in information-processing ability. The test has been used for evaluation of patients with traumatic brain injuries (Sohlberg and Mateer 1989). Lezak (1995) cautioned that this test is stressful even for neuropsychiatrically normal subjects. The test is influenced by age in adults but generally is not strongly associated with measures of intelligence (Brittain et al. 1991; Spreen and Strauss 1991); it is, however, associated with levels of education (Delaney et al. 1988). Weber (1986) found that the score on the Paced Auditory Serial Addition Test was highly correlated with the subject's ability to add. The correlation with mathematics ability (or at least addition ability) is not a surprising confound for this type of test. Assessment of the meaning of problematic scores on this test needs to take into account the patient's skills in addition and consider whether the results are due to a learning difficulty, an attention difficulty, or both.

A computerized administration of the test is available (Cegalis 1990), which makes the administration timing more regular and standardized.

EVALUATION PROTOCOL FOR ADHD

A clinician assessing a patient for possible ADHD has a multifaceted task. Practice parameters for the assessment and treatment of children, adolescents, and adults with ADHD have been developed by the American Academy of Child and Adolescent Psychiatry (AACAP) (AACAP 1997); these parameters outline the steps recommended for the evaluation and treatment of patients with ADHD. The list is extensive and comprehensive. In the clinical practice environment of the late 1990s, the clinician is faced with the dilemma of evaluating all the many conditions affecting the patient—both those pertinent to ADHD and those related to comorbid disorders and to alternative disorders that can involve symptoms similar to those of ADHD—and doing so in a cost-effective fashion that addresses the constraints of managed care. The following is recommended as a supplement to the AACAP practice parameters.

Initial Evaluation Interviews

Any evaluation begins with an interview that not only covers the symptoms with which the patient presents, the symptoms and affected areas of ADHD, and possible comorbid or alternative diagnoses, but also involves the observation of the patient and family. The clinician, in assessing ADHD and related conditions, not only faces the usual challenges of clinical evaluation of patients and relatives who may report information partially and selectively, but also must take into account the fact that patients with ADHD and their families are often unaware of critical aspects of functioning that are related to the disorder. Multiple sources of data are important not only with children, who clearly are unable to report the full range of symptoms and conditions, but also with adolescents and adults, who bring their own unique observations and interpretations. ADHD can differ from setting to setting, and collecting observations from multiple settings, including the clinician's office, is crucial to the comprehensive evaluation of the patient.

No diagnostic instrument, test, or procedure can circumvent the need for a skilled, informed clinician knowledgeable about not only ADHD but also general psychopathology. The clinician may want to begin with one of the structured or semistructured interview schedules to ensure that the relevant areas for evaluation are covered. As recommended in the AACAP practice parameters, the initial interview begins with both a history of the presenting symptoms and the patient's psychiatric/psychological history (including previous evaluations, treatments, and interventions), developmental history (including school functioning), medical history, family psychiatric/psychological history (covering both ADHD and comorbid conditions), and social functioning. Areas of strengths are important to assess as well.

If the patient has not had a recent medical evaluation, one should be arranged as part of the overall evaluation; the medical evaluation should include assessment of overall health status and evaluation for special conditions that can affect attention and affective symptoms (e.g., lead levels in children at risk).

Information from family, spouse, teachers, and/or others familiar with the patient is an important addition to the information about the patient. Checklists of ADHD symptoms represent a beginning in obtaining such information. When it is practical to do so, significant others should be interviewed as well.

Mental Status

Determination of the patient's mental status goes beyond but includes the areas of the traditional mental status examination. Medical practitioners are more typically familiar with this aspect of evaluation; nonmedical practitioners need to be alert to the cues that can be obtained in evaluating the patient's responses to a range of questions and observations of attention, memory, judgment, and cognition that can be gleaned from a mental status examination.

Psychological Testing

Psychological testing contributes considerable information that cannot be obtained in any other fashion. Previous psychological testing, whether as part of a school evaluation or as part of a previous clinical evaluation, frequently contributes valuable information about history and functioning. Nonpsychologists typically will arrange with a psychologist colleague for evaluations of cognitive functioning, including intelligence, memory, academic skills and abilities, and (as assessed with specialized instruments) attention, other aspects of executive functioning, and affect.

Psychological assessment begins with assessment of intelligence, but it does not end there. The goal of intellectual assessment is not only to obtain the patient's IQ—although knowledge of the levels of the various spheres of abilities is important in gauging the degree of realization of the patient's capabilities—but also to compare functioning in areas relatively unaffected by ADHD with functioning in areas that are highly sensitive. In addition to IQ scores, indexes of the different areas of functioning reveal important information for the diagnosis. Assessment of memory and concentration is a critical aspect of a psychological evaluation for patients with ADHD. Such an assessment must go beyond the brief and simple assessments of functions to include more extended testing of memory and concentration, such as with the Logical Memory section of the Wechsler Memory Scale—III. Further memory tests are helpful in severe or equivocal cases—for example, the Wide Range Assessment of Memory and Learning or Children's Memory Scale for younger patients, the balance of the Wechsler Memory Scale–III, the California Verbal Learning Test, or one of the sentence memory tests for adults.

Academic skills are important to assess over and above the areas covered by intelligence tests. Not only are ADHD patients more likely to present with significant learning problems (cf. discussion by Rosemary Tannock in Chapter 4, this volume), but they also frequently have specific difficulties in areas such as reading, in which problems emerge in the sustained attention and concentration required for comprehension of extended reading material. A reading test that extends beyond word pronunciation or brief closure items—for example, the Comprehension section of the Nelson-Denny Reading Test (Hammill et al. 1994)—is particularly helpful with older patients. Further assessment of academic skills in mathematics (with, e.g., the Woodcock-Johnson subtests for written calculation, word-problem solving, and quantitative concepts [Woodcock and Johnson 1989]) is a useful addition.

Specialized tests of attention and executive functioning are useful when interview results either suggest a severe disorder or are equivocal. One of the CPT measures (e.g., Conners rating scale or Test of Variables of Attention), will give a useful and well-normed estimate of sustained attention. Careful behavioral observation of the patient as the test is taken adds important information to understanding how and why difficulties are experienced. The Stroop test and the Wisconsin Card Sorting Test give information on the extent of inhibition and conceptual flexibility or rigidity. The Rey-Osterreith Complex Figure gives a useful picture of organization and planning as well as of retention of complex visual material.

Further assessment of comorbid conditions is indicated when the initial interview and reports indicate one or more comorbid conditions or suggest the possibility of an alternative diagnosis. Although the self-report checklists for anxiety and depression are widely used, the limitations of an ADHD patient's use of rating scales need to be kept in mind. The Minnesota Multiphasic Personality Inventory–2 (Butcher et al. 1989) provides a wealth of useful scales for older subjects, but the cooperation of a patient who shows problems with long and repetitive tasks requiring sustained concentration and reading need to be considered. Projective testing—both the Rorschach (Rorschach 1921) and the Thematic Apperception Test (Murray and Bellak 1973)—gives the patient an open-ended opportunity to respond, an approach that often reveals capacities or limitations in imaginative productions, as well as yields the wealth of clinical information such instruments can produce when administered and interpreted by a well-trained practitioner.

CLINICAL EVALUATION FOR ADHD

The steps in an evaluation of ADHD are outlined in the appendix to this chapter. The first portion of the outline comprises the steps for a child or adolescent, and the remaining portion deals with assessment of older adolescents and adults. The decision as to which procedure to use depends on the age of the patient, the maturity of the patient, the availability and willingness of the parent to be involved, and the willingness of the patient to have his or her parent involved. This approach assumes a transition at age 16 years. Some of the measures (e.g., the Wechsler intelligence scales) use different forms for patients above or below this age. Clinicians should feel free to follow procedures and to select measures from either part as appropriate for the patient.

At some points in the outline, a number of alternative measures that my colleagues and I have found useful are listed. One of these measures is usually sufficient. There are many more measures than the ones listed. Inclusion of a measure is not an endorsement, and omission is not a negative comment. There are too many measures in this area to list. Clinicians should evaluate the validity, reliability, and usefulness of the information provided by the measure used.

Children and Adolescents

For younger patients, the initial interview with the patient and parent is usually preceded by gathering information in the referral process. An early decision that must be made pertains to the order in which to interview the patient and the parent (or other collateral informant). For older adolescents, interviewing the patient first can be useful in establishing rapport. When the patient can work collaboratively with the parent, a joint interview with the patient and parent has the advantage of providing a built-in check on minimization or exaggeration by either party. With younger children, a separate appointment for the parent alone may be helpful. To have an angry adolescent or anxious child stewing for the length of the interview with the parent may undermine rapport.

Another important aspect of the interview is to explore the areas of felt competence and strengths. The patient may often anticipate yet another recitation of his or her weaknesses and failures. Recognizing strengths, successful coping, and areas of competence can help convey that the purpose of the intervention is to improve coping and adaptation rather than to punish or simply overcome shortcomings. The clinical interview is not simply a fact-finding effort; it is also the beginning of a collaborative endeavor for which the patient's cooperation and involvement are essential.

The areas to be covered in an evaluation are varied and extensive. The purpose of the evaluation is not simply to establish or rule out the presence of ADHD. Developmental events are evaluated not only to search for evidence of ADHD but also to detect the presence of other conditions that can mimic ADHD symptoms and to assess for the presence of comorbid disorders. In addition to establishing the presence of ADHD, the evaluation addresses the areas affected by the disorder and degree of impairment in these areas. Determination of effective interventions depends on knowledge of where assistance is needed. It is easy to focus on academic areas, but determination of the effects of ADHD on social, nonacademic, and familial functioning is also important for assessment and intervention.

The social and developmental history is gathered for establishing the early signs of ADHD and also for evaluating the patient for other conditions emerging early in childhood. Illnesses, head injuries, and atypical development are important elements in the assessment. Sadly, children with ADHD are all too often the targets of abuse. It is also important to evaluate for other conditions that can produce the symptoms observed or that are exacerbated by ADHD.

Academic history is often a telling component of the evaluation. Grade reports and teachers' comments are useful for assessing the degree to which the patient is able to translate abilities into achievement. All too often, there is a wide discrepancy between potential and realized achievement. School assessments for learning disabilities can be particularly useful but often need to be supplemented by testing. There is a high degree of comorbidity between ADHD and learning disabilities. It is often necessary to determine whether the learning disability is an outgrowth of the ADHD syndrome or a separate problem. Reading disabilities can sometimes appear when the primary problem is difficulty attending to the reading material long enough to understand the meaning.

With the pressures of school budgets, it is not unusual for a patient who is performing below potential to be given no assessments or only cursory ones. Brighter patients often are able to master the demands of early grades, only to "hit the wall" when the transition is made to modular schedules, which make greater demands on organization. In high school, reading and writing demands may finally exceed the limits of concentration and memory.

Comorbid conditions should be screened for routinely. Dysphoric affect, low self-esteem, anxiety, and obsessional traits are often found in patients with a primary attention-deficit disorder, but they can also occur as separate conditions. The order of onset of ADHD and the comorbid condition is particularly important. When the condition occurs before the onset of attentional, concentration, or hyperactivity issues, careful consideration needs to be given as to whether the presenting problem is alternative diagnosis or a comorbid condition. Onset of ADHD symptoms well before other conditions tends to point to primary ADHD; onset after the comorbid condition raises the possibility that the attention, hyperactivity, and impulsivity symptoms are an outgrowth of the primary disorder. Frequently, it is not possible to obtain firm time sequences, and conclusions about the diagnosis are then more tentative.

Gathering data from external sources is crucial for documenting the impact of the condition. Disagreement between parents and teachers is not uncommon. At times, a child is able to maintain a reasonable semblance of focus and attention in the structured setting of the classroom but shows the full range of symptoms in more unstructured settings such as in the home or during social interactions. At other times, the concentration demands of the classroom elicit the symptoms, but a less demanding setting may allow him or her to maintain a more normal level of activity outside school. Checklists from a teacher, especially a teacher who sees the child over the course of the day, are often quite helpful. When multiple teachers are involved, it is worth noting if there are specific areas that are more affected—for example, subjects with a high demand for reading or independent work, mathematics, or subjects like foreign languages that have a high demand for memorization. Nonacademic areas such as sports and music may reflect functioning in areas with different levels of demand. Broad-band instruments help the clinician to document the degree to which other behavior problems are involved and to assess for possible comorbid disorders.

A cognitive evaluation is important for documenting the degree of impairment in intellectual functioning. Although psychological tests without the interview and informant data usually are not sufficient for establishing a diagnosis, such testing can document the degree to which basic cognitive functions are affected. Memory and processing speed are frequently affected. Working verbal memory represents a source of difficulty for complex tasks (e.g., reading, writing, memorization of the vocabulary and grammar of a foreign language). Impulsivity is often observed during a variety of assessment tasks. Slow motor speed may represent a compensation for impulsive activity, and high motor speed relative to the speed in other performance skills can reveal impulsivity. Careless errors may arise from impulsive efforts or distraction. In an evaluation, the observations of how the patient completes the test are often as important as the resulting scores.

An evaluation should also include assessment of learning skills. When such evaluations have been conducted in the school, the data should be incorporated into the evaluation. It is sometimes necessary to supplement the school evaluations with other tests. For example, reading is often evaluated with tests that do not assess comprehension of more extended reading material and that may not include an evaluation of memory. It is often useful to include a test of arithmetic calculation so as to be able to observe the patient when working at arithmetic and to observe the care and precision used in making computations. A writing sample will sometimes reveal an underlying difficulty in expressive language, either as a separate learning deficit or as an outgrowth of impatience and impulsivity. In testing learning skills, it is important to differentiate problems arising from the ADHD symptoms and those that represent a separate learning deficit.

Adults

Adults present somewhat different tasks in evaluation. One challenge is to establish the age at onset of difficulties. The patient's recollection of early experiences is not necessarily reliable; it can be helpful to interview a parent or sibling. Problems of historical accuracy after a long period of time are not readily resolved. This applies to parent, sibling, and patient reports. In examining early records and recollections, the evaluator contends with the fact that problems of attention and concentration are often recalled or recorded in terms of the patient's being "unmotivated," able "to do better if he/she really tried," or, more colloquially, "lazy," "careless," or "willful." Behavior and disciplinary problems may be indications of hyperactive/impulsive symptoms.

Current problems and symptoms are more readily documented. A spouse is often the motivating force for an evaluation. Alternatively, repeated difficulties at work may motivate the patient to seek an evaluation. Adults often present pictures that are complicated by attempts to cope on the one hand and by emerging comorbid conditions on the other. At times, a sympathetic employer can be a helpful adjunct to the evaluation; at other times, the employer represents a party who will be asked to make accommodations and the patient may not want to involve his or her boss, supervisor, or other persons on the job. Similarly, input from spouses or significant others may represent a helpful complement to the data, or the patient's relationship with the spouse or significant other may be so strained that the patient may not want to involve him or her. The clinician may be placed in a role of educating the spouse or significant other as well as the patient.

Evaluation of comorbid conditions is especially important with adult patients. The years of coping with an unrecognized condition often leaves psychological scars. Both adaptive and maladaptive coping strategies can appear as specific conditions (e.g., depression, anxiety, a high level of substance use or dependence) or as generalized personality traits that are attributed to other sources with negative labels such as "lazy," "spacey," and "unmotivated." Quite often, the clinician's job includes overcoming stereotypes held by both the patient and the significant figures around him or her. Implementation of a comprehensive treatment plan needs to take into account the multiple settings in the patient's daily life and the multiple other behaviors, traits, and characteristics that have emerged as a result of living with diagnosed or undiagnosed ADHD.

Cognitive testing with adult patients is often very helpful. The setting in which the patient is placed may involve many implicit, unspoken accommodations and adjustments. More successful patients may meet the demands of the workplace only with intense effort and at the expense of the ability to find enjoyment in other areas (e.g., personal relationships). The relatively standard conditions of the cognitive testing can uncover underlying deficits and reveal modes of adaptation that need to be acknowledged and at times reworked.

The *integration of data*—often diverse and contradictory data—is the skill one seeks in a well-trained clinician. When the clinician collaborates with another practitioner, such as when a psychologist cooperates with a psychiatrist, it is important to discuss the patient's functioning before the testing as well as afterward, beyond the report itself, in order to use the information fully. Under what conditions does the patient do well, and under what conditions does he or she do poorly? What is the congruence or disparity between abilities and test scores on the one hand and realized achievement on the other? Any collaborative arrangement between clinicians requires full and complete communication, but the kinds of anomalies and inconsistencies found with ADHD patients make such active collaboration essential if the patient's interests are to be served.

Assessment is the beginning of a treatment relationship, but the assessment process does not end with the initial report and diagnosis. Selection of treatments—medical, behavioral, and educational—requires the full use of the assessment information. Treatment of the conditions requires ongoing assessment, even in straightforward and apparently effective interventions. Once improvement in the initial level of difficulties occurs, the clinician must ask himself or herself what skills, abilities, and problems remain for continued work or additional interventions and what additional problems will emerge as the patient begins to face the developmental tasks that were not fully completed because of the ADHD and other conditions. Assessment is part of the continuing relationship between patient and clinician and forms an important evaluation of the efficacy of the treatments used. The challenges of assessing and treating patients with ADHD are both complex and rewarding.

REFERENCES

Achenbach TM: Integrative Guide for the 1991 CBCL14–18, YSR, and TRF Profiles. Burlington, University of Vermont, Department of Psychiatry, 1991a

Achenbach TM: Manual for the Teacher's Report Form and 1991 Profile. Burlington, University of Vermont, Department of Psychiatry, 1991b

Achenbach TM: Youth Self-Report Form and Profile for Ages 11–18 (YSR/11–18). Itasca, IL, Riverside, 1991c

Achenbach TM, Edelbrock CS: Psychopathology of childhood. Annual Review of Psychology 35:227–256, 1984

Adams W, Sheslow D: The Wide Range Assessment of Memory and Learning. Wilmington, DE, Jastak Assessments, 1990

American Academy of Child and Adolescent Psychiatry: Practice parameters for the treatment of children, adolescents, and adults with attention-deficit/hyperactivity disorder. American Academy of Child and Adolescent Psychiatry. J Am Acad Child Adolesc Psychiatry 36 (10, suppl):85S–121S, 1997

American Psychiatric Association: Diagnostic and Statistical Manual of Mental Disorders, 3rd Edition, Revised. Washington, DC, American Psychiatric Association, 1987

American Psychiatric Association: Diagnostic and Statistical Manual of Mental Disorders, 4th Edition. Washington, DC, American Psychiatric Association, 1994

Anastasi A: Psychological Testing, 6th Edition. New York, Macmillan, 1988

Anderson SW, Damasio H, Jones RD, et al: Wisconsin Card Sorting Test performance as a measure of frontal lobe damage. J Clin Exp Neuropsychol 13:909–922, 1991

Babcock H: An experiment in the measurement of mental deterioration. Archives of Psychology 117:105, 1930

Banken JA: Clinical utility of considering digits forward and digits backward as separate components of the Wechsler Adult Intelligence Scale—Revised. J Clin Psychol 41:686–691, 1985

Bannatyne A: Diagnosis: a note on recategorization of the WISC scaled scores. Journal of Learning Disabilities 7:272–274, 1974

Barkley RA (ed): Attention Deficit Hyperactivity Disorder: A Handbook for Diagnosis and Treatment. New York, Guilford, 1990

Barkley RA: Attention Deficit Hyperactivity Disorder: Clinical Workbook. New York, Guilford, 1991

Barkley RA: Behavioral inhibition, sustained attention, and executive functions: constructing a unifying theory of ADHD. Psychol Bull 121:65–94, 1997

Barkley RA, Edelbrock CS: Assessing situational variation in children's behavior problems: the Home and School Situations Questionnaires, in Advances in Behavioral Assessment of Children and Families, Vol 3. Edited by Prinz R. Greenwich, CT, JAI Press, 1987, pp 157–176

Barkley RA, Murphy KR: Attention-Deficit Hyperactivity Disorder: A Clinical Workbook. New York, Guilford, 1998

Barkley RA, McMurray MB, Edelbrock CS, et al: The response of aggressive and nonaggressive ADHD children to two doses of methylphenidate. Journal of the American Academy of Child Psychiatry 28:873–881, 1989

Beck AT: Beck Anxiety Inventory. San Antonio, TX, Psychological Corporation, 1990

Beck AT, Steer RA, Brown GK: Beck Depression Inventory–II. San Antonio, TX, Psychological Corporation, 1996

Bennett GK, Seashore HG, Wesman AG: Differential Aptitude Tests, 5th Edition. San Antonio, TX, Psychological Corporation, 1990

Benton AL, Hamsher K DeS: Multilingual Aphasia Examination. Iowa City, IA, AJA Associates, 1989

Berg EA: A simple objective treatment for measuring flexibility in thinking. Journal of General Psychology 39:15–22, 1948

Biggs SH: Neuropsychological and educational testing in the evaluation of the ADD adult, in A Comprehensive Guide to Attention Deficit Disorder in Adults. Edited by Nadeu KG. New York, Brunner/Mazel, 1995, pp 109–134

Black FW: Digit repetition in brain-damaged adults: clinical and theoretical implications. J Clin Psychol 42:770–782, 1986

Black FW, Strub RI: Digit repetition performance in patients with focal brain damage. Cortex 14:12–21, 1978

Bohnen N, Jolles J, Twijnstra A: Modification of the Stroop Color Word Test improves differentiation between patients with mild head injury and matched controls. The Clinical Neuropsychologist 6:178–184, 1992

Brittain JL, La Marche JA, Reeder KP, et al: The effects of age and IQ on the Paced Auditory Serial Addition Test (PASAT) performance. The Clinical Neuropsychologist 5:163–175, 1991

Brown JI, Fishco VV, Hanna G: Nelson-Denny Reading Test. Chicago, IL, Riverside, 1993

Brown TE: Brown Attention-Deficit Disorder Scales. San Antonio, TX, Psychological Corporation/Harcourt Brace Jovanovich, 1996a

Brown TE: Brown ADD Diagnostic Form. San Antonio, TX, Psychological Corporation/Harcourt Brace Jovanovich, 1996b

Brown TE: Brown ADD Scales for Children. San Antonio, TX, Psychological Corporation (in press)

Butcher JN, Dahlstrom WG, Graham JR, et al: MMPI-2. Manual for Administration and Scoring. Minneapolis, University of Minnesota, 1989

Cegalis J: Paced Auditory Serial Attention Task (Computer Version). San Antonio, TX, Psychological Corporation, 1990

Cohen M: Children's Memory Scale. San Antonio, TX, Psychological Corporation, 1997

Conners CK: The computerized continuous performance test. Psychopharmacol Bull 21:891–892, 1985

Conners CK: Conners Rating Scales—Revised. North Tonawanda, NY, Multi-Health Systems, 1997

Conners CK, Erhardt D, Sparrow E: Conners Adult ADHD Rating Scales. North Tonawanda, NY, Multi-Health Systems, 1999

Connolly AJ: The KeyMath Diagnostic Arithmetic Test—Revised. Circle Pines, MN, American Guidance Service, 1988

Corkum PV, Siegel LS: Is the continuous performance test a valuable research tool for use with children with attention-deficit-hyperactivity disorder? J Child Psychol Psychiatry 34:1217–1239, 1993

Corwin J, Bylsma FW: Translations of excerpts from Andre Rey's "Psychological Examination of Traumatic Encephalopathy" and F. A. Osterreith's "The Complex Figure Copy Test." The Clinical Neuropsychologist 7:3–15, 1993

Delaney RC, Prevey ML, Cramer L, et al: Test-retest comparability and control subject data for the PASAT, Rey-AVLT, and Rey-Osterreith/Taylor figures (abstract). J Clin Exp Neuropsychol 10:44, 1988

Delis DC, Kramer J, Kaplan E, et al: California Verbal Learning Test. New York, Psychological Corporation, 1987

Delis DC, Kramer J, Kaplan E, et al: California Verbal Learning Test—Children's Form. New York, Psychological Corporation, 1994

Derogatis LR: Symptom Checklist-90—Revised (SCL-90-R). Minneapolis, MN, NCS Assessments, 1975

Dyer FN: The Stroop phenomenon and its use in the study of perceptual, cognitive, and response processes. Mem Cognit 1:106–120, 1973

Gadow KD, Sprafkin J: Child Symptom Inventories Manual. Stony Brook, NY, Checkmate Plus, 1994

Gadow KD, Sverd J, Sprafkin J, et al: Efficacy of methylphenidate for attention-deficit hyperactivity disorder in children with tic disorder. Arch Gen Psychiatry 52:444–455, 1995

Gadow KD, Sprafkin J, Nolan EE: AD/HD School Observation Code Manual. Stony Brook, NY, Checkmate Plus, 1996

Golden CJ: Stroop Color and Word Test: A Manual for Clinical and Experimental Use. Chicago, IL, Stoelting, 1978

Gordon M: How is a computerized attention test used in the diagnosis of attention deficit disorder? Journal of Children in Contemporary Society 19(1–2):53–64, 1986

Goyette CH, Conners CK, Ulrich RF: Normative data on Revised Conners Parent and Teacher Rating Scales. J Abnorm Child Psychol 6:221–226, 1978

Graffman J, Jonas BS, Salazar A: Wisconsin Card Sorting Test performance based on localization following penetrating head injury in Vietnam veterans. Brain 111: 169–184, 1990

Grant DA, Berg EA: A behavioral analysis of reinforcement and ease of shifting to new responses in a Weigl-type card-sorting problem. Journal of Experimental Psychology 38:404–411, 1948

Greenberg LM, Waldman ID: Developmental normative data on the Test of Variables of Attention (T.O.V.A.). J Child Psychol Psychiatry 4:1019–1030, 1993

Gronwall D: Paced auditory serial addition task: a measure of recovery from concussion. Percept Mot Skills 44:367–373, 1977

Gronwall D, Sampson H: The Psychological Effects of Concussion. Auckland, New Zealand, University Press/Oxford University Press, 1974

Gronwall D, Wrightson P: Memory and information processing capacity after closed head injury. J Neurol Neurosurg Psychiatry 44:889–895, 1981

Hallowell EM, Ratey JJ: Driven to Distraction: Attention Deficit Disorder in Children and Adults. New York, Pantheon, 1994

Hammill DD, Brown VL, Larsen SC, et al: Test of Adolescent and Adult Language, 3rd Edition (TOAL-3). Austin, TX, Pro-Ed, 1994

Hayslip B Jr, Kennelly KJ: Short-term memory and crystallized-fluid intelligence in adulthood. Paper presented at the 88th annual convention of the American Psychological Association, Montreal, Canada, August 1980

Heaton RK: A Manual for the Wisconsin Card Sorting Test. Odessa, FL, Psychological Assessment Resources, 1981

Heaton RK, Chelune GJ, Talley JL, et al: Wisconsin Card Sorting Test Manual: Revised and Expanded. Odessa, FL, Psychological Assessment Resources, 1993

Janowsky JS, Shimamura AP, Kritchevsky M, et al: Cognitive impairment following frontal lobe damage and its relevance to human amnesia. Behav Neurosci 103: 548–560, 1989

Kaplan E, Fein D, Morris R, et al: WAIS-R as a Neuropsychological Instrument. San Antonio, TX, Psychological Corporation, 1991

Kaufman AS, Kaufman NL: Kaufman Brief Intelligence Test (K-BIT). Circle Pines, MN, American Guidance Service, 1990

Klein RG, Abikoff H, Barkley RA, et al: Clinical trials in children and adolescents, in Clinical Evaluation of Psychotropic Drugs: Principles and Guidelines. Edited by Prien RF, Robinson DS. New York, Raven, 1994, pp 501–546

Lezak MD: Neuropsychological Assessment. New York, Oxford University Press, 1983

Lezak MD: Emotional impact of cognitive inefficiencies in mild head traumas (abstract). J Clin Exp Neuropsychol 13:23, 1991

Lezak MD: Neuropsychological Assessment, 3rd Edition. New York, Oxford University Press, 1995

Lezak MD, Whitham R, Bourdette D: Emotional impact of cognitive inefficiencies in multiple sclerosis (MS) (abstract). J Clin Exp Neuropsychol 12:50, 1990

Loney J, Milich R: Hyperactivity, inattention and aggression in clinical practice. Journal of Developmental Behavioral Pediatrics 3:113–147, 1982

Losier B, McGrath PT, Klein RM: Error patterns of the Continuous Performance Test in non-medicated and medicated samples of children with and without Attention Deficit Hyperactivity Disorder: a meta-analytic review. J Child Psychol Psychiatry 37:971–987, 1996

McFie J: Psychological testing in clinical neurology. J Nerv Ment Dis 131:383–393, 1960

Milner B: Effects of different brain lesions on card sorting. Arch Neurol 9:90–100, 1963

Murray H, Bellak L: Thematic Apperception Test. San Antonio, TX, Psychological Corporation, 1973

Orvaschel H, Puig-Antich J: Schedule for Affective Disorders and Schizophrenia for School-Age Children: Epidemiologic Version. Fort Lauderdale, FL, Nova University, Center for Psychological Study, 1987

Osterreith PA: Le test de copie d'une figure complexe (The test of copying a complex figure). Archives de Psychologie 30:206–256, 1944

Pelham WE, Milich R, Murphy DA, et al: Normative data on the IOWA Conners Teacher Rating Scale. J Clin Child Psychol 18:259–262, 1989

Power TJ: Contextual factors in vigilance testing of children with ADHD. J Abnorm Child Psychol 20:579–593, 1992

Quinlan DM, Brown TE: Type of memory impairments in persons with superior IQ and ADHD. Presentation at symposium "Individuals With ADD and Superior IQ: Unique Risks" at the annual meeting of the American Academy of Child and Adolescent Psychiatry, Toronto, Ontario, October 1997a

Quinlan DM, Brown TE: Working memory functions in adults with ADHD. Paper presented at the annual convention of the American Psychological Association, Chicago, IL, August 1997b

Rapaport DO, Gill MM, Shafer R: Diagnostic Psychological Testing, Revised Edition. Edited by Holt RR. New York, International Universities Press, 1968

Rey A: L'examen psychologique dans les cas d'encephalopathie traumatique (Psychological testing in cases of traumatic encephalopathies). Archives de Psychologie 28(112):286–340, 1941

Reynolds CR, Kamphaus RW: Behavior Assessment System for Children. Circle Pines, MN, American Guidance Service, 1992

Robinson AL, Heaton RK, Lehman RAW, et al: The utility of the Wisconsin Card Sorting Test in detecting and localizing frontal lobe lesions. J Consult Clin Psychol 48:605–614, 1980

Rorschach H: Psychodiagnostics. Bern, Medizinicher Verlag Hans Huber [New York, Psychological Corporation]. Available from The Psychological Corporation, San Antonio, TX

Seidman LJ, Biederman J, Faraone SV, et al: Toward defining a neuropsychology of attention deficit-hyperactivity disorder: performance of children and adolescents from a large clinically referred sample. J Consult Clin Psychol 65:150–160, 1997

Shue KL, Douglas VI: Attention deficit hyperactivity disorder and the frontal lobe syndrome. Brain Cogn 20:104–124, 1992

Sohlberg MM, Mateer CA: Introduction to Cognitive Rehabilitation. New York, Guilford, 1989

Sprafkin J, Gadow KD: Early Childhood Inventories Manual. Stony Brook, NY, Checkmate Plus, 1996

Spreen O, Strauss E: A Compendium of Neuropsychological Tests. New York, Oxford University Press, 1991

Tannock R, Ickowicz A, Schachar R: Differential effects of methylphenidate on working memory in ADHD children with and without comorbid anxiety. J Am Acad Child Adolesc Psychiatry 34:886–896, 1995

Teicher MH, Ito Y, Glod CA, et al: Objective measurement of hyperactivity and attentional problems in ADHD. J Am Acad Child Adolesc Psychiatry 35:334–342, 1996

Thorndike RL, Hagen EP, Sattler JM: The Stanford-Binet Intelligence Scale, 4th Edition. Chicago, IL, Riverside Publishing, 1986

Trommer BL, Hoeppner JB, Lorber R, et al: Pitfalls in the use of a continuous performance test as a diagnostic tool in attention deficit disorder. J Dev Behav Pediatr 9:339–345, 1988

Waber DP, Holmes JM: Assessing children's copy productions of the Rey-Osterreith Complex Figure. J Clin Exp Neuropsychol 7:264–280, 1985

Ward MF, Wender PH, Reimherr FW: The Wender Utah Rating Scale: an aid in the retrospective diagnosis of childhood attention deficit hyperactivity disorder. Am J Psychiatry 150:885–890, 1993

Watkins MJ: Concept and measurement of primary memory. Psychol Bull 81:695–711, 1974

Weber AM: Measuring attentional capacity. Unpublished doctoral dissertation, University of Victoria, Victoria, Canada, 1986

Wechsler D: Wechsler Adult Intelligence Scale—Revised. San Antonio, TX, Psychological Corporation, 1981

Wechsler D: Wechsler Memory Scale—Revised. New York, Psychological Corporation, 1987

Wechsler D: Wechsler Preschool and Primary Scale of Intelligence—Revised. San Antonio, TX, Psychological Corporation, 1989

Wechsler D: Manual for the Wechsler Intelligence Scale for Children, 3rd Edition. San Antonio, TX, Psychological Corporation, 1991

Wechsler D: Wechsler Adult Intelligence Scale–III. San Antonio, TX, Psychological Corporation, 1997a

Wechsler D: Wechsler Memory Scale–III. San Antonio, TX, Psychological Corporation, 1997b

Wender PH: The Hyperactive Child, Adolescent and Adult. New York, Oxford University Press, 1987

Witkin HA, Dyk RA, Faterson HF, et al: Psychological Differentiation: Studies of Development. New York, Wiley, 1962

Woodcock RW, Johnson MB: Woodcock-Johnson Psycho-Educational Battery—Revised. Allen, TX, DLM Teaching Resources, 1989

Woodcock RW, McGrew K, Werder J: Mini-Battery of Achievement. Chicago, IL, Riverside, 1994

Zajano MJ, Gorman A: Stroop interference as a function of percentage of congruent items. Percept Mot Skills 63:1087–1096, 1986

Zametkin AJ, Nordahl TE, Gross M, et al: Cerebral glucose metabolism in adults with hyperactivity of childhood onset. N Engl J Med 323:1361–1366, 1990

APPENDIX
OUTLINE OF AN ASSESSMENT FOR ADHD

Clinical Evaluation of Children and Adolescents

I. Clinical interview—patient

   A. Presenting problem(s)

      1. Why does the patient think he/she is coming for an evaluation?
      2. What are the difficulties the patient notices that may suggest a problem?
      3. What are the problems others have pointed out?
      4. When was the presenting problem(s) first noticed?

   B. Strengths and favorite activities

      1. Hobbies and sports
      2. Friends
      3. Favorite activities
      4. Favorite school subjects

   C. School experience

      1. Best subjects and activities
      2. Difficult subjects and activities

   D. Parents, siblings, relatives

II. Clinical interview—parents

A. Presenting problem(s)

1. What are the symptoms observed?
2. What are the current effects of the presenting problem(s)?
3. Who referred the patient?
4. When did the problems appear?
5. What are the current effects on the patient's work/school, social/family, and personal activities?
6. What evaluations have been done for this problem or related problems?

B. Social and developmental history

1. Circumstances of birth: problems with pregnancy, delivery, early infancy
2. Developmental milestones—motor and speech
3. Family environment and interactions with siblings
4. Health history
    a. Major illnesses, especially with high fever
    b. Injuries, especially head injuries
    c. Episodes of seizures and/or loss of consciousness
    d. Allergies and other chronic illnesses
    e. Current medications and purpose of medications
    f. Vision and hearing
    g. Previous experience with psychotropic medications, stimulants
    h. Immunizations and level of medical care
    i. Lead exposure and evaluations

C. Academic history

1. Preschool experience (e.g., nursery school)
2. Early school grades
3. Middle and later school grades
4. Identified learning problems and interventions
5. Strengths and accomplishments
6. School evaluations and placement; ADHD, learning disabilities, special or remedial training or tutoring, other educational interventions

D. Review of DSM-IV criteria

III. Assessment of other conditions

A. Other conditions to be evaluated

1. Depression
2. Anxiety, panic disorder, agoraphobia
3. Aggressive behavior: conduct disorder, oppositional defiant disorder
4. Obsessive-compulsive disorder
5. Pervasive developmental disorders
6. Neurological conditions
7. Tics, Tourette syndrome symptoms
8. Other psychiatric disorders
9. Current pattern and history of alcohol and substance use
10. Mood pattern: mood tone, temper, sensitivity to criticism

IV. Obtaining information from school and other environments

A. Teacher-completed checklists (see Section V below)

B. Other environments

1. Preschool
2. Sports
3. Tutors
4. Music teachers, scout leaders, etc.

V. Tools for evaluation

A. Semistructured interviews (select one of the following)

1. Barkley Clinical Interview Form (Barkley and Murphy 1998)
2. Brown ADD Diagnostic Form for Adolescents (ages 12–18 years) (T. E. Brown 1996b) or Diagnostic Form for Children (ages 3–12 years) (T. E. Brown, in press)

B. Checklists

1. Broad-band assessment (select one of the following)
   a. Child Behavior Checklist (Teachers and Parents) (Achenbach 1991a, 1991b); Youth Self-Report (Adolescents) (Achenbach and Edelbrock 1984; Achenbach 1991c)
   b. Behavior Assessment System for Children (BASC) (Teachers, Parents, and Self-Report) (Reynolds and Kamphaus 1992)
   c. Child Symptom Inventories (Gadow and Sprafkin 1994)

2. ADHD checklists (children and adolescents) (select one of the following)
    a. Barkley's scales (Barkley 1991; Barkley and Murphy 1998)
        i. Disruptive Behavior Rating Scale (Parent and Teacher forms)
        ii. Home Situations Questionnaire
        iii. School Situations Questionnaire
        iv. Issues Checklist for Parents and Teachers
    b. Brown ADD Scales (Child, Parents, Teacher) (T. E. Brown 1996a, 1996b; T. E. Brown, in press)
    c. Conners Parent Rating Scale (Goyette et al. 1978)

V. Cognitive evaluation

A. Ability assessment (select one of the following)

1. Wechsler Intelligence Scale for Children–III (WISC-III; Wechsler 1991)
    a. Verbal, Performance, and Full Scale IQ
    b. Index scores
        i. Verbal Comprehension (WISC-III and Bannatyne Indexes)
        ii. Perceptual organization
        iii. Freedom From Distractibility (working memory)
        iv. Perceptual Speed
2. Stanford-Binet Intelligence Scale, 4th Edition (Thorndike et al. 1986)
3. Kaufman Brief Intelligence Test (Kaufman and Kaufman 1990)

B. Memory testing: Children's Memory Scale (Cohen 1997), Wide Range Assessment of Memory and Learning (Adams and Sheslow 1990)

1. Logical Memory/Story Memory
2. Verbal Memory
3. Visual Memory

C. Academic skills assessment

1. Reading, especially reading comprehension
    a. Nelson-Denny Reading Test (grades 9 and higher) (J. I. Brown et al. 1993)

b. Woodcock-Johnson—Revised Tests of Achievement (Woodcock and Johnson 1989)
c. Mini Battery for Achievement (Woodcock et al. 1994)

2. Mathematics/arithmetic (e.g., Woodcock-Johnson—Revised Tests of Achievement, KeyMath Diagnostic Arithmetic Test—Revised [Connolly 1988])

D. Continuous performance tests (CPTs) (select one of the following)

1. Conners CPT (Conners 1985)
2. Test of Variables of Attention (Greenberg and Waldman 1993)
3. Gordon Diagnostic System (Gordon 1986)

Clinical Evaluation of College Students and Adults

I. Clinical interview

A. Presenting problem(s)

1. Why is the patient coming for an evaluation?
2. Who referred the patient?
3. What are the problems the patient notices that may suggest a problem?
4. What are the problems others have pointed out?
5. When were the presenting problems first noticed?

B. Current effects of the presenting problem(s)

1. What are the current effects on the patient's work/school, social/family, and personal activities?
2. What evaluations have been done for this or related problems?

C. Social and developmental history (interview a parent when practical)

1. Circumstances of birth: problems with pregnancy, delivery, early infancy
2. Developmental milestones—motor and speech
3. Health history
   a. Major illnesses, especially with high fever
   b. Injuries, especially head injuries
   c. Episodes of seizures and/or loss of consciousness
   d. Allergies and other chronic illnesses
   e. Current medications and purpose of medications
   f. Vision and hearing

g. Previous experience with psychotropic medications, stimulants
h. Immunizations and level of medical care
i. Lead and toxic chemical exposure and evaluations
j. Previous experience with psychotropic medications, stimulants
k. Current medications and purpose of medications

D. Academic and occupational history

1. Current status—grade, school, occupation, position
2. Early academic experience—separation, early reading, writing, mathematics
3. Academic performance (elementary, high school, college, further training, graduate/professional schooling)
4. School evaluations and placement; ADHD, learning disabilities, special or remedial training or tutoring, other educational interventions
5. Military service, if applicable
6. Plans for future education
7. Work history (positions, dismissals, difficulties in positions, accomplishments and promotions)

E. Social and familial interaction

1. Friendship patterns, current and past
2. Interpersonal style, strengths and difficulties
3. Intimate relationships (parents, spouse, girlfriends/boyfriends)
4. Description of parents, siblings, spouse/significant other
   a. Academic history, presence of ADHD or learning problems
   b. Other personal characteristics—depression, anxiety, substance use, and other psychiatric diagnoses and symptoms
5. Legal difficulties, motor vehicle violations

F. Interviews with spouse, parent, significant other

G. ADHD symptoms

1. Current symptoms, including review of DSM-IV criteria
2. Past symptoms, patterns of change
3. Effect of ADHD symptoms on functioning

II. Assessment of comorbid and other conditions

   A. Depression

   B. Anxiety, panic disorder, agoraphobia

   C. Aggressive behavior: antisocial, oppositional defiant disorder

   D. Obsessive-compulsive disorder

   E. Pervasive developmental disorders

   F. Neurological conditions—head injuries, seizures, high fevers with delirium

   G. Tics, Tourette syndrome symptoms

   H. Bipolar disorder, cyclothymic personality

   I. Other psychiatric disorders

   J. Current pattern and history of alcohol and substance use

   K. Mood pattern: mood tone, temper, sensitivity to criticism

III. Tools for evaluation

   A. Semistructured interviews (select one of the following)

      1. Barkley clinical interview forms (Barkley and Murphy 1998)
         a. Adult interview
         b. Developmental, employment, health, and social history forms
      2. Brown ADD Diagnostic Form—Adult (T. E. Brown 1996b)

   B. Checklists

      1. Broad-band scales
         a. Minnesota Multiphasic Personality Inventory-2
         b. Symptom Checklist-90—Revised (Derogatis 1975)
         c. Beck Depression Inventory (Beck 1990),
            Beck Anxiety Inventory (Beck et al. 1996)
      2. ADHD checklists for adults (select one of the following)
         a. Barkley's scales (Barkley and Murphy 1998)
            i. Current Symptoms Scale—Self Report Form, Other Report Form
            ii. Childhood Symptoms Scale—Self Report Form, Other Report Form

b. Brown Attention Deficit Disorder Rating Scales (T. E. Brown 1996a)
c. Conners Adult Attention Rating Scales (Conners et al. 1999)

IV. Cognitive evaluation

A. Ability assessment

1. Wechsler Adult Intelligence Scale–III (Wechsler 1997a)
   a. Verbal, Performance, and Full Scale IQ
   b. Index scores
      i. Verbal Comprehension (WAIS-III and Bannatyne Indexes)
      ii. Perceptual organization
      iii. Working Memory
      iv. Processing Speed
2. Stanford-Binet Intelligence Scale, 4th Edition

B. Memory testing: Wechsler Memory Scale–III

1. Logical Memory/Story Memory
2. Other Verbal Memory subtests
3. Visual memory

C. Academic skills assessment

1. Reading, especially reading comprehension
   a. Nelson-Denny Reading Test
   b. Woodcock-Johnson—Revised Tests of Achievement
   c. Mini Battery for Assessment
2. Mathematics/arithmetic (e.g., Woodcock-Johnson—Revised Tests of Achievement, Differential Aptitude Test—Numerical Ability [Bennett et al. 1990])

D. Continuous performance tests (select one of the following)

1. Conners CPT
2. Test of Variables of Attention
3. Gordon Diagnostic System

16 Pharmacotherapy of Attention-Deficit/Hyperactivity Disorder

Timothy E. Wilens, M.D.
Thomas J. Spencer, M.D.
Joseph Biederman, M.D.

With the increasing recognition and knowledge of the complexity of the presentation of attention-deficit/hyperactivity disorder (ADHD) across the life span, there is a need to develop effective pharmacotherapeutic strategies. While there is a robust literature guiding the pharmacological treatment of ADHD in school-age children, there is relatively less known about the pharmacological treatment of this disorder in preschoolers, adolescents, and adults (Spencer et al. 1996). In this chapter, guidelines for the pharmacotherapy of ADHD are delineated, the available information on the use of medications for ADHD is reviewed, and pharmacological strategies suggested for managing ADHD symptoms with accompanying comorbid conditions are discussed.

ASSESSMENT AND DIAGNOSTIC CONSIDERATIONS

Pharmacotherapy should be part of a treatment plan in which consideration is given to all aspects of the patient's life. Hence, it should not be used exclusive of other interventions. The administration of medication to a patient with ADHD should be undertaken as a collaborative effort with the patient and family (or other caregivers), with the physician guiding the use and management of agents shown to be effective in the treatment of ADHD.

The use of medication should follow a careful evaluation of the patient, including psychiatric, social, and cognitive assessments as indicated. Diagnostic information should be gathered from the patient and, whenever possible, from significant others such as parents, partners, and siblings. If ancillary data are not available, information from an adult is acceptable for diagnostic and treatment purposes, since adults with ADHD, as with other disorders, are usually appropriate reporters of their own condition. Careful attention should be paid to the onset of symptoms, longitudinal history of the disorder, and differential diagnosis, including medical/neurological as well psychosocial factors contributing to the clinical presentation.

With the patient with ADHD, issues of comorbidity with learning disabilities and other psychiatric and substance use disorders need to be addressed. Since learning disabilities do not respond to pharmacotherapy, it is important to identify these deficits so as to help define remedial interventions. Since alcohol and substance use disorders are encountered among adolescents and adults with ADHD, a careful history of substance use should be completed. Patients with ongoing abuse or dependence of psychoactive substances generally should not be treated until appropriate addiction treatments have been undertaken and a drug- and alcohol-free period has been maintained (see Chapter 9, this volume). Other concurrent psychiatric disorders also need to be assessed, and, if possible, the relationships of the ADHD symptoms with these other disorders need to be delineated.

MANAGEMENT

The patient and family need to be familiarized with the risks and benefits of pharmacotherapy, the availability of alternative treatments, and the likely adverse effects. Certain adverse effects can be anticipated on the basis of known pharmacological properties of the drug (i.e., appetite change, insomnia), whereas other, more infrequent effects are unexpected (idiosyncratic) and are difficult to anticipate from the properties of the drug. Short-term adverse effects can be minimized by introducing the medication at low initial doses and titrating slowly. Idiosyncratic adverse effects generally require drug discontinuation and selection of alternative treatment modalities.

Patient expectations need to be explored and realistic goals of treatment need to be clearly delineated. Likewise, the clinician should review with those involved in the treatment the various pharmacological options available and note that each will require systematic trials of the anti-ADHD medications for a reasonable duration of time and at clinically meaningful doses. The potential need for adjunctive treatment and agents also should be explained in advance. Individuals with ADHD with significant psychological distress related to their ADHD (i.e., self-esteem issues, self-sabotaging patterns, interpersonal disturbances) should be directed to appropriate psychotherapeutic intervention with clinicians who are knowledgeable in the treatment of ADHD. For example, significant improvement in ADHD and associated symptoms has been reported in adults after administration of cognitive therapies (Wilens et al. 1999b; see also Chapter 18, this volume).

Medications appear to be a mainstay of treatment for ADHD in a wide range of age groups, from school-age youths to adults. Medications used for ADHD include the psychostimulants, antidepressants, and antihypertensives, with some ongoing work on the cognitive enhancers (Table 16–1).

PHARMACOTHERAPY

Stimulants

The stimulant medications are generally the first-line medications for children, adolescents, and adults with ADHD. Stimulants are sympathomimetic drugs structurally similar to endogenous catecholamines (e.g., dopamine and norepinephrine). The most commonly used compounds in this class include methylphenidate (Ritalin), dextroamphetamine sulfate (Dexedrine), amphetamine compounds (Adderall), and pemoline (Cylert). Methylphenidate and dextroamphetamine are both short-acting compounds with an onset of action within 30–60 minutes and a peak clinical effect usually seen 1–2 hours after administration and lasting 2–5 hours. The amphetamine compounds (Adderall) and sustained-release preparations of methylphenidate and dextroamphetamine are intermediate-acting compounds with an onset of action within 60 minutes and a peak clinical effect usually seen from 1 to 3 hours after administration and maintained for up to 8 hours (Swanson et al. 1998a). Pemoline is a long-acting compound with an onset of action within 1 hour and a peak clinical effect usually seen in 1–3 hours and maintained for up to 12 hours (Sallee et al. 1985).

Table 16–1. Psychotropic agents used in the treatment of ADHD

Medication (brand name)	Total daily dose	Daily dosage schedule	Common adverse effects
Stimulants			
Methylphenidate (Ritalin)	0.25–2.0 mg/kg	Two or three times	Insomnia, decreased appetite, weight loss, dysphoria Possible reduction in growth velocity with chronic use Rebound phenomena
Amphetamines	0.15–1.5 mg/kg		
Dextroamphetamine sulfate (Dexedrine)			
Amphetamine compound (Adderall)			
Methamphetamine hydrochloride (Desoxyn Gradumet)			
Pemoline (Cylert)	1.0–3.0 mg/kg	One time	Same as those of other stimulants Abnormal liver function tests
Antidepressants			
Tricyclic antidepressants	2.0–5.0 mg/kg	One or two times	Dry mouth, constipation Weight loss Vital signs and ECG changes
Desipramine, imipramine			
Nortriptyline	1.0–3.0 mg/kg		
Bupropion hydrochloride (Wellbutrin)	3.0–6.0 mg/kg	Three times	Irritability, insomnia Risk of seizures (in doses >6 mg/kg) Contraindicated for patients with bulimia
Venlafaxine hydrochloride (Effexor)	0.5–3.0 mg/kg	Two or three times	Nausea Sedation Gastrointestinal distress

(continued)

Table 16–1. Psychotropic agents used in the treatment of ADHD *(continued)*

Medication (brand name)	Total daily dose	Daily dosage schedule	Common adverse effects
Antihypertensives			
Clonidine hydrochloride (Catapres)	3–10 μg/kg	Two or three times	Sedation, dry mouth, depression
			Confusion (with high dose)
			Rebound hypertension
			Localized irritation (with patch)
Guanfacine hydrochloride (Tenex)	30–100 μg/kg	Two times	Similar to those of clonidine, but less sedation
			Insomnia, irritability reported

Note. ECG = electrocardiogram.

Although there are more than 250 controlled studies of stimulants in the treatment of attention-deficit disorders, involving more than 6,000 children, adolescents, and adults, the vast majority of the studies were limited to latency-age Caucasian boys treated for no longer than 2 months. These studies documented the short-term efficacy and safety of stimulants in all age groups but more clearly in latency-age children. Despite the findings on the efficacy of the stimulants, studies have also reported consistently that, on average, as many as 30% of children with ADHD (Barkley 1977; Gittelman 1980; Wilens and Biederman 1992) and 50% of adults (Wilens et al. 1998) do not respond to these drugs.

Although methylphenidate is by far the best-studied stimulant, the literature suggests more similarities than differences in response to the various available stimulants (Pelham et al. 1990). However, some patients who do not respond or cannot tolerate one stimulant may respond favorably to another (Arnold et al. 1978; Elia et al. 1991). This difference in response is not surprising because the various classes of stimulants have slightly different mechanisms of action (Arnold et al. 1978; Elia et al. 1991; Wilens and Spencer 1998). For example, whereas methylphenidate and pemoline are specific for blockade of the dopamine transporter protein, amphetamines, in addition to blocking the dopamine transporter protein, release dopamine stores and cytoplasmic dopamine directly into the synaptic cleft (for review, see Wilens and Spencer 1998). Moreover, amphetamines release serotonin and norepinephrine to a greater extent than other stimulants (Wilens and Spencer 1998).

More recently, a preparation of amphetamine compounds (Adderall) has emerged as another-stimulant-class agent approved for the treatment of ADHD. Because this compound has four different preparations of amphetamine (including three dextro forms and one levo form), its pharmacokinetic and pharmacodynamic profile is different from that of the other stimulants. Initial studies of Adderall indicate that this compound, like dextroamphetamine, is approximately twice as potent as methylphenidate (Swanson et al. 1998a, 1998b). Studies by Swanson and colleagues with school-age youths suggest that the behavioral and cognitive effects of this compound have an onset within 1 hour and last 6–8 hours (Swanson et al. 1998a, 1998b). Adverse effects appear to be similar to those of dextroamphetamine.

Although the efficacy of stimulants in the treatment of ADHD is most clearly documented for latency-age children, a more limited literature reveals a good response in both preschool-age children and adolescents. Studies in preschool-age children report improvement in structured tasks as well as mother-child interactions (Barkley 1988; Barkley et al. 1984; Conners 1975; Mayes et al. 1994; Musten et al. 1997; Schleifer et al. 1975). Similarly, in adolescents, response has been reported as moderate to robust, with no abuse or tolerance noted (Brown and Sexson 1988; Coons et al. 1987; Evans and Pelham 1991; Klorman et al. 1987; Lerer and Lerer 1977; MacKay et al. 1973; Safer and Allen 1975; Varley 1983). In adults, response has been variable, with this variation largely related to definition of outcome and dosing of the stimulants (Gualtieri et al. 1985; Iaboni et al. 1996; Mattes et al. 1984; Shekim et al. 1990; Spencer et al. 1995; Wender et al. 1981, 1985a; Wilens et al. 1999a; Wood et al. 1976).

Areas of controversy and concern about stimulant use include long-term efficacy concerns (Gillberg et al. 1997), growth suppression in children (Safer et al. 1972; Mattes and Gittelman 1983), the development of tics (Lowe et al. 1982), drug abuse (Drug Enforcement Administration 1995; Jaffe 1991), use in adolescents and adults (Evans and Pelham 1991), and symptom rebound (Johnston et al. 1988). Although stimulants routinely produce anorexia and weight loss, their effect on growth in height is less certain. Although initial reports suggested that there was a persistent stimulant-associated decrease in growth in height in children (Mattes and Gittelman 1983; Safer et al. 1972), other reports have failed to substantiate this finding (Gross 1976; Satterfield et al. 1979). Ultimate height appears to be unaffected (Gittelman and Mannuzza 1988). However, no studies have examined the effects of stimulants on growth in children treated continually from childhood through adolescence and young adulthood. Moreover, the literature on stimulant-associated growth deficits did not examine the possibility that growth deficits may represent maturational delays related to ADHD itself (i.e., dysmaturity) rather than to stimulant treatment. In a recent report using data from a longitudinal study of children with ADHD, Spencer et al. (1998) suggested that growth deficits in children with ADHD may represent a temporary delay in the tempo of growth but that final height is not compromised. They suggested that this effect is mediated by ADHD and not by stimulant treatment.

Media attention, coupled with case reports of stimulant abuse by inhalation (Jaffe 1991), has highlighted uncertainties about the abuse potential of stimulants in individuals with ADHD. Despite the knowledge that ADHD is an independent risk factor for later substance abuse in adolescents and young adults (see Chapter 9, this volume), there is a paucity of scientific data showing that children with ADHD being treated with a stimulant abuse the prescribed medication or demonstrate a later sensitivity or abuse preference for stimulant-class agents. In fact, the predominant literature suggests the opposite—namely, that adolescents sucessfully treated with stimulants are less likely to demonstrate subsequent illegal drug use (Biederman et al. 1999; Kramer et al. 1981; Loney et al. 1981). However, anecdotal and systematically derived data do indicate that diversion of stimulants from ADHD to non-ADHD youths continues to be a problem (Drug Enforcement Administration 1995). Practitioners should advise youths with ADHD and parents about the potential for theft and resale of stimulants and the need for careful storage and monitoring of these medications.

Antidepressants

The antidepressants are generally considered second-line drugs of choice in the treatment of ADHD. The tricyclic antidepressants (TCAs) include the tertiary amines amitriptyline, protriptyline, and imipramine and the secondary amines desipramine and nortriptyline. The mechanism of action of TCAs in the treatment of ADHD appears to involve primarily the blocking effects of these drugs on the reuptake of central nervous system neurotransmitters, especially norepinephrine. However, these agents also have variable effects on pre- and postsynaptic neurotransmitter systems, and this results in differing positive and adverse effect profiles. Unwanted side effects may emerge from activity at histaminic sites (sedation, weight gain), cholinergic sites (dry mouth, constipation), α-adrenergic sites (postural hypotension), and serotonergic sites (sexual dysfunction). In general, the secondary amines are more selective (noradrenergic) than the tertiary amines and have fewer side effects—an important consideration in sensitive juvenile populations.

TCAs, especially imipramine and desipramine, are the second most studied compounds in the pharmacotherapy of ADHD after the stimulants. Thirty-one studies (19 controlled; 12 open) have evaluated TCAs in 1,060 children and adolescents and 63 adults with ADHD. Almost all these studies (93%) reported at least moderate improvement. As with the stimulants, however, the majority of studies included primarily latency-age children. Similar effectiveness of these agents has been shown in both short- (weeks) and long-term (<2 years) studies. Despite assertion to the contrary, evidence exists that improvement of ADHD symptoms can be maintained when daily doses of TCAs are titrated upward over time (Gastfriend et al. 1985; Wilens et al. 1993). For example, studies using aggressive doses of TCAs reported sustained improvement for up to 1 year with desipramine (>4 mg/kg) (Biederman et al. 1986; Gastfriend et al. 1985) and nortriptyline (2 mg/kg) (Wilens et al. 1993).

In the largest controlled study of a TCA in children, our group reported favorable results with desipramine in 62 clinically referred children and adolescents with ADHD (Biederman et al. 1989). Clinically and statistically significant differences in behavioral improvement were found with desipramine compared with placebo, at an average daily dose of 5 mg/kg. Our group obtained similar results in a similarly designed controlled clinical trial of desipramine in 41 adults with ADHD (Wilens et al. 1996c). Desipramine, at an average daily dose of 150 mg (average serum level of 113 ng/mL), was statistically and clinically more effective than placebo. In both pediatric and adult studies, 68% of desipramine-treated patients, compared with fewer than 10% of the placebo-treated patients, had a response—a response rate that places the effectiveness of desipramine below that of the stimulants. Because of cardiac concerns about desipramine ("Sudden Death in Children Treated With a Tricyclic Antidepressant." *The Medical Letter* 1990), recent attention has been paid to other TCAs, including protriptyline and nortriptyline.

Open trials and case series of nortriptyline in heterogeneous populations of children and adolescents with ADHD have yielded uniformly positive responses (Kurtis 1966; Spencer et al. 1993; Watter and Dreifuss 1973; Wilens et al. 1993). In a prospective, placebo-controlled discontinuation trial, we recently demonstrated the efficacy of nortriptyline in daily doses of up to 2 mg/kg daily in 35 school-age youths with ADHD (Prince et al., in press). In that study, 80% of youths responded by week 6 in the open phase. During the discontinuation phase, the subjects randomized to placebo showed a rapid loss of the effect, in contrast to those receiving nortriptyline, in whom a robust anti-ADHD effect was maintained. ADHD youths receiving nortriptyline were also found to have significant reductions in oppositionality and anxiety. Nortriptyline was well tolerated, with weight gain being a desirable adverse effect. Because of its similarities to nortriptyline, its long half-life, and its stimulant-like properties, we also evaluated protriptyline for ADHD. In a systematic report on 14 youths with treatment-refractory ADHD receiving protriptyline (mean total daily dose = 30 mg), we found that only 45% of the youths responded favorably or could tolerate protriptyline secondary to adverse effects (Wilens et al. 1996a).

Taken together, the available literature suggests that TCAs are effective in controlling abnormal behaviors and improving cognitive impairments associated with ADHD but that they are less effective than the majority of stimulants (Gualtieri and Evans 1988; Quinn and Rapoport 1975; Rapport et al. 1993; Werry 1980). Our data suggest differences in ADHD efficacy of the various TCAs, with desipramine and imipramine being considered more effective relative to nortriptyline and amitriptyline, and protriptyline the least effective of the TCAs.

The potential benefits of TCAs in the treatment of juvenile ADHD have been clouded by concerns about the safety of these agents stemming from older reports of sudden unexplained death in four children with ADHD who were treated with desipramine ("Sudden Death in Children Treated With a Tricyclic Antidepressant" 1990). However, the causal link between desipramine and those deaths remains uncertain. A recent report estimated that the magnitude of desipramine-associated risk of sudden death in children may not be much larger than the baseline risk of sudden death in this age group (Biederman et al. 1995). Moreover, these deaths have been difficult to reconcile with the rather extensive literature evaluating cardiovascular parameters in TCA-exposed patients of all ages and the magnitude of worldwide use of TCAs in all age groups. In most studies, TCA treatment has been associated with asymptomatic, minor, but statistically significant increases in heart rate and electrocardiographic measures of cardiac conduction times consistent with those reported in the adult literature (Wilens et al. 1996b). Given their efficacy, monitoring, adverse effects, and theoretical risk concerns, TCAs should be used only after stimulants have been tried for ADHD in juveniles. Electrocardiographic monitoring at baseline and therapeutic dosing are suggested but not mandatory.

Bupropion hydrochloride is a novel aminoketone antidepressant related to the phenylisopropylamines but pharmacologically distinct from available antidepressants (Casat et al. 1989). Although bupropion possesses both indirect dopaminergic and noradrenergic agonist effects, its specific site or mechanism of action remains unknown. Bupropion was reported to be superior to placebo in reducing ADHD symptoms in two controlled studies in children: a multisite study (*N* = 72) (Casat et al. 1987; Conners et al. 1996a) and a comparison study with methylphenidate (*N* = 15) (Barrickman et al. 1995). In an open study of 19 adults treated with an average total daily dose of 360 mg of bupropion for 6–8 weeks, Wender and Reimherr (1990) reported a moderate to marked response in 74% of the subjects, with sustained improvement at 1 year noted in 53% of the subjects. The response of ADHD to bupropion appears to be rapid and sustained. Dosing of bupropion for ADHD is similar to that recommended for depression. Based on anecdotal reports of anti-ADHD effectiveness at low dosing (i.e., total daily dose <75 mg) in a minority of patients, it is recommended that the treatment be initiated at 37.5 mg and titrated upward every 3–4 days until an effective dose is reached. Bipolar patients with ADHD also benefit from the use of low dosing of bupropion, which reduces the risk for manic activation. Maximal dosing in youths is not established; however, we employ a total daily dose of 300 mg in younger children and 450 mg in older children as parameters for upward dosing. Given its utility in reducing cigarette smoking, improving mood, lack of monitoring requirements, and paucity of adverse effects, bupropion is often used as a first-line agent for patients with complex cases of ADHD in which there is comorbid substance abuse or an unstable mood disorder (Riggs 1998; Wozniak and Biederman 1996).

Preliminary studies suggest that monoamine oxidase inhibitors (MAOIs) are effective in the treatment of juvenile and adult ADHD. In a recent open study (Jankovic 1993), selegiline (L-deprenyl), a specific MAO-B inhibitor at low dose, was evaluated in 29 children with both ADHD and tics. Results indicated that 90% of the children showed improvement in their ADHD symptoms with no serious adverse effects and with only two patients showing an exacerbation of tics. In a 12-week double-blind, cross-over trial using two MAOIs—clorgiline (a specific MAO-A inhibitor) and tranylcypromine (a mixed MAO-A/B inhibitor)—in 14 hyperactive children, Zametkin et al. (1985) reported significant and rapid reduction in ADHD symptoms with minimal adverse effects. In open and controlled studies of adult ADHD, marginal improvements were reported in studies with pargyline and selegiline, along with associated adverse effects (Ernst et al. 1996; Wender et al. 1983, 1985b). A major limitation to the use of MAOIs is the potential for hypertensive crisis (treatable with verapamil) associated with dietetic transgressions (tyramine-containing foods, such as most cheeses) and drug interactions (such as with pressor amines, most cold medicines, and amphetamines).

Although not systematically evaluated, the serotonin reuptake inhibitors do not appear to be useful for ADHD. Although a small open study (Barrickman et al. 1991) suggested that fluoxetine may be beneficial in the treatment of children with ADHD, extensive clinical experience at our center with children, adolescents, and adults does not support the usefulness of these compounds in the treatment of core ADHD symptoms. Venlafaxine, an atypical serotonin reuptake inhibitor with noradrenergic reuptake inhibition, may have some efficacy in the treatment of ADHD. Preliminary results from open studies of venlafaxine in children and adults with ADHD and prominent conduct or mood symptoms indicated moderate improvement with this agent; however, a sizable minority of treated patients could not tolerate the adverse effects (Adler et al. 1995; Findling et al. 1996; Reimherr et al. 1995).

Clonidine

Clonidine is an imidazoline derivative with α-adrenergic agonist properties that has been used primarily in the treatment of hypertension. Clonidine is a relatively short-acting compound, with a plasma half-life ranging from approximately 6 hours (in children) to 9 hours (in adults) (Hunt et al. 1985). Usual daily dose ranges from 3 to 10 μg/kg (ca. 0.05 mg–0.6 mg), given generally in divided doses up to four times daily. Clonidine has been used for the treatment of ADHD as well as associated tics, aggression, and sleep disturbances (Fankhauser et al. 1992; Hunt et al. 1986; Leckman et al. 1991), particularly with younger children. In the treatment of patients with psychiatric disorders in which ADHD was part of the clinical picture, there have been over 30 studies (more than six of which were controlled trials), involving more than 500 children and adolescents, assessing its efficacy (Wilens and Spencer 1999). In the vast majority of these studies, clonidine was reported to be associated with a clinically significant improvement as derived from open or retrospective chart reviews or it was demonstrated to be superior to placebo in controlled investigations.

Coadministration of clonidine and other agents such as the stimulants, despite a lack of controlled data, is prescribed for ADHD youths with aggression, hyperactivity/impulsivity, and sleep disturbance. For example, an improved response was reported in 41 children with ADHD who were receiving the combination of methylphenidate and clonidine compared with either agent alone (Comings et al. 1990). Observations from large case series indicate that methylphenidate and clonidine improved behavioral functioning and concomitantly led to a 40% reduction in methylphenidate dose (Hunt 1989). Our group previously reported the results of a large systematic chart review in which 85% of 62 children receiving clonidine (42 receiving stimulants in combination) at a mean follow-up of 3 years reported improvement in their sleep (Prince et al. 1996).

More recently, four cases of death in children who had received clonidine plus other medications, including methylphenidate, have raised concern about the cardiovascular safety of clonidine. Three of these cases were captured by the Food and Drug Administration (FDA) (Fenichel 1995), and one was captured through another source (Cantwell et al. 1997). In review of these cases, converging evidence from independent investigation (Popper 1995), the FDA (Fenichel 1995), and the National Heart, Lung, and Blood Institute of the National Institutes of Health (Diane Atkins, M.D., Chair, Special Emphasis Panel on Cardiac Arrhythmias in Children, August 29, 1996) indicated that many mitigating and extenuating circumstances were operative, making these cases uninterpretable (Wilens and Spencer 1999). For example, in one of the cases, a 9-year-old child who was receiving promethazine, clonidine, methylphenidate, and fluoxetine died after multiple symptoms, including seizures. Autopsy revealed extraordinarily high blood levels of fluoxetine and promethazine, with the death being ascribed to overdose. Moreover, in studies monitoring the adverse effects of clonidine, no clinically meaningful electrocardiographic changes have been identified.

Antipsychotics

Although earlier studies indicated the efficacy of the antipsychotic agents for ADHD, these studies focused on the behavioral ramifications of ADHD and neglected the cognitive aspects of the disorder. Furthermore, the short- and long-term adverse effects of these agents preclude their use except in cases of refractory ADHD. More recently, the atypical antipsychotics (olanzapine, risperidone, quetiapine) have been employed in the treatment of ADHD and associated behavioral disturbances. Although controlled data are lacking, we recently reviewed the course of 25 children and adolescents treated with risperidone in our clinic for a variety of psychiatric disorders (Frazier et al. 1999). In the majority of youths receiving risperidone, marked diminution in mood lability and outbursts was observed; however, only 10% of those with ADHD were found to have clinically meaningful improvement in their ADHD symptoms.

Alternative Psychoactive Agents

There has been long-standing interest in alternative psychoactive agents for the treatment of ADHD. Among these compounds, amino acids and cognitive enhancers have been systematically assessed. Although, anecdotally, the herbal remedies ginkgo, blue-green algae, and pycnogenol have been advanced for ADHD, no systematically derived data on their effectiveness are available.

Amino Acids

Trials with amino acids were undertaken, in part, with the assumptions that ADHD may be related to a deficiency in the catecholaminergic system and that administration of precursors of these systems would reverse these deficits. The results of open studies of L-dopa and L-tyrosine and controlled studies of phenylalanine in adults with ADHD have generally been disappointing despite robust dosing and adequate trial duration (Reimherr et al. 1987; Wood et al. 1982, 1985). In these studies, transient improvement in ADHD was lost after 2 weeks of treatment.

Nicotine

More recently, the relationship of nicotine and ADHD has attracted attention, yielding, among others, findings of higher-than-expected overlap of cigarette smoking among children with ADHD (Milberger et al. 1997) and adults (Pomerleau et al. 1996). One small study of brief duration showed a significant reduction in ADHD symptoms and improvement in working memory and neuropsychological function in adults wearing standard-sized nicotine patches (Conners et al. 1996b). Moreover, we have observed the efficacy of the nicotine patch in reducing ADHD symptoms in smokers who report the emergence of ADHD symptoms with cigarette cessation.

Other Cognitive Enhancers

Other cholinergic-based cognitive enhancers have also been evaluated for ADHD. We recently completed a 7-week, double-blind, placebo-controlled, randomized, cross-over trial comparing a transdermal patch of ABT-418, a novel cholinergic activating agent with structural similarities to nicotine, with placebo in 32 adults with ADHD. A significantly higher proportion of subjects were considered improved while receiving ABT-418 than while receiving placebo (40% vs. 13%; $P < 0.05$). Similarly, a significantly greater proportion of patients manifested improvement in ADHD symptoms of 30% or more during the ABT-418 phase compared with the placebo phase (47% vs. 22%; $P < 0.03$). Although only a modest reduction was observed in the ADHD symptom checklist scores during the ABT-418 phase relative to the placebo phase ($P = 0.056$), this effect was more robust in milder cases ($P = 0.025$).

ABT-418 was relatively well tolerated, with dizziness, skin irritation, nausea, and headaches the side effects most frequently reported. The cognitive-enhancing cholinergic agent donepezil hydrochloride (Aricept), which has been shown to have efficacy in the treatment of patients with Alzheimer's disease, is the subject of a multisite study in adults with ADHD, but the results remain to be reported.

PSYCHIATRIC COMORBIDITY

Aggression

Several controlled studies reported improvement in ADHD and aggressive symptoms in ADHD subjects treated with stimulants (Cunningham et al. 1991; Gadow et al. 1990; Hinshaw et al. 1989, 1992; Kaplan et al. 1990; Klorman et al. 1988, 1989, 1994; Pelham et al. 1990). Stimulants suppressed physical and nonphysical aggression in these children both at home and in school in a dose-dependent fashion (Gadow et al. 1990; Hinshaw et al. 1989; Murphy et al. 1992). In fact, a recent study demonstrated methylphenidate efficacy for youths with conduct disorder independent of ADHD status (Klein et al. 1997). Stimulants also reduced negative social interactions (Whalen et al. 1987) and covert antisocial behavior (stealing, destroying property, but not cheating) (Hinshaw et al. 1992). Four studies of antidepressants for ADHD children with comorbid conduct disorder also indicated improvement in ADHD (Biederman et al. 1993; Simeon et al. 1986; Wilens et al. 1993; Winsberg et al. 1972) and aggressive symptoms in these subjects (Simeon et al. 1986; Winsberg et al. 1972). Clonidine has been shown to be useful in aggressive patients and patients with developmental disorders for controlling aggression directed at self and others (Fankhauser et al. 1992; Kemph et al. 1993; Schvehla et al. 1994).

Motor Tics

Although stimulants have been thought to precipitate or exacerbate tic symptoms in children with ADHD who have a personal or family history of tics, the extant literature on the subject is equivocal. For example, although new onset of tics has been noted in prospective acute-treatment studies of youths with ADHD (Barkley et al. 1990; Borcherding et al. 1990), retrospective chronic treatment studies of children with ADHD failed to document such an association (Denckla et al. 1976; Lipkin et al. 1994). Similarly mixed is the literature on stimulant exacerbation of preexisting tics in children with ADHD. Although more recent controlled studies reported limited exacerbation of tics in children with ADHD and comorbid tics who were exposed to stimulants (Gadow et al. 1995; Sverd et al. 1989, 1992), numerous earlier studies documented exacerbation of tics in up to 31% of children with ADHD who had preexisting tics (Caine et al. 1984; Comings and Comings 1988; Denckla et al. 1976; Erenberg 1982; Erenberg et al. 1985; Golden 1977, 1982; Konkol et al. 1990; Price et al. 1986; Shapiro and Shapiro 1981). The only prospective longitudinal study of its kind reported that 30% of children with ADHD and comorbid tics had to discontinue stimulant treatment because of worsening of the tics (Castellanos et al. 1997).

In a large, controlled, longitudinal naturalistic study of youths with ADHD, we found a significant overrepresentation of tic disorders in referred boys with ADHD compared with a control sample of boys without ADHD. However, the rates of new onset of tics emerging during the follow-up period, as well as the rates of cessation of tics, were identical in ADHD probands with tic disorders receiving medication and those not receiving medication for ADHD; this suggests that the use of stimulants in this sample of children with ADHD had no discernible effect on the course of the tics (Spencer et al. 1999). Although our findings and those of others are reassuring, group data need to be interpreted with caution: although group data do not show a high prevalence of stimulant-associated tics, at the individual level such tics can be severe and incapacitating. Thus, clinicians should carefully monitor the course of stimulant treatment in children with ADHD who show signs of a tic disorder.

Anxiety and Mood

Little is known about the pharmacotherapy of ADHD and comorbid anxiety or mood disorders in children, adolescents, and adults. Of nine stimulant studies in children with ADHD and comorbid anxiety or depression, the majority reported a diminished response to stimulants in those patients (DuPaul et al. 1994; Pliszka 1989; Swanson et al. 1978; Tannock et al. 1995; Taylor et al. 1987; Voelker et al. 1983). Since stimulants are thought to be anxiogenic and depressogenic, caution should be used in the treatment of individuals with ADHD and comorbid anxiety and mood disorders. In contrast, in the TCA studies that examined the effect of medication on comorbid symptoms, TCA treatment improved both ADHD and anxiety (Prince et al., in press) and depressive symptoms (Biederman et al. 1993; Garfinkel et al. 1983; Wilens et al. 1996c).

Despite increasing recognition of the co-occurrence of ADHD and bipolar disorder (West et al. 1995; Wozniak et al. 1995), little is known about the pharmacotherapy of the combined condition. In a systematic assessment of youths with bipolar disorder, we recently reported little activation of mania with stimulants or TCAs when the youths were receiving mood stabilizers (Biederman et al., in press). Moreover, we also found that success of controlling ADHD symptoms in youths with bipolar disorder is highly dependent on appropriate mood stabilization: in those youths who were judged to have low mood lability, TCAs and stimulants were effective in reducing the ADHD. On the other hand, in those youths with an unstable mood or who were reported to have experienced a relapse in their moodiness, ADHD treatment was unsuccessful (Biederman et al., in press). These findings further the important notion of careful attention to mood status prior to intervention for ADHD.

Substance Abuse

For youths with ADHD and comorbid substance abuse, increasing interest has been paid to the treatment of the ADHD while minimizing the likelihood of abuse of the medication or craving exacerbation (see Chapter 9, this volume). Until more data are available for adolescents and young adults, it has been recommended that treatment should utilize antidepressants (bupropion or TCAs) as first-line agents followed by stimulant medications (Riggs 1998; Wilens et al. 1996d) if antidepressants prove to be ineffective.

COMBINED PHARMACOTHERAPY

Despite evidence that in clinical practice many patients with ADHD are receiving multiple treatments, the literature on combined pharmacotherapy is sparse and does not permit the development of clear therapeutic guidelines. In contrast to polypharmacy, rational combined pharmacological approaches can be used for the treatment of comorbid ADHD—as augmentation strategies for patients with insufficient response to a single agent, as way to effect pharmacokinetic synergism, and for the management of treatment-emergent adverse effects (Wilens et al. 1994). Examples of the rational use of combined treatment include the use of an antidepressant plus a stimulant in the treatment of ADHD and comorbid depression (Gammon and Brown 1993), use of clonidine to ameliorate stimulant-induced insomnia (Prince et al. 1996), use of an ADHD medication to heighten the response to another (i.e., desipramine plus methylphenidate) (Rapport et al. 1993; Wilens et al. 1993), and use of a mood stabilizer plus an anti-ADHD agent to treat ADHD comorbid with bipolar disorder (Biederman et al., in press).

TREATMENT-REFRACTORY ADHD

Despite the availability of various agents for ADHD, a number of individuals appear to be either nonresponsive to or intolerant of the adverse effects of medications used to treat the ADHD. In managing patients with apparent medication nonresponse, several therapeutic strategies are available. If adverse psychiatric effects develop concurrent with a poor medication response, alternative treatments should be pursued. Individuals who are nonresponsive to one stimulant should be considered for another stimulant trial (Elia et al. 1991). If two stimulant trials are unsuccessful, bupropion and the TCAs are reasonable second-line agents. Antihypertensive agents may be useful for younger children or for children with prominent hyperactivity, impulsivity, and aggressiveness. MAOIs and cognitive activators (donepezil) may be considered for youths with highly refractory cases. Combined stimulant/antidepressant/antihypertensive regimens may accentuate the response to monotherapy.

Psychiatric symptoms that emerge during the acute phase can be problematic, irrespective of the efficacy of the medications for ADHD. These symptoms may require reconsideration of the diagnosis of ADHD and careful reassessment of the presence of comorbid disorders. If reduction of dose or change in preparation (i.e., regular vs. slow-release stimulants) does not resolve the problem, consideration should be given to alternative treatments. Concurrent use of the newer antidepressants, mood stabilizers, benzodiazepines, and neuroleptics may be necessary in complex cases. Nonpharmacological interventions such as behavioral and cognitive therapies may assist with symptom reduction.

CONCLUSION

ADHD is increasingly recognized as a heterogeneous disorder that persists in a substantial number of cases into adult years. The scope of comorbidity has expanded to include not only conduct disorder and oppositional defiant disorder but also mood, anxiety, and substance use disorders. If not recognized and attended to, the combination of comorbid symptoms and ADHD may lead to high morbidity and disability with poorer long-term prognosis. Emerging research findings support a genetic and neurobiological basis for ADHD, with catecholaminergic dysfunction as a central finding.

An extensive literature supports the short- and long-term effectiveness of pharmacotherapy not only for the core behavioral symptoms of ADHD but also for linked impairments, such as impairments in cognition, social skills, and family function. The armamentarium of anti-ADHD compounds includes not only the stimulants but also several antidepressants and other medications such as clonidine and guanfacine. Stimulant medications continue to be the first-line drugs of choice for uncomplicated ADHD in individuals of all ages, with TCAs and bupropion for patients who do not respond or who have concurrent psychiatric disorders. Current clinical experience suggests that multiple agents may be necessary for successful treatment in some cases of complex ADHD in which the patients have partial responses or psychiatric comorbidity.

REFERENCES

Adler L, Resnick S, Kunz M, et al: Open-label trial of venlafaxine in attention deficit disorder. Paper presented at the New Clinical Drug Evaluation Unit Program, Orlando, FL, 1995

Arnold LE, Christopher J, Huestis R, et al: Methylphenidate vs dextroamphetamine vs caffeine in minimal brain dysfunction. Arch Gen Psychiatry 35:463–473, 1978

Barkley RA: A review of stimulant drug research with hyperactive children. J Child Psychol Psychiatry 18:137–165, 1977

Barkley RA: The effects of methylphenidate on the interactions of preschool ADHD children with their mothers. J Am Acad Child Adolesc Psychiatry 27:336–341, 1988

Barkley RA, Karlsson J, Strzelecki E, et al: Effects of age and Ritalin dosage on mother-child interactions of hyperactive children. J Consult Clin Psychol 52: 750–758, 1984

Barkley RA, McMurray MB, Edelbrock CS, et al: Side effects of methylphenidate in children with attention deficit hyperactivity disorder: a systematic, placebo-controlled evaluation. Pediatrics 86:184–192, 1990

Barrickman L, Noyes R, Kuperman S, et al: Treatment of ADHD with fluoxetine: a preliminary trial. J Am Acad Child Adolesc Psychiatry 30:762–767, 1991

Barrickman L, Perry P, Allen A, et al: Bupropion versus methylphenidate in the treatment of attention-deficit hyperactivity disorder. J Am Acad Child Adolesc Psychiatry 34:649–657, 1995

Biederman J, Gastfriend DR, Jellinek MS: Desipramine in the treatment of children with attention deficit disorder. J Clin Psychopharmacol 6:359–363, 1986

Biederman J, Baldessarini RJ, Wright V, et al: A double-blind placebo controlled study of desipramine in the treatment of attention deficit disorder, I: efficacy. J Am Acad Child Adolesc Psychiatry 28:777–784, 1989

Biederman J, Baldessarini RJ, Wright V, et al: A double-blind placebo controlled study of desipramine in the treatment of attention deficit disorder, III: lack of impact of comorbidity and family history factors on clinical response. J Am Acad Child Adolesc Psychiatry 32:199–204, 1993

Biederman J, Thisted R, Greenhill L, et al: Estimation of the association between desipramine and the risk for sudden death in 5- to 14-year-old children. J Clin Psychiatry 56(3):87–93, 1995

Biederman J, Wilens T, Mick E, et al: Pharmacotherapy of attention-deficit/hyperactivity disorder reduces risk for substance use disorder. Pediatrics 104(2):e20 [available at http://www.pediatrics.org/egi/content/full/104/2/e20]

Biederman J, Mick E, Bostic JQ, et al: Pharmacologic treatment of ADHD in youth with severe mood instability: a systematic chart review. J Child Adolesc Psychopharmacol (in press)

Borcherding BG, Keysor CS, Rapoport JL, et al: Motor/vocal tics and compulsive behaviors on stimulant drugs: is there a common vulnerability? Psychiatry Res 33: 83–94, 1990

Brown RT, Sexson SB: A controlled trial of methylphenidate in black adolescents. Clin Pediatr 27:74–81, 1988

Caine E, Ludlow C, Polinsky R, et al: Provocative drug testing in Tourette's syndrome: d- and l-amphetamine and haloperidol. J Am Acad Child Adolesc Psychiatry 23:147–152, 1984

Cantwell D, Swanson J, Connor D: Case study: adverse response to clonidine. J Am Acad Child Adolesc Psychiatry 36:539–544, 1997

Casat CD, Pleasants DZ, Van Wyck Fleet J: A double-blind trial of bupropion in children with attention deficit disorder. Psychopharmacol Bull 23:120–122, 1987

Casat CD, Pleasants DZ, Schroeder DH, et al: Bupropion in children with attention deficit disorder. Psychopharmacol Bull 25:198–201, 1989

Castellanos FX, Giedd JN, Elia J, et al: Controlled stimulant treatment of ADHD and comorbid Tourette's syndrome: effects of stimulant and dose. J Am Acad Child Adolesc Psychiatry 36:589–596, 1997

Comings DE, Comings BG: Tourette's syndrome and attention deficit disorder, in Tourette's syndrome and Tic Disorders: clinical Understanding and Treatment. Edited by Cohen DJ, Bruun RD, Leckman JF. New York, Wiley, 1988, pp 119–136

Comings D, Comings B, Tacket T: The clonidine patch and behavior problems (letter). J Am Acad Child Adolesc Psychiatry 29:667–668, 1990

Conners CK: Controlled trial of methylphenidate in preschool children with minimal brain dysfunction. International Journal of Mental Health 4:(1–2):61–74, 1975

Conners CK, Casat CD, Gualtieri CT, et al: Bupropion hydrochloride in attention deficit disorder with hyperactivity. J Am Acad Child Adolesc Psychiatry 35:1314–1321, 1996a

Conners CK, Levin ED, Sparrow E, et al: Nicotine and attention in adult attention deficit hyperactivity disorder. Psychopharmacol Bull 32:67–73, 1996b

Coons HW, Klorman R, Borgstedt AD: Effects of methylphenidate on adolescents with a childhood history of ADHD, II: information processing. J Am Acad Child Adolesc Psychiatry 26:368–374, 1987

Cunningham C, Siegel L, Offord D: A dose-response analysis of the effects of methylphenidate on the peer interactions and simulated classroom performance of ADD children with and without conduct problems. J Child Psychol Psychiatry 32:439–452, 1991

Denckla MB, Bemporad JR, MacKay MC: Tics following methylphenidate administration: a report of 20 cases. JAMA 235:1349–1351, 1976

Drug Enforcement Administration: Methylphenidate Review Document. Washington, DC, Drug Enforcement Administration, Office of Diversion Control, Drug and Chemical Evaluation Section, October 1995

DuPaul G, Barkley R, McMurray M: Response of children with ADHD to methylphenidate: interaction with internalizing symptoms. J Am Acad Child Adolesc Psychiatry 33:894–903, 1994

Elia J, Borcherding BG, Rapoport JL, et al: Methylphenidate and dextroamphetamine treatments of hyperactivity: are there true nonresponders? Psychiatry Res 36:141–155, 1991

Erenberg G: Stimulant medication in Tourette's syndrome (letter). JAMA 248:1062, 1982

Erenberg G, Cruse RP, Rothner AD: Gilles de la Tourette's syndrome: effects of stimulant drugs. Neurology 35:1346–1348, 1985

Ernst M, Liebenauer L, Jons P, et al: Selegiline in adults with attention deficit hyperactivity disorder: clinical efficacy and safety. Psychopharmacol Bull 32:327–334, 1996

Evans SW, Pelham WE: Psychostimulant effects on academic and behavioral measures for ADHD junior high school students in a lecture format classroom. J Abnorm Child Psychol 19:537–552, 1991

Fankhauser MP, Karumanchi VC, German ML, et al: A double-blind, placebo-controlled study of the efficacy of transdermal clonidine in autism. J Clin Psychiatry 53(3):77–82, 1992

Fenichel RF: Combining methylphenidate and clonidine: the role of post-marketing surveillance. J Child Adolesc Psychopharmacol 5:155–156, 1995

Findling R, Schwartz M, Flannery D, et al: Venlafaxine in adults with ADHD: an open trial. J Clin Psychiatry 57:184–189, 1996

Frazier JA, Meyer MC, Biederman J, et al: Risperidone treatment for juvenile bipolar disorder: a case series. J Am Acad Child Adolesc Psychiatry 38:960–965, 1999

Gadow KD, Nolan EE, Sverd J, et al: Methylphenidate in aggressive-hyperactive boys, I: effects on peer aggression in public school settings. J Am Acad Child Adolesc Psychiatry 29:710–718, 1990

Gadow K, Sverd J, Sprafkin J, et al: Efficacy of methylphenidate for ADHD in children with tic disorder. Arch Gen Psychiatry 52:444–455, 1995

Gammon GD, Brown TE: Fluoxetine and methylphenidate in combination for treatment of attention deficit disorder and comorbid depressive disorder. J Child Adolesc Psychopharmacol 3:1–10, 1993

Garfinkel BD, Wender PH, Sloman L, et al: Tricyclic antidepressant and methylphenidate treatment of attention deficit disorder in children. J Am Acad Child Adolesc Psychiatry 22:343–348, 1983

Gastfriend DR, Biederman J, Jellinek MS: Desipramine in the treatment of attention deficit disorder in adolescents. Psychopharmacol Bull 21:144–145, 1985

Gillberg C, Melander H, Knorring A, et al: Long-term stimulant treatment of children with ADHD symptoms: a randomized, double-blind, placebo-controlled trial. Arch Gen Psychiatry 54:865–870, 1997

Gittelman R: Childhood disorders, in Drug Treatment of Adult and Child Psychiatric Disorders. Edited by Klein D, Quitkin F, Rifkin A, et al. Baltimore, MD, Williams & Wilkins, 1980, pp 576–756

Gittelman R, Mannuzza S: Hyperactive boys almost grown up, III: methylphenidate effects on ultimate height. Arch Gen Psychiatry 45:1131–1134, 1988

Golden G: The effect of central nervous system stimulants on Tourette syndrome. Ann Neurol 2:69–70, 1977

Golden G: Stimulant medication in Tourette's syndrome (letter). JAMA 248:1063, 1982

Gross M: Growth of hyperkinetic children taking methylphenidate, dextroamphetamine, or imipramine/desipramine. J Pediatr 58:423–431, 1976

Gualtieri CT, Evans RW: Motor performance in hyperactive children treated with imipramine. Percept Mot Skills 66:763–769, 1988

Gualtieri CT, Ondrusek MG, Finley C: Attention deficit disorder in adults. Clin Neuropharmacol 8:343–356, 1985

Hinshaw S, Buhrmester D, Heller T: Anger control in response to verbal provocation: effects of stimulant medication for boys with ADHD. J Abnorm Child Psychol 17:393–407, 1989

Hinshaw S, Heller T, McHale J: Covert antisocial behavior in boys with attention-deficit hyperactivity disorder: external validation and effects of methylphenidate. J Consult Clin Psychol 60:274–281, 1992

Hunt R: Advances in pediatric psychopharmacology. Presentation at the annual meeting of the American Academy of Child and Adolescent Psychiatry, New York, October 1989

Hunt RD, Minderaa RB, Cohen DJ: Clonidine benefits children with attention deficit disorder and hyperactivity: report of a double-blind placebo-crossover therapeutic trial. J Am Acad Child Adolesc Psychiatry 24:617–629, 1985

Hunt RD, Minderaa RB, Cohen DJ: The therapeutic effect of clonidine and attention deficit disorder with hyperactivity: a comparison with placebo and methylphenidate. Psychopharmacol Bull 22:229–236, 1986

Iaboni F, Bouffard R, Minde K, et al: The efficacy of methylphenidate in treating adults with attention-deficit/hyperactivity disorder. Poster presented at the annual meeting of the American Academy of Child and Adolescent Psychiatry, Philadelphia, PA, October 1996

Jaffe SL: Intranasal abuse of prescribed methylphenidate by an alcohol and drug abusing adolescent with ADHD. J Am Acad Child Adolesc Psychiatry 30:773–775, 1991

Jankovic J: Deprenyl in attention deficit associated with Tourette's syndrome. Arch Neurol 50:286–288, 1993

Johnston C, Pelham WE, Hoza J, et al: Psychostimulant rebound in attention deficit disordered boys. J Am Acad Child Adolesc Psychiatry 27:806–810, 1988

Kaplan SL, Busner J, Kupietz S, et al: Effects of methylphenidate on adolescents with aggressive conduct disorder and ADDH: a preliminary report. J Am Acad Child Adolesc Psychiatry 29:719–723, 1990

Kemph JP, DeVane CL, Levin GM, et al: Treatment of aggressive children with clonidine: results of an open pilot study. J Am Acad Child Adolesc Psychiatry 32:577–581, 1993

Klein RG, Abikoff H, Klass E, et al: Clinical efficacy of methylphenidate in conduct disorder with and without attention deficit hyperactivity disorder. Arch Gen Psychiatry 54:1073–1080, 1997

Klorman R, Coons HW, Borgstedt AD: Effects of methylphenidate on adolescents with a childhood history of attention deficit disorder, I: clinical findings. J Am Acad Child Adolesc Psychiatry 26:363–367, 1987 [published erratum appears in J Am Acad Child Adolesc Psychiatry 26:820, 1987]

Klorman R, Brumaghim JT, Salzman LF, et al: Effects of methylphenidate on attention-deficit hyperactivity disorder with and without aggressive/noncompliant features. J Abnorm Psychol 97:413–422, 1988

Klorman R, Brumaghim JT, Salzman LF, et al: Comparative effects of methylphenidate on attention-deficit hyperactivity disorder with and without aggressive/noncompliant features. Psychopharmacol Bull 25:109–113, 1989

Klorman R, Brumaghim J, Fitzpatrick P, et al: Clinical and cognitive effects of methylphenidate on children with attention deficit disorder as a function of aggression/oppositionality and age. J Abnorm Psychol 103:206–221, 1994

Konkol R, Fischer M, Newby R: Double-blind, placebo-controlled stimulant trial in children with Tourette's syndrome and ADHD (abstract). Ann Neurol 28:424, 1990

Kramer J, Loney J, Whaley-Klahn M: The role of prescribed medication in hyperactive youths' substance use. Poster presented at the annual convention of the American Psychological Association, Los Angeles, 1981

Kurtis LB: Clinical study of the response to nortriptyline on autistic children. International Journal of Neuropsychiatry 2:298–301, 1966

Leckman JF, Hardin MT, Riddle MA, et al: Clonidine treatment of Gilles de la Tourette's syndrome. Arch Gen Psychiatry 48:324–328, 1991

Lerer RJ, Lerer MP: Responses of adolescents with minimal brain dysfunction to methylphenidate. Journal of Learning Disabilities 10:223–228, 1977

Lipkin P, Goldstein I, Adesman A: Tics and dyskinesias associated with stimulant treatment in attention-deficit hyperactivity disorder. Arch Pediatr Adolesc Med 148:859–861, 1994

Loney J, Kramer J, Milich RS: The hyperactive child grows up: predictors of symptoms, delinquency and achievement at followup, in Psychosocial Aspects of Drug Treatment for Hyperactivity. Edited by Gadow K, Loney J. Boulder, CO, Westview Press, 1981, pp 381–415

Lowe TL, Cohen DJ, Detlor J: Stimulant medications precipitate Tourette's syndrome. JAMA 247:1168–1169, 1982

MacKay MC, Beck L, Taylor R: Methylphenidate for adolescents with minimal brain dysfunction. New York State Journal of Medicine 73:550–554, 1973

Mattes JA, Gittelman R: Growth of hyperactive children on maintenance regimen of methylphenidate. Arch Gen Psychiatry 40:317–321, 1983

Mattes JA, Boswell L, Oliver H: Methylphenidate effects on symptoms of attention deficit disorder in adults. Arch Gen Psychiatry 41:1059–1063, 1984

Mayes S, Crites D, Bixler E, et al: Methylphenidate and ADHD: influence of age, IQ and neurodevelopmental status. Dev Med Child Neurol 36:1099–1107, 1994

Milberger S, Biederman J, Faraone SV, et al: ADHD is associated with early initiation of cigarette smoking in children and adolescents. J Am Acad Child Adolesc Psychiatry 36:37–44, 1997

Murphy D, Pelham W, Lang A: Aggression in boys with attention deficit-hyperactivity disorder: methylphenidate effects on naturalistically observed aggression, response to provocation, and social information processing. J Abnorm Child Psychol 20:451–466, 1992

Musten LM, Firestone P, Pisterman S, et al: Effects of methylphenidate on preschool children with ADHD: cognitive and behavioral functions. J Am Acad Child Adolesc Psychiatry 36:1407–1415, 1997

Pelham W, Greenslade K, Vodde-Hamilton M, et al: Relative efficacy of long-acting stimulants on children with attention deficit-hyperactivity disorder: a comparison of standard methylphenidate, sustained-release methylphenidate, sustained-release dextroamphetamine, and pemoline. Pediatrics 86:226–237, 1990

Pliszka SR: Effect of anxiety on cognition, behavior, and stimulant response in ADHD. J Am Acad Child Adolesc Psychiatry 28:882–887, 1989

Pomerleau O, Downey K, Stelson F, et al: Cigarette smoking in adult patients diagnosed with ADHD. J Subst Abuse 7:373–378, 1996

Popper CW: Combining methylphenidate and clonidine: pharmacologic questions and news reports about sudden death. J Child Adolesc Psychopharmacology 5:157–166, 1995

Price AR, Leckman JF, Pauls DL, et al: Gilles de la Tourette's syndrome: tics and central nervous system stimulants in twins and nontwins. Neurology 36:232–237, 1986

Prince J, Wilens T, Biederman J, et al: Clonidine for ADHD related sleep disturbances: a systematic chart review of 62 cases. J Am Acad Child Adolesc Psychiatry 35:599–605, 1996

Prince J, Wilens T, Biederman J, et al: A controlled trial of nortriptyline for children and adolescents with ADHD. J Child Adolesc Psychopharmacol (in press)

Quinn PO, Rapoport JL: One-year follow-up of hyperactive boys treated with imipramine or methylphenidate. Am J Psychiatry 132:241–245, 1975

Rapport MD, Carlson GA, Kelly KL, et al: Methylphenidate and desipramine in hospitalized children, I: separate and combined effects on cognitive function. J Am Acad Child Adolesc Psychiatry 32:333–342, 1993

Reimherr FW, Wender PH, Wood DR, et al: An open trial of L-tyrosine in the treatment of attention deficit hyperactivity disorder, residual type. Am J Psychiatry 144:1071–1073, 1987

Reimherr FW, Hedges D, Strong R, et al: An open-trial of venlafaxine in adult patients with attention deficit hyperactivity disorder. Poster presented at the New Clinical Drug Evaluation Unit Program, Orlando, FL, 1995

Riggs P: Clinical approach to treatment of ADHD in adolescents with substance use disorders and conduct disorder. J Am Acad Child Adolesc Psychiatry 37:331–332, 1998

Safer DJ, Allen RP: Stimulant drug treatment of hyperactive adolescents. Diseases of the Nervous System 36:454–457, 1975

Safer DJ, Allen RP, Barr E: Depression of growth in hyperactive children on stimulant drugs. N Engl J Med 287:217–220, 1972

Sallee F, Stiller R, Perel J, et al: Oral pemoline kinetics in hyperactive children. Clinical Pharmacological Therapy 37:606–609, 1985

Satterfield JH, Cantwell DP, Schell A, et al: Growth of hyperactive children treated with methylphenidate. Arch Gen Psychiatry 36:212–217, 1979

Schleifer N, Weiss G, Cohen N, et al: Hyperactivity in preschoolers and the effect of methylphenidate. Am J Orthopsychiatry 45:38–50, 1975

Schvehla TJ, Mandoki MW, Sumner GS: Clonidine therapy for comorbid attention deficit hyperactivity disorder and conduct disorder: preliminary findings in a children's inpatient unit. South Med J 87:692–695, 1994

Shapiro AK, Shapiro E: Do stimulants provoke, cause, or exacerbate tics and Tourette syndrome. Compr Psychiatry 22:265–273, 1981

Shekim WO, Asarnow RF, Hess E, et al: A clinical and demographic profile of a sample of adults with attention deficit hyperactivity disorder, residual state. Compr Psychiatry 31:416–425, 1990

Simeon JG, Ferguson HB, Van Wyck Fleet J: Bupropion effects in attention deficit and conduct disorders. Can J Psychiatry 31:581–585, 1986

Spencer T, Biederman J, Wilens T, et al: Nortriptyline treatment of children with attention deficit hyperactivity disorder and tic disorder or Tourette's syndrome. J Am Acad Child Adolesc Psychiatry 32:205–210, 1993

Spencer T, Wilens TE, Biederman J, et al: A double-blind, crossover comparison of methylphenidate and placebo in adults with childhood-onset attention deficit hyperactivity disorder. Arch Gen Psychiatry 52:434–443, 1995

Spencer T, Biederman J, Wilens T, et al: Pharmacotherapy of attention-deficit hyperactivity disorder across the life cycle. J Am Acad Child Adolesc Psychiatry 35:409–432, 1996

Spencer T, Biederman J, Wilens T: Growth deficits in ADHD children. Pediatrics 102 (suppl 2):501–506, 1998

Spencer T, Biederman J, Coffey B, et al: The 4-year course of tic disorders in boys with ADHD. Arch Gen Psychiatry 56:842–847, 1999

Sudden death in children treated with a tricyclic antidepressant. The Medical Letter 32(816):37–40, 1990

Sverd J, Gadow KD, Paolicelli LM: Methylphenidate treatment of attention-deficit hyperactivity disorder in boys with Tourette's syndrome. J Am Acad Child Adolesc Psychiatry 28:574–579, 1989

Sverd J, Gadow K, Nolan E, et al: Methylphenidate in hyperactive boys with comorbid tic disorder, I: clinic evaluations. Adv Neurology 58:271–281, 1992

Swanson J, Kinsbourne M, Roberts W, et al: Time-response analysis of the effect of stimulant medication on the learning ability of children referred for hyperactivity. Pediatrics 61:21–24, 1978

Swanson J, Wigal S, Greenhill L, et al: Analog classroom assessment of Adderall in children with ADHD. J Am Acad Child Adolesc Psychiatry 37:519–526, 1998a

Swanson J, Wigal S, Greenhill L, et al: Objective and subjective measures of the pharmacodynamic effects of Adderall in the treatment of children with ADHD in a controlled laboratory classroom setting. Psychopharmacol Bull 34:55–60, 1998b

Tannock R, Ickowicz A, Schachar R: Differential effects of methylphenidate on working memory in ADHD children with and without comorbid anxiety. J Am Acad Child Adolesc Psychiatry 34:886–896, 1995

Taylor E, Schachar R, Thorley G, et al: Which boys respond to stimulant medication? A controlled trial of methylphenidate in boys with disruptive behaviour. Psychol Med 17:121–143, 1987

Varley CK: Effects of methylphenidate in adolescents with attention deficit disorder. Journal of the American Academy of Child Psychiatry 22:351–354, 1983

Voelker SL, Lachar D, Gdowski LL: The personality inventory for children and response to methylphenidate: preliminary evidence for predictive validity. J Pediatr Psychol 8:161–169, 1983

Watter N, Dreifuss FE: Modification of hyperkinetic behavior by nortriptyline. Virginia Medical Monthly 100(2):123–126, 1973

Wender PH, Reimherr FW: Bupropion treatment of attention-deficit hyperactivity disorder in adults. Am J Psychiatry 147:1018–1020, 1990

Wender PH, Reimherr FW, Wood DR: Attention deficit disorder ('minimal brain dysfunction') in adults: a replication study of diagnosis and drug treatment. Arch Gen Psychiatry 38:449–456, 1981

Wender PH, Wood DR, Reimherr FW, et al: An open trial of pargyline in the treatment of attention deficit disorder, residual type. Psychiatry Res 9:329–336, 1983

Wender PH, Reimherr FW, Wood D, et al: A controlled study of methylphenidate in the treatment of attention deficit disorder, residual type, in adults. Am J Psychiatry 142:547–552, 1985a

Wender PH, Wood DR, Reimherr FW: Pharmacological treatment of attention deficit disorder, residual type (ADDRT, "minimal brain dysfunction," "hyperactivity") in adults. Psychopharmacol Bull 21:222–232, 1985b

Werry J: Imipramine and methylphenidate in hyperactive children. J Child Psychol Psychiatry 21:27–35, 1980

West S, McElroy S, Strakowski S, et al: Attention deficit hyperactivity disorder in adolescent mania. Am J Psychiatry 152:271–274, 1995

Whalen C, Henker B, Swanson J, et al: Natural social behaviors in hyperactive children: dose effects of methylphenidate. J Consult Clin Psychol 55:187–193, 1987

Wilens TE, Biederman J: The stimulants. Psychiatr Clin North Am 15:191–222, 1992

Wilens T, Spencer T: Amphetamine pharmacology, in Handbook on Substance Abuse: Neurobehavioral Pharmacology. Edited by Tarter R, Ammerman R, Ott P. New York, Plenum, 1998, pp 501–513

Wilens T, Spencer T: Combining methylphenidate and clonidine: a clinically sound medication option. J Am Acad Child Adolesc Psychiatry 38:614–619, 1999

Wilens TE, Biederman J, Geist DE, et al: Nortriptyline in the treatment of attention deficit hyperactivity disorder: a chart review of 58 cases. J Am Acad Child Adolesc Psychiatry 32:343–349, 1993

Wilens T, Spencer T, Biederman J, et al: Combined pharmacotherapy: an emerging trend in pediatric psychopharmacology. J Am Acad Child Adolesc Psychiatry 34: 110–112, 1994

Wilens TE, Biederman J, Abrantes AM, et al: A naturalistic assessment of protriptyline for attention-deficit hyperactivity disorder. J Am Acad Child Adolesc Psychiatry 35:1485–1490, 1996a

Wilens TE, Biederman J, Baldessarini RJ, et al: Cardiovascular effects of therapeutic doses of tricyclic antidepressants in children and adolescents. J Am Acad Child Adolesc Psychiatry 35:1491–1501, 1996b

Wilens T, Biederman J, Prince J, et al: A double-blind, placebo-controlled trial of desipramine for adults with ADHD. Am J Psychiatry 153:1147–1153, 1996c

Wilens TE, Biederman J, Spencer T: Attention deficit hyperactivity disorder and the psychoactive substance use disorders, in Pediatric Substance Use Disorders. Edited by Jaffee S. Philadelphia, PA, WB Saunders, 1996d, pp 73–91

Wilens TE, Biederman J, Spencer TJ: Pharmacotherapy of attention deficit hyperactivity disorder in adults. CNS Drugs 9:347–356, 1998

Wilens T, Biederman J, Spencer T, et al: Controlled trial of high doses of pemoline for adults with attention-deficit/hyperactivity disorder. J Clin Psychopharmacol 19:257–264, 1999a

Wilens T, McDermott S, Biederman J, et al: Cognitive therapy for adults with ADHD: a systematic chart review of 26 cases. Journal of Cognitive Psychotherapy: An International Quarterly 13, No. 3, 1999b

Winsberg BG, Bialer I, Kupietz S, et al: Effects of imipramine and dextroamphetamine on behavior of neuropsychiatrically impaired children. Am J Psychiatry 128: 1425–1431, 1972

Wood DR, Reimherr FW, Wender PH, et al: Diagnosis and treatment of minimal brain dysfunction in adults. Arch Gen Psychiatry 33:1453–1460, 1976

Wood D, Reimherr J, Wender PH: Effects of levodopa on attention deficit disorder, residual type. Psychiatry Research, 6:13–20, 1982

Wood DR, Reimherr FW, Wender PH: The treatment of attention deficit disorder with d,l-phenylalanine. Psychiatry Res 16:21–26, 1985

Wozniak J, Biederman J: A pharmacological approach to the quagmire of comorbidity in juvenile mania. J Am Acad Child Adolesc Psychiatry 35:826–828, 1996

Wozniak J, Biederman J, Kiely K, et al: Mania-like symptoms suggestive of childhood-onset bipolar disorder in clinically referred children. J Am Acad Child Adolesc Psychiatry 34:867–876, 1995

Zametkin A, Rapoport JL, Murphy DL, et al: Treatment of hyperactive children with monoamine oxidase inhibitors, I: clinical efficacy. Arch Gen Psychiatry 42:962–966, 1985

17 Psychosocial Interventions for Attention-Deficit Disorders and Comorbid Conditions

Thomas E. Brown, Ph.D.

NATURE AND USES OF PSYCHOSOCIAL INTERVENTIONS

Psychosocial interventions for attention-deficit disorders (ADDs) and comorbid disorders include a wide variety of social and behavioral activities. Included in this broad category are almost all interventions used to treat ADDs and comorbid conditions except for interventions involving the chemical actions of medications. Psychosocial interventions include conversations between a clinician and a patient, instructional sessions for parents about behavior management strategies to use with their children, individual coaching of adults who are seeking to improve their workplace efficiency, conjoint family therapy to improve communication between adolescents and their parents, and many other types of interpersonal interaction, some of which are also discussed in other chapters in this volume.

Psychosocial interventions have a variety of purposes:

- Educate patients and families about the nature, causes, and course of ADDs and comorbid disorders and the benefits and risks of available treatment options for these conditions
- Monitor patients and adjust treatments they are receiving
- Teach management skills and advocacy skills to patients with ADD and their families
- Provide therapy and support for patients with ADD and their families

Psychosocial interventions alone usually do not provide the most effective treatment for ADDs and comorbid disorders. The recent National Institute of Mental Health multisite Multimodal Treatment Study of Children With AD/HD (MTA) (MTA Cooperative Group, in press) provided clear evidence to confirm that the most effective treatment for most persons with ADDs is a well-tailored ongoing course of stimulant medication. Psychosocial interventions alone do not come close to alleviating the symptoms of ADDs as effectively as does appropriate medication, carefully prescribed and consistently monitored, for those 70%–80% of persons with ADD who respond to medication treatment. Yet medication is not effective for 20%–30% of persons with ADDs (Spencer et al. 1996); for these persons, other treatments are critically important. And even for those persons who can benefit from medication treatment, psychosocial interventions play a very important role.

Psychosocial interventions can be powerfully helpful to individuals with ADDs and their families. They can provide a beginning point for understanding the nature of ADDs and comorbid conditions, which can serve as an antidote to the sense of isolation and helplessness that demoralizes so many individuals and families affected by ADDs. Psychosocial interventions are the vehicle for communicating accurate information about treatment possibilities, which may kindle enough hope for persons to seek evaluation and treatment for ADD symptoms and related problems that they had previously felt so hopeless about or considered so shameful that they never sought assistance.

Without psychosocial interventions, the benefits of treatment with medication may never be experienced by a person with an ADD. Pills alone cannot effectively treat an ADD. The whole process of medication prescription and use is inextricably enmeshed in psychosocial processes. Without effective psychosocial interventions to adequately assess the patient, to educate the patient and family about the disorder and its treatments, to elicit from the patient accurate reports about side effects and benefits and limitations of his or her medication use, and to provide support for related problems, it is unlikely both that the medication will be appropriately tailored to the individual patient and that it will be consistently taken. Medication cannot produce therapeutic effects if it is not taken correctly and consistently.

Even when medication treatment is being used effectively, psychosocial interventions may play a critical role in helping patients with ADDs and their families to address aspects of the impairments associated with these disorders that are not sufficiently changed by medication alone. When a student is diagnosed and begins treatment for an ADD, even if the medication is very effective, it does not teach the student how to study effectively or how to make up for academic skills that were inadequately learned because of an untreated ADD. Nor does the medication teach the student how to cope with peers who want to borrow the medication or tease him or her for being "one of those ADD kids."

Moreover, a student's taking medication for an ADD does not help parents implement necessary changes in their attempts to micromanage the student's homework. Nor does the medication provide parents with strategies to modify their long-standing pattern of arguing over whether their child should be given more or less opportunity to use the family car. Nor does the medication give parents answers as they respond to their uninformed neighbors or relatives who are persistently critical, asking, "Why are you giving your child that dangerous medication instead of just making her shape up?"

Some psychosocial interventions are directed specifically to the child, adolescent, or adult diagnosed with an ADD; other psychosocial interventions are more focused on parents, siblings, spouses, or other family members who frequently interact with the individual diagnosed with an ADD; still other psychosocial interventions may be directed at teachers, school counselors, athletic coaches, employers, or others who may play a pivotal role in helping or hindering the individual's efforts in trying to meet the challenge of living with an ADD in the world beyond the immediate family.

Psychosocial interventions are delivered in a variety of ways. Sometimes psychosocial interventions are implemented face to face in one-on-one conversations, conjoint couple or family meetings, small group meetings, or large convention gatherings. At other times psychosocial interventions may be offered more indirectly via telephone conversations, e-mail, Internet communication, radio or TV shows, videotapes, books, pamphlets, or newspaper or magazine articles. Any of these modalities may offer a particular individual or family critically important support, information, insight, or suggestions to help them recognize, understand, and more adequately respond to the ADD and related impairments that they or their family member or friend experience.

Sometimes psychosocial interventions are delivered in very systematic ways—for example, in a structured program of treatment sessions or training workshops provided in a scheduled, carefully planned way over an extended period of time. Sometimes they are chance encounters—brief conversations in a supermarket checkout line or on a commuter train. The impact of these interactions is not always directly proportional to the amount of time involved. Sometimes engaging in one brief conversation or reading a single article may open a person's awareness to the possibility that problems with which they or a loved one has been struggling for many years could be due to a neurochemical problem that may be effectively treated. That single conversation or article might then lead that person to seek an evaluation and perhaps find treatment that could positively change the course of his or her entire lifetime.

INTERVENTIONS TO EDUCATE ABOUT ADDS AND COMORBID CONDITIONS

Perhaps the most important psychosocial interventions are those that help to educate people about ADDs and comorbid conditions. Individuals with undiagnosed and untreated ADDs encounter, often from their earliest years, extraordinarily frequent experiences in which they are being corrected for misunderstanding what was said to them, for doing the wrong thing at the wrong time, or for failing to do what they are expected to do. Accumulating experiences of failure or frustration can lead these individuals to think of themselves as hopelessly lazy, stupid, or inadequate, even though at times they may perform very well.

Often these demeaning self-perceptions are reinforced by well-meaning but uninformed parents, teachers, spouses, friends, or others who respond with nagging, ridicule, or persistent criticism of discrepancies between the individual's apparent abilities and his or her actual achievements. "Why do you keep making these same stupid mistakes when you clearly know better?" "I get so sick of telling you the same things over and over again!" "Do you want to be a loser all your life?" "You could do so much better if only you would try harder or be more consistent!" The net effect of such criticism, however well intentioned, is that the individual with an ADD learns to think of himself or herself as suffering from some fundamental and persistent character flaw that could be easily overcome if he or she only would put forth more effort.

Education about the nature, causes, and course of ADDs and comorbid conditions can offer an alternative viewpoint for persons with ADDs—a perspective that helps to explain why they, more than most of their peers, are so often inconsistent in their performance, so inattentive, or so impulsive or hyperactive, even when they are trying hard to do the right thing. Education about ADDs should not be an excuse for poor effort. Instead, it should help to clarify why, for some individuals, even strenuous efforts may not bring about the usually expected results. It may help to explain how individuals with the impairments of ADDs can be helped significantly to modify the persisting impairments in self-management that they experience.

The most fundamental element of education about ADDs is an attitude of respect and empathy for the individual who suffers from an ADD and for those who suffer with him or her. Often the person with an ADD has learned to criticize himself or herself excessively or to feign indifference or denial about problems that have brought excessive frustration, embarrassment, failure, or shame. If the clinician or other information-giver can convey an attitude of respect for the person with ADD, this attitude may provide a beginning point for development of a more positive self-understanding in the patient. One specific way in which this respect can be shown by the clinician is by explicit recognition of the positive step the individual has taken in seeking an evaluation.

It is no small step for most people to ask for or comply with being evaluated by a clinician for problems with their cognitive, emotional, or behavioral functioning. Many people struggle intensively with themselves and their friends or family members for many weeks, months, or years over whether they should seek an evaluation for a possible ADD diagnosis. They may worry about how intrusive or humiliating the evaluation process may be. They may feel extreme embarrassment about recognizing and disclosing the many ways in which they are unable to meet their own expectations or those of others. They may be ashamed of how they have misrepresented themselves or cheated to cover over their weaknesses, or they may be afraid that the evaluator will find them even more impaired or hopeless than they have seen themselves.

The prospective patient may also fear disappointment in the evaluation: perhaps the clinician may conclude that the patient's chronic problems are not due to an ADD but to a lack of ability or effort. Or a course of treatment may be recommended and tried, yet yield only adverse effects with no significant benefits. Making a phone call to schedule an evaluation and then showing up to face the evaluator is a step that requires considerable courage and determination as well as hope. Anyone who undertakes an evaluation for themselves or their child is deserving of sincere respect. Likewise, although children and adolescents are usually brought by parents for evaluation, and do not seek it themselves, the child's willingness to endure the evaluator's questioning about embarrassing problems and to cooperate with the necessary testing is deserving of respect.

In addition to respect, however, the clinician ought to demonstrate empathy. One way to do this is to provide some opportunity for the patient and family seeking evaluation to describe how they decided to seek the evaluation and what hopes, fears, and aims they bring to it. Helping the patient and family explicitly to state their mixed feelings and to describe their specific struggles in deciding to get the evaluation helps them to show themselves and the clinician what they have already accomplished in beginning to actively confront their problems. On the basis of this understanding the clinician can respond more sensitively to communicate specific empathy and respect for those who seek and/or cooperate with an evaluation.

Another way in which the evaluating clinician may help to alleviate the excessive burdens of self-criticism usually carried by those who seek an evaluation for an ADD is to recognize explicitly the adaptive strengths demonstrated by the person being evaluated. Often when someone seeks a clinical evaluation, they, and those reporting about them, tend to be so focused on weaknesses and failures that they do not think about or mention their strengths and accomplishments. Any sensitive clinician will elicit from each patient information about activities they enjoy and in which they do well and about skills or accomplishments in which they can take legitimate pride. The child who is getting failing grades in school may be the best pitcher on his little league team or the best artist in her class or an exceptionally skilled designer of Lego constructions. A woman who dropped out of high school may be a very skilled worker on her job and/or a sensitive, hard-working, and loving mother. The clinician's interest in and acknowledgment of these positive aspects of the person being evaluated may be an important antidote to the poison of excessive self-criticism.

A third way in which the clinician may help to alleviate a patient's excessive self-criticism is by providing accurate information about aspects of ADDs and comorbid conditions about which this particular person may need to know. Often patients and their families come with insufficient, inaccurate information or mistaken assumptions about the problems they are facing. They may assume that ADD symptoms are a consequence of inadequate prenatal care or poor parenting or insufficient effort or lack of "willpower." They may assume that individuals who receive an ADD diagnosis are doomed to a life of chronic academic and vocational failure or that they will eventually have all the same problems of a severely disturbed individual who was in their school class or lived in their neighborhood and was rumored to have an ADD. A sensitive clinician will elicit conversation from the patient and family members to learn about what they know and have heard about ADDs and related problems, attending carefully to implicit attitudes or fears that may need to be addressed. Robin, in his book *ADHD in Adolescents* (1998a), includes a chapter on educating families about ADDs that offers a useful format for providing basic information about these disorders and addressing explicitly some of the assumptions that patients and their families may bring to the evaluation.

Patients and their family members often need education about comorbid disorders as well as about ADDs. Parents of a child whose ADD symptoms are accompanied by an urgent, persisting need to report excessive worries to teachers and family members many times a day may need education about the nature and treatment of obsessive-compulsive disorder (OCD) comorbid with an ADD. An adult whose ADD is accompanied by unpredictable swings between episodes of severe depression and manic elation with racing thoughts and self-destructive behavior is likely to need education about the nature and treatment of bipolar disorder concurrent with that of ADD. An adolescent who is extremely avoidant of peers and extracurricular activities while experiencing apparently irremediable cluelessness in social interactions may need education for himself and his family about the nature and course of Asperger's disorder concurrent with that of ADDs.

Any time the diagnostic process indicates that an individual with an ADD has a comorbid disorder, the clinician has an obligation to help the patient and involved family develop an appropriate, adequate understanding of the comorbid disorder as well as the ADD. If the evaluating clinician is not sufficiently familiar with the possibly comorbid disorder to provide adequate evaluation and education, a referral to a more appropriately equipped clinician is indicated. Such a referral will allow the consulting clinician to provide appropriate education about the possible comorbidity, evaluate whether the comorbidity is present, and recommend any additional treatment that may be appropriate.

INTERVENTIONS TO EDUCATE ABOUT TREATMENTS FOR ADDS AND COMORBID CONDITIONS

After a patient and family undergoing an initial evaluation have been provided basic information about the nature of ADDs and a diagnosis that includes an ADD has been made, the clinician faces a major educational task: providing information about treatment options and recommendations. It is very important that patients and family members understand the nature of ADD impairments, the contribution of neurochemical factors to ADD symptoms, and the fact that ADDs, though superficially appearing to be the result of a lack "willpower," are not caused by a lack of willpower and are not cured by exercise of willpower. Usually the patient and family need to understand these basic facts about the nature of ADDs before they can be ready to collaborate fully and effectively in the process of treatment.

Often patients and their families bring to the evaluation many assumptions and strong feelings about the nature of ADDs and various modes of treatment, particularly those involving medications. They may come with expectations that a few doses of medication will quickly cure all the problems of the individual that are attributed to the ADD. They may come fearing that any medication prescribed for ADDs is dangerous and should be avoided at all costs. Whether they are expecting medication to be a magical panacea or a dangerous threat, the patient and the family need to be educated about the scientific realities, the uses and limitations, and the risks and the benefits of medication treatments for ADDs.

Parents bringing their son or daughter for assessment of a possible ADD may approach the initial evaluation with explicit fears about the possibility that stimulant medication will be recommended. They may state strong preferences against medications and for use of dietary restrictions, diet supplements, biofeedback techniques, or other treatment strategies not, at present, adequately supported by scientific research. Ingersoll and Goldstein (1993) have discussed some of these more controversial treatments. When patients or their family members indicate any fears or hesitations about treatments being recommended, it is critically important that the clinician encourage them to express their specific concerns so that the concerns can be explicitly understood and reasonably addressed.

Sometimes clinicians who have seen the benefits of medication treatment for ADDs are too quick to try to persuade a person with an ADD to begin medication treatment or to try to encourage parents to try medication treatment for their child with an ADD. Although these clinicians may operate with good intentions, they may abandon their usual clinical sensitivity and willingness to try to understand reasons underlying a patient's resistances to a particular course of action. The insensitive clinician may unintentionally take on the role of a salesman trying to argue away any hesitations, pressing to close a deal to begin the proposed treatment plan. When parents or patients are hesitant about any particular treatment, it is especially important that the clinician maintain empathy and clinical curiosity to try to understand the particular reasons, explicit and implicit, that these particular parents or this particular patient feels hesitant about accepting the clinician's recommendations for treatment. Only after these reasons have been recognized, clarified, and addressed to the satisfaction of all persons involved can reasonable planning for effective, sustained treatment be accomplished.

In the course of educating patients and families about ADD treatment options, especially about medications, it is important that the clinician not imply a promise for more benefits than can be delivered. For example, when discussing medications useful for treatment of ADD, it is important to make clear from the outset that medication treatments are not tolerable or effective for every person diagnosed with an ADD. Most studies indicate that medication treatments currently available are effective for approximately 70%–80% of children, adolescents, and adults diagnosed with ADD. These are very good odds for those who fall into the fortunate 70%–80%; they are not good odds for those in the remaining 20%–30% for whom these medications produce intolerable side effects or are simply not effective.

Patients need to be adequately informed about potential side effects and how they may or may not be effectively managed. They should be told about how the currently available treatments produce amazingly positive results in some ADD patients, substantial but not amazing results in others, and much more modest improvements in still others. They need to be made aware of the variability among persons in the size and timing of doses that work best for them and of the need for "fine-tuning," sometimes over a protracted period, to ascertain the most effective dosing strategy with the minimum of adverse effects for a particular patient. Patients and families who agree to undertake a trial of medication treatment after they have been adequately prepared with accurate, understandable information about the nature and causes of ADDs, about how the medication is presumed to act on the body to alleviate ADD symptoms, and about the risks and potential benefits of the treatment proposed are more likely to persevere with the clinician in the sometimes frustrating task of developing, implementing, and fine-tuning an appropriate plan of treatment.

When a patient has a more complicated ADD, one with comorbid conditions requiring more complex interventions (e.g., multiple medications, concurrent remediation for a learning disorder, 12-step recovery program for substance abuse), the need for adequate education of the patient and family about the treatment options is even greater. It is necessary that the patient and family recognize the multifaceted aspects of the patient's difficulties and the proposed treatments; they should be helped to understand at whatever level of detail they need and can comprehend. They need to know what the target symptoms are, why the more basic treatment is not sufficient, how the additional treatments are expected to be helpful, and what additional risks and potential benefits can be expected. Complex cases, especially those in which there is no response to the usual first-line treatments, may present a challenge to the clinician's educational skills as much as to his or her diagnostic and treatment planning skills. If the clinician is not careful to help the patient and family develop a clear, shared understanding of how the problems being faced by the patient are related to the treatment interventions proposed, compliance with the treatment is likely to be lost. This educational work is likely to be the work of ongoing conversation between patient and clinician.

Conversation between a clinician and the patient in the presence and absence of family members is but one of many ways in which education about

ADDs and comorbid disorders can be provided. Such conversation is important because it can be tailored to the specific clinical situation of the patient and can be enriched by the clinical skills and experience of the psychologist, psychiatrist, or other professional. Yet even when individualized clinical consultation is provided, additional educational materials or resources can be useful.

Carefully selected reading materials or videotapes can provide valuable information to which patients and family members can repeatedly refer as questions arise. Twelve-step programs like Alcoholics Anonymous have long made good use of bibliotherapy to educate and support their members' understanding of addiction and recovery. In a similar way, clinicians often provide handouts of selected articles or information sheets to patients newly diagnosed with an ADD or another disorder; they may offer book lists from which they recommend to patients books that the patients or their family members may find helpful. Recommended books may help adults or older children to better understand the nature of ADDs and comorbid conditions and the wide variety of ways in which they manifest.

Books like Hallowell and Ratey's *Driven to Distraction: Attention Deficit Disorder in Children and Adults* (1994), Solden's *Women With Attention Deficit Disorder* (1995), Hallowell's *When You Worry About the Child You Love* (1996), and Dendy's *Teenagers With ADD: A Parents' Guide* (1995) have been very helpful introductory resources for many individuals and families. Wilens' *Straight Talk About Psychiatric Medications for Kids* (1999) is a useful source of accurate information about medications for ADDs and other comorbid disorders. Additional resources for education about ADDs and comorbid disorders are described in relevant professional journals and in magazines such as *ATTENTION,* published by CHADD (Children and Adults With Attention Deficit/Hyperactivity Disorder), or publications of other national support organizations. Clinicians should be alert for publications that might be useful to patients with specific combinations of needs so they can offer reading lists or make suggestions that will be up-to-date and useful. At this point, suffice it to say that the task of educating patients and families about the nature of ADDs and comorbid conditions is a critically important aspect of intervention and is ongoing throughout the course of treatment.

INTERVENTIONS TO MONITOR AND ADJUST THE COURSE OF TREATMENT

Evaluation is never a one-shot process in good clinical work. Evaluation is needed at the outset to help the clinician, patient, and family understand the presenting problems of the patient and the psychological, physiological, and social contexts in which they occur. The initial assessment is the basis on which the working diagnosis is formulated and from which the initial treatment plan is developed. From that starting point evaluation continues as the clinician, patient, and others who may be involved (e.g., parents, teachers) monitor and assess responses of the patient to the ongoing treatment, weighing positive and negative aspects to determine how best to shape interventions to minimize adverse effects and to maximize treatment benefits.

There are many ways in which treatment interventions may fail; one of the most common is lack of compliance or follow-through from the patient. This is a major problem in many aspects of general medicine as well as in treatment of ADDs and other psychiatric disorders. Stine (1994) reviewed literature indicating that, in general, no more than 50% of patients in adult or pediatric medical populations are compliant with treatment regimens extending beyond 6–9 months. When the patient is a child or adolescent, the possibilities for noncompliance are multiplied by the need for cooperation from both the child and various family members who are directly or indirectly involved. There are many points at which the process of moving from diagnosis to implementation of treatment can break down.

For example, prescription of medications to treat ADD symptoms does not mean that the patient will take the medications long enough or consistently enough even to assess effectiveness of the medication. Sherman and Hertzig (1991) surveyed records of all prescriptions for methylphenidate written for children in one New York county within a full year. Their analysis indicated that 52% of the children in this sample who received prescriptions for methylphenidate that year received only one prescription during the entire year. Since federal regulations limit each prescription for methylphenidate to a one month's supply with no refills, this research finding indicates that a majority of children for whom met

hylphenidate was prescribed did not follow through with that medication long enough to extend the coverage into a second month within the same year. It would appear that they never completed titration trials to become stabilized for more than 1 month on this medication.

Careful guidance and monitoring of responses are especially important in the early phases of titration trials with stimulant medications for ADD. The short half-life and wide variability among patients in the size of effective dosing make fine-tuning of stimulant dosage considerably more complicated than adjustment of doses for many other types of medications. Sometimes patients are resistant to using specific medications to treat their ADD because the medication causes uncomfortable adverse effects or seems simply not to be bringing any noticeable improvement in the target symptoms. Since patient's age, weight, body mass, symptom severity, and medication serum levels are not useful guides to an appropriate dose of stimulants for ADD, trial and error is the primary way to establish an effective dose regimen. Careful monitoring of the patient's positive and negative responses to a gradually increasing dose regimen is critically important to effective titration.

More than with any other aspect of treatment for an ADD, except, perhaps, in the initial evaluation, the clinician who is monitoring medication response needs to be what Jackson (1992) has described as a "listening healer"—one who listens with carefully tuned empathy to the complexities of the patient's description of his or her personal experience and perspectives.

No laboratory tests or imaging techniques can adequately assess the subtleties of how a particular medication treatment is affecting the patient with an ADD. Minimizing adverse effects and maximizing therapeutic benefits while tailoring dose and timing to fit the schedule and activities of a particular individual with his or her own idiosyncratic bodily reactions is a difficult task that requires considerable sophistication in interviewing skills, as well as thorough knowledge of the wide diversity of ways these medications can affect different individuals.

Since stimulant medications have short half-lives and often require several doses daily, assessing positive and negative effects of these medications requires that the clinician query the patient with reference to very specific time frames. Only by inquiring very specifically about baseline symptoms and by learning exactly when each dose is taken and when various positive and negative effects occur can the clinician determine how the target symptoms are affected by the medication and how the medication may or may not be causing various adverse effects during its time of ingestion, absorption, onset, and duration of action or in rebound as it wears off. Such assessment is even more complicated if the patient is taking more than one medication simultaneously.

This detailed information about positive and negative effects of medication treatments for ADD is not easy to obtain. Often patients are very global in reporting their impressions—"I feel a lot better since I started taking this medicine" or "I don't like the way this medicine makes me feel"—without discriminating between times this short-acting medication is and is not active. Moreover, many patients are hesitant to report that medication a clinician has provided for them is making them uncomfortable or seems not to be working. They may, correctly or incorrectly, assume that the clinician will be disappointed or frustrated if they do not report positive results; they may minimize mention of adverse effects, fearing that the clinician will react with annoyance or consider them ungrateful for the prescription.

Without the patient's supplying information about persisting headache or stomachache, excessive appetite suppression or insomnia, muted affect, excessive irritability or rebound fatigue, and so forth, the clinician cannot know what adjustments need to be made to alleviate such adverse effects. Without specific, accurate information about timing and degree of persistence or alleviation of target symptoms, the clinician cannot adequately assess effectiveness of current dosing and suggest alterations that might improve medication effects.

Skilled clinicians learn how to reduce implicit "demand" for only positive responses in their inquiries of patients; they actively invite negative reports from the patient, inviting him or her to function as a needed collaborator in monitoring treatment problems and effectiveness. This process might include explicitly telling the patient at the outset of treatment that accurate reporting of negative effects is required to adequately monitor treatment and adjust dosages for treatment effectiveness. When lack of positive effects or presence of negative effects is unreported, the clinician does not have the information needed to correct the difficulties. The persisting problems are likely to cause frustration and discouragement that may lead the patient to quietly discontinue taking prescribed medication and perhaps to give up on treatment.

In addition to lack of effects or adverse effects of medication, patients may have other reasons to avoid taking prescribed medications. Stine (1994) described the wide variety of psychosocial and psychodynamic factors that may affect compliance with psychostimulant treatment of a child with ADD. He described psychosocial factors such as the child's passivity or oppositionality, parental concerns about medication safety, reactions of patient or family members to the illness, media misinformation, and the perceived or actual stigma of medication treatment. Stine also discussed various psychodynamic meanings of medication that may interfere with particular individuals' consistently following recommendations for medication treatment.

In addition to factors described by Stine, clinicians need also to take into account the possible conflicts between family members concerning treatment compliance. Often significant disagreements about the validity and appropriateness of ADD diagnosis and treatment arise between parents or between parents and grandparents or other extended family members. Sometimes these disputes arise when one parent is well informed about ADDs and their treatment, while the other is operating without much factual information, with a viewpoint possibly biased by insufficient or inaccurate information. In other situations disputes between parents or between parents and other family members may have little to do with the specific facts of the ADD diagnosis and treatment. Conflicts between parents over whether their child has an ADD or should use a specific treatment for the ADD may be secondary to chronic marital conflicts in which each parent is irrationally opposed to any viewpoint or plan proposed by the other party. In such situations the clinician may need to spend considerable time helping parents to disentangle their marital conflicts from the specific issues related to ADD diagnosis and treatment of their child.

As the research of Strupp et al. (1977) indicated, evaluation of treatment effects needs to be considered simultaneously from several different perspectives: the viewpoints of the patient, of others in the patient's environment, and of the treating clinician all need to be taken into account. For example, a specific regimen of stimulant medication administered in early morning and at noon may lead a child's teacher to report marked improvement in work output and behavior. Yet if the child is enduring persistent headaches or frequent teasing from peers for having to go to the nurse daily for medication, that child may refuse to continue with the medication. Or if parents are experiencing daily episodes of unprecedentedly hostile or aggressive behavior from their son or daughter on rebound from medication after school, they may conclude that the medication is worsening their child's condition and decide that the treatment should be stopped. Adequate monitoring of medication effects requires eliciting subjective and objective data from the relevant sources. For an adult all the necessary information may be accessible from self-report as the clinician inquires about subjective impressions, work output, comments from co-workers or supervisors, reactions of family members, and so forth. Yet in some instances it may be useful to get additional perspectives by encouraging an adult patient to bring a spouse, co-worker, or friend in to discuss his or her impressions of the patient's ADD symptoms when on and off the medications. Information gained and education given in such conjoint sessions may be helpful to the patient, the collateral participant, and the clinician.

For children and adolescents being treated for an ADD, impressions of teachers are often solicited by clinicians assessing the effectiveness of treatment; teacher reports, often just a few checkmarks on a rating scale, are sometimes used as the sole source of data for making important decisions about adjusting dose, timing, and so forth. Such an approach may overvalue teacher input and ignore the importance of the parents and the patient, who can offer critically important information about aspects of treatment response, favorable or not, at times and in settings and domains not accessible to teachers.

Teacher-report data may be especially limited for older students (e.g., those in junior high or high school, who no longer spend most of their school day with just one teacher who has the opportunity to observe them in many types of tasks and interactions. When a student is dealing with five to seven different teachers, each of whom is dealing with four to five large classes daily, the capacity of any one teacher to offer very substantial information to assess treatment effectiveness may be quite limited. Often the adolescent student or parents can provide much useful information about functioning in class, homework completion, extracurricular activities, and so forth. This information may be augmented by reviewing graded papers, tests, written progress reports, and report cards or by telephone or face-to-face conferences with teachers and/or school counselors.

Ultimately the task of evaluating the effectiveness of medications or any other treatment interventions involves three phases: 1) eliciting a variety of information to illuminate the positive and negative aspects of treatment from a variety of perspectives (e.g., patient, family, school or work, social relationships) regarding all the relevant domains of the patient's functioning (e.g., eating, sleeping, overall health, subjective feelings, school or work, interpersonal relationships); 2) integrating and weighting the various types of data to form a clear impression of the ongoing process of treatment and to identify factors that are facilitating and/or impeding its effectiveness; and 3) formulating a plan to sustain the benefits and minimize the problems so the patient will gain maximum benefit over the longer term. Doing this monitoring effectively and using it to shape and guide the treatment process are critical and ongoing aspects of effective clinical work.

INTERVENTIONS TO TEACH MANAGEMENT SKILLS TO PATIENTS WITH ADDS OR THEIR FAMILIES

Another important aspect of psychosocial interventions for ADDs and comorbid disorders is to provide to patients and/or their families instruction in management skills that will be helpful to them. Often parents seek treatment for their child because they have found that their existing strategies are not working to encourage their child to behave appropriately; the child may be so consistently impulsive, inattentive, or oppositional that the parents are chronically frustrated, alternating between intense rage at their misbehaving child and intense guilt that they themselves have not been successful in getting the child to behave, at least as well as most of his or her peers.

When parents present themselves seeking help for such difficulties, the initial task is an evaluation to determine as clearly as possible the nature of the difficulties and to ascertain what factors within the child, the household, and the wider setting (e.g., school, neighborhood, extended family) may be contributing to the problems that led them to seek treatment. If an ADD with or without comorbid problems appears to be an aspect of the situation, then this should be explained to all those involved. As discussed earlier, the process of educating the identified patient and others involved about the nature of the disorders and the range of possible treatment options is an important and often not easy task. One option to be considered might be medication, but, regardless of whether medication is used, instruction about how to guide and shape specified behavioral responses might be very useful.

Sometimes it is assumed that every parent has intuitive knowledge about how best to manage the behavior of his or her children in an effective way—that the parent knows his or her own child intimately and therefore will know how best to manage the child. This assumption ignores the fact that many parents are very limited in their parenting skills. Some have grown up in families in which their own parents were not very effective modelers of parenting skills. Some parents have endured a childhood history characterized by chronic and severe conflict among family members or by vacillation between excessive indulgence or neglect and episodes of harsh, inconsistent, demeaning, or abusive treatment at the hands of their own parents. Others have grown up with parents who were, for any of many possible reasons, not able to be very effective at the often difficult task of childrearing. Even when there is no history of parental mistreatment or when their own parents provided very good examples of parenting skills, many parents are bewildered by the task of parenting their own children. This bewilderment and the resulting fears and frustration may be greatly magnified when a parent has to deal with the exceptionally problematic behaviors and reactions of a child with an ADD, especially if the ADD problems are compounded by comorbid oppositional defiant behavior or a mood disorder or aggression. Sometimes parents have been quite successful in raising several other children but find themselves chronically frustrated by one child whose behavior is extraordinarily difficult to manage.

For parents whose children's behavior is exceptionally difficult to manage, learning basic principles of behavior modification can be quite helpful. At the least, they can learn how to avoid unwittingly reinforcing the difficult behaviors of their child that they are trying to change. At best, they may be able to develop more consistent and effective patterns of interacting with their child that will reduce unnecessary conflict and support appropriate behaviors.

Barkley (1998) has developed a very useful, systematic approach to teaching child management skills to parents of children with ADDs and oppositional, aggressive behavior problems; his recently revised training program helps parents to learn techniques of behavior modification useful for dealing with their defiant children. Kazdin (1997) has evaluated evidence, outcomes, and issues for a variety of approaches to parent management training.

Although behavior management techniques can be very useful in helping parents and teachers to manage more effectively the problematic behaviors of children with ADDs, these methods may not be equally effective at all ages. Dishion and Patterson (1991) and Ruma et al. (1996) have reported data suggesting that parent training for behavior management may be less effective in alleviating behavioral problems of adolescents than it often is with younger children. Robin (1998a) described techniques for facilitating negotiation between parents and adolescents that may be a more effective strategy for this often problematic age group.

For clinicians who want to review research and basic principles to develop programs for behavior modification in families, classrooms, or other settings, the classic text is Kazdin's *Behavior Modification in Applied Settings* (1994), now in its fifth edition. Specific applications of these principles to training of parents are described in two chapters of Barkley's recently revised handbook (Barkley 1998). There, Anastopoulos et al. (1998) describe a clinical approach to parent counseling, and Cunningham (1998) provides information about a large-group community-based approach to training of parents in behavioral management techniques of parenting. In another volume, Braswell and Bloomquist (1991) describe applications of cognitive-behavioral interventions with children who have ADDs. An excellent chapter by Robin (1998b) on training sessions for families with adolescents who have attention-deficit/hyperactivity disorder (ADHD) is provided in the Barkley handbook.

Although several excellent programs for parent training are available and may be quite useful to many parents, it is important to avoid simplistic models of providing such services. As Patterson and Chamberlain (1994) described, there are many ways resistance to change may impede parents' utilization of new parenting skills they are taught. Therapists attempting to provide these interventions need to remember that ignorance of effective techniques is not the only factor that may hold parents back from being more effective in managing their child's behavior. As Kazdin and Kagan (1994) explained, dysfunction in parenting, individual, and family functioning is often embedded in complex, dynamic "packages" of social and psychological factors that are not easy to analyze, especially with single-dimension models, and are often quite resistant to change. Even when changes are accomplished with specific interventions, the benefits may not be persistent over time unless "booster sessions" or other maintenance strategies are provided. Eyberg et al. (1998) described the formidable obstacles to maintaining therapeutic gains of parent training in families with more problematic, chronic impairment. Not all families with chronic dysfunction are amenable to quick and lasting improvement with psychosocial interventions or any other techniques.

In his book *The Explosive Child,* Greene (1998) described a type of child who often does not respond well to conventional behavior modification approaches, for whom standard behavioral interventions may exacerbate "meltdown" of the child's ability to function, possibly leading to extremes of outrageously provocative and sometimes dangerous behavior. Greene described these dilemmas and suggested more flexible and realistic options for parents who are forced to deal with the severely distressing behaviors of these children, many of whom might be diagnosed as having ADD with concurrent bipolar disorder or pervasive developmental disorder or Asperger's disorder. Cases described in Greene's book are a useful reminder of the need to adapt intervention strategies to a specific child and family rather than attempting to work with generic interventions for particular types of problems. Psychosocial interventions need at least as much "tailoring" for the particular persons involved as do psychotropic medication treatments.

A more comprehensive approach that integrates multiple behavioral interventions for ADHD has been described by Pelham and Waschbusch (1999). This approach utilizes parent training with intensive school interventions, direct child interventions, and, often, careful medication management, all concurrent, often over periods of 2 years or more, followed by maintenance and relapse prevention services.

In a comprehensive treatment program, the parent training might include therapist-directed weekly group sessions to deal with problematic behaviors of the ADHD child and with emotional and behavioral problems of the parents and/or other family members. School interventions might include frequent consultations between the classroom teacher and a clinician experienced in behavioral treatment techniques for ADHD. These consultations might focus not only on academic difficulties but also on peer interaction problems. Direct services for the ADHD child might include an intensive summer day camp treatment program followed in the school year by daily report cards, behavioral contracts, after-school tutoring, and recreational sessions with a paraprofessional.

These integrated, highly structured, closely monitored contingency management programs can be quite potent interventions for ADHD, but the skilled personnel and other resources needed to implement such comprehensive programs are not readily available or feasible in many communities. Moreover, most research on these behavioral methods, including the recent MTA study (MTA Cooperative Group, in press), indicate that behavioral treatments for ADHD usually work best when combined with appropriate medication treatment. For relatively uncomplicated cases of ADHD, addition of behavioral treatments may not substantially improve outcome beyond what is usually accomplished with appropriate medication management treatment. Yet in some cases, particularly those in which there are substantial comorbid behavior problems, addition of carefully tailored behavioral treatment techniques to medication treatment regimens may be quite helpful.

The potential usefulness of behavior modification strategies is not limited to children. Older adolescents and adults with ADDs sometimes seek behavioral intervention guidelines to use to improve their functioning in school, work, family, or social relationships; they want to develop more effective self-management techniques. Nadeau (1995, 1996, 1997) described a number of attitude strategies and organizational techniques often useful to adults with ADDs as they seek to manage themselves more effectively in the various domains of their work and social relationships. Nadeau's book *Comprehensive Guide to Attention Deficit Disorder in Adults* includes useful chapters by Murphy, Hallowell, Nadeau, Dixon, Ratey, Richard, Latham and Latham, Kelly, and others discussing psychosocial interventions for a variety of issues in family and social relationships and in work and career development of adults with ADDs.

One limitation of some of the guidebooks for adolescents and adults seeking to improve their self-management skills is that the problems considered are generally assumed to be those of "ADD simplex," uncomplicated by comorbid conditions. For example, many articles and books encourage persons with an ADD to clean out their "clutter" in home and workplace, advocating a systematic plan for removing mountains of objects and papers stored in piles throughout one's workspace or home. For some persons with ADDs a rational explanation of the values of discarding unneeded papers and junk followed by suggestions for how to do it might be very helpful. Yet some other persons with ADDs who complain of persisting problems with excessive "clutter" are suffering not from ignorance of the values of tidiness but from a type of OCD characterized by hoarding. For these individuals, the prospect of discarding piles of old newspapers and unworn clothing or household goods may be fearful and overwhelming. They may need more specific therapeutic interventions to assess and treat their OCD before they can even approximate the increased efficiency and household organization advocated by guidelines for adults with ADDs who have excessive clutter.

Similarly, although many publications offer advice and strategies for persons with ADDs who have difficulties in their social relationships, these difficulties in social functioning may be caused by more complicated factors that just an ADD. It is true that some individuals with ADDs have problems in their social functioning that are directly related to their ADD symptoms—for example, they may irritate others with chronic tardiness for appointments, lack of attention to details that are very important to others, failure to fulfill commitments, or excessively impulsive verbal or behavioral responses to frustration. Medication for ADDs may help to alleviate some of these problems that negatively affect others; psychoeducation about strategies for more successful social functioning also may be useful in helping persons with these difficulties to be more fully aware of how their attitudes and behaviors may affect others.

Yet social problems of persons with ADDs may not simply be due to the ADDs. As described in other chapters of this volume, some individuals with ADDs also have comorbid anxiety disorders that make them phobic about social interactions outside their closest circle of companions. Others are insensitive to social cues and often may behave in socially inappropriate ways because their ADD is complicated with Asperger's disorder or another severe disorder of social functioning. Attwood (1998) provided an excellent description of the multiple domains of impairment characteristic of persons with Asperger's disorder, a severe disorder of cognitive and social functioning that is often accompanied by ADDs; his description includes suggestions about how family members and teachers may assist the person with Asperger's disorder to function more effectively with others. Psychosocial interventions may be useful to these individuals if the interventions are appropriately informed by clear understanding not only of ADDs but also of Asperger's disorder. Providing effective education about management skills for ADD patients and families often requires information and strategies for dealing with not only the ADD but also comorbid disorders.

INTERVENTIONS TO EQUIP PATIENTS WITH ADDS AND THEIR FAMILIES FOR SELF-ADVOCACY

One other domain in which specific information may be helpful to persons with ADDs is that of self-advocacy, particularly for seeking appropriate accommodations in schools, in colleges and universities, and in the workplace.

In the United States a number of federal laws provide that individuals with disabilities are entitled to certain protections and accommodations to ensure that they are not unfairly discriminated against because of their disabilities. These laws apply to a wide variety of physical, mental, and learning disabilities; most also have been held to extend these protections, under stipulated conditions, to persons with ADDs. Such protections are not currently available in some other countries.

Some individuals with ADDs and their families are unaware of their eligibility for these legal protections. They do not know that with proper documentation of diagnosis of ADD they may be eligible to have extended time to take standardized examinations such as the SAT, ACT, MCAT, LSAT, GRE, or other tests required for admission to colleges, universities, or professional schools. Some persons with ADD impairment who graduate from these programs are not aware that they may be eligible to have extended time to take medical board, law board, or other such examinations required for initial admission or advanced status in their professional fields.

Extended time for tests and examinations, probably the most widely used of accommodations provided by law for persons with documented ADD and/or learning disabilities, is important to many students who have the slowed processing time and weaknesses in working memory common in ADDs. Without extended time, many ADD students are unable to demonstrate on a test the full extent of what they know. Impaired by their need to reread, often many times, passages that most of their peers fully grasp in a single reading, by chronic difficulties in organizing their written responses, and by their need to recheck their answers to correct for excessive impulsivity, students with ADD often score quite poorly on time-limited examinations; yet they often are able to perform quite well on the same examination if they are allowed a reasonable extension of time to take the test. Such accommodations seem quite reasonable for those with such impairments, especially when rapid processing of information is not an essential aspect of the skills or work for which the examination is a prerequisite.

Many students with ADDs and their parents may be unaware of other accommodations that may be available for those with diagnosed ADDs while they are enrolled in elementary schools, high schools, or colleges or universities: extended time for taking all examinations, preferential seating close to the instructor, assistance in taking notes in lecture classes, opportunity to tape-record class sessions for later review, books on tape, supportive tutoring, and so forth. For students in elementary and secondary schools, federal law also provides for special education services and a variety of related services when they are needed.

Eligibility for these accommodations and supportive services is not automatic upon receipt of a diagnosis of an ADD or learning disorder. Most educational settings and examining boards have established procedures for determining eligibility of a student or graduate for legally mandated accommodations intended for those with disabilities. Such screening is needed to maintain fairness so that individuals are given accommodations that they truly need and are not given an unfair advantage. It is important for those diagnosed with ADDs to have accurate information about what protections are available to them, what accommodations might be appropriate to their specific impairments, and how they can provide the necessary information to the appropriate authorities to gain the support and accommodations to which they are entitled.

For adolescents and adults with ADDs who need and want to utilize accommodations and protections granted under the Americans With Disabilities Act and related legislation, there are specified procedures for establishing adequate documentation of disability. Latham and Latham (1995, 1996) are attorneys who have published useful summaries and explanations of relevant laws and case precedents to guide persons with ADDs or learning disorders and the professionals who work with them. Gordon and Keiser (1998) have edited a volume elaborating specifically on accommodations in higher education, particularly the more complex and controversial issues of accommodations for students with ADD impairments who are relatively high functioning. Information about laws and procedures relevant to education for children and for adolescents still in secondary school is provided in the chapter by DuPaul and Power in this volume (see Chapter 19).

It is important that parents of children in elementary and secondary schools be well informed about the protections, accommodations, and, when needed, special education services provided by law for those diagnosed with ADDs, learning disorders, and related impairments. Armed with this information parents can work more effectively with local school authorities to make certain that their child with ADD, with or without comorbid disorder, receives what he or she needs and is legally entitled to. When relevant literature is not available or is insufficient, it may be useful for parents to contact the national office or website of CHADD or the Learning Disabilities Association of America to inquire about local resources for assistance and advocacy.

Although there is a well-established system to guide educational interventions for children with disabilities in elementary and secondary schools, at least in the United States, the provision of services and accommodations for postsecondary students is not automatic. Students in colleges and universities need to overcome their own resistances, to seek out appropriate resources, to obtain required evaluations for documentation of eligibility, and often to deal with many bureaucratic frustrations in order to avail themselves of services and accommodations for which they might be eligible on the basis of an ADD or learning disorder diagnosis. This process can be difficult for anyone; it is especially difficult for persons with ADDs, particularly when they are under the stresses of leaving a familiar setting and of trying to adjust to a new one.

Thus, to utilize the opportunities and protections provided by law, a college or university student must learn how to self-advocate effectively, just as parents of younger students with ADDs or a learning disorder need to learn to negotiate and advocate to obtain needed accommodations and services for their children in elementary and secondary schools. To become equipped for such advocacy, individuals need accurate information about what they are and are not entitled to. They need to understand the processes and procedures needed to negotiate the relevant bureaucracies, and they need support to maintain hope and determination in the face of the frustrations that often arise, especially in the initial phases of seeking out and determining eligibility for appropriate services.

Similar, and potentially more difficult, dilemmas face adults with ADDs or learning disorders who may wish to invoke for themselves in the workplace those legal protections or accommodations provided by the Americans With Disabilities Act. This law is relatively new legislation with only a small body of case law interpretations thus far to guide its applications. Some adults with ADDs have read or heard about some provisions of this law and then impulsively have demanded accommodations from their employers, occasionally threatening to take legal action against the employer if these demands are not promptly met. Such actions have sometimes had disastrous consequences, with the employee experiencing unforeseen negative consequences on the job, in some instances being fired, because of direct or indirect fallout from inappropriate demands or threats against an employer.

The legal protections provided under the Americans With Disabilities Act and related legislation have been very helpful in protecting many persons with disabilities in the workplace. Yet those with impairment due to an ADD or learning disorder who wish to avail themselves of these protections and services need to prepare carefully and to have access to accurate information relevant to their specific situation if they are going to be equipped adequately to advocate for themselves with their employers. Further information about these matters is provided in a series of papers and handbooks by Latham and Latham at the National Center for Law and Learning Disabilities (P.O. Box 368, Cabin John, MD 20818). Additional information on relevant issues may be obtained from the national offices of CHADD or the National Attention Deficit Disorder Association.

INTERVENTIONS TO PROVIDE THERAPY AND SUPPORT TO PATIENTS WITH ADDS AND THEIR FAMILIES

For some patients with ADDs and their families, education about the disorder, appropriate accommodations, and training in various management skills are not sufficient. The patients' symptoms and situation may be too complicated, and their individual and family resources too depleted, for them to make effective use of interventions that may be quite adequate for others. For these people, more individualized psychosocial interventions—coaching, individual psychotherapy, conjoint psychotherapy in couple or family units, and/or small group psychotherapy—may be needed.

ADD Coaching

ADD coaching refers to an individualized relationship between someone diagnosed with an ADD, usually an adult or late adolescent, and someone else who agrees to function for a limited time as a mentor to assist with efforts to change life patterns related to the ADD. Sometimes the coach may be simply an unpaid friend who is very familiar with ADDs and willing, for a time, to offer intensive support but who lacks any specialized training. More often, the coach is a social worker, psychologist, educator, or other professional person who charges for this service and has taken specialized workshops and supervision to learn how to provide coaching assistance to persons with ADDs. In either case, the quality and effectiveness of the client-coach relationship depend heavily on the competence of the coach, the motivation of the client, and the quality of the personality fit between the two.

In some ways, receiving ADD coaching may be similar to working with a coach or trainer one might employ for assistance in starting and monitoring a program of physical fitness. However, one difference is that ADD coaching focuses not on physical fitness, but on helping a person with an ADD, usually after that person has been stabilized on an effective course of treatment for ADD symptoms, to identify and modify problematic personal behaviors and to develop more effective self-management skills. Typically, coaching involves an initial assessment of problematic behavior patterns that the client wants to change—for example, chronically disorganized, cluttered household and work space, chronic lateness and inefficient work behavior, poor financial planning and personal bookkeeping, excessive procrastination in seeking a new job, and so forth. The coach then collaborates in developing a plan, offering appropriate cautions to remain realistic and providing very direct and explicit suggestions for modifying relevant patterns of behavior. Perhaps most important, the coach collaborates with the client in maintaining a scheduled program of frequent client-coach contacts for the client to report progress and receive encouragement and "helpful reminders" from the coach.

Thus far there has not been much research on the practice or outcomes of ADD coaching; most of the available data are anecdotal. Some persons with ADDs report that frequent face-to-face and/or telephone contact with their coach for monitoring and encouragement of progress on the behavioral goals has been very helpful in their efforts to modify long-standing, problematic behavioral patterns. For some, participating in the circumscribed collaborative relationship that they chose to develop with a coach works more successfully than trying to make the same changes on their own or with solicited or unsolicited assistance from close friends, co-workers, or family members. After a time of working with the coach, they may develop skills and routines for organizing their workload—utilizing a daytimer book to manage their time, setting up a more reasonable system to keep their household routines organized, and so forth—which they are then able to maintain for themselves with diminished or curtailed coaching support. Others report that they began coaching relationships with high hopes but quickly found that they got caught up in the same problematic patterns with their coach that they had previously encountered with family members or others to whom they turned for help. Systematic research might help to clarify the types of behavioral change and the types of client-coach interactions that tend to be most helpful for various types of persons with ADDs.

Psychotherapeutic Interventions

Many individuals and families have ADD-related problems that are not helped sufficiently by comprehensive assessment and the usual treatments of education and medication for ADD symptoms. These individuals may seek additional assistance from psychologists, psychiatrists, clinical social workers, or other professional psychotherapists who offer counseling or psychotherapy for persons with ADDs and related problems. Psychotherapy alone is not recognized as offering effective alleviation of the primary symptoms of

ADDs, but it may be useful in providing more adequate clarification of the specific ADD problems or other psychiatric problems or other difficulties that interfere with the adaptive functioning of the patient. It also may help to facilitate and support behavioral change. Hallowell (1995) discussed some adaptations of traditional psychotherapeutic techniques for treatment of persons with ADDs, and McDermott, in his chapter in this volume (see Chapter 18), describes adaptations of cognitive-behavioral therapy techniques that have been effective for treatment of adults with ADDs.

These more individualized and more expensive psychotherapeutic resources may be needed only briefly at the outset of the evaluation and diagnostic process or at a specific time of crisis, or they may be needed for intermittent monitoring or at times of transition or other individual/family stresses. For example, when a child is brought for an initial assessment for an ADD and/or comorbid disorders, there may be intense conflict between separated or divorced parents or between parents and members of the extended family about the validity of the diagnosis or the appropriateness of the recommended treatments. If family conflict over such issues becomes too intense or complicated, therapeutic intervention may be needed to disentangle the issues and help in developing understanding and effective collaboration.

Another example of a possible need for psychotherapeutic intervention occurs when a young student with an ADD anticipates the transition into junior high school or high school, where there is a need to relate not just to one classroom teacher, with whom one remains most of the day, but to multiple teachers in different classrooms, each of whom is seen for only one class period each day. The student and his or her parents may need some therapeutic assistance to deal with transitional worries and to develop effective strategies to deal with problems of homework management, medication administration, arrangement of accommodations for extended time for taking tests, and so forth.

For other families, intense, persistent conflicts may develop between parents and an adolescent son or daughter with an ADD who refuses to take prescribed medications for the ADD or a comorbid disorder, is unwilling or unable to organize and complete homework required to get acceptable grades, or demands permission to get a driver's license or to drive the family car before the parent is willing to allow it. Such conflicts are commonplace in many families and are usually resolved more or less adequately. But in some families these matters may be complicated considerably by an adolescent's severe ADD symptoms regardless of whether a mood disorder or substance abuse is present. Or the family problems may be further complicated by a parent's also having an ADD, a mood disorder, or a substance abuse problem, treated or untreated. In these situations, the ADD symptoms offered as the presenting complaint may be the smallest of the difficulties faced by the family; the ADD may simply function as the "ticket" to get the family members inside the therapist's door.

Interaction of parent and child problems can chronically skew family interaction and can exacerbate routine parent-adolescent conflicts into bitter, protracted, and destructive family wars. Sometimes in families seeking help for dealing with the problematic ADD symptoms of one family member, severe, complicated problems will be present in several members of the family or in the family system itself. In such situations, a clinician who understands ADDs and other psychiatric disorders as well as how to evaluate and intervene effectively in family interaction processes may be able to assist by providing parent counseling, adolescent counseling, and/or conjoint family therapy.

Sometimes intensive psychotherapeutic intervention is sought because of a crisis. For example, a college student may return home after being put on probation or expelled from college or university because of academic failure or excessive behavior problems. Such occasions are generally fraught with complicated emotional reactions within the student and between the student and other family members. The excitement and high hopes of high school graduation are suddenly exchanged for a mix of shame over failure, resentment and disappointment over wasted resources, and the bewildering uncertainties of finding another school or a job and needing to develop a revised plan for entering the adult world. In such a situation, psychotherapeutic assistance for student and parents, both separately and conjointly, may be useful to fully assess the situation and to facilitate realistic and appropriate plans that will avert the likelihood of one failure giving rise to another.

Regardless of whether the ADD and/or comorbid disorders contributed to the failure in college, the problems associated with the ADD and comorbid disorder should be taken into account as parents and their son or daughter try to cope with such a situation. If, for example, the student developed a severe depression or anxiety disorder or substance abuse problem while at college, those difficulties should be evaluated and appropriate treatment should be provided. If the college failure was due to the student's inability to meet the academic demands of college, questions about whether the ADD was correctly evaluated and appropriately treated, whether medications were taken as prescribed, whether there may be an unrecognized learning disorder, or whether unrealistic goals were being pursued, and so forth, need to be raised and suitably addressed with appreciation both for the limitations that the ADD or comorbid difficulties may create and for all the many other factors that need to be considered.

Other crisis situations may arise if parents separate or divorce or if a family member is arrested, runs away from home, loses a job, becomes suicidal, has a serious motor vehicle accident, develops an addiction, and so forth. In such situations clinicians should be careful to avoid attributing too much blame for problems to ADD impairments in one or more family member. Careful assessment requires taking into account all the intrapersonal, interpersonal, family, and wider social system factors that might be contributing to the difficulties. In such situations, ADD may be one contributing factor among many that have shaped the problem.

Some individuals and families seem to live in chronic crisis; at least one family member seems always to be in serious difficulty. In families in which severe stresses and very limited emotional-social resources persist, there may be a long-continuing need for therapeutic assistance or intervention over protracted periods. As Cornsweet (1990) has observed, when multiple psychiatric comorbidities are present, there is often greater biological, familial, and socioeconomic disadvantage as well. In these markedly more severe and complex situations, more sustained psychotherapy and many other types of interventions may be needed to assess and address multiple individual and family problems intertwined with or exacerbating ADD symptoms of the identified patient.

Decisions about when more intensive interventions are needed and who should be directly involved in which treatments and for how long are often complex. Jensen and Abikoff, in their chapter in this volume (see Chapter 20), discuss the multiple factors that should be taken into account in tailoring treatment plans for specific individuals and families. The main point here is that various types of psychosocial intervention often play a critical role in developing and implementing effective treatment for individuals with ADDs and their families.

One of the most important contributions that can result from effective psychosocial interventions is the development of realistic hope that supports and nurtures the efforts of patients and their families to work for constructive change. Unfortunately, some who speak and write about ADDs, and some who provide treatment services for persons affected by ADDs, attempt to encourage hope in unrealistic ways. They recognize the persistent demoralization that often arises in persons with ADDs and in their families; they empathize with the chronic discouragement. They try to dispel this hopelessness by offering blanket reassurances about the dramatic life-transforming improvements that stimulant medications and psychosocial interventions may bring to persons with ADDs and their families. They suggest or imply that emotional and practical effects of years of frustration and failure from untreated ADD symptoms can be suddenly undone by instituting appropriate treatment. Change is rarely that simple or complete.

In providing excessively simplistic, overly optimistic reassurance, helpers may ultimately cause even more devastating hopelessness in the patient and family. Searles (1979) described how therapists, in their own human limitations, sometimes encourage patients to expect too much too quickly or to overlook the painful reality of constraints and obstacles to desired changes in themselves or others. If excessive promises are implied and the treatment interventions are not quickly, substantially, and persistently effective, those who have been encouraged in unrealistic hopes for specific interventions are likely to give up hope and to be less willing to make further efforts. It is important that therapists help their patients and others involved to nurture realistic hope.

In cultivating realistic hope in the therapist and patient, it is important for both to avoid overly simplistic formulations of complex problems. Kazdin and Kagan (1994) provided a thoughtful assessment of the multiple positive and negative factors usually involved in the "packages" of influences that shape longer-term outcomes of individual and family problems. Recognition of these complexities does not make hope impossible, and it may help to keep expectations more realistic and to support the combined efforts of therapists and their patients so they can sustain the difficult and often frustrating work of changing destructive effects of complex ADDs and comorbid disorders.

Self-Help and Advocacy Groups

In addition to coaching and psychotherapeutic treatments, patients with ADD and their families may find important social support and practical assistance in various self-help and advocacy groups. Some such groups are specifically oriented toward ADDs: CHADD and the National Attention Deficit Disorder Association are two national groups that support websites, publications, and conferences to provide useful information and support for those affected by ADD.

Persons with ADDs with comorbid disorders may find it useful to assess resources not only in organizations specifically focused on ADDs but also in groups focused on other particular disorders with which they are concerned. Individuals affected by ADDs with substance abuse might benefit from seeking information available from Alcoholics Anonymous, Narcotics Anonymous, Al-Anon, and so forth. Those concerned with learning disorders might find useful information available from the Learning Disabilities Association of America and related organizations. Others more concerned with OCD or Tourette syndrome can find assistance through the Obsessive-Compulsive Foundation and Tourette Syndrome Association, respectively. Locations and directions to contact these and a myriad of other organizations that offer rich stores of information, often without charge, can be readily located on the Internet or from a local public library.

For some, the primary usefulness of these organizations is as a source of accurate, up-to-date information about the disorder, resources for learning more about it, and information on how to access services. This information is often available from the organizational websites or in packets of information or periodical publications often available in response to a postcard or phone call. For others, it may be helpful to seek out and attend local meetings of affiliated groups or to attend a regional or national convention, where more information can be obtained and it is possible to meet and learn from others affected by the disorder. Participation in such meetings may significantly help to alleviate the bewilderment and intense feelings of isolation that may be experienced when one has no contact with others who struggle with a similar set of problems.

Ultimately, the most important psychosocial intervention for ADDs and related problems may be making a connection with a competent professional who can provide needed evaluation and treatments, as well as with some peers who have struggled with similar problems and are willing to share accurate information and emotional support. Often these support organizations can help to open doorways to both types of relationships. Local chapters of support and advocacy groups like CHADD, the National Attention Deficit Disorder Association, and the Learning Disabilities Association of America often maintain and make available lists of medical, psychological, and educational professionals who have been helpful in providing evaluations, education, and treatment about ADDs and/or learning disorders to people in their community.

In many communities, including in the United States, where ADDs are rapidly gaining wider recognition, individuals with ADDs and their families need to expend considerable effort to develop adequate support networks and to locate needed professional services for psychosocial and medical interventions. Yet, through the efforts of many, national, regional, and international resources are being more widely developed to facilitate sharing of accurate information and to establish more adequate resources for persons with ADDs and their families.

REFERENCES

Anastopoulos AD, Smith JM, Wien EE: Counseling and training parents, in Attention-Deficit Hyperactivity Disorder: Handbook for Diagnosis and Treatment, 2nd Edition. Edited by Barkley RA. New York, Guilford, 1998, pp 373–393

Attwood T: Asperger's Syndrome. London, Jessica Kingsley, 1998

Barkley RA (ed): Attention-Deficit Hyperactivity Disorder: Handbook for Diagnosis and Treatment, 2nd Edition. New York, Guilford, 1998

Braswell L, Bloomquist ML: Cognitive-Behavioral Therapy With ADHD Children: Child, Family and School Interventions. New York, Guilford, 1991

Cornsweet C: A review of research on hospital treatment of children and adolescents. Bull Menninger Clin 54:64–77, 1990

Cunningham CE: A large-group community-based, family systems approach to parent training, in Attention-Deficit Hyperactivity Disorder: Handbook for Diagnosis and Treatment, 2nd Edition. Edited by Barkley RA. New York, Guilford, 1998, pp 394–412

Dendy CAZ: Teenagers With ADD: A Parents' Guide. Bethesda, MD, Woodbine House, 1995

Dishion TJ, Patterson GR, Stoolmiller M, et al: Family, school, and behavioral antecedents to early adolescent involvement with antisocial peers. Dev Psychol 27:172–180, 1991

Eyberg SM, Edwards D, Boggs SR, et al: Maintaining the treatment effects of parent training: the role of booster sessions and other maintenance strategies. Clinical Psychology: Science and Practice 5:544–554, 1998

Gordon M, Keiser S (eds): Accommodations in Higher Education Under the Americans With Disabilities Act. New York, Guilford, 1998

Greene RW: The Explosive Child. New York, HarperCollins, 1998

Hallowell EM: Psychotherapy of adult attention deficit disorder, in Comprehensive Guide to Attention Deficit Disorder in Adults: Research, Diagnosis and Treatment. Edited by Nadeau KG. New York, Brunner/Mazel, 1995, pp 146–167

Hallowell EM: When You Worry About the Child You Love. New York, Simon & Schuster, 1996

Hallowell EM, Ratey JJ: Driven to Distraction: Attention Deficit Disorder in Children and Adults. New York, Pantheon, 1994

Ingersoll B, Goldstein S: Attention Deficit Disorder and Learning Disabilities: Realities, Myths and Controversial Treatments. New York, Doubleday, 1993

Jackson SW: The listening healer in the history of psychological healing. Am J Psychiatry 149:1623–1632, 1992

Kazdin AE: Behavior Modification in Applied Settings, 5th Edition. Belmont, CA, Wadsworth Press, 1994

Kazdin AE: Parent management training: evidence, outcomes, and issues. J Am Acad Child Adolesc Psychiatry 36:1349–1356, 1997

Kazdin AE, Kagan J: Models of dysfunction in developmental psychopathology. Clinical Psychology: Science and Practice 1:35–52, 1994

Latham PS, Latham PH: Legal rights of the ADD adult, in Comprehensive Guide to Attention Deficit Disorders in Adults: Research, Diagnosis and Treatment. Edited by Nadeau KG. New York, Brunner/Mazel, 1995, pp 337–351

Latham PS, Latham PH: Documentation and the Law: For Professionals Concerned With ADD/LD. Washington, DC, JKL Publications, 1996

MTA Cooperative Group: Fourteen-month randomized clinical trial of treatment strategies for attention-deficit/hyperactivity disorder. Arch Gen Psychiatry (in press)

Nadeau KG (ed): Comprehensive Guide to Attention Deficit Disorder in Adults: Research, Diagnosis and Treatment. New York, Brunner/Mazel, 1995

Nadeau KG: Adventures in Fast Forward: Life, Love and Work for the ADD Adult. New York, Brunner/Mazel, 1996

Nadeau KG: ADD in the Workplace: Choices, Changes and Challenges. New York, Brunner/Mazel, 1997

Patterson GR, Chamberlain P: Functional analysis of resistance during parent training therapy. Clinical Psychology: Science and Practice 1:53–70, 1994

Pelham WE, Waschbusch DA: Behavioral intervention in attention-deficit/hyperactivity disorder, in Handbook of Disruptive Behavior Disorders. Edited by Quay HC, Hogan AE. New York, Kluwer Academic/Plenum, 1999, pp 255–278

Robin AL: ADHD in Adolescents. New York, Guilford, 1998a

Robin AL: Training families with ADHD adolescents, in Attention-Deficit Hyperactivity Disorder: Handbook for Diagnosis and Treatment, 2nd Edition. Edited by Barkley RA. New York, Guilford, 1998b, pp 413–457

Ruma PR, Burke RV, Thompson RW: Group parent training: is it effective for children of all ages? Behavior Therapy 27:159–170, 1996

Searles HF: Development of mature hope in the therapist-patient relationship, in Countertransference and Related Subjects. New York, International Universities Press, 1979, pp 479–502

Sherman M, Hertzig ME: Prescribing practices of Ritalin: The Suffolk County, New York Study, in Ritalin: Theory and Patient Management. Edited by Greenhill LL, Osman BB. New York, Mary Ann Liebert, 1991, pp 187–193

Solden S: Women With Attention Deficit Disorder. Grass Valley, CA, Underwood Books, 1995

Spencer TJ, Biederman J, Wilens T, et al: Pharmacotherapy of attention-deficit hyperactivity disorder across the life cycle. J Am Acad Child Adolesc Psychiatry 35:409–432, 1996

Stine JJ: Psychosocial and psychodynamic issues affecting noncompliance with stimulant treatment. J Child Adolesc Psychopharmacol 4:75–86, 1994

Strupp HH, Hadley SW, Gomez-Schwartz B: Psychotherapy for Better or Worse: The Problem of Negative Effects. New York, Jason Aronson, 1977

Wilens TE: Straight Talk About Psychiatric Medications for Kids. New York, Guilford, 1999

18 Cognitive Therapy for Adults With Attention-Deficit/Hyperactivity Disorder

Stephen P. McDermott, M.D.

Attention-deficit/hyperactivity disorder (ADHD) is a prevalent disorder estimated to affect 2%–9% of school-age children (Anderson et al. 1987; Bauermeister et al. 1994; Safer and Krager 1988). (ADHD, as used in this report, refers to previous definitions of the disorder as well as the current DSM-IV definition.) Although, historically, ADHD was not thought to continue beyond adolescence (Laufer and Denhoff 1957), prospective, long-term follow-up studies have shown the persistence of the syndrome in approximately 50% of young adults diagnosed as having ADHD in childhood (Mannuzza et al. 1991, 1993; Weiss and Hechtman 1986). Recent epidemiologically derived data suggest that as many as 5% of adults may have ADHD (Murphy and Barkley 1996).

Studies of adults with ADHD have demonstrated high rates of comorbidity with depression, anxiety, substance use, and conduct/antisocial personality disorders (Biederman et al. 1993; Shekim et al. 1990). It is not surprising that studies indicate that 20%–25% of adult outpatients with depression or substance abuse also have ADHD (Alpert et al. 1996; see also Chapter 9, this volume).

Further, many authors describe problems associated with ADHD in adults

---

The author wishes to acknowledge gratefully Timothy E. Wilens, M.D., Andrew Butler, Ph.D., and Aaron T. Beck, M.D., for their generous editorial assistance.

that are due to neither the core symptoms of ADHD nor distinct comorbid disorders. Adults with ADHD are often described as having problems with procrastination, boredom intolerance, frustration intolerance, and disorganization. They also have been shown to have more relationship difficulties, as well as academic and occupational underachievement despite adequate intellectual abilities (Biederman et al. 1993; Mannuzza et al. 1993). Ratey et al. (1992) noted that "associated problems" and comorbid disorders often cause more distress and dysfunction for adults with ADHD than the core symptoms themselves and are often the reasons these patients seek treatment.

Little information exists in the literature on the use of psychotherapies for adults with ADHD (Bemporad and Zambenedetti 1996; Hallowell 1995; Ratey et al. 1992). In a retrospective assessment of the histories of 60 adults with ADHD, Ratey et al. (1992) reported that the majority of the patients in their sample did not respond favorably to adequate psychotherapeutic treatment delivered by experienced psychotherapists through both short-term focused and long-term unstructured psychotherapies. However, these retrospective patient accounts were limited to descriptions of diverse, broadly defined psychotherapeutic interventions. Moreover, these adults did not receive a diagnosis or treatment for their ADHD at the time of their psychotherapeutic involvement.

Cognitive-behavioral interventions have emerged as one of the most efficacious psychotherapeutic interventions in the treatment of children and adolescents with ADHD (Barkley 1990; Hinshaw and Erhardt 1991). The theoretical construct of cognitive therapy addresses the interaction of cognition, behavior, and affect (McDermott and Wright 1992)—areas that are thought to be dysregulated in ADHD (Hinshaw and Erhardt 1991). Cognitive therapy has demonstrated efficacy in the treatment of major depression (Hollon and Najavits 1988) and anxiety (Sokol et al. 1989) and shows promise in the treatment of substance abuse (Najavits and Weiss 1994)—disorders that are highly comorbid with ADHD in adults.

The proactive, focused, structured, and goal-directed nature of cognitive therapy is compelling, given the nature of the disturbances in ADHD (Bemporad and Zambenedetti 1996; Hallowell 1995). Cognitive therapy shares many characteristics with psychotherapies used in pediatric ADHD groups—namely, training in self-evaluation, social skills, and anger and impulse management, as well as self-instruction that includes coping skills and problem-solving (Barkley 1990). Yet, these protocols may not be directly adaptable to adults with ADHD, given the reliance of these psychotherapies on parental involvement for structure and motivation.

This chapter presents an adaptation of Beck's cognitive therapy for use with adults with ADHD. In the following sections, the theoretical model, as well as the modification of basic cognitive therapy techniques addressing specific ADHD symptoms, associated problems, and comorbid disorders, is described.

COGNITIONS, EMOTIONS, BEHAVIORS, AND BELIEFS

The cornerstone of A. T. Beck's cognitive therapy is the interplay among cognitions, emotions, behaviors, and beliefs. Beck suggests that specific cognitions, emotions, and behaviors in a given situation are linked, with each affecting, and being affected by, the others (A. T. Beck et al. 1990). Although some thoughts (e.g., "I can't concentrate in class") are rather specific to ADHD, many more are seen in other emotional disorders. For example, "I can't do it" or "I'm annoying her" are thoughts that commonly cause problems for adults with ADHD. These, or similar thoughts, are also seen frequently in disorders such as depression and social phobia.

Although some behaviors (e.g., severe hyperactivity) occur most frequently in ADHD, many other symptoms of ADHD are common in a variety psychiatric disorders. Fidgeting is seen in anxiety disorders, procrastination is not uncommon in depression, and impulsivity is a frequent occurrence in bipolar disorders.

Many beliefs of adults with ADHD also occur in patients with other disorders. Beck's theory focuses on specific cognitions that occur in particular situations. These thoughts arise from beliefs that cut across many different, but related, situations (e.g., interactions with authority figures, events requiring assessment of one's competency) (A. T. Beck et al. 1990).

Beliefs tend not to form as discrete, isolated entities, but rather to occur in relationship to similar beliefs, which can be more or less specific. These hierarchical collections of interrelated beliefs are called *schemas* (A. T. Beck 1996; A. T. Beck et al. 1990). Each belief in a schema may affect, and be affected by, similar beliefs (Segal et al. 1996). Because of the interplay among related beliefs in schemas, beliefs that arise because of specific effects of ADHD can be generalized to areas outside of ADHD.

The Case of Jack

Jack was a very bright, likeable 19-year-old college sophomore who was referred for treatment of recently diagnosed ADHD and a first episode of depression in the setting of difficulty with school.

Jack had done relatively well in grade school and high school despite his undiagnosed ADHD. He was intelligent and learned material quickly, and this allowed him to compensate for his inefficient studying. He could often deduce material he missed in lectures from the content that preceded and followed it.

Jack was generally well liked but felt he had to work harder at maintaining relationships because he was somewhat socially awkward, because of his impulsive behavior. This became particularly more noticeable as he grew older and his classmates became increasingly more mature.

Because of the increased productivity demands of high school, Jack started to have problems meeting deadlines. For the first time in his academic career, he had to study hard for tests. He oftened procrastinated. He found it difficult to study because of his attention problems. Still, he was able to do reasonably well on tests by "cramming" but noticed he seemed to have more trouble studying than most of his friends. His grades started to drop. He recognized he was somehow "different" from his friends, who generally were able to maintain the good grades they had been achieving earlier in school.

He began to worry about his ability to do well in college. He had thoughts such as "If I keep messing up like this in high school, how will I ever be able to handle college? Maybe I'll screw it up. Maybe I'm not cut out for college." He felt anxious, sad, and somewhat ashamed when he had these thoughts, but he usually found them fairly easy to dismiss. He told himself, "This is ridiculous. I've always done well in school. I'll just have to work a little harder and be more organized."

These thoughts and feelings had appeared in the past when he failed to accomplish a task such as submitting a paper on deadline or applying in a timely and organized way for a college interview. Eventually, painful cognitions and emotions would arise when he merely considered attempting such tasks, making it more difficult just to start them.

These thoughts and feelings had never interfered with his studying. He had always considered himself to be "bright enough to get by" until his freshman year in college, when the work demands overwhelmed his attentional and organizational abilities. For the first time, he failed a test and did poorly in several courses that he found uninteresting.

Increasingly, Jack had difficulty studying even the courses he liked. He was often distracted by thoughts such as "I'll do poorly in this test," "I only did well in high school because it was easy," and "I'm too far behind to get a decent grade in this course." He was troubled by shameful images of telling his parents and friends he was flunking out of college. He started to withdraw socially and emotionally from family and friends and became more isolated.

He always considered studying to be somewhat difficult, but he now thought of productive studying as nearly impossible. When he even thought of studying, his cognitions were likely to be "Even if I try to study, it won't do me any good" or, more simply, "I can't study." As he began to avoid studying, his grades fell even more. He became more anxious, depressed, and ashamed, and his concentration worsened further.

His worsening grades led him to develop the (distorted) belief that he could not learn at all. He believed that he would never succeed at school or in a career. He presumed he would fail at anything he held to be important in his life. He sought professional help when he received notice that his school was putting him on "academic probation."

Jack's narrow beliefs about his difficulty with studying became more generalized. The belief "Studying is harder for me than for other students" became linked with other specific beliefs about school, such as "I don't do my work on time" and "I'm more disorganized than other students." This led to the broader belief "I'm not a legitimate student."

He interpreted this as further support for his belief "I am different," which had developed much earlier in his life because of his social awkwardness. The belief "I am different" to him was synonymous with "I am abnormal." As this broad schema, "I'm different," became activated, his mind would be filled with images of past examples of being different ("abnormal") in many different circumstances, academic or otherwise. He would be left with thoughts of "I'm incompetent" and "I'm a failure," accompanied by a profound sense of sadness and shame.

Jack's generalization of specific beliefs over time occurred because of interrelated schemas (see the discussion of attention and perception in the next section). The beliefs, thoughts, emotions, and behaviors were all integrally linked and reinforced each other. This may be why psychotherapeutic approaches that focus on only a portion of this system—such as emotions and beliefs, or cognitions and behaviors—may be ineffective.

Because of the chronicity of ADHD in adults, long-standing dysfunctional beliefs can be extremely persistent and quite powerful. As Spencer and colleagues (1994) noted:

> This disorder is not benign. . . . Given the longer duration of psychopathology and the increased demands for independent functioning,

> the level of dysfunction may be even more severe in adults than in children. A lifetime of interpersonal, academic, and occupational failure may be qualitatively and quantitatively different than a limited experience in childhood in a more protected family setting. (p. 333)

The cognitive therapy of ADHD strongly emphasizes belief change, much as in the cognitive therapy of other chronic disorders such as chronic depression, substance abuse, and personality disorders. This emphasis may be different from the relatively greater focus on thoughts, feelings, and behaviors in the cognitive therapy of anxiety or depression (in patients with relatively good intermorbid functioning).

What may be striking in this example of a patient with ADHD is the similarity between his cognitions, emotions, and beliefs and those of patients with other disorders, such as anxiety and depression. These nonspecific cognitions, emotions, and beliefs can affect more ADHD-specific features, like distractibility and impulsivity. Trying to separate the "ADHD-related" thoughts and beliefs from the "non–ADHD-related" ones may become an artificial, unproductive exercise because of the tight integration of belief systems. Yet, this similarity of cognitions, emotions, and beliefs between ADHD and other disorders may cause clinicians to overlook important differences that impede the effective use of the usual cognitive and behavioral techniques. To understand these differences, one must look at the next level in the model: the roles of attention and perception.

ATTENTION AND PERCEPTION

As recently reported, prominent symptoms of inattention and distractibility are found in the vast majority of clinically referred ADHD adults (Millstein et al. 1997; Wilens et al. 1998). Although the general level of distractibility in adults with ADHD may be notable, these adults are not easily distracted in all situations. When Jack is sitting around with his friends watching their favorite football teams, he may be as attentive and engaged in the game as they. The football game is inherently interesting to all of them and attracts (or "grabs") their attention.

The difference between Jack and his friends with no ADHD becomes apparent when they are in a classroom or other work setting dealing with material that is not inherently interesting. It is much more difficult for Jack to pull his attention away from more attractive stimuli (like the whispered conversation of the students sitting behind him) and to keep it on the less interesting physics lecture. (What makes one stimulus more or less "inherently attractive" than others is discussed below.)

This attentional dyscontrol is characteristic of an adult with ADHD. These persons may attend to certain attractive stimuli more intently than may individuals without ADHD and may show a deficit of attention only when trying to sustain their attention on a stimulus that is less attractive than competing stimuli. Adults with ADHD often have difficulty focusing their attention where they want it to be rather than where it tends to be drawn naturally.

To see how the attentional dyscontrol of ADHD affects individuals, one must first understand how attention and perception are influenced by beliefs in individuals without ADHD (or in adults with ADHD independent of their attention problems). In any given situation, many complex, conflicting, and ambiguous stimuli are present. One's beliefs about the situation, oneself, and others involved determine which stimuli are relevant for decision making (and thus should be attended to) and which are extraneous or inaccurate (and therefore should be ignored).

Beliefs that are activated more frequently tend to develop lower thresholds (i.e., to be activated with weaker stimuli) (Segal et al. 1996). These beliefs are likely to be activated more quickly in situations that might activate several competing beliefs. Also, their responses tend to be more powerful (relative to the response of other beliefs for a given stimulus). In addition, specific beliefs that are frequently activated tend to generalize. They more predictably and strongly activate related beliefs that previously had not been associated with the belief. This process is referred to as, "spreading activation" (Segal et al. 1996).

Beliefs that are more quickly, strongly, and broadly activated have greater influence on an individual's attention and perception in a given situation. This, in turn, increases the likelihood that stimuli will be perceived that support the belief, activating it further. This self-reinforcing process is referred to as *sensitization* (A. T. Beck 1996; Segal et al. 1996).

An individual's perception of a situation can be biased if the activated belief is particularly strong or has no contradictory beliefs to compete with it for control of the individual's attention. This can result in a "feed-forward" cycle of biased perceptions reinforcing the beliefs from which they arise, which in turn makes these same biased perceptions and assessments more likely in the future (A. T. Beck 1996).

Activated beliefs and the resulting thoughts and moods also influence the memories that one selectively recalls to process ambiguous situations. Those memories that are congruent with the activated belief tend to be perceived as more relevant to the assessment of the situation, and therefore are more likely to be attended to, than those that are contradictory to it (Segal et al. 1996; Williams 1996).

The emotional consequences of the activation of schemas can also influence one's attention. Powerful negative beliefs can give rise to excruciating sadness, anxiety, or shame. In trying to avoid the triggers of these painful emotions, individuals may pay much more attention to the negative aspects of a situation than to the less-threatening, positive aspects. They may exaggerate the likelihood or result of adverse outcome and/or underestimate their resources for dealing with the situation or its emotional consequences.

The hurtful aspects of situations may have stronger control of one's attention, or are "more inherently attractive," than the positive or neutral components. The inherent attractiveness of a stimulus is merely a description of its ability to strongly activate a belief (relative to other stimuli in the situation). "Attractiveness" does not refer to how pleasant, alluring, or appealing the stimulus is. For example, automobile accidents can be inherently attractive to passersby. Belief systems do not necessarily "control" one's attention. They only determine the inherent attractiveness of stimuli, thereby influencing which stimuli one attends to.

The concept of inherent attractiveness is extremely important in the cognitive therapy of ADHD, because it allows one to predict the ways in which one's attention may be influenced in a situation. It also gives one new tools for controlling one's attention that are not commonly considered in the treatment of ADHD—that is, techniques for dealing with cognitions, emotions, and beliefs, in addition to the more typical behavioral and environmental interventions.

The degree of an individual's emotional arousal is a useful measure of the degree of activation of a belief and, therefore, of its control of the person's attention. The degree of emotional arousal associated with a particular stimulus (i.e., how much it is "imbued" with emotion) will correlate with its inherent attractiveness (i.e., how tightly it will capture and hold one's attention). As the degree of emotional arousal increases in a situation, one's attention is focused more strongly on those features of the situation that are congruent with the emotion (e.g., potentially dangerous stimuli when one is feeling anxious). There is, consequently, a greater exclusion of competing stimuli. The result is both a more intensely emotional perception and a more narrow one.

The concepts outlined above are crucial to understanding the causes and treatments of the emotional sequelae of ADHD (discussed in the next section).

In summary, the proportional activation of competing beliefs, with their concomitant emotional arousal, influences attention. Attention, in turn, controls what is perceived. This perception of the situation strengthens relevant beliefs, further amplifying the influence of these beliefs on subsequent attention and perception. The increased activation of the beliefs makes it more likely these beliefs will be stronger in their responses and easier to activate the next time a relevant situation is perceived (Figure 18–1).

The feed-forward cycle of increasing activation and reinforcement of a belief system can be counteracted by competing (contradictory) beliefs of similar strength. When individuals find their perceptions of situations being pulled in one direction (e.g., "I'll do poorly this semester because I never do well on tests, and there's nothing I can do about it"), they can recruit competing beliefs (and the thoughts that arise from them) to steer their attention and perception in another direction (e.g., "I have had trouble with tests in some subjects in the past because of my anxiety, but it's early in the semester, and I've learned several new ways to deal with my anxiety"). This not only leads to a more balanced perception of the given situation but also prevents one belief from becoming relatively predominant by balancing it with the activation of the competing beliefs.

This model of attention and perception applies to all individuals. What distinguishes persons with ADHD is their inability to pull their attention away from more inherently attractive stimuli. This creates more intense and

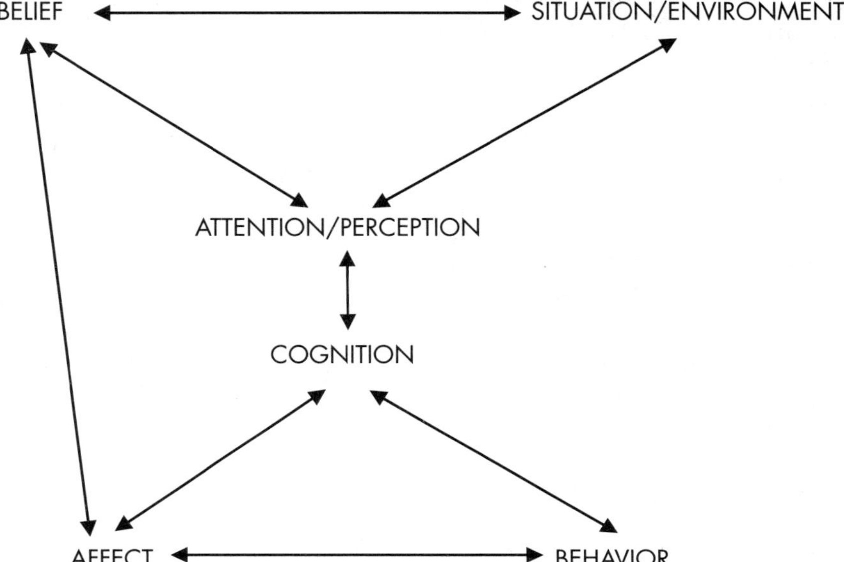

Figure 18–1. Interactions among components of the psychological system.

labile affect than might be expected in a given situation. It also distorts their perceptions of situations by focusing and maintaining their attention on maladaptive components of the situation while consequently making more difficult the recruitment of adaptive competing beliefs. A more balanced perspective of the situation (which is required for rational responding and other core cognitive therapy techniques) becomes increasingly difficult to achieve and maintain, even temporarily. The continuing focus on negative aspects of the situation further strengthens the maladaptive schemas.

EMOTIONAL SEQUELAE OF ADHD

The attentional dyscontrol of ADHD individuals has important specific emotional and cognitive sequelae. The pattern of interactions among cognitions, emotions, attention, and beliefs in ADHD discussed in previous sections gives rise to two prominent emotional sequelae: downward spirals and cognitive avoidance.

Once a powerful belief system is activated, it creates an "affective-cognitive feedback loop" (A. Butler and A. T. Beck, personal communication, 1997) or "cognitive-affective vicious cycle" (Segal et al. 1996), which generates progressively more affect. This further narrows the focus of attention on the activating stimuli, increasing the activation of the belief and related schemas. Persons with ADHD can show a pattern of relatively brief periods of rapidly intensifying, usually painful dysphoric emotions called *downward spirals.* (Segal et al. [1996, p. 375] use this term to describe a similar, but much slower, process.) A balanced appraisal of the situation may be difficult because thoughts that are more rational may not be sufficiently powerful to attract and anchor the ADHD individual's attention away from more emotional stimuli in order to break the cycle.

Downward spirals can continue until interrupted by more powerful stimuli, or "distractors." Adults with ADHD use distractors that can become dysfunctional in and of themselves. Common examples include binge eating, exercise, sex, computer games, and social interactions. Strong, positive stimuli can break the downward spirals by pulling the individual's attention away from less-intense negative stimuli. Some individuals also use sleep to break the downward spirals.

Although downward spirals are typically painful, spirals of intense, pleasurable emotions occur as well. Positive spirals may prompt adults with ADHD to focus on promising aspects of a situation to the exclusion of harmful ones, resulting in potentially detrimental or dangerous courses of action.

Risk-taking behaviors are often labeled as "self-destructive" behaviors. They might better be understood as the distorted assessment of risks versus benefits in the emotionally charged moments in which the actions are contemplated (see also discussion of problems with perspective and cognitive impulsivity in the next section).

Adults with ADHD also may prevent downward spirals by using cognitive avoidance, the process of actively avoiding thoughts (and therefore, behaviors) that might provoke painful emotional responses. Individuals who frequently use cognitive avoidance become adept at monitoring their emotions. When their moods take a more negative turn, they focus their attention on more neutral or positive thoughts. This occurs early in the emotional response, before the activation of the negative schema increases to such an extent that it becomes difficult for the individual to "grab control" of his or her attention and the downward spiral occurs.

The thoughts and beliefs behind cognitive avoidance are usually related to helplessness (e.g., "I can't do it"), affect intolerance (e.g., "I'll feel terrible if I try"), and hopelessness (e.g., "I will always fail, so I shouldn't put myself through the misery of trying").

Often, patients avoiding situations imagine dreadful consequences of their emotions, such as becoming increasingly sad and eventually killing themselves, or becoming so anxious they have a heart attack or "go crazy." Embarrassment and shame are particularly common emotions that can cause cognitive avoidance.

Cognitive avoidance is a major source of disorganization for individuals with ADHD and can be a serious impediment to their treatment. Cognitive avoidance leads to procrastination when adults with ADHD delay even contemplating a task. They do not actively decide *not* to do the chore, because that would require them to think about it, which could provoke a downward spiral. Initially, they simply "push aside" the thoughts, saying to themselves they will do the task at another time (which is usually unspecified). Eventually, they may actively distract themselves from these cognitions by doing other work instead. When circumstances finally force them to confront the avoided task, they may begin it with insufficient preparation or, in the extreme, decide they are unable even to attempt it. This increases the likelihood they will be disappointed with the results of their labors, reinforcing their negative predictions and increasing the probability that they will avoid similar situations in the future.

> While studying in the library, Jack was distracted by painful cognitions and emotions. This reinforced his belief "Studying is difficult and un-

productive (because I have problems with concentration)." The distressing emotional state also gave rise to the belief "Studying is onerous (because I can't tolerate the agonizing feelings that arise)." As these two beliefs strengthened, he predicted ever more strongly that studying would be excruciating and unproductive. He started to avoid the library. This usually diminished or eliminated the tormenting thoughts he had when he even anticipated schoolwork.

When he avoided studying instead of learning to overcome the suffering, these two beliefs became broader and more powerful, eventually generalizing to the belief "I can't study." The more strongly he believed he could not study, the more his motivation to push past the pain was diminished. This increased the probability he would avoid his assignments, diminishing the likelihood of his success and further reinforcing his belief that he could not study.

As his grades worsened, his belief "I can't study" broadened further to the more powerful schema "I'm a bad student." This, in turn, made his strategy of withdrawal from academic situations even more likely.

Patients with cognitive avoidance can be difficult to treat with medications as well. They can be exquisitely sensitive to minor side effects (or even therapeutic effects) of medications. These sensations activate painful underlying beliefs about having a disorder (e.g., "I'm defective"), being on medications (e.g., "I'm weak"), and being unable to tolerate side effects (e.g., "I'm having a bad reaction to the medication"). The distressing thoughts and emotions engender diminished compliance when patients "forget" to take their medications regularly. They also can amplify the attention patients pay to the negative aspects of the medications, making "side effects" even more likely.

COGNITIVE SEQUELAE OF ADHD

The cognitive sequelae commonly seen in individuals with ADHD are grouped in three major categories: difficulty with perspective, cognitive impulsivity, and obsessiveness.

Difficulty with perspective describes the problems adults with ADHD have in "getting the big picture" or "seeing the forest for the trees." This occurs when their attention gets pulled to one part of a situation before they can accurately assess the whole. This cognitive error occurs when an attractive component of a situation pulls and holds the attention to the detriment of other aspects (including a perception of the situation as a whole). This can be especially problematic when individuals try to solve problems in which one aspect is strongly emotion-provoking but assessment of the less emotional aspects is necessary to put the overall problem in perspective and to understand their resources for dealing with the problem.

Difficulty with perspective can also create problems with prioritizing. To prioritize, one needs to perceive different parts of a situation and at the same time see where each fits relative to the other parts and the whole. If any particular subset of these components holds one's attention excessively, it becomes difficult to place the items in their proper context. When adults with ADHD try to prioritize, their attention may become locked on one option or may jump from option to option without their ever understanding the interrelationships between the parts and the whole.

Cognitive impulsivity refers to the tendency of some adults with ADHD to analyze or interpret only part of a situation before jumping to a conclusion about it. This occurs when dysfunctional beliefs are more quickly and strongly activated than adaptive ones. Cognitive impulsivity makes alternative interpretations or solutions more difficult to produce.

Obsessiveness is the relative inability to stop thinking about distressing topics or repeating nonproductive behaviors in difficult situations. Adults with ADHD often describe this as "getting stuck." The patient's inability to pull his or her attention away from emotional cognitions may be the basis of the repetitious thoughts and behaviors.

> Jack bought a new computer. When he was assembling it, he had to input a certain code. He typed the code, but nothing happened. He typed it again but saw no results. He became more frustrated and found himself repeatedly entering the code, banging on the keyboard harder and harder, as if this would somehow allow the machine to better understand him. A friend came to his door, interrupting him. After he spoke with her briefly, he went back to the computer, and as he sat down, he noticed a switch had not been thrown on the keyboard. He threw it, entered the code, and received the desired results.

OVERDEVELOPED AND UNDERDEVELOPED STRATEGIES

The beliefs and processes that underlie the cognitive and emotional sequelae of ADHD may result in the development of overdeveloped and underdeveloped strategies (A. T. Beck et al. 1990). Patterns of behaviors that are habitual responses to similar situations are called *strategies.* Patients with chronic and severe disorders, such as personality disorders, use many of the strategies that people without disorders use, but use them excessively. When strategies are used to an extreme degree, they are called *overdeveloped strategies.*

Certain pathological mechanisms can propel individuals toward more extreme or maladaptive behaviors or can impede the use of more moderate, or counter-balancing, behaviors (i.e., the underdeveloped strategies). These mechanisms can be beliefs or other aspects of ADHD. Impulsivity and frustration intolerance can lead to aggression and hostility as one's primary response to conflict, while at the same time hindering the individual's ability to use behaviors that require restraint and emotional tolerance, such as diplomacy or assertiveness.

For individuals with ADHD, these moderate patterns of behavior may be difficult to learn because they require nonimpulsive responses to emotional situations. Therefore, even when the underlying mechanisms (e.g., impulsivity and frustration intolerance) are ameliorated, the individual still may not have the skills necessary to implement the underdeveloped strategies (e.g., assertiveness skills).

PROBLEMS ASSOCIATED WITH ADHD

Not all problems related to ADHD in adulthood relate to the comorbid disorders or core symptoms of ADHD. Associated problems are conceptualized in this model as combinations or "final common pathways" of other components of the model rather than distinct entities of their own.

For example, procrastination can be caused by many different mechanisms in adults with ADHD. Distraction can delay completion of a task, as can cognitive avoidance, yet each might be treated in very different ways (as discussed in the next section). Some adults with ADHD deliberately postpone starting certain tasks, such as studying, because doing them closer to the final deadline seems to focus their attention better than if the tasks are performed without time pressure. If this coping strategy is effective for them, interventions to change it might be counterproductive.

One or several of these mechanisms might contribute to procrastination in different situations in the same individual. The patient and the cognitive therapist must sort out the different components of the associated problem in each particular situation rather than attempt to use one intervention to treat them all.

COGNITIVE THERAPY OF ADHD IN ADULTHOOD

The cognitive therapy of ADHD differs from the cognitive therapy of other disorders in its greater emphasis on direct intervention on emotions, the focus of attention, and the activation of the belief systems, and less emphasis on thoughts and behaviors.

The components of the cognitive therapy of ADHD for the purposes of this chapter are separated into three areas: general issues (addressing the therapeutic relationship and the structure of the therapy), model-specific targets (techniques for treating the emotional and cognitive sequelae of ADHD), and standard treatment targets (with notations about impediments to standard interventions).

General Issues

The Therapeutic Relationship

Collaboration between therapists and patients about treatment decisions makes patients more active in treatment and less dependent on their therapists. It also enhances patients' beliefs that they are partners in their treatment, and this allows them to tolerate active and focused interventions that otherwise might seem oppressive.

Such a situation occurs when the therapist needs to interrupt the patient. Patients can become so engrossed in telling their stories that the session can be devoted to just one or two anecdotes. Interrupting may activate patients' beliefs about being incompetent (or being seen by their therapists as incompetent). Instead, therapists can explain that overly detailed stories and explanations are common manifestations of ADHD and are understood by the therapist as such and not as a personality flaw or "resistance." Therapist and patient can discuss this as an impediment to the therapy and solve the problem together.

The problem-solving, to be successful, needs to be truly collaborative. The patient and therapist may agree that the therapist should gently interrupt the patient when the therapist believes she has heard enough of a story to understand its meaning. She can test out her hypothesis by summarizing the main points for the patient. If the patient believes the therapist did not understand the main points or important details, or merely feels that it is important to share the rest of the story with her, he can continue. Otherwise, they will move on.

Thus, the therapist assumes responsibility for her part of the dilemma (interrupting and summarizing), while the patient assumes responsibility for his portion of the problem (identifying his own main points and agreeing or disagreeing with the summary). The patient and therapist can feel better about seeing the interruption as a collaborative solution to a common problem.

Structure of the Therapy

Cognitive therapy is active and focused to a large extent because it is goal oriented. The patient and therapist work together on treatment goals that are set mutually. The goals are specific, concrete, and presented in behavioral terms so that both patient and therapist know when the goal has been reached.

Not all goals in the treatment will be related to the ADHD. It may be important for the patient to develop skills for dealing with comorbid disorders such as depression, anger, or anxiety before focusing on the more typically ADHD-related problems. Associated problems, such as procrastination or poor social skills, also need to be addressed. Such "comorbid treatments" can be handled much more seamlessly in Beck's cognitive therapy because all these treatments share the same underlying model (McDermott and Wright 1992).

Patients with ADHD need to understand the chronic nature of the disorder. The adaptive strategies they learn must be continually practiced and reinforced or relapse is likely. Because patients with ADHD are often attracted to novel circumstances and lose the ability to stay on target as the situation loses its novelty, the therapist needs to stress that new skills can be lost if not used regularly. It is important to systematically review with patients on a regular basis how well they are maintaining their skills.

Patients may be encouraged to have a subset of skills listed on a *daily list of skills*—a card with activities that they will carry out on a daily basis until the activities are adequately incorporated into their daily routine. At that point, the activities will go onto the patients' lists of skills they review weekly. If they notice any skills are "slipping," they can put them back on their daily skills list.

One tool for keeping therapy on track collaboratively is the *session agenda.* This listing of topics to be covered is set by both the patient and the therapist at the beginning of the session. The agenda and concrete goals provide structure for the therapy overall and, in so doing, model for patients the advantages of setting short-term goals and providing greater structure to their lives.

The agenda can prevent the therapy from becoming focused on a "crisis du jour," whereby therapists deal only with the crises and catastrophes that patients bring into the session each week. Patients do not develop the week-to-week continuity they need to solidly acquire a set of skills. Further, they can develop the belief that they cannot learn problem-solving skills themselves but instead need to rely on the therapist to solve their problems. To guard against this possibility, the therapist should set aside time to deal with "the crisis" but also should allot time to continue the work begun the previous week.

One common mistake of novice cognitive therapists is the decision to abolish the structure (e.g., the agenda) in the face of a crisis. It is precisely in a crisis that a patient needs to be able to pull back and use a structured, standardized approach to his or her problems.

Ultimately, patients need to develop their skills until the skills become "second nature." It is important for therapists to discuss with their patients the benefits of developing a "routine," the habits used by individuals without ADHD to accomplish repetitive tasks without constantly needing to plan for them.

Model-Specific Techniques

Techniques for Treating the Emotional Sequelae

The individual with downward spirals may have difficulty benefiting from the usual cognitive and behavioral techniques used with patients with dysfunctional moods, such as rational responding and relaxation techniques.

> Jack had problems working with his classmates on group projects. As their discussions progressed, any disagreements he had with the group would trigger thoughts that the others were seeing him as unintelligent. Initially, these thoughts were not intense, but they still distracted him from the group process. They also became progressively more generalized and powerful, evolving to "They think I'm stupid" and "I'll never fit in—I'm not a legitimate student like they are." Jack became increasingly anxious, sad, and self-loathing but refused to leave the group for fear he would only confirm more strongly what the others must be thinking. He quickly learned to avoid not only group situations but also being around other students all together, even to the point of having difficulty sitting alone at a table in the library if other students were nearby.

To set the stage for other techniques to work, the activation of the beliefs generating the strong emotion has to be dealt with directly. The individual's attention needs to be interrupted in order to decrease the stimulation of the activated belief. As the predominant belief becomes less activated, other, more positive or neutral beliefs can be recruited to develop a more balanced view of the situation and options for dealing with it.

One useful technique for accomplishing this is the SPEAR (Stop, Pull-back, Evaluate, Act, and Re-evaluate) technique.

1. *Stop* refers to breaking the connection between the patient's attention and the emotion-provoking situation. Patients might say aloud, "Stop!" (as in the thought-stopping technique), or temporarily remove themselves from the situation.

Jack broke his concentration on the self-critical thoughts by excusing himself from the group and going to the restroom.

2. *Pull-back* refers to continuing the process of deactivating the predominant belief and attempting to put oneself in a more emotionally neutral state (i.e., calmer or less sad). The patient uses the intensity of the emotion as a gauge of how activated the belief remains. Relaxation techniques or imagery techniques may be helpful. They often are not effective, however, until distraction is used to decrease the activation of the predominant belief to the point at which the attention can be more firmly anchored in the calmer images and self-statements required by these techniques.

Jack used the time alone in the restroom to calm himself and collect his thoughts. He used coping cards with calming statements that he developed in therapy to rationally respond to his negative thoughts. At times, he was also able to use relaxation techniques briefly.

3. *Evaluate* refers to the process of re-examining the situation once the patient is in a calmer state. Patients can use many of the problem-solving skills normally taught in cognitive therapy, such as rational responding, because in the more emotionally neutral state, they have access to more neutral or positive belief systems with which they can better assess the situation, generate alternative hypotheses, and develop multiple options for solutions.

Since students could arrange their own groups, Jack always attended groups in which his friends Bill or Mary participated. He felt comfortable that they did not see him as stupid. He reminded himself that he frequently "felt stupid" in groups, but when he checked out his thoughts with Mary or Bill, the thoughts proved to be unfounded.

4. *Act* refers to patients beginning to resolve the problem on the basis of the results of their evaluation. Teaching the patient to use graded tasks (i.e., breaking large, overwhelming tasks into smaller, more manageable parts) may be particularly helpful in this step (A. T. Beck et al. 1979).

Jack returned to the group and resolved just to listen until he felt comfortable participating more actively again.

5. *Re-evaluate* refers to the process of continually alternating between small actions and reassessing one's emotional state before acting further. Patients, while acting on their evaluation, should not allow themselves to return to the previously highly charged emotional state. Re-evaluation prevents one's mood from rising again to extremes. It does not mean that one takes a complete series of actions and then re-evaluates the results of one's strategy.

Jack focused his attention on Bill, Mary, or anyone else in the group who seemed to be responding positively to him and diverted his attention away from those who seemed at all negative. He rationally responded to negative thoughts that arose. He sometimes needed to take another break from the group when he noticed his anxiety increasing.

Cognitive avoidance needs to be addressed with the patient in an open, nonjudgmental manner. The treatment of cognitive avoidance must become a priority in therapy, because it can slow progress to such an extent that the therapy ceases or becomes interminable.

Over the course of therapy, Jack came to understand that much of his inability to get a job was due to cognitive avoidance. Whenever he thought about applying for a job, he had images of interacting with his co-workers. He was flooded with thoughts such as "I won't fit in with the others" and "They'll think I'm different (i.e., strange)." He avoided starting the tasks needed to seek a job. He eventually decided that he could not work for someone else; he concluded he should seek a business of his own. When he considered his options for such businesses, however, he was filled with thoughts such as "That job would be be-

> neath me. People will think I just can't handle a better job." It was at this point he decided to become a lawyer.

In some cases, cognitive avoidance may not be readily apparent to individuals because of their habitual use of it. In others, avoidance may be quite deliberate. These patients may have difficulty discussing the avoidance because of their concern that their therapists will perceive it and react to it negatively.

Graduated task assignments can be useful for dealing with cognitive avoidance (A. T. Beck et al. 1979). The task may be started in the therapy session, but it is often completed for homework. Such homework, no matter how simple it seems to the therapist, requires adequate preparation in the therapy session. Rehearsing the steps of the graduated task assignment during the therapy session not only ensures a greater understanding of what is required of the patient but also confronts the thoughts that the patient is trying to avoid about the likelihood of failure, the consequences of failure, and the emotional aftermath of contemplating these thoughts. The patient might not discuss these thoughts otherwise, even if asked directly about impediments to doing the assignment.

The major modification of the graduated task assignment for patients with cognitive avoidance, however, is that the primary task is simply to attempt to *start* any part of it (including just thinking about beginning it). In doing so, the patients will be confronting the thoughts that have prevented them from starting, or even thinking about, the task. At the same time, they will be testing out their beliefs about dealing with these thoughts (e.g., "I get so anxious thinking about this, I'll fall apart"). If they do any activity toward their goal, they should give themselves credit for having successfully started the assignment.

> Jack often had difficulty studying because he was overwhelmed by thoughts (including images) that he would surely fail, and he avoided the affect that accompanied such thoughts. Eventually, he put off even attempting to study. He and his therapist agreed that if he could not study in the library for a few hours (which was typical for him previously), he would attempt to study for just 15 minutes. If he could not study even for 15 minutes, he would give himself credit for just going to the library, turning around, and returning home. If he could not get to the library, he was encouraged just to pack up his books, head to the bus stop, and return. In each case, he was told to pay attention to the task-interfering thoughts and write them down. If he could not respond to them at that time, he would bring them to therapy, where he and his therapist would deal with them together.

Thus, the assignment of the homework became a win-win situation: When he completed the task, he got closer to his goal. If, however, he could not complete the task but caught the automatic thoughts that interfered with his doing so, he achieved a greater understanding of what had been preventing him from accomplishing his task. He and his therapist could work on this further.

Sometimes patients have to be encouraged to "just do it" and not give themselves the option of avoiding a task. This should be done only after careful preparation and after other cognitive therapy techniques have failed.

Strong encouragement should not be a replacement for more traditional cognitive therapy techniques. If it fails, the failure can increase the patient's sense of hopelessness and introduce concerns about "disappointing" the therapist. If it succeeds, the success may be seen as a result of the therapist's efforts instead of the patient's new skills. Rather, the successful use of encouragement should become further evidence that the patient can confront and get past his or her cognitive avoidance. This bolsters the patient's confidence, and the patient often finds that the task he or she was avoiding is less onerous than the avoidance itself.

As a last resort, the therapist may need to discuss stopping therapy (for a certain period of time or even permanently) until the patient can learn to get past the avoidance. Otherwise, the therapy can become an endless exploration of possibilities without creating any concrete change in the patient's life.

Techniques for Treating Cognitive Sequelae

The treatment of cognitive distortions is well described (A. T. Beck et al. 1979; McDermott and Wright 1992). Cognitive distortions can be difficult to treat in adults with ADHD and *cognitive impulsiveness.* These individuals have difficulty pulling their attention away from emotion-laden, distorted thoughts in order to attend to the less-emotional, rational responses. Even when one can temporarily focus one's attention away from the distorted thoughts, the dysfunctional beliefs, because of their lower thresholds, may reactivate before more rational beliefs, which require a higher threshold for activation, can operate.

Imagery techniques can be a useful way of blending problem-solving strategies with strong positive emotions as a counterbalance to the intense negative emotions of dysfunctional beliefs. The following example illustrates how the powerful positive feelings patients have for close friends may allow them to engage in helping strategies that they would otherwise have difficulty using.

> Jack had difficulty calling a young woman to ask her for a date. He could recite a list of reasons she might want to go out with him, but these seemed "rather hollow" to him. His attention kept getting pulled to the thought "Who are you kidding? She'll laugh at you when you call, and if she doesn't, it's only because she feels sorry for you." He felt extremely anxious and embarrassed when he even thought about phoning.
>
> Jack remembered asking women for dates in college. His roommate used to give him "pep talks" before he called. He believed his friend's positive comments because he knew his roommate genuinely liked him.
>
> Before Jack tried to phone the young woman, he imagined what his roommate would say if he were there with him. Many of the comments were the same ones that seemed "hollow" before. But in the image, they seemed much more "realistic," and he felt more confident proceeding with the phone call.

Patients can also use images to access their problem-solving skills by imagining helping a friend with a similar problem. Seeing the problem resolve in their image can allow some of their hopelessness and helplessness to diminish as well. Patients can ask themselves, "If I can use this technique to help my friend, can't I also use it to help myself?"

Treatment interventions that help manage affect, such as medications, SPEAR, and other distraction techniques, can help increase the effectiveness of the cognitive interventions. The medications that ameliorate behavioral impulsivity in patients with ADHD (i.e., stimulants and antidepressants) can also help lessen their cognitive impulsivity as well.

Patients can use distractors, particularly the SPEAR technique, to help pull their attention away from inherently attractive thoughts that cause obsessiveness. Such techniques can be helpful in dealing with repetitious behaviors as well.

Individuals can learn to prioritize by adopting a simpler task than prioritizing the unit as a whole. They list items on individual 3 × 5 cards and arrange the cards in front of them. Then they select the single most important item in the group. They put it aside and again select the single most important item out of those left. They repeat this sequence until they have gone through the pile of cards. This allows them to build up a prioritized sequence of items by choosing the single most important item (which often stands out as the most attractive) without distraction from other ones.

Miscellaneous Techniques

Forgetfulness is a common complaint of adults with ADHD. They frequently describe losing things or forgetting what they are doing in the middle of a task. These situations may appear to be due to short-term memory difficulties, but testing the patient's short-term memory may reveal no discernible deficits. Often, "forgetfulness" may be related to two different problems:

1. *Distractibility.* Individuals without ADHD keep track of commonly misplaced items in two ways. One is to note to themselves (ever so briefly) where they are putting the car keys when they put them down. They are ensuring that the spot where they left the keys enters their short-term memory. Frequently, persons with ADHD are distracted (by their own thoughts or by external stimuli) before they note where they place something. They can often decrease their frequency of losing things by learning to deliberately notice where they place them before proceeding to their next task. This "sets" the location of the object more firmly in their short-term memory. This can also be helpful for patients who complain of "forgetting what I wanted to do by the time I get to where I was going."
2. *Disorganization.* Another way individuals without ADHD prevent losing things is through organization and structure. This is sometimes described as "a place for everything and everything in its place." They do not have to remember the location of their keys if they already have a well-developed strategy of putting them in the same place every time they enter their residence.

People with ADHD have greater difficulty building and maintaining such organizational structures. These structures depend on habitual behaviors or "routines" for their maintenance, but actions that are routine are less inherently attractive. Organizational structures, such as consistently using specific places to keep commonly misplaced things, need to be built one task at a time. Otherwise, the novelty of learning newer routines will distract from solidifying older ones. Patients then add other organizational tasks, with the understanding that they need to maintain the previous ones.

Scheduling can be another extremely difficult task for patients. Some scheduling skills patients may need to develop are

1. Breaking big tasks into smaller units that can be handled at separate (i.e., noncontiguous) times (because people often need to work on several projects at once).

2. Learning to interrupt activities at appropriate points to maintain a schedule and keep to a timetable or to see if other tasks have become more urgent.
3. Learning to assertively defend their schedules from intrusions by others.
4. Prioritizing (discussed earlier in this section).

Patients also may have scheduling difficulties because they overextend themselves. They impulsively accept new, more novel tasks before other work is completed, or they have problems with assertiveness. Thoughts such as "People will like me more if I do this job for them" often are related to negative beliefs such as "I'm inherently unlikeable (so I must do things for other people or I'll be rejected)."

Standard Treatment Targets and Impediments

The exaggerated attentional dyscontrol of adults with ADHD in emotional situations explains the difficulty of using standard cognitive and behavioral techniques with this population. This subsection addresses the impediments created by ADHD for typical treatment targets and techniques in cognitive and behavioral therapies.

Behavior

The ultimate test of any cognitive or behavioral therapy is its ability to produce meaningful changes in significant observable behaviors. Simple behaviors related directly to the core ADHD symptoms of impulsivity, distractibility, and hyperactivity seem to respond best to medications. The medications most commonly used in ADHD are stimulants and tricyclic or nonserotonergic antidepressants (Wilens et al. 1995; see also Chapter 16, this volume).

The complex dysfunctional behaviors seen in problems associated with ADHD (e.g., aggression as the primary response to conflict) may have components related to one or more underlying mechanisms:

- Core symptoms of ADHD (e.g., impulsivity)
- Emotions (e.g., affect intolerance)
- Perception/attention (e.g., difficulty in pulling one's attention from anger-provoking aspects of the situation to look for other interpretations of the conflict)
- Beliefs (e.g., "If I back down from a fight, I'll prove I'm weak")

The treatment of complex dysfunctional behaviors first requires dealing with the underlying mechanisms. Adults with ADHD then can learn and practice skills needed for the development of more adaptive competing behaviors (i.e., underdeveloped strategies such as negotiation skills and diplomacy). At the same time, they need to keep in check the use of overdeveloped strategies when uncomfortable situations recur.

Impediments to standard techniques. Because behavior is influenced by all the other components in the model, simple behavioral interventions may not be effective for adults with ADHD. (The impediments to behavioral change are discussed in each of the subsections below.)

Emotions

Overabundant emotions create the same problems for ADHD patients as they do for individuals with other psychiatric disorders. In addition, the exaggerated emotional response of the downward spirals is thought to underlie cognitive avoidance.

Medications such as anxiolytics or selective serotonin reuptake inhibitors (SSRIs) may be the most effective treatments for the excessive emotional reactions seen in these patients. Although tricyclic antidepressants are traditionally prescribed for mixed ADHD and depression (Spencer et al. 1996), SSRIs are used preferentially in this protocol for their effectiveness with a broader spectrum of emotional disorders (i.e., depression, anxiety, and anger) (Baldessarini 1996). Cognitive and behavioral techniques designed to control anxiety, depression, and anger also may be helpful.

Impediments to standard techniques. Because of the episodic nature of the emotional responses, they may be difficult to detect, even when they are extreme (e.g., the patient denies a baseline feeling of depression, but upon questioning admits to periods of intense sadness with suicidal ideation when dealing with failure).

Cognitive and behavioral techniques often rely on the patient's distancing from automatic thoughts in order to use interventions such as rational responding and relaxation techniques. The "magnifying" effect of intense emotion on the attentional dyscontrol makes attending to these less emotional stimuli much more difficult, and thus these techniques are rendered less effective.

Attention/Perception

The attentional dyscontrol of adults with ADHD can create major disorganization in their lives. It also may serve as the basis for downward spirals, which can lead to cognitive avoidance, another major source of dysfunction.

Medications to improve the attentional dyscontrol are crucial. Cognitive/behavioral interventions to interrupt the effect of emotions on attention or to refocus attention may be beneficial. Psychoeducation designed to help adults with ADHD change their environment to decrease competing stimuli may be useful but has certain limitations (see discussion of the environment later in this section).

Impediments to standard techniques. Medications, such as stimulants, and cognitive or behavioral techniques aimed at refocusing attention may have little effect in the presence of intense affect or beliefs. For example, it is difficult to focus one's attention away from thoughts about perfection when starting a task if one truly believes this is a crucial requirement for success.

Cognitions

Frequently, adults with ADHD can be distracted in a task by their own cognitions. Rationally responding to distorted automatic thoughts can be used to limit the degree to which the negative cognitions interfere with the task. Responding in this way can also control emotional and behavioral responses to situations and forms the early foundation for changing dysfunctional beliefs.

Impediments to standard techniques. Rational responding to distorted cognitions usually requires distancing one's attention from emotion-laden thoughts and replacing them with more rational, less emotional thoughts. This can make rational responding extremely laborious and rather ineffective for adults with ADHD until the emotion and attention components are controlled more directly—usually with medications and, to a lesser extent, with cognitive and behavioral strategies.

Environment

Psychoeducational, cognitive, and behavioral techniques can help individuals change their environments. Such interventions can decrease distracting stimuli and reduce stressful situations that tend to activate dysfunctional schemas, increase negative emotions, or have a deleterious effect on their support systems. They also can increase positive situations that build up positive emotions, schemas, and support systems.

Impediments to standard techniques. It can be arduous for individuals to restructure their environments when such efforts compete with firmly held beliefs. For example, it is difficult for patients to deal with being overextended in their commitments if they believe they are worthwhile only when they do things of value to others.

Beliefs

The foundation of Beck's cognitive therapy is that long-term improvement comes about only with changes in one's belief systems. Cognitive therapy focused on the long-term change in beliefs (known as *schema work*) uses cognitive and behavioral techniques to tear down negative belief systems and, at the same time, build up competing positive schemas (A. T. Beck et al. 1990).

Short-term belief change can be crucial for controlling the dysfunctional emotions, cognitions, and cognitive avoidance that are major impediments to therapeutic success. Patients may be willing to briefly test beliefs in limited, well-defined homework assignments, called *behavioral experiments.* The suspension of specific, narrow beliefs may be seen by the patient as having less drastic consequences than the examination of broader, more powerful beliefs. The narrow beliefs might be related to an impediment in treatment (e.g., "I shouldn't tell my therapist when I'm upset with him"), or they may seem peripheral to the treatment (e.g., beliefs about people who are not involved in the individual's life). In any event, patients learn that there are benefits to changing beliefs, and they develop the skills required to change them.

Initially, successes in such endeavors are seen merely as exceptions to an otherwise legitimate rule. As patients perceive an increasing number and scope of situations in which their beliefs are inaccurate and/or maladaptive, the broader belief can weaken to the point where it can be challenged more directly with the standard cognitive and behavioral techniques of schema work.

Managing patients' expectations may directly diminish their reluctance to engage in behavioral change. In some situations this means increasing the prediction of success. In others, diminishing unreasonable positive or negative expectations is required.

Novice therapists sometimes focus on strong, broad beliefs at the beginning of treatment. Doing so can exacerbate the pain and dysfunction of patients before they have the skills and insights they require to manage their maladaptive thoughts, emotions, and behaviors. These cognitive, behavioral, and affective management skills are acquired when patients learn the standard cognitive and behavioral techniques. Once these basic skills are developed, therapists can begin schema work with weaker, more narrow beliefs.

Impediments to standard techniques. There is an optimal level of activation of schemas (i.e., an optimal range of emotion) when one is doing beliefs work. In order for schema change to occur, the dysfunctional beliefs must be activated; otherwise, interventions may yield only intellectualization. Too much activation can be painful, and adults with ADHD may respond with cognitive avoidance, which makes schema work strenuous and potentially ineffective. Before schema work can commence, the individual must be able to deal with the strong emotions, cognitions, and behaviors that occur when these powerful negative belief systems are activated.

Some maladaptive beliefs are specific to ADHD. Jack, the subject of the case study introduced earlier in this chapter, had the belief "If I'm doing something and I think of something else to do, I need to stop what I'm doing and go on to the other task so I don't forget it." He interrupted his tasks so frequently, he rarely completed any of them in one sitting. He was even more inefficient when he returned to the task and tried to pick up where he left off.

Other beliefs may relate more generally to the treatment of ADHD. Jack had difficulty engaging in therapy because of beliefs such as "Normal people don't have to make schedules, keep priority lists, etc." This resulted in painful affect and thoughts, such as "This just proves how defective I really am," whenever he attempted his homework assignments. The result was noncompliance with his treatment plan.

Some particularly important beliefs relate to what it means for the individual to have ADHD. These beliefs can make dealing with ADHD in the therapy session more difficult to tolerate. For example, patients sometimes learn the concept of *self-sabotaging*—dysfunctional behaviors that result from a motivation to hurt oneself. This conceptualization can often have a deleterious effect on the patient with ADHD, as shown in the following example (Figure 18–2):

1. The patient is dealing with a difficult situation.
2. Beliefs about the situation engender thoughts that lead to depression, anxiety, or anger in the patient.
3. In order to deal with the painful affect, the patient uses his typical coping strategy of distractors such as binge eating, sleep, sex, or substance abuse.
4. The patient does not see the distractors as dysfunctional coping strategies for which he needs to substitute more adaptive coping strategies. Rather, he believes the distractors are evidence of self-sabotaging—that is, another example of his underlying motivation to hurt himself.
5. Misinterpreting the function of the distractors increases the patient's belief "I'm defective (because normal people don't do things to hurt themselves)."

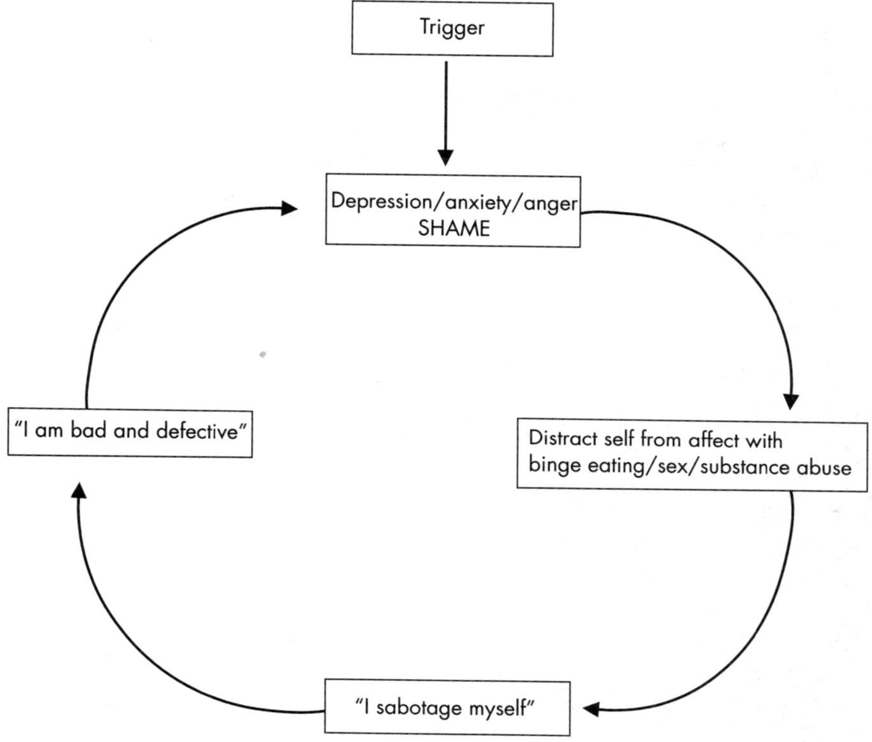

Figure 18–2. The vicious cycle of the "self-sabotage" belief.

6. The patient's belief that he or she is "defective" increases his anxiety, depression, anger, and shame, strengthening his urge to use the distractors and perpetuating the cycle.

The result is that the patient feels even more certain he is "defective" and becomes even more hopeless about changing.

Some beliefs relate more generally to the individual and are not specific to ADHD. These include broadly based "core beliefs" that serve as the basis for many other beliefs. Examples of these are "I'm weak and helpless" and "I'm inherently unlovable." Such beliefs are associated with particularly powerful thoughts, emotions, and behaviors. (For a more detailed discussion of core beliefs, see A. T. Beck et al. 1979; J. Beck 1995; Leahy 1996.)

The Treatment Sequence

Exclusively focusing treatment interventions on any one element of the model can be ineffective. Therapists may need to deal with several components simultaneously (or in short succession) in order to help the patient achieve successful behavioral change. Before a behavioral intervention is attempted, therapists may need to attain limited modification of related beliefs and/or regulate affect generated by contemplating the action. The timing of procedures is determined by the following treatment guidelines:

1. *Medication stabilization.* Medication initiation and stabilization start at the beginning of treatment because of the central role of medications in dampening exaggerated affective response and in allowing greater regulation of attentional dyscontrol.
2. *Psychoeducation.* Psychoeducation about ADHD and its effects on adults, and about the overall treatment plan, begins, as does medication stabilization, with initiation of treatment. Patients begin to put their ADHD in proper perspective (i.e., as a disorder instead of a series of character flaws) and start to challenge maladaptive beliefs (e.g., "I'm just lazy," "I'm just stupid").
3. *Modified standard cognitive therapy.* After basic psychoeducation about the disorder with which they present, patients begin standard cognitive therapy (with modifications as discussed), including setting concrete treatment goals, learning about collaboration in the therapeutic relationship, and learning basic strategies and techniques for dealing with their dysfunctional thoughts, emotions, and behaviors.
4. *Cognitive avoidance.* Cognitive avoidance can occur at any point in the therapy. It is crucial for the clinician to recognize the sometimes subtle signs of this process and to discuss it with the patient in a supportive, firm, and nonconfrontational way. Cognitive avoidance can severely impede or completely derail the treatment.
5. *Schema work.* As standard cognitive therapy and medications allow patients to have better control over their thoughts, emotions, behaviors, and attention, the therapy moves toward dealing with changing the beliefs that underlie much of the dysfunction in these processes.
6. *Environment.* Environmental restructuring encompasses goals as specific as modifying where a student studies or developing daily and weekly routines to those as broad as effecting more extensive career or lifestyle changes. Such restructuring is often best achieved in small steps spread out over time. Therapists should be aware of opportunities to introduce

environmental change as they arise in the context of other therapeutic goals (e.g., learning to maintain a schedule when dealing with work problems, or developing a filing system when working on financial difficulties).

Therapists should not work on more than one or two environmental modifications at a time. Patients need time to incorporate each modification into the routines of their lives before going on to new ones. If new changes are attempted before older ones are solidified, patients will see a pattern of gains and regressions and may believe consistent, long-term progress is not possible. Instead, they need to learn that maintaining small behavioral changes can lead to major improvements in the quality of their lives.

Some therapists attempt environmental modification too early in the treatment. Patients must have the attention, behavior, and affective controls necessary to maintain environmental changes. If they do not, attempts at environmental change will only increase their sense of helplessness and hopelessness. It is often most effective to begin environmental restructuring after patients learn to modify their basic beliefs.

7. *Relapse prevention.* The final phase of the protocol helps patients develop *treatment plans* for dealing with possible relapses after therapy. Relapse prevention has four stages:

    a. Patients reexamine the problems that brought them to treatment but conceptualize them from a cognitive therapy perspective. "I couldn't study" now is understood as "It's always been difficult for me to study because I'm easily distracted because I have ADHD (not because I'm 'abnormal'). Still, I did well enough in elementary school and high school. I didn't start having significant problems with school until I started believing I was incapable of studying, because I was 'different' from other students. That's when I started to avoid studying, and my grades plummeted."

    b. Patients review how they successfully dealt with the initial problems. "I learned that I was avoiding school-related situations because I was afraid of feeling 'abnormal.' My avoidance was making the situation much worse. Once I was able to push past it, the feelings weren't as bad as I had imagined. I learned to catch the thoughts that were making me feel bad and answer back to them. Then I started to feel better and my studying improved. My medication makes studying easier and more productive than before, but it's still harder for me than for most people. That doesn't make me 'abnormal.' I need to make accommodations for my distractibility, but I still can accomplish what I want. It just may take a little more time."

c. Patients use the conceptualization of their initial problems to predict circumstances that might be difficult in the future. "When I start my new job, or have other major life changes, I'll probably compare myself with others to see if I'm 'normal.' This is a set-up for me to become self-critical and to start avoiding situations in which I might be evaluated. I'll then have even more problems than I would otherwise."

d. Patients develop strategies for preventing or dealing with the potential problems. "I need to have realistic, measurable goals that are appropriate for me, not focused on others. I also need to recognize my avoidance earlier, when it's easier to deal with. If I don't, the negative beliefs behind it will continue to grow and make me feel (and behave) worse."

Treatment Termination

Therapists and patients can use the lists of problems and goals developed at the beginning of therapy to determine when to end treatment. The objective is not for the therapy to eliminate all the patient's dysfunctional thoughts. Rather, patients work on problems in therapy in order to develop skills for overcoming these difficulties and those yet to come. The focus throughout treatment must be on skills acquisition and not just problem-solving with the therapist, for there will always be new obstacles after termination of treatment.

Patients and therapists need to develop realistic, not idealistic, endpoints for treatment. Some patients with ADHD become so focused on their "deficiencies" that they neglect concentrating on their strengths. Their goals can attain special, symbolic meanings. Success in a particular career may be seen as a way to "undo" a sense of underachievement or incompetency, even though other careers might be better suited to the person's particular strengths.

A student with a great deal of disorganization and distractibility may need to reconsider becoming an accountant. An extraordinary amount of work may be required for her to achieve even the minimal standards of organized precision demanded by this field. This may impair her satisfaction with other important areas of her life. She might be happier in a more conceptual, project-oriented field, such as marketing. It may be difficult for her to adequately assess this option, however, if she has spent years reassuring herself that "once I become a CPA, I'll feel good about myself."

Obviously, therapists cannot impose these judgments on patients. Rather, it is through their collaborative exploration of options (and of the meanings behind them) that they come to conclusions together. Patients may need to try out certain alternatives even if they conclude the chances of success are low.

> Jack successfully completed all but one of the courses required for law school admission. While in therapy, however, he concluded that although he believed he could get into law school, being an attorney would not make him happy. Indeed, he realized that a good career alone was insufficient for his well-being. He began to date, but later ended the relationship when he realized it was not meeting his needs. He began to get together with old friends and asked them to introduce him to some of their female friends.
>
> Jack was quite proficient at woodworking, a skill he had always considered "unimportant." As therapy ended, he was applying to apprenticeship programs for professional furniture makers. For the first time, he was leaving the area where he grew up.

Patients must understand that they need to practice their skills continuously or they will lose them. Therapists need to deal with patients' beliefs about how difficult maintaining their skills may be. Some patients may always have more difficutly than others doing certain tasks, but they need to remember that just because an undertaking is more difficult does not mean it is impossible.

Discussions about treatment endpoints often reveal beliefs about "relative normality," such as "I wouldn't have to work this hard if I were a 'normal person.'" Behind such beliefs, often, is the belief "Tasks are more difficult for me because I have ADHD, so if I didn't have ADHD, they wouldn't be difficult at all." Individuals with these beliefs often have an exaggerated sense of how much easier tasks are for people without ADHD and therefore may have unrealistic treatment expectations.

> A young graduate student in history was recently diagnosed with ADHD. She had trouble reading the large volumes of material required because it was difficult for her to sit for more than 15 minutes at a time. The patient started a stimulant medication and returned 2 weeks later. She stated, "Well, I'm doing better, but I still have a long way to go." She now could read complicated material for an hour at a time with good comprehension, take a break for about 15 minutes, and then read for

> another hour. She was doing this for about 6 hours a day.
>
> When her psychiatrist asked her how long other graduate students were reading, she said she did not know exactly. She guessed they studied for about 8 hours solidly, took about a 20-minute break for a meal, and studied for another 6 hours. She imagined they would eat dinner briefly and then study for 5 or 6 hours after that. As she said this, she realized it was exaggerated.
>
> She checked with her classmates and found that many of them were using a schedule similar to hers. There were some, however, who could study for longer periods of time without a break. She was closer to the "relative normal" (i.e., average) student than she thought, and she learned she had to question her thoughts about her "deficits" relative to others.
>
> As the issue of her "normality" resolved, it became easier for her to accept a new belief. She decided that the more important assessment was whether her abilities were "good enough" to accomplish what she wanted and not how they compared with those of others. She concluded that, although perhaps not "ideal," the study schedule she maintained was sufficient for her to complete her coursework.

Adults with ADHD who have an underlying belief such as "If I'm not normal, I'm defective" may have trouble maintaining skills and routines that have been beneficial.

> Jack found that keeping a "to do" list was helpful for organizing his day. He eventually discontinued the practice but wasn't sure why he stopped. For homework, he restarted his "to do" lists but also paid close attention to his thoughts when he used the lists. He discovered thoughts such as "The only reason I have to keep 'to do' lists is because I have ADHD. Normal people don't need 'to do' lists. If I were 'normal,' I wouldn't have to use them." Then he felt ashamed. Soon, he noticed the thought "Maybe I don't need these lists anymore" and felt the urge to stop using them. Jack was able to determine that most busy people he knew kept "to do" lists, and he then felt better about using them again.

An important part of relapse prevention is discussing with patients the probability that at some point after therapy they will have a "lapse," or stray from the routine and skills they have developed. This lapse is likely to include their routine of catching and responding to maladaptive thoughts. Patients need to understand that a lapse does not have to become a "relapse" into disorganized ADHD. That is, the therapist "decatastrophizes" the lapse by noting that it is typical to stray from a routine now and then.

People with ADHD need to return to their routines as soon as they recognize they have lapsed from them, because patients with ADHD are at greater risk for becoming disorganized and dysfunctional. This risk seems to increase the longer they avoid their routines.

Therapists need to emphasize to patients the disadvantages of their castigating themselves for lapsing. Self-criticism rarely helps patients return to their routines; it instead fuels the maladaptive beliefs and the dysfunctional thoughts, feelings, and behaviors that follow from those beliefs. Instead, the lapse is framed as an opportunity to observe the subtle remnants of previously powerful beliefs that make relapse more likely. When Jack and his therapist saw that his belief "If I'm not normal, I'm defective" was responsible for his avoiding "to do" lists, they briefly reexamined the schema work they had previously done on it.

Preliminary Outcome Data

Wilens et al. (in press) evaluated the potential benefit of this adapted form of Beck's cognitive therapy for adults with ADHD. Twenty-six consecutive adult outpatients with a DSM-III-R diagnosis of ADHD were treated naturalistically with cognitive therapy by an experienced Beckian cognitive therapist. The patients were evaluated for response to treatment on the basis of multiple variables assessed both prospectively and by retrospective review of the medical charts.

The results showed all 26 adults with ADHD had received prior psychotherapy, 96% (lifetime) had a psychiatric disorder comorbid with ADHD, and 85% were receiving medications in combination with cognitive therapy. The patients were treated, on average, for nearly a year (mean ±SD = 11.7 months ±8 months), with a mean (±SD) number of sessions of 36 (±24). Treatment was associated with significant improvements in ADHD, anxiety, and depressive symptoms, as well as overall global functioning ($P < 0.01$ for each of these associations). Overall, 69% of the adults with ADHD were considered to have much to very much improvement in their ADHD at the end of treatment.

The authors suggested that cognitive therapy, generally used in conjunction with medications, appears to be useful for adults with ADHD. They conclude that, within the limitations of a naturalist chart review, these pilot data suggest the need for further controlled investigations.

CONCLUSION

Adults with attention-deficit/hyperactivity disorder represent a challenging treatment population, in that the disorder often is refractory to traditional forms of psychotherapy. When standard cognitive therapy treatments are modified to take into account the specific effects of the disorder, treatment of these patients may become more productive.

Controlled trials of cognitive therapy for reducing the core symptoms of ADHD, its associated problems, and its comorbid disorders need to be completed. From these, more specific changes in the cognitive therapy for ADHD, mediated by outcomes of improvement in the functioning and quality of life, need to be undertaken.

REFERENCES

Alpert J, Maddocks A, Nierenberg A, et al: Attention deficit hyperactivity disorder in childhood among adults with major depression. Psychiatry Res 62:213–219, 1996

Anderson J, Williams S, McGee R, et al: DSM-III disorders in preadolescent children. Arch Gen Psychiatry 44:69–76, 1987

Baldessarini RJ: Chemotherapy in Psychiatry. Cambridge, MA, Harvard University Press, 1996

Barkley RA (ed): Attention-Deficit Hyperactivity Disorder: Handbook for Diagnosis and Treatment. New York, Guilford, 1990

Bauermeister JJ, Canino G, Bird H: Epidemiology of disruptive behavior disorders. Child Adolesc Psychiatr Clin North Am 3:177–194, 1994

Beck AT: Beyond belief: a theory of modes, personality, and psychopathology, in Frontiers of Cognitive Therapy. Edited by Salkovkis PM. New York, Guilford, 1996, pp 1–25

Beck AT, Rush AJ, Shaw BF, et al: Cognitive Therapy of Depression: A Treatment Manual. New York, Guilford, 1979

Beck AT, Freeman A, and Associates: Cognitive Therapy of Personality Disorders. New York, Guilford, 1990

Beck J: Cognitive Therapy: Basics and Beyond. New York, Guilford, 1995

Bemporad J, Zambenedetti M: Psychotherapy of adults with attention deficit disorder. J Psychother Pract Res 5:228–237, 1996

Biederman J, Faraone SV, Spencer TJ, et al: Patterns of psychiatric comorbidity, cognition, and psychosocial functioning in adults with attention-deficit hyperactivity disorder. Am J Psychiatry 150:1792–1798, 1993

Hallowell EM: Psychotherapy of adult attention deficit disorder, in A Comprehensive Guide to Attention Deficit Disorder in Adults: Research, Diagnosis, and Treatment. Edited by Nadeau KG. New York, Brunner/Mazel, 1995, pp 146–167

Hinshaw S, Erhardt D: Attention deficit hyperactivity disorder, in Child and Adolescent Therapy: Cognitive-Behavioral Procedures. Edited by Kendall P. New York, Guilford, 1991, pp 98–122

Hollon SD, Najavits L: Review of empirical studies on cognitive therapy, in American Psychiatric Press Review of Psychiatry, Vol 7. Edited by Frances AJ, Hales RE. Washington, DC, American Psychiatric Press, 1988, pp 643–666

Laufer MW, Denhoff E: Hyperkinetic behavior syndromes in children. J Pediatr 50:463–474, 1957

Leahy R: Cognitive Therapy: Basic Principles and Applications. Northvale, NJ, Jason Aronson, 1996

Mannuzza S, Klein RG, Bonagura N, et al: Hyperactive boys almost grown up, V: replication of psychiatric status. Arch Gen Psychiatry 48:77–83, 1991

Mannuzza S, Klein RG, Bessler A, et al: Adult outcome of hyperactive boys: educational achievement, occupational rank, and psychiatric status. Arch Gen Psychiatry 50:565–576, 1993

McDermott SP, Wright FD: Cognitive therapy: long-term outlook for a short-term psychotherapy, in Psychotherapy for the 1990's. Edited by Rutan JS. New York, Guilford, 1992, pp 61–99

Millstein R, Wilens TE, Biederman J, et al: Presenting symptoms of ADHD in clinically referred adults with ADHD. Journal of Attention Disorders 2:159–166, 1997

Murphy K, Barkley RA: Prevalence of DSM-IV symptoms of ADHD in adult licensed drivers: implications for clinical diagnosis. Journal of Attention Disorders 1:147–161, 1996

Najavits LM, Weiss RD: The role of psychotherapy in the treatment of substance-use disorders. Harv Rev Psychiatry 2:84–96, 1994

Ratey JJ, Greenberg MS, Bemporad JR, et al: Unrecognized attention-deficit hyperactivity disorder in adults presenting for outpatient psychotherapy. J Child Adolesc Psychopharmacol 2:267–275, 1992

Safer DJ, Krager JM: A survey of medication treatment for hyperactive/inattentive students. JAMA 260:2256–2258, 1988

Segal Z, Williams J, Teasdale J, et al: A cognitive science perspective on kindling and episode sensitization in recurrent affective disorder. Psychol Med 26:371–380, 1996

Shekim WO, Asarnow RF, Hess E, et al: A clinical and demographic profile of a sample of adults with attention deficit hyperactivity disorder, residual state. Compr Psychiatry 31:416–425, 1990

Sokol L, Beck AT, Greenberg RL, et al: Cognitive therapy of panic disorder: a nonpharmacological alternative. J Nerv Ment Dis 177:711–716, 1989

Spencer TJ, Biederman J, Wilens TE, et al: Is attention deficit hyperactivity disorder in adults a valid diagnosis? Harv Rev Psychiatry 1:326–335, 1994

Spencer TJ, Biederman J, Wilens TE, et al: Pharmacotherapy of attention deficit disorder across the life cycle. J Am Acad Child Adolesc Psychiatry 35:409–432, 1996
Weiss G, Hechtman LT: Hyperactive Children Grown Up. New York, Guilford, 1986
Wilens TE, Spencer TJ, Biederman J: Pharmacotherapy of adult ADHD, in A Comprehensive Guide to Attention Deficit Disorder in Adults: Research, Diagnosis, and Treatment. Edited by Nadeau KG. New York, Brunner/Mazel, 1995, pp 168–188
Wilens TE, Biederman J, Spencer TJ: Pharmacotherapy of attention deficit hyperactivity disorder in adults. CNS Drugs 9:347–356, 1998
Wilens T, McDermott S, Biederman J, et al: Cognitive therapy for adults with ADHD: a systematic chart review of 26 cases. Journal of Cognitive Psychotherapy (in press)
Williams JMG: Memory processes in psychotherapy, in Frontiers of Cognitive Therapy. Edited by Salkovkis PM. New York, Guilford, 1996, pp 97–113

19 Educational Interventions for Students With Attention-Deficit Disorders

George J. DuPaul, Ph.D.
Thomas J. Power, Ph.D.

One of the greatest complications associated with attention-deficit disorders (ADDs) is academic underachievement and scholastic failure (e.g., Barkley et al. 1990b; Weiss and Hechtman 1993). In fact, as Tannock and Brown (Chapter 7, this volume) and Denckla (Chapter 8, this volume) point out, the combination of an ADD and learning disorders is common and often persists into adulthood. Beyond the nearly 30% of individuals with ADDs who have a learning disorder, most children, adolescents, and adults with an ADD have some degree of academic impairment (Cantwell and Baker 1991). Presumably, the poor academic performance of these individuals is due to their low levels of active engagement in academic work and inconsistent work productivity (DuPaul and Stoner 1994). Given the high risk for educational impairment in individuals with ADDs, clinicians must design interventions that enhance academic performance as well as reduce the behavioral manifestations of the disorder.

The purpose of this chapter is threefold. First, we delineate federal guidelines for determining the eligibility of individuals with ADDs for educational modifications and provide clinicians with a strategy for making eligibility decisions. Second, we provide an overview of educational interventions for students with ADDs. Finally, we discuss how clinicians can collaborate effectively with educators in assisting students with ADDs.

FEDERAL GUIDELINES FOR PROVIDING SERVICES TO STUDENTS WITH ADDS

Before 1991, students with ADDs were not eligible for special education services or educational modifications unless they qualified for such services on the basis of having a designated educational disability, such as a learning disability or a serious emotional disturbance. Following the reauthorization of the Individuals with Disabilities Education Act (IDEA) by Congress in 1990, a joint memorandum was issued by the U.S. Department of Education Office of Special Education and Related Services and the Office of Civil Rights that specified three possible conditions under which students with ADDs may be eligible for modifications to educational programming (Davila et al. 1991). The first possibility is the same as under previous federal regulations. If a student with an ADD is found to have a comorbid educational disability like a learning disability, then that student is eligible for special education services on the basis of the aforementioned educational disability, not on the basis of having the ADD.

Even in the absence of a comorbid educational disability, a student with an ADD may be eligible for special education under the "Other Health Impaired" category of Part B of the IDEA. This category is described as follows:

> The term "other health impaired" includes chronic or acute impairments that result in limited altertness, which adversely affects educational performance. Thus, children with ADD should be classified as eligible for services under the "other health impaired" category in instances where the ADD is a chronic or acute health problem that results in limited alertness, which adversely affects educational performance. In other words, children with ADD, where the ADD is a chronic or acute health problem resulting in limited alertness, may be considered disabled under Part B solely on the basis of this disorder within the "other health impaired" category in situations where special education and related services are needed because of the ADD. (Davila et al. 1991, p. 3)

Several components of this definition need to be considered. First, the clinician must establish that the individual has a chronic or acute health problem that results in limited alertness. By definition, an ADD is a chronic health problem wherein the individual exhibits problems with attention (American Psychiatric Association 1994). As such, if a student is diagnosed with an ADD, then this first criterion should be met automatically. Second, the ADD must adversely affect educational performance. Clearly, if one defines educational performance as the student's ability to consistently meet the work demands of the classroom, most students with ADDs would be eligible under this provision. Finally, the clinician must establish whether the student with an ADD needs special education or related services or whether interventions in the general education classroom will be sufficient. In the absence of definitive guidelines from federal agencies, we offer suggestions later in this chapter on how to make this determination.

The third and final provision outlined by Davila et al. (1991) is related to Section 504 of the Rehabilitation Act of 1973. This is a civil rights law that states that schools must address the needs of children considered to be handicapped as competently as the needs of nonhandicapped students. A "handicapped person" is defined as "any person who has a physical or mental impairment which substantially limits a major life activity" (Davila et al. 1991, p. 6). A number of life activities, including learning, are listed. If a student is found to be handicapped, then he or she is eligible for educational modifications that may or may not include special education services. The most prominent life activity that could be affected by an ADD is learning, and, as such, the clinician must determine whether the student's ADD substantially limits learning (i.e., academic performance). Thus, even individuals who are not eligible for special education services under the IDEA could be considered in need of individualized interventions and educational modifications on the basis of being handicapped in accordance with Section 504.

Zirkel (1992; see appendix to that article) has designed a checklist for determining the legal eligibility for special education services and educational modifications in accordance with the regulations outlined above. Figure 19–1 provides a decision-making flowchart, adapted from Zirkel's checklist, that can be used as a guide to determine eligibility for educational modifications as specified by IDEA or Section 504, as follows:

1. Conduct a multimodal and comprehensive evaluation for ADDs and associated comorbid conditions as described by Quinlan (see Chapter 15, this volume). If the student is found to have both an ADD and an educational disability such as learning disability or serious emotional disturbance, then he or she is eligible for special education services under the IDEA.
2. If the student does not have a comorbid educational disability, his or her eligibility under the "Other Health Impaired" category should be assessed. First, if the student has an ADD, then by definition he or she has a

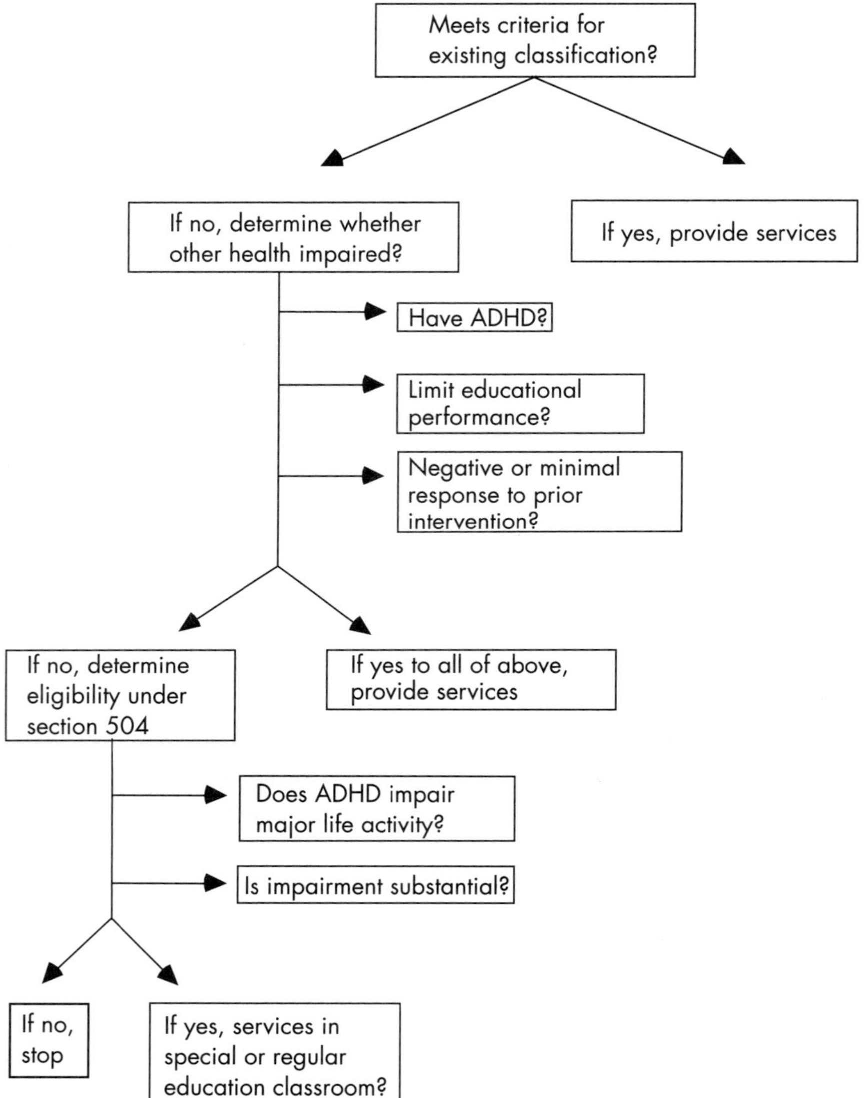

Figure 19–1. Decision tree for determining the eligibility of students with attention-deficit disorders (ADDs) for educational modifications and/or special education.
Source. Reprinted from DuPaul GJ, Stoner G: *ADHD in the Schools: Assessment and Intervention Strategies.* New York, Guilford, 1994. Copyright 1994, Guilford Press. Used with permission.

chronic health condition that significantly limits alertness. Second, the degree to which the student's ADD limits his or her educational performance must be determined. In the absence of definitive federal or state guidelines to make this determination, the clinician can consider several sources of data. The results of educational achievement tests (e.g., Woodcock-Johnson) may be illustrative of educational deficiencies related to the student's ADDs. It should be noted, however, that many students with ADDs (particularly those who do not have comorbid learning disability) obtain scores in the average range on individual achievement tests (e.g., Barkley et al. 1990a). The more fruitful line of investigation is to examine the student's daily academic performance in the classroom. That is, how productive and accurate is the student relative to his or her classmates and/or grade-level expectations? The academic impairment most often associated with ADDs is below-average performance on the day-to-day tasks assigned by the teacher.

When impairment in educational performance is established, a school-based team (in concert with the clinician) must ascertain whether special education services are necessary. Although a student may be performing poorly academically, it is possible, in some instances, that modifications to instruction in the general education classroom (e.g., reduction in workload, preferential seating, untimed tests) may be sufficient. Alternatively, some students with ADDs will be educationally impaired to the extent that they will require special education services either in the general education classroom or in a segregated setting.

The problem is that there are no clear-cut guidelines for determining the necessity of special education services other than the severity of the student's educational impairment. If the school-based team and clinician are unsure of the need for such services, the best option is to design interventions (as described later in the chapter) that can be implemented in the general education classroom for a trial period. If, after these interventions have been implemented, the student does not show improvement, then more restrictive procedures (i.e., special education) may be necessary (Gresham 1991) and an individualized educational plan (IEP) is developed. Baseline data should be collected on key behaviors (e.g., completion and accuracy of classwork) prior to implementing a specific intervention. After making educational or other modifications for a specified period of time, data are collected again to enable assessment of possible changes in performance. If improvements are not evident, the school-based team and clinician may recommend a) changes to the intervention plan in the general education classroom, b) provision of special education or related services, or c) both changes to the general education plan and implementation of special education services.

3. Typically, a school-based team comprising an administrator, special education teacher, school psychologist, school nurse, regular educator, and the student's parent will evaluate IDEA eligibility, as described earlier. If the student with an ADD is deemed ineligible for special education services under the IDEA guidelines, this same team or another group of school-based professionals will meet to examine the student's eligibility for educational modifications under Section 504. First, the team must decide whether the student's ADD impairs a major life activity (e.g., learning). We recommend using classroom academic performance data to make this determination. Second, the team must establish whether this impairment is substantial by addressing the question of how far below the student's peers or grade-level expectations is he or she functioning. Of course, it becomes a subjective, team-based decision as to whether a given impairment level is substantial. Finally, the team must decide what modifications are necessary to address the impairment in learning and whether placement in special education will be required to implement these modifications. A written service agreement is developed that includes goals and educational modifications. In most cases, modifications are made to instruction and assignments in the general education classroom.
4. Whether or not special education services are provided, interventions addressing the student's ADDs must be designed. The efficacy of both general and special education interventions should be evaluated on a continuous basis to determine whether changes in educational programming and/or placement are necessary.

Most elementary and secondary school students with ADD are placed in general education classrooms (Reid et al. 1994). It is our belief that this is appropriate for most students with this disorder provided that *effective interventions and modifications are implemented by the general education teacher.* In fact, there is no guarantee that special education will be effective for these students, as research reviews have documented equivocal efficacy for such programs (Kavale 1990). The critical determinant of successful outcome is not so much the placement of the student (i.e., general vs. special education classroom), but rather what the teacher does or does not do in the classroom. In the next section, we describe educational and school-based interventions that have been successful for students with attention disorders.

EDUCATIONAL INTERVENTIONS

A recent meta-analysis has indicated that, on average, school-based interventions for students with ADDs are effective in ameliorating both the behavioral and academic deficits associated with this disorder (DuPaul and Eckert 1997). In general, interventions have focused primarily on reducing ADD symptoms and, less frequently, on enhancing academic performance. Thus, we review treatment strategies that address both the behavioral and educational performance of students with ADDs in school settings. (For a more comprehensive review of behavioral and academic interventions, see Fiore et al. 1993 and DuPaul and Eckert 1998, respectively.) For discussion purposes, educational interventions are categorized according to whether they are parent-mediated, teacher-mediated, peer-mediated, or self-directed (Table 19–1). Further, an attempt has been made to describe exemplary strategies for elementary, secondary, and postsecondary students with ADDs.

Teacher-Mediated Strategies

Teachers can have an effect on student performance and behavior in two general ways: 1) by strategically modifying methods of instruction/evaluation or 2) by managing the contingencies (consequences) for desirable and undesirable behavior.

Table 19–1. Educational interventions for students with an ADD

Strategy	Children	Adolescents	Adults
Parent-mediated	Goal setting Contracting Home-based reinforcement Parent tutoring	Negotiating Contracting Home-based reinforcement	—
Teacher-mediated	Strategic instruction Contingency management	Study skills instruction Contracting	Modifications to assignments
Peer-mediated	Peer tutoring Cooperative learning	Peer coaching Peer mediation	Coaching
Self-directed	Self-monitoring	Self-monitoring Self-reinforcement	Self-monitoring Self-help groups Bibliotherapy

Modification of Instruction/Evaluation

Student attention and learning are greatly affected by the extent of match between student skills and the level of difficulty of instructional materials. On-task behavior and rates of task completion and comprehension have been shown to vary as a function of instructional match. In a study of young elementary school students with significant reading problems, Gickling and Armstrong (1978) found that the level of on-task behavior and rates of task completion and comprehension were very low when students were requested to work on curricular materials that were clearly too difficult for them (i.e., fewer than 70% of the items on seatwork assignments were familiar to the child). In contrast, when students were taught at the proper instructional level (i.e., the answers to about 80% of the items on seatwork tasks were already known), levels of attention, productivity, and accuracy improved dramatically. Furthermore, when students were provided with material that was too easy for them (i.e., more than 97% of the items on seatwork assignments were known), task completion and comprehension were high but on-task behavior declined dramatically.

This research strongly suggests that a mismatch between student skills and the level of difficulty of curricular materials can create or exacerbate attention problems. In subsequent research, Gickling and his colleagues provided preliminary evidence that altering instructional materials so that there is a more favorable match between student skills and curriculum can reduce the inattentiveness of students with ADDs (Gickling and Thompson 1985). These findings highlight the importance of assessing instructional match in students with attention deficits and making modifications in instructional procedures and learning materials when students demonstrate insufficient familiarly with curricular requirements.

Students with ADDs are able to sustain attention for longer periods of time when tasks are presented in a novel manner. For instance, Zentall and colleagues have shown that students with ADD were able to pay attention longer and were less hyperactive when stimuli were presented in color as opposed to black-and-white (Zentall and Dwyer 1988; Zentall et al. 1985). In addition, attention span can be improved and hyperactivity can be reduced by students' being provided with tasks that require an active, motoric response (Zentall and Meyer 1987) and frequent opportunities to receive high-interest feedback for performance, such as those provided by computer-assisted learning activities. Although research regarding the efficacy of computer-assisted instruction for students with ADDs is lacking, this type of instruction generally has been found to increase on-task behavior and academic skills in students with learning problems and is a promising avenue of intervention for children with ADDs (DuPaul and Eckert 1998).

A number of other task and/or instructional modifications can be made to enhance the academic performance of students with ADDs. First, a mixed rate of presentation of educational material that is varied in response to the skills and interests of the student appears to be optimal for learning (Conte et al. 1987). Second, direct instruction in note-taking, study, and test-taking skills should be provided to adolescents and young adults with ADD. For example, Evans et al. (1995) found that teaching a structured, systematic approach to note taking (i.e., Directed Notetaking Activity [Spires and Stone 1989]) was effective in increasing the notebook quality, on-task behavior, and accuracy on academic assignments of several adolescents with ADD. Finally, students with this disorder are more likely to follow through on academic tasks that they have chosen rather than on work that is assigned by the teacher (Dunlap et al. 1994). More specifically, students could be presented with a menu of possible assignments, all of which provide them with an opportunity to practice specific academic skills (e.g., working with a written sheet of addition problems, completing problems on a computer, or taking turns practicing problems with a classmate).

At the postsecondary level, a number of accommodations should be made by the instructor (see McCormack and Leonard 1994). For example, in lecture classes, the student should be allowed to use other students' notes or be assigned a notetaker. Students could be provided with extra time to complete writing assignments. The success of the latter is enhanced when the student is allowed to submit drafts of the paper prior to the final deadline in order to receive feedback from the instructor. Extra time should be provided for written examinations as well. Altering the format (e.g., allowing the student to give oral rather than written responses or having the student complete small components of the examination on successive days) of examinations also may be helpful. Finally, students should be allowed to use auxiliary aids (e.g., textbooks on tape, calculator) for the completion of assignments. The overriding goal at the postsecondary level is to provide students with accommodations that are practical and useful not only for fostering educational progress but for promoting lifelong learning.

Managing Consequences

Systematically manipulating the contingencies or consequences of behavior can be a powerful tool in changing the behavior and performance of children with ADDs. The strategic use of teacher praise and attention repeatedly has been found to improve the behavior of students in classroom settings. More specifically, praising students frequently for desirable behavior and ignoring them consistently for undesirable behavior generally will improve the performance of students with conduct problems (Madsen et al. 1968). However, the strategic use of praise and attention with students who have ADDs is not sufficient (Pfiffner and O'Leary 1993). Students with ADDs require more intensive programs of behavior modification involving very frequent and immediate feedback through a combination of enhanced positive reinforcers and strategic use of negative consequence interventions.

One method of enhancing the effects of a positive reinforcement system is to provide more concrete reinforcers (e.g., access to special privileges or activities) contingent on the performance of specified target behaviors, such as paying attention during class instruction or completing 90% of seatwork. Often it is impractical to offer concrete reinforcers frequently and immediately after a student emits target behaviors. A more efficient means of providing enhanced positive reinforcement is to introduce *tokens* (e.g., stars, stickers, points) that can be accumulated and exchanged for backup reinforcers of greater value (e.g., five stars can be exchanged for 10 minutes of computer time at the end of the school day). The advantage of tokens is that they can be distributed frequently, immediately, and inexpensively. Enhanced positive reinforcement systems such as these have been shown to be much more effective in increasing on-task behavior and academic accuracy than interventions involving the use of verbal praise alone (Pfiffner et al. 1985).

The effects of token systems sometimes are enhanced through group contingencies, involving the provision of positive reinforcement to a group of students when the targeted student is able to achieve a stated goal (Rosenbaum et al. 1975). Group contingencies appear to be particularly useful when responses from the peer group are contributing to the maintenance of a student's problem.

The choice of target behaviors is important in designing systems of behavior modification. Research has shown that when academic productivity and accuracy are targeted, token systems often result in an improvement in academic performance and a reduction in disruptive behavior. However, when disruptive behavior is the target of intervention, improvements are often demonstrated in behavior but not in academic performance (Pfiffner and O'Leary 1993). We recommend applying the "dead man's rule" (Lindsley 1991) in deciding on targets for intervention. This rule, simply stated, is that if a dead man can earn reinforcement, then the behavior is not a good target for treatment. Thus, for example, asking students to sit still or refrain from calling out violate the dead man's rule. Alternatively, targeting active appropriate responding such as completion and accuracy of work is in keeping with the spirit of this rule. Identifying critical, keystone target behaviors can enable clinicians to design interventions that are not only effective but also efficient to use.

Teachers frequently report that token systems work for short periods of time and then lose their effectiveness. One reason for this is that the value of reinforcers declines when they are used repeatedly, and this appears to be particularly true for their use with students with ADDs. Thus, when designing behavior modification plans, it is important to vary reinforcers frequently and randomly (Rhode et al. 1992).

The use of an all-positive system of contingency management is usually not sufficient to improve the performance and behavior of students with ADDs. The strategic provision of negative consequences generally is very useful in developing behavior modification programs for these youngsters. Verbal reprimands, a mild form of punishment, are very commonly used by teachers and can be effective if delivered properly. A series of studies has shown that reprimands can be effective if they are short, firm, immediate, and consistent (see Abramowitz and O'Leary 1991). In addition, research suggests that when rules are taught to children through a combination of verbal praise and reprimands, it may be possible to maintain the effects of the intervention with an all-positive token system (Pfiffner and O'Leary 1987). It should be noted that it is easy to overuse verbal reprimands with a child who is impulsive and/or inattentive. A helpful rule of thumb for teachers is to provide positive reinforcement at least three times more often than verbal reprimands or other forms of negative consequences.

Many students with ADDs require an enhanced system of negative consequences to modify their performance and behavior. One method of enhancing a system of negative consequences is *response cost,* which involves the withdrawal of a reinforcer contingent on inappropriate or unproductive behavior. Rapport et al. (1982) found that response cost was very effective in improving the on-task behavior and academic performance of students with ADDs. In their study, students lost a minute of recess each time the teacher observed them to be off-task. The response-cost procedures developed by Rapport and colleagues have been used to develop the Attention Training System (Gordon 1988), a remote-control electronic mechanism that has been field tested with children with ADDs and shown to be useful in increasing on-task behavior, improving academic performance, and reducing disruptive behavior (DuPaul et al. 1992). Although response-cost interventions can be highly effective, there are potential side effects associated with their use. Response cost is a form of punishment; if response-cost procedures are not embedded in a system of behavior modification that is primarily positive, students may become discouraged and behavior change may be minimal. It is essential that students earn points at a faster rate than they lose them. Teachers may need to modify the criteria used to take points away to ensure that students do not lose points too frequently (DuPaul and Stoner 1994).

Time-out has been demonstrated repeatedly to be effective in reducing the occurrence of inappropriate behaviors (Brantner and Doherty 1983). Time-out involves the systematic withdrawal of sources of positive reinforcement (e.g., teacher attention, peer attention, curricular materials) contingent on maladaptive behavior. Time-out procedures vary in their level of restrictiveness. Examples of time-out ordered from least restrictive to most restrictive are the following: ignoring, removing reinforcing stimuli, excluding from the group, and removing from class. In general, it is recommended that teachers employ the least restrictive method of time-out that is effective and that they refrain from using isolation by removal from the classroom if possible (Lentz 1988). Time-out is effective only when there is a clear contrast between the positive reinforcement received when a student is behaving appropriately (time-in) and the lack of positive reinforcment experienced when the child misbehaves (time-out). Time-out is not effective when the student receives as much or more positive reinforcement in the time-out area as in the general classroom setting (Shriver and Allen 1996). For example, if the student is sent to the principal's office as punishment but then receives verbal attention from the school secretary, this might actually be rewarding rather than punishing to the student. The duration of time-out should be relatively brief (e.g.,1–4 minutes); for many students with ADDs long time-outs can be difficult to enforce and may be counterproductive.

Contracting involves a process of negotiation between a student and teacher that stipulates in specific terms 1) behaviors targeted for change, 2) goals for behavior, and 3) consequences for attaining goals. Contracts are designed mutually by the student and teacher through a process of collaboration, and they generally result in written agreements that include specific details of the behavioral plan (Rhode et al. 1992). Involving students in the process of designing behavioral interventions generally is a wise practice because it is likely to result in treatments that are viewed by students as fair and reasonable. Contracting is particularly well suited for adolescents and adults who place a high value on being autonomous and desire some measure of control over decisions made about their lives. Behavioral interventions with adolescents are much more likely to be effective if students express a willingness to change certain behaviors, have input into goals for future behavior, and specify short-term and long-term positive consequences they can earn for attaining goals. Contracts sometimes fail to be effective with students who have ADDs when goals are stated in general, ambiguous terms or are too lofty to be attained a high percentage of the time. Also, the effectiveness of contracts can be mitigated by delays in providing consequences for behavior (DuPaul and Stoner 1994).

Designing educational interventions for adolescents with ADDs can be complicated in that these students usually relate to several teachers during the course of a day. Teachers in middle school, high school, and college settings may have fewer opportunities to observe students and understand their unique learning needs than teachers in preschool and elementary environments. Teachers working with adolescents generally instruct many more students per day than teachers who instruct younger students; in some cases, this may reduce their willingness to employ intensive behavior modification strategies often required by students with ADDs. In addition, teachers in middle school and beyond often expect a level of independence, responsibility, and organization that many students with ADDs have difficulty assuming (Shapiro et al. 1996). One method that has been used to help an adolescent with an ADD to adjust in school is to establish a *mentoring or coaching system* (see Guare and Dawson 1995). The mentor is an adult within the school (e.g., teacher, counselor, coach) whom the student believes could be helpful and who has the time and willingness to commit to the mentoring process. The role of the mentor includes 1) developing a trusting and supportive relationship with the student, 2) designing strategies to assist the student with organization of materials and assignments, 3) negotiating detailed behavioral contracts with the student, 4) monitoring student performance carefully by meeting with the student frequently and checking with teachers on a regular basis, 5) holding the student accountable to the terms of the behavioral contract, and 6) consulting regularly with teachers to design helpful classroom interventions. Many schools lack the knowledge and resources to design effective mentoring programs for adolescents with ADDs, so consultation from clinicians external to the system may be needed to design such interventions.

The success of educational interventions depends not only on the potential effectiveness of the treatments being used but also on teachers' perceptions of the acceptability of the intervention program. Treatment acceptability has been defined as judgments by consumers about whether intervention procedures are fair and reasonable (Kazdin 1981). In general, teachers prefer interventions that use positive as opposed to negative consequences and treatments that require a relatively short time to implement, although the severity of a student's problem has been shown to be an important mediating variable (Witt et al. 1984). Research regarding treatments for ADDs has demonstrated that teachers vary greatly in their attitudes about the use of behavioral interventions, but, in general, they prefer token economy over response-cost interventions (Power et al. 1995). Acceptability of treatment procedures may be enhanced if the teacher is provided with information about ADDs and successful interventions for this disorder. Several books (e.g., Parker 1992; Pfiffner 1996) may be helpful in this regard. Before a course of treatment is initiated, it is recommended that clinicians assess teachers' attitudes about proposed interventions. When teachers convey ambivalent attitudes about the use of negative consequence procedures, a time-efficient, primarily positive-consequence intervention could be initiated at the outset. Response-cost components can then be added to the intervention program if a primarily positive system of behavior management is not sufficient to treat the problems.

Parent-Mediated Strategies

Parents can assist children with ADDs with their education in several ways, including the use of homework strategies such as goal setting with contingency contracting, home-based consequences for school performance and behavior, parent tutoring, and negotiating.

Goal Setting With Contingency Contracting

Students with ADDs frequently have problems completing homework assignments (DuPaul and Stoner 1994). Several interventions have been designed to assist students with homework problems, including having students complete homework assignment sheets and requesting teacher verification for accuracy, structuring the home environment, and providing positive reinforcement contingent on cooperative behavior and the completion of homework (Olympia et al. 1992). An approach to homework intervention that appears particularly promising is goal setting with contingency contracting. In a study conducted by Kahle and Kelley (1994), each parent-child dyad was trained to divide homework assignments into small, manageable units of work. For each unit the child and parent were requested to agree on a goal for time spent on task, number of items to be completed, and number of items to be completed accurately. The child was instructed to work for the specified amount of time and, upon expiration of the time limit, to evaluate performance with regard to work completion and accuracy. The child was reinforced for goal attainment in accordance with a contract that had been negotiated by the parent and child. This intervention was found to be quite effective in improving rates of homework completion and accuracy, and parents reported that the procedures were useful and easy to implement.

Home-Based Reinforcement Systems

A commonly used intervention for improving children's performance and behavior in school is a school-home note with home-based consequences (Kelley 1990). These procedures have been found to be helpful in working with students diagnosed with ADD (O'Leary et al. 1976). This intervention involves having teachers evaluate students on one or more target behaviors at least once per day. Target behaviors might include completion of work, attention to instruction, and speaking at appropriate times. Teachers often use a 3-point scale to evaluate each behavior (0 = work harder, 1 = OK, 2 = good job!). At the end of the school day, the student is instructed to take the note home for parental review. Parents are guided in setting reasonable goals for performance and rewarding the child for goal attainment. When this intervention is used with students who have ADDs, it is often necessary for teachers to provide feedback to students several times during the course of the day (e.g., at the end of each class period). The delay of reinforcement involved with this procedure may diminish its effectiveness. In these cases, it may be helpful to supplement home-based contingencies with a school-based system of consequences. Also, children with ADDs may benefit from including a response-cost component in the school-home note. For instance, the loss of a point in school could result in the subtraction of a minute of special playtime with the parent in the evening.

Parent Tutoring

A majority of children with ADDs are underachievers and have academic skills deficits. Teacher-mediated and peer-mediated interventions have been shown to be quite effective in addressing the needs of children with academic deficits. Parent tutoring of academic skills also has been found to be effective in enhancing student performance (Graue et al. 1983; Hook and DuPaul 1999). For instance, parents have been successfully trained to use paired reading strategies (Topping 1987) and interactive book reading techniques (Taverne and Sheridan 1995). Parent tutoring strategies to improve spelling and math skills also have been developed (Bowen et al. 1994).

When it is not possible to provide parents with sufficient training to provide parent tutoring at home, community members have been enlisted by the school to provide daily tutoring to students in a school setting (Power et al. 1996). In tutoring children with ADDs, the use of reinforcement procedures to enhance attention and motivation often is necessary. Because parent tutoring entails making additional demands on the child for academic work, the use of these techniques is generally not recommended until the child is able to complete homework in a reasonable amount of time.

Negotiating

When children enter adolescence, it is important that they assume increasing control over interventions used on their behalf (Robin and Foster 1989). Thus, when parent-mediated strategies are being designed, the perceptions and wishes of adolsecents need to be given serious consideration. For instance, with homework interventions the adolescent with an ADD needs to play an active role in setting goals for performance. By the same token, these individuals, at times, may be unrealistic with regard to goal setting, and in these instances parents need to provide guidance and negotiate reasonable performance standards. Also, during the homework evaluation stage of treatment, adolescents can be given responsibility for determining rates of completion and accuracy, but parents of teens with ADDs often need to check to make sure the evaluation is conducted accurately. In this case, bonus points can be provided to the youth for accurate self-evaluation, and over time it may be possible to gradually decrease the frequency of parental checks (Smith et al. 1988).

In addition, the adolescent must have input into short- and long-term reinforcers for attaining established goals. However, parents must be included in this determination and agree that the reinforcers are reasonable and feasible to administer on an ongoing basis. Adolescents with ADDs often have problems accepting the consequences of failing to achieve stated goals; it may be useful for the parents and youths to negotiate how parents should react when their sons or daughters defy attempts to enforce mutually established contingencies for performance.

Peer-Mediated Strategies

Peers can play a role in implementing several of the strategies discussed in the foregoing sections on teacher- and parent-mediated strategies. For example, peer coaching would involve a peer or older student's employing the methods described for teacher coaching (i.e., helping the student with an ADD to set, monitor, and carry out school-related goals; see Dawson and Guare 1998). Also, peer mediation could be used to help an adolescent with an ADD negotiate with adults or peers with whom he or she is experiencing problematic interactions.

The peer-mediated strategy that has been most successful in working with students with ADDs has been peer tutoring. Peer tutoring can be defined as any instructional strategy wherein two students work together on an academic activity, with one student providing assistance, instruction, and/or feedback to the other (Greenwood et al. 1991). Peer tutoring models vary with respect to instructional focus (acquisition vs. practice), structure (reciprocal vs. nonreciprocal), and procedural components (e.g., number of sessions per week, methods of pairing students, type of reward system used) (for review, see Fuchs et al. 1995). Despite these procedural differences, peer tutoring models share instructional characteristics that are known to enhance the sustained attention of students with ADDs. These characteristics include 1) one-to-one work with an instructor, 2) instructional pace determined by the learner, 3) continuous prompting of academic responses by the instructor, and 4) frequent, immediate feedback about quality of performance from the instructor (Pfiffner 1996; Pfiffner and Barkley 1990).

The most widely known and used form of peer tutoring is ClassWide Peer Tutoring (CWPT; Greenwood et al. 1988), which has been found to enhance the mathematics, reading, and spelling skills of students of *all* achievement levels (for review, see Greenwood et al. 1991). This form of peer tutoring includes the following steps:

1. The class is divided into two teams.
2. Within each team, classmates form tutoring pairs.
3. Students take turns tutoring each other.
4. Tutors are provided with academic scripts (e.g., math problems with answers).
5. Praise and points are contingent on correct answers.
6. Errors are corrected immediately, and students are provided with an opportunity to practice the correct answer.
7. Teacher monitors tutoring pairs and provides bonus points for pairs that are following prescribed procedures.
8. Points are tallied by each individual student at the conclusion of each session.

Tutoring sessions typically last 20 minutes, with an additional 5 minutes allowed at the end of the session for charting progress and putting materials away. Points earned in the CWPT program are used to document academic progress and are paired with praise from the teacher; typically, no backup rewards are necessary.

In two separate investigations, CWPT was found to enhance the task-related attention and academic accuracy of elementary school students with ADDs (DuPaul and Henningson 1993; DuPaul et al. 1998). Similar, positive changes in behavior and academic performance were exhibited by randomly selected students without ADDs, confirming the findings of Greenwood et al. (1993) that CWPT is helpful for all students, not just those who are experiencing difficulties. Further, the teachers and students participating in these investigations rated CWPT as effective, practical, and highly acceptable.

Peer tutoring provides another way for students with ADDs, who usually have problems completing independent assignments, to practice and refine their academic skills. Peer-mediated interventions, such as peer tutoring and cooperative learning (three to five children complete an assignment in a collaborative fashion [Slavin et al. 1985]), are not meant to take the place of other forms of instruction (e.g., teacher-led lesson, group discussion). It also is important to note that the behavioral improvements obtained during peer tutoring sessions typically do not carry over to other classroom activities and that, therefore, it is necessary to use other interventions (e.g., the teacher-mediated strategies discussed earlier). At the present time, the most prudent conclusion is that peer tutoring can be an effective intervention to enhance sustained attention and academic performance, at least over the short term, especially when combined with other treatment strategies.

Self-Directed Strategies

One of the primary treatment goals is for students with ADDs to gain more control over their behavioral conduct and academic performance while relying on less support from teachers, parents, and peers (i.e., to gain independence). Barkley (1989) outlined three major self-directed strategies that have been used with this population: self-instruction, self-monitoring, and self-reinforcement. Although these techniques possess strong face validity, empirical investigations have yet to consistently support their efficacy in work with this population (Abikoff 1985).

Self-instruction typically involves a series of one-to-one training sessions with a therapist directed toward the goal of getting the student to "stop, look, and listen" in the context of completing school tasks (Braswell and Bloomquist 1991). Training steps include 1) therapist modeling a reflective task approach by stating thoughts aloud prior to each action, 3) having the student imitate this strategy by stating thoughts aloud while completing a task, 3) having the student gradually reduce the volume of thought statements, and 4) asking the student to engage in reflective thought covertly while completing work. Unfortunately, strong empirical support for self-instruction has not been gathered to date. The most pressing issue has been the degree to which gains made in therapy sessions can be generalized to task performance in the natural environment (e.g., classroom). In the absence of prompts and reinforcement from the teacher, students are unlikely to use the self-instructional skills on their own.

Self-monitoring involves students observing and recording the occurrence of their own behaviors (Barkley 1989). In the most common application of this technique, a student will be cued (e.g., hear an audiotaped signal) periodically to record whether or not he or she was paying attention during an assigned task. Other variations of this procedure are to have the student self-monitor the amount of work produced (i.e., task completion) or percentage of work completed correctly. Self-monitoring strategies have been found effective for increasing on-task behavior and academic performance among children with attention problems (Maag et al. 1993). For students whose ADD symptoms are in the clinical range, self-monitoring appears to be more effective when combined with self-reinforcement (e.g., Barkley et al. 1980).

Probably the most effective self-directed strategy is *self-reinforcement,* wherein the student is taught to monitor and evaluate his or her performance and based on this evaluation provide feedback to himself or herself (Barkley 1989; Shapiro and Cole 1994). For example, Rhode et al. (1983) described a procedure for students with "behavioral handicaps" that involves several steps. First, the teacher develops a set of criteria for rating student performance in both academic and behavioral domains (Table 19–2). Second, the student is taught how to evaluate himself or herself with these criteria by receiving reinforcement for matching teacher ratings. If the student's rating is within 1 point of the teacher's rating, a bonus point is earned. During the third stage of this treatment, the frequency of teacher matching challenges is gradually and systematically reduced, such that the student rates himself or herself in the absence of external feedback. Finally, the student is asked periodically to provide a verbal report about his or her performance to the teacher.

In addition to some early work that documented the success of self-reinforcement in the treatment of ADDs (Barkley et al. 1980; Hinshaw et al. 1984), more recent case studies have highlighted the potential effectiveness of this technique with both elementary school and middle school students (Hoff and DuPaul 1998; Shapiro et al. 1998). For this technique to be successful, consistent teacher feedback must be provided to the student during the initial stages of training. Further, it is important that teacher feedback is gradually reduced rather than abruptly discontinued, because students with ADDs need ongoing support in order to accurately self-evaluate on a consistent basis.

Table 19–2. Self-management criteria for rating student performance in following classroom rules

5 = Followed classroom rules (see below) entire interval

4 = Minor infraction of rules (e.g., talked out of turn); followed rules remainder of interval

3 = Did not follow all rules for entire time, but no serious offenses

2 = Broke one or more rules to extent behavior was unacceptable (e.g., physically aggressive with classmate), but followed rules remainder of interval

1 = Broke one or more rules almost entire interval or engaged in higher degree of inappropriate behavior most of the time

0 = Broke one or more rules entire interval

Classroom rules

1. Talking to classmates is allowed only during group discussions.
2. Keep hands to self and own property unless you ask for teacher permission.
3. Follow teacher directives.

Source. Reprinted from DuPaul GJ, Hoff K: "Attention/concentration problems," in *Child Behavior Therapy: Ecological Considerations in Assessment, Treatment, and Evaluation.* Edited by Gresham F, Watson TS. New York, Plenum, 1998, pp. 99–126. Copyright 1998, Plenum Press. Used with permission.

Self-monitoring interventions also can be used to help adults with ADDs, particularly in situations in which the individual is attempting to sustain attention to lengthy, effortful tasks such as studying, reading textbooks, and completing written assignments. In addition, self-help groups and bibliotherapy may aid adults in understanding the disorder and its impact on their educational functioning and to adopt strategies that will enhance their performance (e.g., time management) (Murphy and Levert 1995).

Combining Interventions

Behavioral interventions are usually helpful in working with students who have ADDs, but the behavior and performance of these children generally cannot be normalized with behavioral interventions alone (Pelham et al. 1993). Stimulant medication often is needed to enable children with ADDs to function adaptively in educational settings. By the same token, stimulant medication often is not sufficient to normalize the academic and behavioral functioning of children with ADDs. In a study involving a large sample of children, Rapport et al. (1994) examined the effects of four doses of methylphenidate (5 mg, 10 mg, 15 mg, 20 mg) on teacher ratings of attention and behavior, direct observations of on-task behavior, and academic efficiency on seatwork tasks. These researchers found that the optimal dose of medication for each student resulted in the following rates of normalization on each outcome measure: 78% for teacher ratings of behavior, 72% for direct observations of attention, and 53% for academic efficiency in classwork. They determined that the following percentages of children displayed no change on outcome measures: 7% for teacher ratings, 24% for observations of attention, and 50% for classwork efficiency. These findings confirm the efficacy of stimulant medication with children who have ADDs but highlight the limits of medication, particularly with regard to improving academic performance. In about half the cases, stimulant medication did not normalize the academic performance of students with ADDs, and alternative procedures, such as the educational interventions outlined earlier in this section, were needed. In addition, a low percentage of children have been found to exhibit side effects in response to medication, necessitating the use of alternative treatments.

Effective educational treatment for ADDs usually involves the use of multimodal interventions, which might include a combination of two or more of the following: teacher-mediated, parent-mediated, peer-mediated, self-directed, and pharmacological interventions. The types of interventions required by an individual to perform well in school depend on multiple factors, including the settings where the impairment is occurring; the level of functional impairment manifested; the resources available in the home, school, and community; the motivation of the student to change; the presence of comorbid psychiatric conditions; and the prior response to educational, behavioral, and/or pharmacological interventions.

COLLABORATION BETWEEN CLINICAL AND EDUCATIONAL PROFESSIONALS

Attention-deficit disorder is a complex constellation of symptoms that generally has pervasive effects on an individual's functioning. As such, multimodal interventions are usually required to successfully address the problems with which these individuals present. The need for multiple interventions requires that professionals from many disciplines be involved in the care of these individuals. Interdisciplinary collaboration is essential to ensure a comprehensive, well-integrated, systematic approach to treatment (DuPaul and Stoner 1994).

Historically, treatment for ADDs has occurred primarily in public or private clinic-based settings. A clinic-based model has several advantages (Table 19–3). Professionals working in clinic settings often have a high degree of expertise regarding ADDs and their comorbid conditions, coordination between health and mental health providers may be feasible to arrange, and child and family rights to privacy can be protected quite readily in clinic settings. However, clinic-based programs for ADDs face several limitations, including problems accessing naturalistic data about academic and peer functioning, the impracticality of collaborating with educators on an ongoing basis, and the inaccessibility of clinic services to some families because of problems with payment, scheduling, or transportation (Power et al. 1994).

Over the past 10 years, the need to develop a school-based model for delivery of services to students with ADDs has become apparent (DuPaul and Stoner 1994; Teeter 1991). The legal mandate to provide school-based services to students with ADDs who display impairments in educational settings, issued by the U.S. Department of Education in 1991, affirmed the importance of a school-based model of programming for these individuals. As outlined in Table 19–3, school-based models of service delivery have some clear strengths: naturalistic information about academic and peer functioning is easy to obtain, ongoing collaboration between educators and school-based consultants (e.g., school psychologist, school nurse, guidance counselor) is feasible to arrange, and school-based services are readily accessible to families living in the

Table 19–3. Characteristics of clinic-based and school-based models of service delivery for students with ADD

Dimension	Clinic model	School model
Assessment	Data about home behavior easy to obtain; data about school behavior less accessible	Data about school behavior easy to obtain; data about home behavior less accessible
Expertise with ADD	Generally strong	Variable
Coordination with health care providers	Health care providers often members of the clinical team	Collaboration with health care providers possibly limited
Collaboration with educators	Consultation with teachers possibly difficult to arrange	Ongoing consultation with teachers feasible
Access to services	Access contingent on payment and transportation issues	Schools accessible to virtually all families
Privacy	Rights to privacy can be protected quite readily	Privacy of schools may be questioned by some families

community. School-based models of service delivery are not without limitations, however, and these may include variable expertise with regard to ADDs and its comorbid conditions, a lack of collaboration between clinic-based health professionals and school personnel, and issues of privacy related to the provision of clinical services in the public world of the school (Power et al. 1994).

Because both clinic-based and school-based models of programming for students with ADDs have their strengths and limitations, a model of service delivery that integrates both approaches has been advocated (Power et al, 1994). Coordinating clinic-based and school-based services requires close collaboration between professionals working in each of these settings. Through ongoing collaboration between clinical and school professionals, clinicians can learn how school personnel can be helpful in addressing the problems of these students; school professionals can gain valuable medical and psychological perspectives and learn efficient methods to report treatment outcome when medication is prescribed. One method to achieve more effective working relationships is for a group of school professionals to collaborate with health and mental health professionals from the departments of psychiatry or pediatrics of a nearby, community-based medical center to organize seminars regarding methods of providing community-based care to families coping with ADDs. Through these training activities, a committee consisting of psychiatrists, pediatricians, clinical psychologists, school psychologists, school administrators, teachers, and parents could emerge to coordinate the efforts of regional clinical and educational professionals regarding optimal methods of service delivery for students with this disorder (Power et al. 1994).

CONCLUSION

Symptoms of attention-deficit disorders significantly compromise academic performance across the lifespan of individuals with this disorder. Consequently, most students with ADDs will require educational modifications in addition to other treatments (e.g., stimulant medication) that are designed to address their disorder. Federal regulations in the areas of special education and civil rights ensure that students with ADDs at all educational levels will be provided with necessary and reasonable accommodations. Effective treatment approaches have been discussed in this chapter in the context of whether the approaches are mediated by teachers, parents, peers, or the students themselves. The specific technique and/or mediator will vary according to the individual strengths and weaknesses of the student. Further, the choice of specific strategies should be made collaboratively among teachers, parents, and students in order to promote greater acceptability of treatment plans and, ultimately, to improve the likelihood that participants will implement the prescribed procedures. Ultimately, the educational achievement of individuals with ADDs is more likely to be improved when teachers, parents, peers, and the students themselves are all involved in the intervention process.

REFERENCES

Abikoff H: Efficacy of cognitive training intervention in hyperactive children: a critical review. Clin Psychol Rev 5:479–512, 1985

Abramowitz AJ, O'Leary SG: Behavioral interventions for the classroom: implications for students with ADHD. School Psychology Review 20:220–234, 1991

American Psychiatric Association: Diagnostic and Statistical Manual of Mental Disorders, 4th Edition. Washington, DC, American Psychiatric Association, 1994

Barkley RA: Attention-deficit hyperactivity disorder, in Treatment of Childhood Disorders. Edited by Mash EJ, Barkley RA. New York, Guilford, 1989, pp 39–72

Barkley RA, Copeland A, Sivage C: A self-control classroom for hyperactive children. J Autism Dev Disord 10:75–89, 1980

Barkley RA, DuPaul GJ, McMurray MB: A comprehensive evaluation of attention deficit disorder with and without hyperactivity as defined by research criteria. J Consult Clin Psychol 58:775–789, 1990a

Barkley RA, Fischer M, Edelbrock CS, et al: The adolescent outcome of hyperactive children diagnosed by research criteria, I: an 8-year prospective study. J Am Acad Child Adolesc Psychiatry 29:546–557, 1990b

Bowen J, Olympia D, Jenson WR: Study Buddies: A Parent-to-Child Tutoring Program in Reading, Math, and Spelling. Longmont, CO, Sopris West, 1994

Brantner J, Doherty M: A review of timeout: a conceptual and methodological analysis, in The Effects of Punishment on Human Behavior. Edited by Axelrod S, Apsche J. New York, Academic Press, 1983, pp 87–132

Braswell L, Bloomquist ML: Cognitive-Behavior Therapy With ADHD Children: Child, Family, and School Interventions. New York, Guilford, 1991

Cantwell DP, Baker L: Association between attention-deficit hyperactivity disorder and learning disorders. Journal of Learning Disabilities 24:88–95, 1991

Conte R, Kinsbourne M, Swanson J, et al: Presentation rate effects on paired associate learning by attention deficit disordered children. Child Dev 57:681–687, 1987

Davila RR, Williams ML, MacDonald JT: Clarification of policy to address the needs of children with attention deficit disorders within general and/or special education. Unpublished letter to chief state school officers, U.S. Department of Education. September 16, 1991

Dawson P, Guare R: Coaching the ADHD Student. North Tonawanda, NY, Multi-Health Systems, 1998

Dunlap G, dePerczel M, Clarke S, et al: Choice making to promote adaptive behavior for students with emotional and behavioral challenges. J Appl Behav Anal 27:505–518, 1994

DuPaul GJ, Eckert TL: School-based interventions for attention-deficit hyperactivity disorder: a meta-analysis. School Psychology Review 26:5–27, 1997

DuPaul GJ, Eckert TL: Academic interventions for students with attention-deficit/hyperactivity disorder: a review of the literature. Reading and Writing Quarterly 14:59–82, 1998

DuPaul GJ, Henningson PN: Peer tutoring effects on the classroom performance of children with attention deficit hyperactivity disorder. School Psychology Review 22:134–143, 1993

DuPaul GJ, Stoner G: ADHD in the Schools: Assessment and Intervention Strategies. New York, Guilford, 1994

DuPaul GJ, Guevremont DC, Barkley RA: Behavioral treatment of attention-deficit hyperactivity disorder in the classroom: use of the Attention Training System. Behav Modif 16:204–225, 1992

DuPaul GJ, Ervin RA, Hook CL, et al: Peer tutoring for attention deficit hyperactivity disorder: effects on classroom behavior and academic performance. J Appl Behav Anal 31:579–592, 1998

Evans SW, Pelham W, Grudberg MV: The efficacy of notetaking to improve behavior and comprehension of adolescents with attention deficit hyperactivity disorder. Exceptionality 5:1–17, 1995

Fiore TA, Becker EA, Nero RC: Educational interventions for students with attention deficit disorder. Exceptional Children 60:163–173, 1993

Fuchs LS, Fuchs D, Phillips NB, et al: Acquisition and transfer effects of classwide peer-assisted learning strategies in mathematics for students with varying learning histories. School Psychology Review 24:604–620, 1995

Gickling E, Armstrong DL: Levels of instructional difficulty as related to on-task behavior, task completion, and comprehension. Journal of Learning Disabilities 11:559–566, 1978

Gickling E, Thompson VP: A personal view of curriculum-based assessment. Exceptional Children 52:205–218, 1985

Gordon M: Attention Training System. DeWitt, NY, Gordon Systems, 1988

Graue ME, Weinstein T, Walberg HJ: School-based home instruction and learning: a quantitative analysis. Journal of Educational Research 76:351–360, 1983

Greenwood CR, Delquadri J, Carta JJ: ClassWide Peer Tutoring. Seattle, WA, Educational Achievement Systems, 1988

Greenwood CR, Maheady L, Carta JJ: Peer tutoring programs in the regular educatio classroom, in Interventions for Achievement and Behavior Problems. Edited b Stoner G, Shinn MR, Walker HM. Silver Spring, MD, National Association School Psychologists, 1991, pp 179–200

Greenwood CR, Terry B, Utley CA, et al: Achievement, placement, and services: middle school benefits of classwide peer tutoring used at the elementary school. School Psychology Review 22:497–516, 1993

Gresham FM: Conceptualizing behavior disorders in terms of resistance to intervention. School Psychology Review 20:23–36, 1991

Guare R, Dawson P: "Coaching" teenagers with attention disorders. NASP Communiqué 24(3):9, 1995

Hinshaw SP, Henker B, Whalen CK: Self-control in hyperactive boys in anger-inducing situations: effects of cognitive-behavioral training and of methylphenidate. J Abnorm Child Psychol 12:55–77, 1984

Hoff K, DuPaul GJ: Reducing disruptive behavior in general education classrooms: the use of self-management strategies. School Psychology Review 27:290–303, 1998

Hook CL, DuPaul GJ: Parent tutoring for students with attention deficit hyperactivity disorder: effects on reading at home and school. School Psychology Review 28: 60–75, 1999

Kahle AL, Kelley ML: Children's homework problems: a comparison of goal setting and parent training. Behavior Therapy 25:275–290, 1994

Kavale K: The effectiveness of special education, in The Handbook of School Psychology, 2nd Edition. Edited by Gutkin TB, Reynolds CR. New York, Wiley, 1990, pp 868–898

Kazdin AE: Acceptability of child treatment techniques: the influence of treatment efficacy and adverse side effects. Behavior Therapy 12:493–506, 1981

Kelley ML: School-Home Notes: Promoting Children's Classroom Success. New York, Guilford, 1990

Lentz FE: Reductive procedures, in Handbook of Behavior Therapy in Education. Edited by Witt JC, Elliott SN, Gresham FM. New York, Plenum, 1988, pp 439–468

Lindsley OR: From technical jargon to plain English for application. J Appl Behav Anal 24:449–458, 1991

aag JW, Reid R, DiGangi SA: Differential effects of self-monitoring attention, accuracy, and productivity. J Appl Behav Anal 26:329–344, 1993

sen C, Becker W, Thomas D: Rules, praise, and ignoring: elements of elementary ssroom control. J Appl Behav Anal 1:139–150, 1968

nack A, Leonard F: Learning accommodations for ADD students, in ADD and ollege Student. Edited by Quinn PO. New York, Magination Press, 1994, pp

Levert S: Out of the Fog. New York, Hyperion, 1995

Pelham WE, Rosenbaum A, et al: Behavioral treatment of hyperkinetic n experimental evaluation of its usefulness. Clin Pediatr 15:510–515,

Olympia D, Jenson WR, Clark E, et al: Training parents to facilitate homework completion: a model for home-school collaboration, in Home-School Collaboration: Enhancing Children's Academic and Social Competence. Edited by Christenson SL, Conoley JC. Silver Spring, MD, National Association of School Psychologists, 1992, pp 309–331

Parker H: The ADD Hyperactivity Handbook for Schools: Effective Strategies for Identifying and Teaching Students With Attention Deficit Disorders in Elementary and Secondary Schools. Plantation, FL, Impact, 1992

Pelham WE, Carlson C, Sams SE, et al: Separate and combined effects of methylphenidate and behavior modification on boys with attention-deficit hyperactivity disorder in the classroom. J Consult Clin Psychol 61:506–515, 1993

Pfiffner LJ: All About ADHD: The Complete Practical Guide for Classroom Teachers. New York, Scholastic, 1996

Pfiffner LJ, Barkley RA: Educational placement and classroom management, in Attention-Deficit Hyperactivity Disorder: A Handbook for Diagnosis and Treatment. Edited by Barkley RA. New York, Guilford, 1990, pp 498–539

Pfiffner LJ, O'Leary SG: The efficacy of all-positive management as a function of the prior use of negative consequences. J Appl Behav Anal 20:265–271, 1987

Pfiffner LJ, O'Leary SG: School-based psychological treatments, in Handbook of Hyperactivity in Children. Edited by Matson JL. Boston, MA, Allyn & Bacon, 1993, pp 234–255

Pfiffner LJ, Rosen LA, O'Leary SG: The efficacy of an all-positive approach to classroom management. J Appl Behav Anal 18:257–261, 1985

Power TJ, Atkins MS, Osborne ML, et al: The school psychologist as manager of programming for ADHD. School Psychology Review 23:279–291, 1994

Power TJ, Hess LE, Bennett DS: The acceptability of interventions for attention-deficit hyperactivity disorder among elementary and middle school teachers. Dev Behav Pediatr 16:238–243, 1995

Power TJ, Andrews TJ, Dowrick PW: Parents as partners: the efficacy of school-based parent tutoring in improving the reading skills of first grade students. Paper presented at the annual meeting of the National Association of School Psychologists, Atlanta, GA, March 1996

Rapport MD, Murphy A, Bailey JS: Ritalin vs. response cost in the control of hyperactive children: a within subject comparison. J Appl Behav Anal 15:205–216, 1982

Rapport MD, Denney C, DuPaul GJ, et al: Attention deficit disorder and methylphenidate: normalization rates, clinical effectiveness, and response prediction in 76 children. J Am Acad Child Adolesc Psychiatry 33:882–893, 1994

Reid R, Maag JW, Vasa SF, et al: Who are the children with attention-deficit hyperactivity disorder? A school-based survey. Journal of Special Education 28:117–137, 1994

Rhode G, Morgan DP, Young KR: Generalization and maintenance of treatment gains of behaviorally handicapped students from resource rooms to regular classrooms using self-evaluation procedures. J Appl Behav Anal 16:171–188, 1983

Rhode G, Jenson WR, Reavis HK: The Tough Kid Book: Practical Classroom Management Strategies. Longmont, CO, Sopris West, 1992

Robin AL, Foster SL: Negotiating Parent-Adolescent Conflict: A Behavioral-Family Systems Approach. New York, Guilford, 1989

Rosenbaum A, O'Leary KD, Jacob RG: Behavioral interventions with hyperactive children: group consequences as a supplement to individual contingencies. Behavior Therapy 6:315–323, 1975

Shapiro ES, Cole CL: Behavioral Change in the Classroom: Self-Management Interventions. New York, Guilford, 1994

Shapiro ES, DuPaul GJ, Bradley KL, et al: A school-based consultation model for service delivery to middle school students with attention deficit disorder. Journal of Emotional and Behavioral Disorders 4:73–81, 1996

Shapiro ES, DuPaul GJ, Bradley KL: Self-management as a strategy to improve the classroom behavior of adolescents with ADHD. Journal of Learning Disabilities 31:545–555, 1998

Shriver MD, Allen KD: The time-out grid: a guide to effective discipline. School Psychology Quarterly 11:67–74, 1996

Slavin R, Sharan S, Kagan S, et al: Learning to Cooperate, Cooperating to Learn. New York, Plenum, 1985

Smith DJ, Young KR, West RP, et al: Reducing the disruptive behavior of junior high students: a classroom self-management procedure. Behavioral Disorders 13: 231–239, 1988

Spires HA, Stone DP: The Directed Notetaking Activity: a self-questioning approach. Journal of Reading 33:36–39, 1989

Taverne A, Sheridan SM: Parent training in interactive book reading: an investigation of its effects with families at risk. School Psychology Quarterly 10:41–64, 1995

Teeter PA: Attention-deficit hyperactivity disorder: a psychoeducational paradigm. School Psychology Review 20:266–280, 1991

Topping K: Paired reading: a powerful technique for parent use. The Reading Teacher 40:608–614, 1987

Weiss G, Hechtman L: Hyperactive Children Grown Up: ADHD in Children, Adolescents, and Adults, 2nd Edition. New York, Guilford, 1993

Witt JC, Martens BK, Elliott SN: Factors affecting teachers' judgments of the acceptability of behavioral interventions: time involvement, behavior problem severity, and type of intervention. Behavior Therapy 15:204–209, 1984

Zentall SS, Dwyer AM: Color effects on the impulsivity and activity of hyperactive children. Journal of School Psychology 27:165–174, 1988

Zentall SS, Meyer MJ: Self-regulation of stimulation for ADD-H children during reading and vigilance task performance. J Abnorm Child Psychol 15:519–536, 1987

Zentall SS, Falkenberg SD, Smith LD: Effects of color stimulation and information on the copying performance of attention-problem adolescents. J Abnorm Child Psychol 13:501–511, 1985

Zirkel PA: A checklist for determining the legal eligibility of ADD/ADHD students. Special Educator 8(7):93–97, 1992

20 Tailoring Treatments for Individuals With Attention-Deficit/Hyperactivity Disorder: Clinical and Research Perspectives

Peter S. Jensen, M.D.
Howard Abikoff, Ph.D.

The essence of clinical skill is the clinician's ability to match the type, timing, and intensity of specific treatments and rehabilitative approaches to the particular clinical needs of the individual patient. In this era of managed care and increasing constraints according to cookbook approaches, careful clinicians must avoid simple solutions of "one size fits all," while also eschewing the muddle-headed notion that suggests that clinicians should be allowed to practice according to "clinical wisdom," unencumbered by rigorous research evidence. Although persons with attention-deficit/hyperactivity disorder (ADHD) have important characteristics in common (e.g., the many symptoms of ADHD), there are multiple aspects and unique characteristics of children and families with ADHD that must also be addressed as a part of successful clinical management.

Unfortunately, the specific need to match treatment approaches to specific patient characteristics, while a laudable goal, suffers at the implementation stage because of the lack of research that has been directed to this area. Although we have ample "clinical" wisdom based on many years of accumulated practice experience to guide these decisions, we cannot rely on solid empirical evidence to guide us, except in a few specific instances.

In this chapter we review some of the major considerations that guide treatment strategies when clinicians are attempting to tailor treatments to the needs of specific patients. We note where research evidence supports such practices, where it does not, and particular areas in which more research is needed. Although we currently lack research evidence to guide most clinical decisions in terms of tailoring treatments to patients' particular clinical needs, the next several years should witness rapid advances in this area, as results from several major clinical trials become available, including those from the two-site Multi-Modal Treatment study of Abikoff and Hechtman (Abikoff and Hechtman 1996; Hechtman and Abikoff 1995) and the six-site Multimodal Treatment Study of Attention Deficit Hyperactivity Disorder (MTA) (Arnold et al. 1997a; MTA Cooperative Group 1999a; Richters et al. 1995). In fact, a major aim of the MTA study was to recruit sufficient sample sizes so that more could be learned about the specific question of which patients are likely to benefit from which specific forms of treatment.

PATIENT CHARACTERISTICS GUIDING CLINICIANS' CHOICE AND TAILORING OF TREATMENTS

A range of child and family characteristics are often used to guide clinicians' decisions about treatments. These include the following:

1. Age and intellectual ability of the child and family
2. Severity and urgency of the condition itself
3. Patient's treatment history and the effects of those treatments
4. Presence of comorbidity or other complicating conditions that also must be addressed as a part of a comprehensive treatment plan
5. Family factors, including the presence of psychopathology in parents and/or other family members
6. The parents' ability and willingness to apply recommended treatments
7. Families' wish for input and preferences about specific treatment types

In addition, the nature of available resources to the family (e.g., insurance, school-based treatment resources within the community) is also likely to guide clinicians' decisions in determining the feasibility of specific treatments.

Child Age and Cognitive Capacity

Frequently, many clinicians will attempt to take the child's age into account in deciding on the particular choice of treatment modalities. For example, very young children who are not yet in school but have significant ADHD symptoms often can be treated with behavioral interventions in the home or in preschool settings (Pisterman et al. 1989). Very young children are often highly motivated by small rewards, such as stickers, "smiley faces," small treats, and adults' praise directed toward particular target behaviors identified for behavioral modification. As a first step, many clinicians prefer behavioral approaches over pharmacological approaches in very young children, since there is less research data to support the use of psychostimulants in these youngsters, and because younger children often have somewhat more frequent difficulties with untoward side effects. Although these side effects (e.g., appetite suppression, insomnia, moodiness, and separation anxiety symptoms) are generally of a modest nature, the general caveat to not use medication when other approaches will suffice seems prudent and appropriately cautious. However, when behavioral approaches alone are insufficient or the child has significant impairment in preschool or home settings as a result of the ADHD symptoms, medications should be considered and can be very helpful. The general assumption that medications may be less often warranted in very young children rests in part on the fact that younger children and preschoolers, compared with older children, frequently have shorter school days, are more easily restructured and directed into activities that they can perform satisfactorily, and have fewer cognitive and performance demands on them.

In school-age children academic and task-related pressures mount, as the child must increasingly master school-related, peer relationship, and/or home-based tasks. While behavioral treatments are clearly efficacious for this age group, as demands on the child increase, assistance for the child and better control of symptoms across multiple settings become increasingly necessary. Particularly in second and third grade, as cognitive and homework-type tasks increase, the child with significant ADHD may fall behind his or her age-mates if significant inattention, impulsivity, and/or motor symptoms interfere with task mastery and performance.

Children up through the end of grade school are generally quite willing to work with both behavioral and medication approaches, and compliance is not usually a major problem. As the child reaches middle school and high school, however, autonomy and self-direction become a sine qua non for good clinical management. The young adolescent may be quite concerned about taking medication during the school day or may be unwilling to take medicine altogether. Major concerns about taking medicine can become a significant obstacle for some adolescents who "just want to be normal" and not be identified as different in any way from peers. It is usually wise and appropriate for the clinician to give the adolescent autonomy in this regard, instead focusing on building a therapeutic alliance and identifying with the adolescent any areas of difficulty he or she may have in performing important age-related tasks, including succeeding in school. Such an approach is vastly preferable to getting into a "power struggle" over whether the child should or should not take medicine.

Strategically, we encourage parents to give an adolescent this right of self-direction, since it is usually most successful first to develop the adolescent's trust in the treating therapist and encourage the adolescent to identify and talk about difficulties he or she has in school and home-related settings and then to encourage the youngster to participate in a "clinical trial" of the potential benefits of the medicine for him or her. Most adolescents, when encouraged in this manner and when power struggles are avoided, will work with the clinician. Once seeing the benefits of medication on performance for themselves, they are more likely to take the medicine themselves without parental or therapist coercion.

In our experience, no child wants to do poorly in school or wants to think of himself or herself as less capable than his or her peers. Self-direction is essential for teenagers, however, and the teenager's wish to avoid the possibility of being identified as different or in need of medication for "mental illness" is paramount. In terms of medication strategies, this consideration frequently requires a choice of agents that have a longer dose-response profile, such that the medicines may be administered exclusively at home (e.g., sustained release forms of dextroamphetamine, or longer-acting agents such as pemoline, tricyclic antidepressants, and so forth).

Although behavioral programs, such as star charts, daily "report cards," and other similar techniques, are frequently effective for elementary school-age children, as children grow older an approach more centered on contract negotiation may be required to enlist the adolescent's willingness to participate in behavior-modification strategies. If power struggles, battles over who is in control, or concerns on the adolescent's part about being manipulated become the dominant themes in the parent-child relationship in terms of how behavioral treatments are administered, problems invariably result. With this point in mind, under these conditions the therapist's role is often more that of a labor-management relations negotiator. Successful use of behavioral contracts in such situations requires careful consideration of appropriate rewards and consequences, tied to some parent-adolescent quid pro quo adjusted for adolescents' need for increasing autonomy and self-direction. Choice and timing of rewards and consequences with a great amount of adolescent input is essential for such programs to succeed. Putting the contract and the rules governing the contract down on paper not only is good practice but may be an important means of establishing trust and a sense of fairness for both parties when working out arrangements. In addition, in our experience, adolescents are also quite capable of employing behavioral self-management, including self-established rewards with behavioral contingencies, use of the Premack principle (using regularly scheduled, necessary daily activities as the reinforcer), and other similar strategies. Behavioral self-management may be used when the need for self-direction is central or when parents' opportunities to provide structure are limited.

Severity of the Presenting Problem

Many times a child or adolescent may present with such severe ADHD symptoms that he or she is in danger of failing in school or of being suspended or expelled or has extremely disturbed relationships in peer, home, or school settings. In such instances, treatment of the ADHD symptoms assumes some urgency. Given the necessary compliance and willingness of the parties involved, including parents and children, in severe or urgent circumstances combined treatment approaches are preferred, beginning simultaneously with medication and behavioral therapeutic approaches.

Very commonly, children with severe forms of ADHD may also have other complicating conditions, such as oppositional defiant disorder, conduct disorder, substance use, related difficulties, or learning disabilities. A comprehensive approach to each of the major areas of difficulties and functioning deficits is essential. Once the overall symptoms are under better behavioral control and the risks for increasing difficulties or irreversible consequences (e.g., school expulsion) have lessened, the clinician and family can more appropriately decide which of the several treatments must remain in place as the overall symptoms subside. In our experience it is often necessary to employ simultaneously pharmacological and behavioral approaches, including home- and school-based behavioral approaches in the treatment of children with severe cases of ADHD.

After parent-child relations have improved, school personnel are reassured, and the child's self-esteem and motivation have shown meaningful gains, it is usually possible to decrease the intensity and number of treatment modalities. For example, once the parents have learned more effective parenting strategies and tensions in the parent-child or child-school relationships have eased, sessions for behavioral treatments may be tapered, with an emphasis more on providing "booster" treatments as needed, along with continuing medication treatment. Similarly, as children increasingly acquire behavioral, academic, and social skills, the dosage of medication can sometimes be reduced or the medication can be eliminated altogether, depending on the needs and the wishes of the particular child and family. Commonly, we find that it is appropriate to reexamine the child's ongoing requirement and benefit from stimulant or other pharmacological approaches shortly after the beginning of a new school year. Although we initially encourage the parent and youngster to begin a new school year on medication, once the youngster has made the successful transition into the school year, we encourage the use of a double-blind, placebo-controlled trial for that individual child, worked out with a local pharmacy able to provide pill and placebo in masked form, in order to determine the child's ongoing benefit and requirement for medication treatment.

Comorbidity

The study of ADHD comorbidity and treatment response is providing further insights and evidence-based guidance concerning tailoring of specific pharmacological approaches when ADHD is comorbid with other conditions. The preceding chapters address these considerations in substantial detail, so readers should carefully note the treatment recommendations when ADHD co-occurs with mood disorders (see Chapter 3, this volume), substance abuse (Chapter 9, this volume), and anxiety disorders (Chapter 4, this volume). A good example of the implications of comorbidity for tailoring of treatment can be seen in recent studies by Pliszka (1989), DuPaul et al. (1994), and Tannock et al. (1995), all of which suggest that children with ADHD comorbid with an anxiety disorder may show somewhat greater likelihood of side effects, including irritability and increased anxiety, when treated with psychostimulants, as well as decreased likelihood of stimulant benefit. Of note, a recent study by Diamond and colleagues (1999) failed to confirm the findings from these earlier reports. Moreover, findings from the MTA study indicate that these children may be particularly likely to respond to treatments that include behavior therapy (either alone or in combination with medication) (MTA Cooperative Group 1999b). Like Diamond et al., the MTA investigators did *not* determine that anxiety predicted a poorer response to stimulants. In sum, these findings do not suggest that medication should not be used; rather, they indicate that behavioral treatments may be especially indicated. In addition, other evidence suggests that these children may also be responsive to tricyclic medications. Likewise, some evidence suggests that children with ADHD and comorbid depression may benefit, in terms of their ADHD and depressive symptoms, when treated with tricyclic medications, although more research is needed to confirm these findings (Biederman et al. 1993; Garfinkel et al. 1983).

Other areas of comorbidity research concern the presence of co-occurring tic disorders. Indeed, recent evidence suggests that children with ADHD and comorbid tic disorders, although they often can be successfully treated with psychostimulants, may show increased tics while under treatment with psychostimulants (Castellanos et al. 1997). Some of these children can nonetheless be successfully treated with stimulants without significant tic exacerbation (Gadow et al. 1995), but it is often necessary to consider other medications as a better treatment alternative. Medications to be considered include tricyclic antidepressants and buproprion (Greenhill et al. 1996; Spencer et al. 1994).

Similarly, some clinicians have advocated the use of clonidine in conjunction with psychostimulants (Hunt et al. 1994). Although this approach has been criticized as being potentially related to some unexplained deaths in children (Cantwell et al. 1997), medication combinations generally have not been well studied, nor are we aware of any controlled trials showing the benefits of medication combinations for ADHD children with or without comorbidity.

Children with ADHD frequently have co-occurring oppositional defiant disorder or conduct disorder. Although psychostimulants have been shown to ameliorate impulsivity and aggressive behavior and reduce symptoms of conduct disorder (Klein et al. 1997), as well as to improve peer, teacher-child, and parent-child relationships, insufficient studies have been conducted to determine how children with this comorbidity should be treated. Clinical experience, as well as uncontrolled research data from Satterfield et al.'s (1987) studies, suggests, however, that combined pharmacological and behavioral and family approaches should be utilized to address the range of these children's difficulties. Given the well-established knowledge concerning malleable risk factors, including lax discipline, exposure to delinquent peers, and coercive parenting, as well as the adverse impact of these factors on the emergence and persistence of conduct disorder, children with comorbid ADHD and oppositional defiant disorder or conduct disorder probably should be treated with combined approaches until research data suggest otherwise. These combined approaches should include pharmacotherapy and behavior management training with parents and/or teachers, depending on the setting(s) in which the child's behavior is problematic. Of note, data from controlled multimodal treatment studies do not support this recommendation (e.g., Abikoff and Hechtman 1996; Hechtman and Abikoff 1995; Horn et al. 1991). While more recent evidence from the MTA study suggests that combined treatments may offer modest advantages over medication-only approaches (MTA Cooperative Group 1999a), individuals with conduct disorder were not differentially responsive to combined treatments. Nonetheless, given the severity and likely tenacity of their difficulties, combined treatments for this group may be especially indicated. Thus, in our view, it is quite likely that the most severely ill children with comorbid ADHD will require an array of medication and psychosocial treatment approaches.

For children with ADHD and comorbid substance abuse, a number of difficulties must be faced by the clinician concerning the possibility that the child or adolescent might abuse or otherwise misuse (e.g., sell) his or her stimulant medication. Schubiner et al. (1995) have developed some clinical recommendations in this arena, recommending that the adolescent first be substance free for several months before beginning stimulant treatments. Obviously, getting the adolescent to this point may require a combination of inpatient, family-based, and behavioral approaches with careful follow-up for potential ongoing substance abuse, as well as careful monitoring of medication and other appropriate behavioral strategies (e.g., urine screens). Although there is little research data supporting the efficacy of behavioral interventions for substance use treatments, until empirical data suggest otherwise, common sense must prevail. Clinicians should treat adolescents with comorbid substance use and ADHD in a "commonsense" fashion: namely, first treat the substance use, establish sobriety or abstinence, and then treat the ADHD symptoms and other related difficulties.

As noted by Clarkin and Kendall (1992), at the same time that comorbid conditions are being increasingly identified, clinicians can rely on fewer available treatment resources and shorter compensable treatment periods because of the growth of managed care. Thus, a clear understanding of comorbidity is necessary to provide the optimal sequence of appropriate intervention targets.

FAMILY FACTORS GUIDING TREATMENT CHOICES

A critical consideration in treating the child with ADHD concerns the caretaking family. Too often, family factors are ignored in the treatment algorithms in extant clinical trials, although clinicians do take better account of these factors as a general rule when determining treatments. In common clinical practice, family preferences and concerns about treatments frequently are factored into treatment plans. For example, if the parent has concerns about medication, the final decision about the use of medication will rest with the parent rather than the physician. Even if the medication is prescribed, the family's compliance and adherence to the treatment regimen will determine whether the treatment is actually delivered as prescribed. Similarly, the family's participation and compliance with any behavioral program are essential ingredients of success.

The wise clinician seeks family input and obtains an understanding of their knowledge of the specific treatments and their views of advantages and disadvantages, including potential misperceptions or lack of knowledge concerning the specific treatments. The parents and family members should first be approached as active collaborators in the treatment, as the clinician, parents, and child together reach agreement about which treatments are most appropriate and in what order. This is usually best considered as a part of an "informed consent process" as the clinician advises parents and families about the advantages and disadvantages about specific treatments. In this regard, we have described the use of "informed consent as a therapeutic strategy" in dealing with the normal therapeutic uncertainty about which treatment works best for which child and the potential risk-benefit ratios for specific treatments (Jensen et al. 1989).

In addition to family factors such as compliance and participation in the treatment, other family factors, including stressors and family psychopathology, should be incorporated into clinicians' considerations concerning treatment strategies. For example, if there are high levels of psychiatric illness in parents or family members such that their ability to participate effectively in treatment is compromised, the treating clinician must account for these factors and consider alternative strategies. In some instances, primary treatment of the parents' difficulties may be necessary before effective treatment of a child can proceed. Quite commonly, parents who themselves have ADHD may have difficulties in administering the behavioral treatments and providing the necessary follow through with behavioral consequences. In our experience, it is sometimes effective in providing some behavioral modification for parents themselves to assist them in monitoring their completion of daily report cards, star charts, or other behavioral modification regimens on behalf of their child.

Evidence for the importance of addressing family factors related to comorbidity can be gleaned from a number of studies. For example, Jensen et al. (1993) compared ADHD children from an ADD clinic with children from community and psychiatric clinic matched control samples in order to examine the role of environmental and psychosocial family risk factors in children diagnosed with ADHD. Comparing the ADHD children with and without comorbid internalizing disorders, the authors found that the children with a comorbid affective/anxiety disorder had experienced significantly higher stress levels during the past year than the children in the "pure" ADHD group. Similarly, mothers whose children had ADHD with comorbid depressive or anxiety disorders reported significantly higher total symptoms for themselves on the Hopkins Symptom Checklist-90 than mothers of children with "pure" ADHD. Biederman et al. (1995) studied the effect of psychosocial and family environmental risk factors on the development of ADHD. Higher scores on an index of family and psychosocial adversity were related to increased ADHD symptoms and to the presence of a range of comorbid psychopathologies, including depression, anxiety, and general psychosocial dysfunction. All in all, these data suggest that ADHD severity and internalizing comorbidity are related to both family psychosocial and environmental factors, a finding also demonstrated in earlier studies (e.g., Barkley et al. 1989). Presumably, the clinician must address these related factors and associated comorbidities if interventions are to succeed.

When there is significant or severe parental psychopathology, "workarounds" of obstacles may have to be developed if the parent cannot be an effective treatment ally or, in some instances, may actually be undermining the treatment. For example, if one parent is a "nonbeliever" in ADHD or of certain treatment approaches, more exclusive work with the other parent may be necessary, as long as this parent has effective and primary responsibility for the parenting and day-to-day management of the child. Alternatively, if the parents are divided as to the best approaches to treatment, it may be necessary first to deal with the parental disagreement about the choice and use of particular therapeutic modalities, their differences in perceptions about the nature of the child's difficulties, and so forth. Obviously, severe disagreement on the part of parents concerning the management of their child's ADHD circumscribes and sets an upper limit on the benefit of any therapies.

In other instances of severe parental psychopathology, referral of the parent for treatment outside of the treatment arrangements for the child may be necessary. Special concerns may be warranted when one of the parents has a history of substance abuse so as to ensure that medications are not diverted into the parent's substance use.

Very commonly, once an effective therapeutic alliance has been formed with the parent, obstacles to full implementation of the various aspects of therapy (e.g., the parent's willingness to consider medication or behavioral treatment) may be alleviated as increasing confidence in the clinician is developed. Commonly, after a period of time in treatment, the parents, now trusting the clinician, may be more willing to consider the very treatments that they initially deemed unacceptable.

FAMILY AND CLINICIAN FACTORS IN THE CHOICE OF TREATMENT

Family Factors

In considering specific treatment modalities for a given patient, practical considerations must be entertained, including the actual costs of the treatment and the resources of the family. Can the family afford to come in and obtain weekly psychotherapy?; can they pay for medication? Has the family had experience with either of these treatments in the past? Have there been side effects during the delivery of any of these treatments such that the family anticipates a negative experience in one way or the other? Not uncommonly, a parent may be skeptical about psychotherapy, about medications, and even about ADHD itself, so addressing parents' concerns and misconceptions or preconceptions about the treatment components becomes necessary. Not uncommonly a child may have experienced side effects with a treatment in the past. Any history of side effects or the actual presence of current side effects will of course guide final decisions about specific treatment choices.

Clinician Factors

A given clinician may have varying degrees of comfort and experience with various therapies. It is unfortunate when such considerations are the sole guiding factor determining which treatments are offered to a given family. However, in some instances the clinician's familiarity with one kind of treatment over another (assuming both are effective) may be a reasonable approach when offering a specific treatment. For example, if the clinician is more familiar with imipramine or nortriptyline, he or she may prefer to offer one of these medications as a first choice when antidepressants are indicated for the treatment of ADHD. But ethically it seems appropriate to advise the parent and family about the risk-benefit ratios of all known and available therapies, including those with which the clinician is not familiar. This increases family autonomy and decision making, should the family decide to pursue other approaches. Similarly, the clinician who has extensive experience in the use of daily report cards in school may prefer these versus a more traditional, "star chart" and behavioral tracking system. Nonetheless, the principles are the same. Effective treatments, however, should always be offered to families, and if the clinician cannot provide effective treatment when indicated, a referral should be made. Clinicians who have insufficient experience in a given area should see that they obtain appropriate training or refer to those who are so trained.

TREATMENT-TAILORING PARAMETERS

Choice and Number of Modalities

The first parameter along which one might consider adjusting treatments for a specific child with ADHD and his or her family concerns the actual selection of which treatment modality, either alone or in combination with other modalities, is most appropriate. Once the clinician decides that multiple modalities are indicated, the order in which they are provided is critical. In every instance it may not be advisable to begin multiple treatments simultaneously, either because of potential burden on the patient/family or because of other clinical considerations, as noted earlier. Consideration of which treatment ought to come first is essential. For example, initially starting with medication treatment may allow a given child and family to take better advantage of the behavioral treatments once such treatments are implemented. On the other hand, beginning a behavioral treatment first may offer the family an area in which they can practice their skills. Treating the child first with medication may so mitigate his or her symptoms that the parents and child may be less motivated to acquire critical behavioral skills. It should be noted that this possibility, while sensible, is not supported by research evidence and should not be a guiding factor in withholding medication.

Other tailoring parameters include the duration and intensity of the selected treatments. Thus, consideration of how frequently sessions are to be conducted, who is involved, and how long the sessions are continued requires strategic decisions. Too often these decisions are left to the vagaries of the families' ability to pay, and, in our experience, it is not uncommon for children with ADHD and their families to receive less-than-optimal length of treatments and intensity.

Research Basis and Evidence for Tailoring Recommendations

Given the above recommendations and clinical considerations to tailor treatments for the specific illness, what can we say we know about these guidelines on the basis of the research evidence? Surprisingly little, except in the area of comorbidity, where research evidence is beginning to provide clues concerning the treatments for ADHD with co-occurring conditions (e.g., anxiety and ADHD). Furthermore, although most clinical practice guidelines suggest that intensive treatments and multimodal treatments are better than less-intensive, unimodal treatments, until the MTA study these clinical assumptions were based on findings from uncontrolled studies (e.g., Satterfield et al. 1987) confounded with subject choice and family characteristics. In fact, as noted earlier, results from randomized trials in children with ADHD indicate only modest advantages to multimodal treatment compared with treatment with stimulants alone (MTA Cooperative Group 1999a, 1999b).

As a general rule, it seems prudent to suggest that in the presence of comorbidity, any treatments that are indicated for the comorbid condition should also be administered, along with the indicated ADHD treatments. Thus, the child with ADHD and comorbid oppositional defiant disorder, depression, conduct disorder, or substance use should receive treatments for these conditions, along with the treatments indicated for the ADHD. When the treatments for the disorders are the same (e.g., imipramine for the depressed child with ADHD), so much the better. At this current point in our knowledge, we must assume that treatment of comorbid conditions requires interventions for both of the conditions. The critical decision to make involves determining the order in which to treat the various combined conditions, if an ordering of treatments is required. In general, the most severe or impairing condition should be treated first, and once that condition is stabilized, the second condition should be addressed.

Another possible area of research comprises clinical trials comparing outcomes with strategies involving family input and choice in the selection of treatment modalities vs. those in which families are randomly assigned to treatments designed without family input. Likewise, it will be necessary to develop additional clinical treatment algorithms for systematic approaches to be compared with each other. These algorithms must address some of the routine clinical factors that occur during practice, such as difficulties with compliance, parental psychopathology, or comorbid conditions, that otherwise would constitute obstacles to the treatment plan (Kazdin et al. 1997b). In other areas we have outlined the development of systematic treatment approaches in this regard (Arnold et al. 1997). We anticipate that this area will become a substantial research agenda that must be addressed to fully meet the needs of providing the necessary and sufficient research evidence on which to base individualized treatments for specific families. Likewise, additional research must address the potential benefits of the effects of adding together specific psychotherapies, alone and in combination with medication.

CONCLUSION

In general, although much is known about certain benefits of medications and behavioral-modification approaches in the treatment of children with ADHD, much less is known about the optimal strategies for tailoring these treatments according to timing, dose, and combination for specific patients and families. Although the field rests largely on "clinical wisdom" at this point, important strides will likely be made in the next few years, and new areas of research are likely to flourish.

REFERENCES

Abikoff H, Hechtman L: Multimodal therapy and stimulants in the treatment of children with ADHD, in Psychosocial Treatment for Child and Adolescent Disorders: Empirically Based Approaches. Edited by Jensen P, Hibbs ED. Washington, DC, American Psychological Association, 1996, pp 341–369

Arnold LE, Abikoff HB, Cantwell DP, et al: NIMH Collaborative Multimodal Treatment Study of Children With ADHD (the MTA): design challenges and choices. Arch Gen Psychiatry 54:865–870, 1997a

Arnold LE, Hoagwood K, Jensen PS, et al: Towards clinically relevant clinical trials. Psychopharmacol Bull 33:145–142, 1997b

Barkley RA, McMurray MB, Edelbrock CS, et al: The response of aggressive and nonaggressive ADHD children to two doses of methylphenidate. J Am Acad Child Adolesc Psychiatry 28:873–881, 1989

Biederman J, Baldessarini RJ, Wright V, et al: A double-blind placebo controlled study of desipramine in the treatment of attention deficit disorder, III: lack of impact of comorbidity and family history factors on clinical response. J Am Acad Child Adolesc Psychiatry 32:199–204, 1993

Biederman J, Millberger S, Faraone SV, et al: Family-environment risk factors for attention-deficit hyperactivity disorder: a test of Rutter's indicators of adversity. Arch Gen Psychiatry 52:464–470, 1995

Cantwell DP, Swanson J, Connor DF: Case study: adverse response to clonidine. J Am Acad Child Adolesc Psychiatry 36:539–544, 1997

Castellanos FX, Giedd JN, Elia J, et al: Controlled stimulant treatment of ADHD and comorbid Tourette's syndrome: effects of stimulant and dose. J Am Acad Child Adolesc Psychiatry 36:589–596, 1997

Clarkin JF, Kendall PC: Comorbidity and treatment planning: summary and future directions. J Consult Clin Psychol 60:904–908, 1992

Diamond I, Tannock R, Schachar R: Response to methylphenidate in children with ADHD and comorbid anxiety. J Am Acad Child Adolesc Psychiatry 38:402–409, 1999

DuPaul GJ, Barkley RA, McMurray MB: Response of children with ADHD to methylphenidate: interaction with internalizing symptoms. J Am Acad Child Adolesc Psychiatry 33:894–903, 1994

Gadow KD, Sverd J, Sprafkin J, et al: Efficacy of methylphenidate for attention-deficit hyperactivity disorder in children with tic disorder. Arch Gen Psychiatry 52: 444–455, 1995

Garfinkel BD, Wender PH, Sloman L: Tricyclic antidepressants and methylphenidate treatment of attention deficit disorder in children. Journal of American Academy of Child Psychiatry 22:343–348, 1983

Greenhill L, Arnold L, Cantwell D, et al: Medication treatment strategies in the MTA study: relevance to clinicians and researchers. J Am Acad Child Adolesc Psychiatry 35:1304–1313, 1996

Hechtman L, Abikoff H: Multimodal treatment plus stimulants vs. stimulant treatment in ADHD children: results from a two-year comparative treatment study. Paper presented at the annual meeting of the American Academy of Child and Adolescent Psychiatry. New Orleans, LA, October 1995

Horn WF, Ialongo NS, Pascoe JM, et al: Additive effects of psychostimulants, parent training, and self-control therapy with ADHD children. J Am Acad Child Adolesc Psychiatry 30:233–240, 1991

Hunt RD, Hoehn R, Stephens KJ, et al: Clinical patterns of ADHD: a treatment model based on brain functioning. Compr Ther 20:106–112, 1994

Jensen PS, Josephson AM, Frey J: Informed consent: legal content versus therapeutic process. Am J Psychother 43:378–386, 1989

Jensen PS, Shervette RS, Xenakis SN, et al: Anxiety and depressive disorder in attention-deficit disorder: new findings. Am J Psychiatry 150:1203–1209, 1993

Kazdin AE, Holland L, Crowley M: Family experiences of barriers to treatment and premature termination from child therapy. J Consult Clin Psychol 65:453–463, 1997

Klein RG, Abikoff H, Klass E, et al: Clinical efficacy of methylphenidate in conduct disorder with and without attention deficit hyperactivity disorder. Arch Gen Psychiatry 54:1073–1080, 1997

MTA Cooperative Group: Fourteen-month randomized clinical trial of treatment strategies for attention deficit hyperactivity disorder. Arch Gen Psychiatry 56: 1073–1086, 1999a

MTA Cooperative Group: Moderator and mediator challenges to the MTA Study: effects of comorbid anxiety, family poverty, session attendance, and community mediation on treatment outcome. Arch Gen Psychiatry 56:1088–1096, 1999b

Pisterman S, McGrath P, Firestone P, et al: Outcome of parent-mediated treatment of preschoolers with attention deficit disorder with hyperactivity. J Consult Clin Psychol 57:628–635, 1989

Pliszka SR: Effect of anxiety on cognition, behavior, and stimulant response in ADHD. J Am Acad Child Adolesc Psychiatry 28:882–887, 1989

Richters J, Arnold LEA, Jensen PS, et al: NIMH Collaborative Multimodal Treatment Study of Children With ADHD, I: background and rationale. J Am Acad Child Adolesc Psychiatry 34:987–1000, 1995

Satterfield JH, Satterfield BT, Schell AM: Therapeutic interventions to prevent delinquency in hyperactive boys. J Am Acad Child Adolesc Psychiatry 26:56–64, 1987

Schubiner H, Tzelepis A, Isaacson JH, et al: The dual diagnosis of attention-deficit/hyperactivity disorder and substance abuse: case reports and literature review. J Clin Psychiatry 56:146–150, 1995

Spencer TJ, Biederman J, Wilens TE: Tricyclic antidepressant treatment of children with ADHD and tic disorders. J Am Acad Child Adolesc Psychiatry 33:1203–1204, 1994

Tannock R, Ickowicz A, Schachar R: Differential effects of methylphenidate on working memory in ADHD children with and without comorbid anxiety. J Am Acad Child Adolesc Psychiatry 34:886–896, 1995

Index

*Page numbers printed in **boldface** type refer to tables or figures.*